ANIMAL
MICROBIOLOGY

ANIMAL MICROBIOLOGY

VOLUME 1

Immunology, Bacteriology, Mycology

Diseases of Fish and Laboratory Methods

A. BUXTON

Ph.D. F.R.C.V.S. F.R.S.E.

Professor of Veterinary Pathology,
Royal (Dick) School of Veterinary Studies, University of Edinburgh

and

G. FRASER

B.Sc. Ph.D. M.R.C.V.S.

Senior Lecturer in Veterinary Microbiology,
Royal (Dick) School of Veterinary Studies, University of Edinburgh

BLACKWELL SCIENTIFIC PUBLICATIONS

OXFORD LONDON EDINBURGH MELBOURNE

First published 1977

British Library Cataloguing in Publication Data
Buxton, A.
    Animal microbiology.
    Vol. 1: Immunology, bacteriology, mycology,
    diseases of fish and laboratory methods.
    1. Micro-organisms, Pathogenic
    I. Title   II. Fraser, G.
    591.2′3   QR175

ISBN 0 632 00690 0

Distributed in the United States of America by
J. B. Lippincott Company, Philadelphia,
and in Canada by
J. B. Lippincott Company of Canada Ltd., Toronto

Typesetting by Dai Nippon Printing Co., Hong Kong, and Printed and bound by T. & A. Constable Limited, Edinburgh

Contents

(Detailed contents are found at the start of each chapter)

VOLUME 1

VOLUME 2

Preface

Our purpose in writing this book has been to collect together information on animal microbiology required both by undergraduates studying for their primary veterinary degrees and
by veterinarians undertaking postgraduate courses. We also hope that the book will be of use
to veterinary surgeons in different walks of professional life as well as being of interest to
medical microbiologists and others requiring information on this subject. To cater for these
various interests we have included discussions on the epidemiology, pathogenesis, clinical
features, diagnosis, control, public health and other aspects of infectious diseases as well as
on purely microbiological matters. We hope that the tables of contents at the beginning of
each chapter, the textual headings and lists of further reading, together with the general
index, will enable the reader to locate easily any required information.

In order to present the subject in a manner equally acceptable to all readers, we have
supported the text with a selection of coloured photographs and drawings as well as mono-
chromes illustrating the appearance of microbiology as seen in a diagnostic laboratory. For
the benefit of postgraduate students, and particularly those in tropical and subtropical
countries, we have tried to maintain a balance between our discussions on microbial diseases
of animals occurring in warmer climates and those in more temperate zones. Consequent
upon the recent expansion of fish farming throughout the world and as a result of the
increasing importance of controlling and preventing diseases of fish, a chapter has been
devoted to this specialist subject.

During the prolonged gestation period of this book we have become increasingly aware of
the difficulties that can beset two authors when trying to ensure that a text covering such a
wide canvas as animal microbiology is up-to-date in all its facets, while simultaneously
avoiding undergraduate indigestion arising from the inclusion of too much detailed information in particular areas. It is inevitable in a first edition of a book of this size that
some errors and omissions will have occurred and we hope that readers will call our
attention to any shortcomings. While the preparation of the whole book has been the
concern of both of us, the senior author has dealt in particular with the introductory
chapters, bacteriology and the appendices and the junior author has been responsible for
the sections on mycotic, rickettsial and viral infections.

During the writing and correction of the text we have received advice and encouragement
from many people, and we should like to mention in particular Dr. G. H. K. Lawson for
information on *Campylobacter*, Dr. W. J. Penhale on Immunology and Dr. J. E. Phillips on
Actinobacillus. We are especially grateful to Dr. W. B. Martin for reading the whole of the
manuscript on Virology and for making many valuable suggestions and corrections.

It is a special pleasure to acknowledge the apparently inexhaustible patience and skill of
Mr. R. C. James, who was responsible for photographing most of the colour plates used in
this book. We also hope that we have done justice to those who have contributed illustrative
material and we accord our thanks to Mr. I. S. Beattie, Mr. K. W. Head and Mr. A. C.
Rowland for allowing us to include some of their coloured transparencies of pathological
lesions in the section on Bacteriology. Recognition of colleagues, research students and
correspondents who have kindly provided us with many of the illustrations in the chapters

dealing with Mycology and Virology is recorded in the captions of the relevant plates. To all those and to others, too numerous to mention individually, who have helped in many ways, large and small, we offer our sincere thanks.

It is a pleasure to record the untiring assistance we have received from Miss M. Millar, who has not only typed the entire manuscript but has also helped in numerous other ways towards the completion of the final text.

Finally, our grateful thanks are due to our publisher, in particular Mr. Per Saugman, who invited us to write the book, and Mr. Nigel Palmer for his constant advice in matters relating to production.

A. Buxton
G. Fraser

Edinburgh, April 1977

CHAPTER 1

HISTORY AND DEVELOPMENT OF MICROBIOLOGY

CHAPTER 1

History and development of microbiology

Bacteriology

From the earliest written records there are references to diseases in animals. For example, Egyptian writings dated between 2000 B.C. and 1500 B.C. refer to descriptions of diseases and attempts to control them which suggest that anthrax, bovine tuberculosis and sheep pox may have been serious problems at that time. Both the Greek and Roman Empires recognized the economic importance of animal health in relation to human food and welfare, and introduced studies into diseases of animals and regulations for their control. However, the effectiveness of these measures in relation to diseases caused by microbes had to await firstly, the development of lenses, microscopes and staining techniques which enabled investigators to observe for the first time the microbes responsible for these diseases; and secondly, the establishment of cultural techniques which provided methods for studying the characteristic properties of growth and metabolism of these organisms.

Lenses and microscopes

Lenses were first made during the thirteenth century but the degrees of magnification they provided were extremely limited and it was not until the end of the sixteenth century that compound lenses were introduced which increased the magnification and formed the basis for the development of the modern microscope. Using this method, Hooke introduced his compound microscope in the middle of the seventeenth century and examined a variety of materials including some moulds, but there is no evidence that he observed bacteria. At about the same time, Antony van Leeuwenhoek, a Dutch merchant, using simple lenses which he ground himself, examined a variety of biological materials, including plants, water, scrapings from teeth, blood and manure. His detailed reports and drawings were submitted to the Royal Society and from these it is possible to recognize the first descriptions of protozoa, including coccidia, and of bacteria which

seem to have included bacilli, cocci and spirochaetes. However, no attempt was made at that time to assess the possible association of these organisms with disease in man and animals, and this significant step was delayed until further developments of compound microscopes had been made.

Staining methods

Initial observations of bacteria under microscopes consisted of examining unstained, moist preparations, and it was soon realized that the application of staining techniques would greatly enhance the facility and quality of such examinations. The preparation of aniline dyes, particularly fuchsin, began in 1856 at about the time when haematoxylin, carmine and other stains were first used for histological examinations of tissues. During the following years, Hoffmann stained bacteria with carmine and fuchsin, Weigert used methyl violet in 1875, and Salomonsen employed a watery solution of fuchsin in 1877. In that year, Koch made a major advance in the technique for examining bacteria by preparing films on cover glasses, drying them, fixing in alcohol and staining with methyl violet, fuchsin or aniline brown. Four years later he used heat for the first time as a fixative for his films. To his delight and surprise, Koch found that the morphology of the bacteria remained unaltered after this treatment and several of his preparations of anthrax and other organisms were photographed. The use of methylene blue was introduced by Ehrlich in 1881, and in the following year was used by Koch when he discovered the tubercle bacillus and found that in the presence of alkali the dye penetrated the organism. This latter observation was the origin for the development of Loeffler's methylene blue which was first introduced in 1884. Koch's method for staining tubercle bacilli was modified by Ehrlich and this formed the basis of the Ziehl–Neelsen staining technique by showing that after staining with an aniline-water solution of methyl violet, the organisms were acid-fast when treated with 30 per cent nitric acid in water. The modification to Ehrlich's technique made by Ziehl was the use of carbolic acid instead of aniline-water, and Neelsen introduced sulphuric acid instead of nitric acid. In 1884, a Danish worker named Christian Gram, experimented with Ehrlich's technique and showed that bacteria could be divided into two groups by staining with a solution of gentian violet in aniline-water, then applying Lugol's iodine solution in potassium iodide, and finally treating the preparation with alcohol. He noted that some organisms retained the dye and that others became decolourised. This significant observation formed the basis of the Gram staining method which, with minor modifications, continues to be widely used today.

Media preparation

At about the same time that staining methods were being introduced, the initial steps were also being taken in the development of media for isolating and growing pure cultures of bacteria on artificial media. Pasteur in 1861 was the first to take important steps in the preparation of fluid media by concocting a mixture of ammonium tartrate, the ashes from yeasts, cane sugar and water for the growth of organisms. This was followed by trials of a host of different fluid media, including Loeffler's preparation in 1881 which consisted of meat infusion, peptone, sodium phosphate and salt. This type of broth was to form the basis of nutrient broth which is so commonly used today, and emphasises how bacteriological media have changed little for almost a century.

The first attempts to prepare solid media using potato and bread began in about 1865, and during the next decade additional ingredients included flour, egg albumen and meat. In 1872, Oscar Brefeld, a mycologist, developed a solid medium by adding gelatin to liquid medium. He also stressed in the detailed reports of his research work the importance of techniques for obtaining pure cultures by inoculating only one spore on to a sterile, transparent medium which had to be maintained free from atmospheric contamination. Some ten years later, Koch applied and improved Brefeld's use of gelatin for the isolation of pure cultures of bacteria, using meat extract and gelatin, and inoculating solid medium with a sterilised platinum needle. He also introduced the use of nutrient gelatin slopes in test tubes with cotton wool bungs, and developed the 'poured plate' technique in which bacteria were mixed with melted gelatin and then poured on to a plate and allowed to set — thus giving an even distribution of the bacterial inoculum throughout the medium. The limitations of this medium, that it did not solidify at body temperature and was liquefied by certain strains of bacteria, were overcome by the introduction of agar-agar on the inspiration

of Frau Hesse, the wife of one of Koch's colleagues. Also in the year 1882, Koch introduced the use of inspissated serum and Petri, another of Koch's colleagues, devised the glass plate with a lid for containing solid media which is now commonly referred to as a Petri plate and continues to be widely used by microbiologists.

Recognition of pathogenic bacteria

The use of the light microscope, the introduction of staining methods for observing bacteria and the development of artificial media capable of supporting the growth of these organisms, led to a period of research and discovery which was to explode the theory of spontaneous generation and to establish the germ theory of disease. Outstanding among those who contributed to this fundamental change in belief were Louis Pasteur and Robert Koch who, with their contemporaries, established the foundations of microbiology as we know it today. During the remarkably short period of little more than a decade commencing in 1874, a variety of microbes were identified and described as the causes of disease in man and animals, including the anthrax bacillus, fowl cholera bacillus, leprosy bacillus, typhoid bacillus, gonococcus, staphylococcus, streptococcus, and the causes of swine erysipelas, actinomycosis, tuberculosis, diphtheria and glanders. This classification of some bacterial species as causal agents of disease, which continued until the early years of this century, was based to a large extent on the development of artificial media and the ability to grow pure cultures of different bacterial strains in the laboratory. On the assumption that growth on artificial media was comparable in all respects to the development of the organisms in host tissues, Koch postulated the properties of pathogenic bacteria as being organisms which must be observed in each case of the particular disease being studied, must be isolated and grown in pure culture on artificial media, and when subsequently inoculated into a susceptible host must be capable of causing the development of that disease and be recovered from the animal.

Although the exciting era of the discovery, description and identification of a variety of bacterial species as the causes of disease in man and animals is now over, it has confronted the bacteriologist of today with some important problems concerning the modes of development of these various infections and of reliable methods for their prevention and control. For example, it has become increasingly clear that the application of Koch's postulates as criteria for the identification of a bacterial species as the cause of a particular disease was not always reliable. As this type of approach to establishing the aetiology of infectious diseases was applied on an increasing scale, it soon became apparent that the cultivation of bacteria in the laboratory on artificial media often resulted in a reduced ability of the organisms to produce disease when subsequently inoculated into susceptible hosts. This alteration in the properties of organisms was demonstrated by experiments which showed that after cultivation in the laboratory, disease may be reproduced in susceptible hosts only after inoculation of excessively large doses of organisms given by an unnatural route, or even a total failure to produce any clinical symptoms of disease by this method. Apparently negative results of this nature can result from either the rapid and total elimination of inoculated organisms by the host from its tissues, or from the maintenance of a proportion of the bacteria for periods of weeks or months when a symbiotic relationship develops between host and parasite leading to a condition known as the 'carrier state'.

Since the beginning of the twentieth century the realisation that potentially disease-producing bacterial species (i.e. pathogenic organisms) can show this important variation in their ability to produce disease has led to investigations related to the study of the properties of bacteria when grown *in vitro* and *in vivo* under a variety of conditions. The main aspects of these studies have been concerned with the chemical and biochemical constitution of bacteria and requirements for their growth, the identification of antigens and toxins and the reactions they produce in host tissues, the production and use of bacteria and their products as immunizing agents (i.e. vaccines) for the control and prevention of disease, and more recently the introduction and use of chemotherapeutic agents as additional tools for disease control and prevention. For the most part the study under defined *in vitro* conditions of factors which affect the growth and ability of bacteria to produce disease remains limited by the media and laboratory techniques used for their cultivation. Apart from the introduction of chemically defined media and preliminary attempts to grow organisms in tissue cultures or in media containing hormones and other substances derived from host tissues, the common methods of bacterial cultivation in various gaseous atmospheres provide conditions far different from those of the microenvironment experienced by bacteria growing in host tissues. Current techniques remain substantially similar to those originally devised by Koch and his contemporaries. It is in this field, particularly, that further advances are required to provide appropriate controlled environments in order to observe more reliably the reactions of pathogenic bacteria to their environments in host tissues, thereby increasing our understanding of the pathogenesis of infections. The development of the broad field of bacteriology has established that only a small proportion of bacterial species are

pathogenic to animals and man, that we cannot eradicate these organisms from our environment, and that we must learn to live with them and continue to improve our methods of prevention and control.

Mycology

Fungi belong to a very large group of microorganisms that are devoid of chlorophyll and are reproduced by spores. They are widely distributed throughout the world and a conservative modern estimate places the number of known species at over 40 000. Most of these are saprophytic but many are parasitic, causing important diseases of man and animals.

Fungi have probably existed since the earliest times and, despite their fragile structure, non-septate hyphae of species resembling the *Phycomycetae* are to be found in plant fossils in the 300 million-year-old Middle Devonian strata in Rhynie, Aberdeenshire. Yeasts, which are generally included with the fungi, have an early origin also and Grüss isolated a yeast which was named *Saccharomyces winlocki*, from 'beer-bread' and from the sediment in a beer-jar in a Theban tomb of the eleventh dynasty (2000 B.C.). Besides the importance of yeasts in such fermentations as baking, brewing and wine-making, their application to the cure of diseases goes back to very early times. Monks are known to have used yeast for curing plague and Hippocrates described its beneficial effects in cases of leucorrhoea.

Prior to the eighteenth century, the only scientific accounts of fungi were almost entirely devoted to illustrations of the gross morphology of the better known species but, in 1729, Micheli not only published one of the first accounts of the microscopical structure of fungi but even attempted to grow them in culture. This important advance in our knowledge of fungi was followed by a period of intense activity and so many descriptive papers were published during the next hundred years that, by the early 19th century, a considerable number of fungi had been described often, unfortunately, with different names for the same species. Although the earliest accepted system of nomenclature was that published by Fries in his *Systema Mycologium* of 1821–32, the culmination of so much descriptive work in the general field of mycology was the massive 25 volume *Sylloge Fungorum* published by Saccardo between 1882 and 1931.

Recognition of fungi as causes of disease

The science of mycology, and of medical mycology in particular, is of such recent development that it is not possible to account for the means by which saprophytic yeasts and fungi arose during the process of evolution and how some members became adapted to growth in the tissues of man and animals. Nor is it known how a few of these parasitic forms succeeded in overcoming the lethal effects of cellular and humoral immunity to become established as potentially pathogenic microorganisms within the animal host.

However closely the theoretical views of Fracastoro, von Plenciz and other eighteenth century writers approached the correct explanation of the nature and causation of infectious diseases, they were unable through lack of experimental facilities, to put their opinions to the test. The first practical demonstration of such a possibility was made by Bassi in 1835 who, in opposition to the beliefs of the time, showed conclusively that the economically important disease of silkworms, called 'calicino' or 'muscardine' is transmissible and that the causative agent is a fungus (*Botrytis bassinia*). Two years after Bassi's classical observations in support of his germ theory of disease, Cagniard-Latour first described the reproduction of yeasts by budding and, in the same year, Schwann described the relationship between yeasts and fermentation, suggesting that yeasts are a type of fungus.

As a result of these discoveries, many other workers were stimulated to examine diseased human and animal tissues for the presence of microorganisms and, within a few years, the existence of many parasitic species was reported in conditions affecting the skin and mucous membranes. Thus, Schönlein (1839) showed that the fungus, now known as *Achorion schonleinii*, is always present in favus or ringworm, and *Oidium albicans* was established as being a human pathogen by Berg (1841) and Gruby (1842). Also in 1842, Muller and Retzius described a mucor mould in the lungs and air sacs of an owl and in 1843–44 Gruby presented detailed accounts of the occurrence of *Microsporum audouini* and *Trichophyton tonsurans* in lesions of human ringworm. Shortly afterwards, mucor moulds were found in the aural passage of a child and in the sputum and lungs of a case of pneumothorax. The parasitic role of fungi gained wide acceptance largely as a result of Robin's *Histoire Naturelle des Végétaux Parasites* published in 1853.

In the 1860s the initial steps were taken in the development of artificial media for the growth of bacteria but the first attempts to prepare solid media for the cultivation of fungi did not begin until about 1870. Pure culture techniques were first used in mycology by Bresfeld (1872) who isolated a single fungal spore and allowed it to develop into a mycelium. Pure cultures of yeasts were first obtained by Hansen (1883) using a modification of Lister's (1878) limiting dilution method.

Other important observations made around the middle of the nineteenth century included confirmation of the phenomenon of 'alteration of generations' whereby one and the same species of fungus can appear in several morphological forms. Also of interest at this time was Metchnikoff's discovery while studying *Monospora tricuspidata* fungus infection of Daphnia, that white cells in non-immunized hosts were capable of ingesting yeast particles. As a result of these findings Metchnikoff proposed that white blood cells and other phagocytes of vertebrates could engulf 'parasites' and act as defensive mechanisms of the body.

Discovery of antibiotic substances

From the end of the nineteenth century onwards, many microbiologists had noted the inhibitory effects of microorganisms on pathogenic bacteria and, in 1929, Fleming published his classical account of the antibiotic, penicillin, which enabled later workers to develop a therapeutic substance for use against a wide range of bacterial infections. Since then many other antibiotics have been discovered and the most important sources are some of the filamentous fungi, particularly species of *Penicillium*, *Aspergillus* and *Actinomyces*.

In recent years antifungal substances were discovered and some have been used successfully to combat fungal and yeast infections in man, animals and also in cell cultures. The most important of these are probably nystatin in candidiasis, emphotericin in systemic fungal infections and griseofulvin in dermatomycosis.

Since the mode of replication of viruses is different from that of bacteria and fungi, antibacterial and antifungal agents are wholly ineffective against viral infections. However, in 1961, an antibiotic named statolon having a wide antiviral spectrum, was isolated from cultures of *Penicillium stoloniferum* and a substance called helenine having similar properties, was obtained from *Penicillium funiculosum*. Both of these substances inhibit the development of certain viruses grown in cell cultures by acting as non-viral inducers of interferon. There is recent evidence, also, that statolon may possess anti-viral activity against a number of oncogenic viruses. If these preliminary observations are confirmed, it is probable that other substances will be discovered that are capable of protecting animals against a wide range of viral infections without causing damage to the host.

Although mycotic infections have been recognised in man and animals for many years their importance in human and veterinary medicine has tended to increase with the widespread use of penicillin and other antibiotics. More recently the risk of fungal infections has risen sharply following the introduction of corticosteroid hormones and other chemotherapeutic agents used in the treatment of chronic and debilitating diseases, and it is a matter of grave concern that this recent increase is particularly striking in patients who have undergone organ transplant surgery.

Virology

Virus diseases have existed since very early times and there is evidence that rabies was recognised by the peoples of India 5000 years ago. There are also Chinese accounts dating from 1700 B.C. which would seem to refer to smallpox and, in the writings of Hippocrates and Aristotle, there are clearly recognizable descriptions of mumps and of the contagious nature of rabies. From ancient times, methods have been devised to increase resistance to infectious agents and there are early reports from China and other Eastern countries that variolation, the deliberate infection with smallpox, had been practised long before vaccination was introduced into England in the eighteenth century.

At least three of the great pestilences of domestic animals, rinderpest, foot-and-mouth disease and sheep pox, have been known throughout the centuries and the description of a virus disease of plants causing 'break' or variegation in the colour of tulips was published in the late sixteenth century. In more recent times, a number of important virus diseases have been described in arthropods and other invertebrate animals (e.g. silkworm jaundice and 'sacbrood' of bees) while the identification of bacterial viruses (bacteriophages) causing lysis of bacterial cultures was discovered little more than 50 years ago.

The viral aetiology of diseases

It is a remarkable fact that the technique used by Jenner in 1796 of inducing resistance to smallpox by injecting people with material from naturally acquired cowpox (vaccination), and Pasteur's outstanding work on rabies immunization were reported before the existence of viruses was known. Credit for the first demonstration of a virus goes to the Russian botanist Ivanowski who showed in 1892, that the symptoms of tobacco mosaic disease could be reproduced in healthy tobacco plants by rubbing their leaves with sap from infected plants after the juice had been passed through a Chamberlain bacteria-proof filter-candle. Six years later, the Dutch microbiologist, Beijerinck, repeated Ivanowski's experiments and extended his investigations to include studies of the diffusion of the infective agent into agar blocks. Although Ivanowski had failed to appreciate the full significance of his findings, Beijerinck quickly realised that a new type of infectious agent had been discovered that was not a tiny bacterium, and which he called a *contagium vivum fluidum*. In the same year that Beijerinck reported on the filterable nature of the agent of tobacco mosaic disease, Loeffler and Frosch showed that bacteria-free filtrates of vesicular fluid from cases of foot-and-mouth disease could induce the characteristic illness when inoculated into susceptible cattle. This first description of an animal virus was followed in 1902 by the report of Reed and his colleagues in America who found that yellow fever in man is caused by a 'filterable' virus carried by mosquitoes. In subsequent years, a wide range of viruses affecting plants, lower animals and man were discovered and, since the existence of these agents was mostly demonstrated by the ability of filtrates to produce clinical diseases in animals, they were termed 'filterable viruses'. Although it was then clearly recognized that viruses were capable of causing infectious diseases, the discovery by Rous in 1911, that certain sarcomas in chickens could be induced with cell-free filtrates of the tumour, passed almost unnoticed until nearly 20 years later when work by Shope (1932), Bittner (1936) and others clearly established that certain viruses are capable of producing tumours in animals and birds.

A new class of viruses was discovered between 1915–17 when Twort in England and d'Herelle in France found that various types of bacteria were susceptible to infection by filterable agents and that a successful replicative cycle usually resulted in lysis and death of the bacterial cell. Since the destructive effects of the agent, bacteriophage, on agar plate cultures of the host bacterium are seen as large clear areas or plaques on the surface of the confluent bacterial growth, a method was quickly devised for studying the mechanisms of infection and reproduction of this class of viruses. Since much of the work was carried out in the days before chicken embryo and cell culture methods became readily available, the growth of bacteriophages was used with considerable success as a model of virus activity, particularly in genetic and other studies of the more complex relationships between animal viruses and their host cells.

The properties of viruses

After a lean period of about 20 years when the accumulation of knowledge about animal viruses was slow, Elford's (1931–33) introduction of a series of collodion membranes of graded porosity was a significant advance towards the study of the physicochemical and biological properties of viruses. Early experiments with membrane filters showed that virus particles range in size from about 20–700 nm and the accuracy of these measurements has been largely confirmed by the more recent techniques of ultracentrifugation and electron microscopy.

Interest in the chemistry of viruses was greatly stimulated in 1935 by Stanley's account of the isolation and purification of tobacco mosaic virus in the form of fine needles or paracrystals and by the discovery of Bawden and Pirie (1937) that the tobacco mosaic virus is a nucleoprotein. The report on the crystallization of tobacco mosaic virus presented the fascinating but seemingly paradoxical situation that a substance which can in one sense be regarded as a molecule can also be accepted as a microorganism. Subsequently, it was found possible to separate the protein and nucleic acid components of this virus, and in 1956 Gierer and Schramm, and independently Fraenkel-Conrat, showed that RNA separated from tobacco mosaic virus is, itself, infectious and can initiate the multiplication of the virus in susceptible host cells. These and later experiments with other simple RNA viruses such as poliovirus, provided direct confirmation of the thesis that nucleic acid, alone, may be the carrier of viral genetic information and that viral nucleic acids represent the chemical counterparts of biological genomes.

Equally exciting was the report by Spiegelman and his colleagues in 1965, of the successful synthesis *in vitro* of a molecule of viral RNA which can infect the viral host, in this case a bacterial cell, and multiply therein. This observation suggests that it may now be possible to synthesise a living organism from synthetic precursors in a test-tube.

The cultivation of viruses
In the early days of virology the presence of a virus could only be detected by its ability to pass through bacteria-proof filter candles of the Chamberland or Berkefeld types and produce clinical disease in susceptible animals. However, in 1931 an important step in the cultivation of viruses was made by Woodruff and Goodpasture who showed that cowpox and some other viruses could be grown in the tissues of the developing chick embryo. The technique was extensively developed by Burnet and his colleagues over the ensuing 20 years and it was found that many animal viruses inoculated by four main routes, namely, allantoic, chorio-allantoic, amniotic and yolk-sac could give rise to the formation of pocks, oedema of the membranes, death, deformities or other abnormalities of the embryo. By 1940 the amniotic and allantoic sacs were being used extensively for the cultivation of human influenza viruses and in the following year Hirst and, later, McLelland and Hare observed that the virus would agglutinate healthy chicken red blood cells. This interesting discovery led to the haemagglutination technique being introduced as a standard method for the titration of myxovirus and many other species of haemagglutinating viruses. At the same time, a simple but highly specific serological test was devised for the detection of haemagglutinin-inhibiting antibodies in the sera of patients recovering from the illness.

Since Pasteur (1885) demonstrated attenuation of rabies virus in the spinal cord of experimentally infected rabbits which he used as a source of vaccine, laboratory animals such as rabbits, ferrets and guinea-pigs have played a key role in the historical development of animal virology. However, their main use today is generally restricted to providing model systems for the study of pathogenic mechanisms, and animals are seldom used for virus isolation. Not until 1948 was another important observation made on the susceptibility of laboratory animals to virus infections. In that year, Dalldorf and Sickler discovered that children suffering from a mild form of poliomyelitis in the American township of Coxsackie, were excreting a virus in the faeces and that this virus was pathogenic for newborn but not for adult mice. This important observation resulted in the recognition of unweaned mice, hamsters and other rodents as being particularly susceptible hosts for a variety of other viruses including reoviruses, togaviruses and the virus of foot-and-mouth disease.

Other important developments in the biological field include the report by Findlay and MacCallum (1937) of interference in monkeys between the serologically unrelated viruses of Rift Valley fever and yellow fever, and the momentous discovery by Isaacs and Lindenmann (1957) of a small protein, named interferon, made in cells in response to virus infection and concerned in halting the replicative cycle of a wide range of viruses.

The earliest recorded attempts to cultivate tissues *in vitro* date from about 1885 when Roux successfully explanted chick embryo tissues into warm saline for several days, but it is only since the advent of antibiotics that cell culture methods have become a matter of simple routine. In 1925 Parker and Nye first showed that vaccinia virus could multiply in tissue culture. However, progress in this new field was limited until 1949 when Enders, Weller and Robbins published their outstanding discovery that poliovirus could be grown in cultured non-neural cells with the production of easily recognizable cytopathic effects. This important landmark in virology stimulated considerable activity in medical and veterinary research until, today, almost every known human and animal virus has been grown in cell cultures. Not only have hundreds of previously unknown viruses been isolated and identified in this way but the method has also revolutionized the diagnosis of viral diseases and the development of viral vaccines. Four years later, Dulbecco and Vogt (1953) described the formation of areas of local destruction in infected monolayer cultures overlaid with agar and showed that the production of the plaques was a valuable method for studying viruses quantitatively. In 1957 Shelokov and Vogel reported that monolayers of cells infected with myxoviruses or other viruses which mature by budding from the cytoplasmic membranes are capable of adsorbing healthy red blood cells added to the culture medium. This phenomenon of haemadsorption has proved of value for the early detection of a number of viruses that do not produce visible cytopathic changes in cell cultures. Another major step in the development of virology was the application of Coons' (1957) immunofluorescence method for the visual detection of viral antigens within infected cells. An extension of the indirect method of fluorescent antibody staining, using ferritin-coupled γ-globulin in electron microscopy, was developed by Morgan and his colleagues in 1962.

Although the electron microscope was first applied to the demonstration of a virus by Kausche, Pfankuch and Ruska in 1939, the method had very little practical application until Williams and Wyckoff (1946) introduced the shadow-casting technique in which an opaque material such as gold or palladium is vaporized at an angle to the plane of the specimen. In recent years, the use of negative staining has enabled many workers including Horne, Almeida, Valentine, Pereira and Wildy to study the ultra-structure of the virion, and their observations have added greatly to our knowledge of the nature of viruses. Electron microscopy of ultra-thin sections of infected cultures is also useful for studying the growth and development of viruses within the cell.

As a result of the widespread application of these newer techniques, the current emphasis in virus research is now changing from one of isolation and identification of causative agents of disease to more fundamental studies of their physicochemical properties and the relationships between viruses and their host cells. A considerable amount of attention is now being paid to latent, persisting and defective infections, chronic and slow virus infections and, in particular, the implications of viral oncogenesis.

Immunology

Foundations of immunology
As soon as pathogenic microbes had been identified as the causes of infectious diseases in man and animals, the early research workers turned their attention to methods for preventing some of the known scourges of those times. The foundations of immunology were laid by Pasteur in his experiments on the prevention of a number of diseases, including anthrax, fowl cholera, swine erysipelas and rabies, and also by Salmon and Theobald Smith in 1884-6 who studied immunological reactions in pigeons using the so-called hog-cholera bacillus. They made the discovery that vaccination of these birds with a killed suspension of the organisms protected them against subsequent infection with the living bacilli. This important observation led quickly to the application of the technique to the study of additional diseases, including human plague, typhoid fever and other infections, all of which may be summarised as the prophylactic approach to immunology.

Humoral and cellular theories
Concurrently with these prophylactic studies, fundamental aspects of immunology were being investigated in an attempt to understand the nature of the processes involved. Two theories were put forward to explain the mechanism; one being the humoral theory suggesting that immunity was due to the presence of substances in the body fluids which prevented microbial infections developing; the other maintained that immunity was due to a cellular mechanism which was strongly held by Metchnickoff, a Russian zoologist. In relation to the humoral mechanism, Nuttall showed in 1888 that blood from various animal species was bactericidal to the anthrax organism and that this property did not last for long in a given sample of blood, and was rapidly destroyed in a few minutes when the sample was heated to 55°C. Two years later, Behring and Nissen showed that whereas the sera from normal guinea-pigs had little or no bactericidal effect on vibrio organisms, sera from immunized guinea-pigs was markedly bactericidal. In the same year, Behring and Kitasato published a particularly important paper showing that the blood sera of rabbits and mice immunized with tetanus organisms, contained a substance which neutralized the toxin produced by the organism, and they referred to this action as 'antitoxic' — a term which has persisted to the present day. This outstanding work together with a similar report by Behring on diphtheria, acted as a stimulus to a great deal of further research along similar lines which included a number of important observations. Outstanding among these was the contribution by Paul Ehrlich who formulated a method for the standardization of bacterial toxins and antitoxins as a result of his work on diphtheria.

Complement
In 1894 Pfeiffer showed that cholera vibrios were dissolved by the serum of immunized guinea-pigs (a process he called 'bacteriolysis'), that the reaction occurred in the absence of cells, that it was highly specific for the cholera vibrio, and that it was inhibited by the previous heating of immune serum to 60°C. Continuing Pfeiffer's experiments, Bordet showed that the addition of normal, unheated serum to heated immune serum resulted in the bacteriolytic properties of the latter being restored. The study of this lytic phenomenon was then applied to red blood cells and many experiments were carried out to

observe the conditions under which immunological haemolysis would occur. As a result of his experiments, Bordet termed the heat-labile substance 'alexine' and the heat-stable material as 'substance sensibilisatrice'. Ehrlich confirmed Bordet's findings and he labelled the two substances 'complement' and 'amboceptor', respectively.

Phagocytosis

While the experiments outlined above were in accord with the general concept of a humoral mechanism of immunity, Metchnickoff was making some important contributions related to his cellular theory, although he ignored earlier observations on cellular reactions made during the previous decade by Birch-Hirschfeld, Panum, Koch and others. Metchnickoff concluded from his experiments that bacteria in the body were destroyed by cells as a result of some form of intracellular digestion, and in 1884 he introduced the term 'phagocytes' to describe the cells which had this property, and the process of digestion he called 'phagocytosis'. As a result of his experiments a great deal of discussion and controversy arose between the protagonists of the humoral and cellular theories of immunity, and it soon became clear from further discoveries that the immune response was a highly complex process which involved both mechanisms. The establishment of a relationship between the two resulted firstly, from further studies on the mode of action of immune sera on bacteria and secondly, on the incorporation of leucocytes into the system and observing the effect of immune sera on the susceptibility of bacteria to phagocytosis.

Agglutinins and precipitins

During the last decade of the nineteenth century some fundamental observations were made on the reactions between immune sera and bacteria which were neither antitoxic nor lytic. Charrin and Roger noted that when *Pseudomonas pyocyaneus* was grown in serum derived from an animal immunized against that organism, the bacteria were not evenly distributed in the fluid medium but formed themselves into clumps. Clumping under similar conditions was observed by Metchnickoff in 1891 when working with vibrio organisms and pneumococci; and a more detailed report of this phenomenon which is now referred to as agglutination, was given by Durham in 1896, following the work he did at Guy's Hospital, London. He also realised the possible value of the agglutination test as a method for diagnosing disease, and this was applied by Widal in the same year to enteric infections and became known as the 'Widal test'. Soon afterwards, Bordet (1899) showed that during the process of agglutination the antibodies were removed from the serum by absorption

and that this process was highly specific for each bacterial species being investigated.

At the same time, the development of the precipitation test was taking place. In 1897 Kraus prepared clear filtrates from a variety of bacterial species, inoculated them into animals, and found that when he mixed the immune sera with the appropriate filtrates, precipitation reactions occurred. In the following years, immunological precipitation was examined in a variety of different systems and the specificity of the reaction between the material inoculated into animals (antigen) and the substances present in the sera (antibodies) was confirmed.

Opsonins and bacteriotropins

At the time when the agglutination and precipitation reactions were being recognised as new systems of antigen–antibody reactions, important observations were being made which were to show the interrelationship between the humoral and cellular theories of immunity. In 1894 two Belgians named Denys and Havit noted that the bactericidal effect of whole blood derived from dogs was greater than the effect of cell-free plasma from the same animals, and that the increased activity of whole blood was due to the presence of leucocytes. These observations were followed up by Wright and Douglas (1903) who showed that substances in serum called 'opsonins' prepared bacteria in some way for phagocytosis, and this established the interrelationship between the humoral and cellular theories of immunity. Later, it was to be shown that specific bacterial antibodies, known as bacteriotropins, developing as a result of artificial immunization or natural infection, enhanced still further the process of phagocytosis.

Modern developments

Thus, by the beginning of this century the foundations of immunology had become established and subsequent developments during the last 25 years have been particularly exciting and far-reaching. During this time the application of physical chemistry and biochemistry and the introduction of new techniques, particularly the antiglobulin test, blood grouping methods, gel precipitation techniques, fluorescence microscopy and the use of radioisotopes, have revealed a host of new facts and stimulated new theories related to an understanding of the many facets of immunopathology, the epidemiology and pathogenesis of diseases, and the various relationships which may develop between hosts and parasites. Some of the important areas of recent research which have been studied are hypersensitivity and related cellular reactions, the origin, structure and function of antibody molecules, the development of immune mechanisms in the young, the recognition and continued study of autoimmunity, the possible association of immune responses with the aetiology of some chronic diseases and tumour formation, and the importance of immunological problems in relation to tissue transplantation.

Contemporary aspects of veterinary microbiology

This brief outline of the history and development of microbiology emphasises the broad scope of the subject as it applies to the veterinarian of today who is concerned with infectious diseases in a variety of host species maintained under widely different conditions of animal husbandry and climatic environments. It also emphasises both the varied technical skills and knowledge of the epidemiology and pathogenesis of infectious diseases of animals which are available to the microbiologist, and indicates the fields of current interest and research which foreshadow some important areas where further knowledge is required to improve our understanding of infectious processes and disease control. Sufficient information is now available for the veterinarian to appreciate that we live in an environment laden with microbes, that many of these are saprophytes and of no consequence as pathogenic entities, that others are essential for the role they play in nutrition, digestive processes and the well-being of healthy animals, and that a relatively small group are pathogens capable of producing disease and which cannot be eradicated from the environment.

At the present time the period of research into the recognition and classification of infective agents is reaching its final stages, and attention is being given on an increasing scale to the pathogenesis of microbial infections. In the field of bacteriology, important areas of study are those concerned with the direct relationships between parasites and hosts developing in animals which either may become temporary carriers of latent but potential pathogens, may act as foci of infection for other susceptible hosts, or suffer serious or even fatal disease from the sudden and overwhelming multiplication of the parasitic organisms. Of similar importance is the relationship between the impact of modern, intensive methods of husbandry on the consequent facility for rapid transfer of pathogens from one host to another, and on the increased susceptibility of animals reared under these conditions to suffer from infectious diseases consequent upon the sudden and rapid multiplication of bacterial species which constitute part of the normal bacterial flora of healthy animals.

Further current problems concern the preparation and application of reliable immunizing agents in relation to the established fact that living, virulent organisms can stimulate a solid immunity at the risk of initiating clinical disease and the spread of infection among susceptible populations, and that attenuated or killed organisms constitute relatively safe immunizing agents which produce only limited degrees of immunity and protection. The veterinarian has to consider the comparable values of antibacterial therapy in relation to the development of resistant strains of microorganisms, the possible interference of such therapy with the development of immunity from natural infection or artificial immunization, the effect on growth and development in young animals, and the economics of therapy in relation to the control of disease in the individual animal or on a herd or flock basis.

In virology recent research has revealed important information on the structure and life cycles of viruses which has emphasised the need to extend our knowledge on the intimate and varied relationships which can exist between viruses and the cells which support their growth, on the effects of different strains of virus on each other in a mixed infection, on the development of variant strains which may cause world-wide epidemics, and on methods for controlling viral diseases by substances which are viricidal and interfere with the normal life cycle of these organisms.

The rapid expansion of immunopathology in recent years has revealed the complexity of the processes involved and also some important fundamental information on the conditions under which the host responds to both foreign and to its own tissue antigens. The extension and application of this knowledge in conjunction with the continued application of biochemical techniques will lead to a better understanding of the pathogenesis of disease, of the fundamental question of how organisms react with tissues to cause disease and the consequent host responses which develop, and of improved techniques for both immunization procedures and diagnosis of infection in the living animal.

Further reading

BROCK T.D. (1961) *Milestones in Microbiology*. Translated by N.J. Englewood. London: Prentice Hall.

BULLOCH W. (1960) *The History of Bacteriology*. London: Oxford University Press.

BURNET SIR MACFARLANE AND WHITE D.O. (1972) *Natural History of Infectious Disease*, 4th Edition. London: Cambridge University Press.

DOBELL C. (ed.) (1932) *Antony van Leeuwenhoek and his Little Animals.* London: John Bale & Sons and Danielsson. Reprint New York: Dover Publications.

FOSTER W.D. (1970) *A History of Medical Bacteriology and Immunology*. London: Heinemann Medical.

KRUIF DE P. (1958) *Microbe Hunters*. London: Hutchinson.

SMITHCORS J.F. (1964) The development of veterinary medical science: Some historical aspects and prospects. *Advances in Veterinary Science*, **9**, 1.

ZINSSER H. (1937) *Rats, Lice and History*. London: Routledge.

CHAPTER 2

CELL STRUCTURE AND FUNCTION

Cell structure and function

During the prolonged earlier development of cellular life, some originally simple forms of cells underwent processes of natural selection and mutation which resulted in the development of relatively complicated structures. A characteristic feature of these more complicated cell types is the enclosure of the nucleus within a clearly defined nuclear membrane, which results in the formation of a true nucleus clearly delineated from the cytoplasm. For this reason, these cells have been termed **eukaryotic** (Gr. *eu* = true; *karyon* = nucleus). Examples of eukaryotic cells are the higher plant and animal cells, including moulds, yeasts, fungi, green algae and protozoa. In contrast, some cell types have not developed into the more complicated structures characteristic of eukaryotic cells, and in particular, they have failed to develop a distinct nuclear membrane. Although the nuclear material is usually concentrated in one mass, it is not separated by a membrane from the cytoplasm of the cell. These relatively simple cells have been termed **prokaryotic** (Gr. *protos* = primitive; *karyon* = nucleus) and include the bacteria.

In the infected host, tissue cells form the micro-environment in which the growth of bacteria and fungi develop, either intracellularly or extracellularly, and they also provide the essential intracellular environment for the development of viruses. For these reasons, the following brief description of an animal cell is given for comparison with a bacterial cell and as an essential background to the later discussion on the life cycle of viruses.

The animal cell

Although the cells of various animal tissues (e.g. the brain and muscle) differ widely in morphology and function, they each have a cell membrane, cytoplasm, and a central nucleus surrounded by a well-defined nuclear membrane (Fig. 2.1). In general, the mammalian cell is approximately 15–20 μm in diameter.

Cell membrane (plasma membrane)

This is the retaining sheath that encloses the cellular constituents, and is composed of a polysaccharide-protein-lipid complex. Under the electron microscope it is seen to have a definite structure consisting of three layers: the outer protein and carbohydrate layer, a middle zone containing lipid molecules and an inner protein layer. The rim of cytoplasm just beneath the limiting membrane may consist of two layers — the gel-like ectoplasm and the more fluid endoplasm. Neuraminic acid is also present in specialised surface areas which act as receptors for certain viruses. The functional properties of the cell membrane include, in some cells at least, the ability to distinguish between potassium and sodium ions although these are alike in size and electrical charge. The membrane assists the entry of the former but opposes the latter whilst, with large molecules, it facilitates their entry into the interior of the cell by a process of mechanical ingestion or engulfment. This process of engulfment of droplets of liquid from the environment by the exposed surfaces of cells is called **pinocytosis**, whereas the ingestion of particulate matter (e.g. bacteria) by a similar process is called **phagocytosis**. Following adsorption of particles, molecules or ions on to the cell surface, the membrane slides or flows forwards forming a deep invagination or vesicle extending towards the inside of the cell. In time, this vesicle becomes 'pinched-off' from the cell surface and a pouch or vacuole appears inside the cytoplasm containing the ingested particle or, in the case of virus infected cells, the virion or virions.

The cell membrane is in continuous motion and as the cell moves, long villi continuously form on the leading edge of the cell, but as soon as it comes into contact with a neighbouring cell these movements cease and adhesion of the two cells takes place. The region of contact may be modified by specialised organelles called desmosomes which reinforce the cells and give greater rigidity to the tissue. This loss of cell movement as a result of

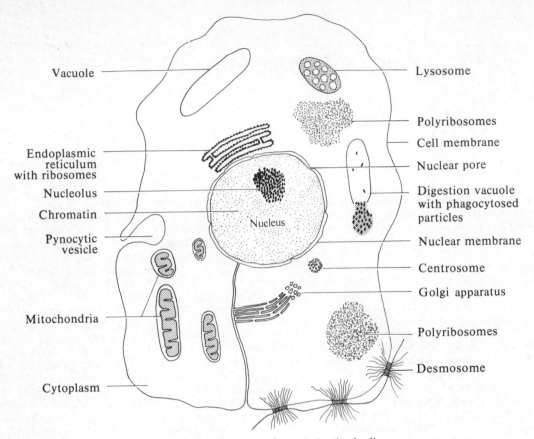

Fig. 2.1. Structure of a typical animal cell.

Labels (left, top to bottom): Vacuole; Endoplasmic reticulum with ribosomes; Nucleolus; Chromatin; Pynocytic vesicle; Mitochondria; Cytoplasm. Centre: Nucleus. Labels (right, top to bottom): Lysosome; Polyribosomes; Cell membrane; Nuclear pore; Digestion vacuole with phagocytosed particles; Nuclear membrane; Centrosome; Golgi apparatus; Polyribosomes; Desmosome.

contact with other cells is called **contact inhibition**. Contact between cells inhibits both motility and mitosis so that in tissue cultures, monolayers of cells are formed on the glass instead of multilayers. Neoplastic cells lack this property of contact inhibition and studies with polyoma virus have shown that after 'transformation' the affected cells continue to move, multiply and pile on top of each other to form well-defined multilayers of cells. (See Chapter 46)

Cytoplasm

Structures to be found within the cytoplasm include the large, sausage-shaped mitochondria, the largest of the cytoplasmic organelles, which act as the 'power houses' of the cell and supply up to 90 per cent of the energy that it requires for viral multiplication. They vary considerably in both size and shape and contain a high concentration of respiratory enzymes. Infoldings of the inner of its two membranes form incomplete compartments within the mitochondrion. Other equally highly organised membrane-bound structures occurring in the cytoplasm are lysosomes. They vary in size and shape but are mostly round bodies about 0·4 μm. They are somewhat smaller than the mitochondria and contain a number of enzymes, including phosphatases, ribonucleases and deoxyribonucleases. These enzymes are capable of breaking down (hydrolysing) large molecules such as those of fats, proteins and nucleic acids into smaller particles capable of being oxidized by the enzymes of the mitochondria. When a cell ingests a virus particle enclosed in a portion of the cell membrane, the vesicle and its contents pass into the cytoplasm where it comes into contact with a lysosome. The membranes of the two structures then meet and fuse to form a 'digestion vacuole' in which the phagocytosed particles are digested by the enzymes of the lysosome.

Other visible particles within the cytoplasm are the centrosomes or centrioles which appear about the time of cell division at the poles of the spindle apparatus that divides the chromosomes. Electron micrographs show that the cytoplasm also contains

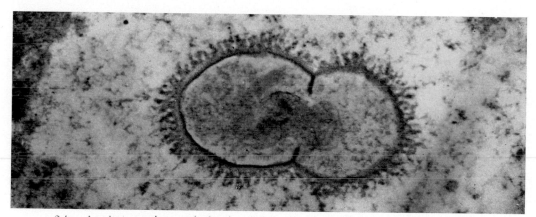

2.1a   An electron micrograph showing division of a coccus by binary fission, × 54 000.

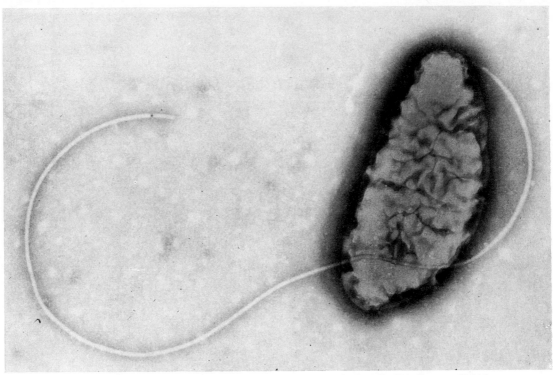

2.1b   An electron micrograph showing a bacillus with a single polar flagellum, × 58 000.

a complicated 'skeleton' or system of internal membranes known as the endoplasmic reticulum and it has been suggested that through the very fine 'caniculi' formed by the membranes, which may be continuous with the external membrane, particles may pass through the cytoplasm to the membrane lining the nucleus.

Also continuous with the endoplasmic reticulum is the Golgi apparatus, a complex of crescent-shaped cisternae lying in the cytoplasm near the nucleus, but whether or not the Golgi bodies are responsible for the production of the smooth-surfaced endoplasmic reticulum is not known. There is some evidence that one of the functions of the Golgi apparatus may be concerned with the combination of carbohydrate components (polysaccharides) with protein molecules to form glycoproteins and mucoproteins. It has also been suggested that lysosomes are formed by budding-off from the Golgi apparatus.

The electron microscope has confirmed that the tubular structures of the endoplasmic reticulum may be either smooth-walled or their outer surfaces may be studded with spiral curved rows of tiny granules called ribosomes. These are mostly small bodies (15–25 nm) each of which consists of a large and small sub-unit, and they occur either fixed or free in the cytoplasm. Although very small, they are exceedingly rich in RNA, intimately associated with protein synthesis and especially prevalent in cells that produce large amounts of protein. In fact, ribosomal RNA accounts for about 90 per cent of the total cellular RNA. The ribosomal subunits are assembled in the nucleus and the nucleolus itself is largely composed of ribosomes. Although it seems likely that the ribosomal proteins are not only assembled but are actually synthesised in the nucleus, they mostly function in the cytoplasm where they usually occur as aggregates of varying sizes, held together by a strand of messenger RNA. These aggregations are termed polyribosomes and constitute the sites where polypeptides are synthesised.

Nucleus

In contrast to bacterial cells, the genetic apparatus of animal cells is separated from the cytoplasm within a specialised organelle, the nucleus, which is usually about 5μm. in diameter. It is bounded by a double membrane which acts as a barrier to the random movement of molecules from the nucleus into the cytoplasm. Nevertheless, in the outer layer there are pores (annuli) open to the cytoplasm through which micromolecules may pass as well as some organelles such as the ribosomes and their subunits. The precise structure of the nuclear pore is not known but electron microscopy suggests that it is in the form of an annulus with eight structural units arranged radially which opens and closes

in the manner of an 'iris' diaphragm. The nuclear membrane disappears during mitosis but is presumed to be subsequently reformed from the cytoplasmic membrane. Within the nucleus are the strands of chromatin which contain almost all of the cell's DNA apart from a very small amount that is associated with the mitochondria. In the resting stage the filaments of chromatin are diffusely distributed throughout the nucleus but immediately before cell division takes place the chromatin threads coil up tightly to form the chromosomes. The chromosomes carry most of the genetic information of the cell and the number of such chromosomes and their structure is a highly characteristic feature of each animal species.

Also inside the nucleus are small spherical bodies, the nucleoli, which are packed with tiny granules that are rich in RNA. The number of nucleoli varies with the cell type and their size increases in cells that are actively synthesising proteins. These granules resemble the ribosomes in the cytoplasm and are active in protein and RNA synthesis. Recent investigations suggest that the nucleus of the cell is the principal centre for the synthesis of nucleic acid (both DNA and RNA) and that the nuclear RNA is capable, in some way, of transferring genetic material from the DNA to the cytoplasm. The cytoplasm on the other hand, and the ribosomes in particular, are thought to be the main sites for the synthesis of proteins including many different types of enzymes.

The bacterial cell

Morphology

Bacteria are microorganisms of relatively simple unicellular structure. Their shapes differ among various genera (Fig. 2.2) and, according to environment, a particular strain may show variations of shape and size. It is a characteristic feature of some bacteria to grow and multiply in filaments, clusters, chains or mycelia. All these morphological properties are of value in the identification and classification of bacteria. During the development of bacteriology the study of morphology was made by microscopical examinations of unstained and stained films, and it is a remarkable fact that the use of more sophisticated instruments, including the electron and phase contrast microscopes, has largely confirmed these earlier observations.

The units of measurement used for recording the sizes of bacteria are as follows:

1 micrometre (μm) ≡ 1 micron (μ) ≡ 1/1000 mm
1 nanometre (nm) ≡ 1 millimicron (mμ)
  ≡ 1/1000 micrometre (micron)
0·1 nanometre ≡ 1 Angström unit (Å or AU)

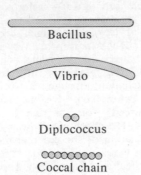

FIG. 2.2. Bacterial morphology.

Bacillus

Vibrio

Diplococcus

Coccal chain

Coccal cluster

Spirillum

Spirochaete

Mycelium

On the basis of their morphology bacteria can be classified as follows:

Bacilli
Rod-shaped (i.e. cylindrical) organisms, usually straight, varying in length from 2–10 μm and breadth from 1–2 μm according to species. (e.g. *Corynebacterium, Erysipelothrix, Clostridium, Bacillus, Salmonella, Escherichia, Brucella, Mycobacterium*).

Vibrios
Rod-shaped (i.e. cylindrical) organisms, usually curved or comma-shaped (e.g. *Vibrio, Campylobacter*).

Spirilla
Spiral-shaped, non-flexuous filaments (e.g. *Spirilla*).

Spirochaetes
Spiral-shaped, flexuous, actively motile filaments (e.g. *Leptospira, Treponema, Borrelia*).

Cocci
Circular- (i.e. spherical) or lanceolate-shaped organisms about 1 μm in diameter occurring in the following characteristic cell groupings: clusters (*Staphylococcus*), chains (*Streptococcus*), pairs (*Diplococcus, Neisseria*), cubical groups (*Sarcina*).

Mycelia
Branching filaments which may tend to fragment (*Actinomyces, Nocardia*) or to remain filamentous (*Streptomyces*).

Structure
In recent years, interest in bacterial cytology has been revived and the application of modern biochemical and microscopical techniques is revealing the detailed structure of these organisms. A bacterial cell consists of a cell wall and within this is the cytoplasmic membrane containing the cytoplasm in which is situated the nuclear body (Fig. 2.3). Other additional features characteristic of some bacterial species are capsules surrounding the cell wall, flagella and fimbriae. The following is a brief account of the structure and properties of the various constituents of bacterial cells.

Cell Wall
This structure surrounds the protoplasm which forms the protoplast or living body of the organism. The cell wall is, itself, a structural unit associated with the shape and rigidity of the whole organism. The main component of the wall is a mucopeptide complex. In addition, there are other substances which vary from one bacterial species to another. For example, the wall of *Staphylococcus pyogenes* contains teichoic acid and glycine which compose 20 per cent by weight of this structure. In *Escherichia coli* some 80 per cent consists of protein and lipopolysaccharide (i.e. somatic antigen). The amino sugar muramic acid and glucosamine are incorporated in the polysaccharide complex and form the substrate with which sensitivity to lysozyme, penicillin and other antibacterial substances is associated.

The wall is intimately concerned with bacterial multiplication. Division of one bacterium into two by binary fission is initiated by a constriction of the wall in the central region of the bacterium. This continues until complete division has occurred, which involves a splitting of the membrane and liberation of two separate bacteria (Plate 2.1a, facing p. 12). On some occasions this final splitting is delayed or fails to occur, in which case cocci will grow in characteristic clumps (*Staphylococcus*) or chains (*Streptococcus*), and bacilli will produce filaments (*Bacillus anthracis, Sphaerophorus necrophorus*).

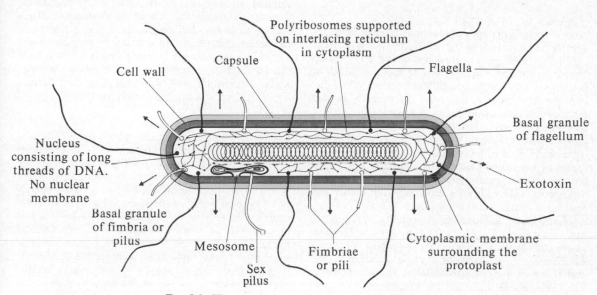

Cell wall

Capsule

Polyribosomes supported
on interlacing reticulum
in cytoplasm

Flagella

Basal granule
of flagellum

Nucleus
consisting of long
threads of DNA.
No nuclear
membrane

Exotoxin

Basal granule
of fimbria or
pilus

Mesosome

Sex
pilus

Fimbriae
or pili

Cytoplasmic membrane
surrounding the
protoplast

FIG. 2.3. The morphological features of a bacterial cell.

Cytoplasmic membrane

Between the cell wall and the cytoplasm is a very thin cytoplasmic membrane which not only surrounds the cytoplasm but also forms folds which penetrate into its substance. These folds have been demonstrated in bacteria grown aerobically, and although they may not always be present they appear to be uniquely characteristic for bacteria.

The cytoplasmic membrane functions as a permeable membrane which allows water and nutrients to pass into the cell and waste products to pass out into the external environment. The membrane contains a complex enzyme system concerned not only with the uptake of soluble nutrients but probably with the formation of the cell wall. Both the cytoplasmic membranes and cell walls vary in their porosity, and this has an important relationship to the Gram-staining reaction. The more porous membranes do not retain methyl violet dye when decolourised by acetone or alcohol and, consequently, the bacteria stain Gram-negative. Conversely, less porous membranes stained with methyl violet retain the dye when decolourising agents are applied and these organisms stain Gram-positive.

Cytoplasm

Bacterial cytoplasm is of a watery, gelatinous consistency containing organic and inorganic solutes, and several thousand ribosomes often occurring in groups (polyribosomes) which are distributed throughout the substance of the cytoplasm as small granules, 10–30 nm in diameter. These ribosomes contain protein and ribonucleic acid (RNA). Nuclear bodies containing chromosomal desoxyribonucleic acid (DNA) are seen in the cytoplasm either as single bodies in resting cells or as two or more bodies in actively dividing cells. Inclusion granules have also been observed in a variety of bacterial species. Volutin granules contain inorganic phosphates and increase in size and number when bacteria are actively growing in a favourable environment. They can be shown characteristically in the diphtheria bacillus and in some other corynebacterial species after staining with Neisser's or Albert's stain. Lipid granules containing β-hydroxybutyric acid have been observed in *Bacillus megaterium*, and in some bacteria polysaccharide granules occur which are presumed to contain glycogen because they stain brown with iodine. In the cytoplasm are often seen invaginations of the cytoplasmic membrane which are called mesosomes. The function of these organelles has not been clearly established but they may correspond to the mitochondria of eukaryotic cells.

Nucleus

The function of the bacterial nucleus is similar to that of the animal cell but differs from it structurally in not possessing either a nuclear membrane or a nucleolus. During the logarithmic phase when bacteria are rapidly multiplying, the nuclei divide by simple fission and two nuclei may often be observed in a single bacterium before complete division of the cell has taken place.

Capsules

Many bacteria produce a gelatinous layer of material on the outer surface of the cell wall which is usually termed the capsule. The thickness of this layer varies considerably and when 0·5 μm or more in width it is easily visible under the light microscope. When the capsule is thinner it has been referred to as the envelope or microcapsule. In the past, a great deal of confusion has arisen over the use of the terms capsule and envelope which have described what were considered to be separate structures. However, recent experimental evidence indicates that the terms envelope and capsule refer to the same structure.

Capsular material varies in composition, consisting mostly of water containing about 1–2 per cent of polysaccharide, polypeptide or protein, according to individual bacterial species. The capsules of *Yersinia pestis* consist of a polysaccharide-protein complex, *Bacillus anthracis* capsules contain a polypeptide, and those of some other bacterial species, notably *Klebsiella*, *Escherichia* and the pneumococcus, consist of polysaccharides. In contrast, the capsules of *Streptococcus pyogenes* contain hyaluronic acid and a protein which can be removed by trypsin digestion without affecting the viability of the organisms. Well-developed capsules are often slimy and this is clearly seen in recently isolated strains of *Actinobacillus equuli* in which the treacle-like consistency of the colonies is a characteristic property of these organisms.

Bacterial capsules seem to be produced as a protective covering by the organism against attack from the defence mechanisms of the body, particularly phagocytic cells and various enzymes. This has been illustrated with *Bacillus anthracis*, *Yersinia pestis*, *Klebsiella pneumoniae* and other bacterial species. Thus, the number of organisms required to initiate disease may be far smaller in the case of capsulated as compared with non-capsulated organisms. Nevertheless, well-developed capsules do not always signify increased virulence since some capsulated strains of *Bacillus anthracis* and *Yersinia pestis* may be relatively susceptible to phagocytosis. Virulence will depend not only on the degree of capsule formation but also on the toxigenic properties of the organisms, the availability of suitable nutrients for bacterial growth and on the immune status of the animal.

Capsules are antigens and when inoculated into animals stimulate the production of specific antibodies. As early as 1896, Roger noted that soon after adding homologous antiserum to *Oidium albicans*, an apparent swelling of the surface layer of the organisms occurred. A similar reaction was observed in 1902 by Neufeld with *Diplococcus pneumoniae*, and this type of reaction has since been applied to various other groups of organisms, including *Haemophilus*, *Klebsiella*, *Pasteurella*, *Streptococcus* and *Bacillus*. Originally, it was thought that the reaction consisted of a marked swelling of the capsular material but more recently it has been shown that it involves a precipitation between antigen (capsule) and antibody (immune serum) which renders the capsule clearly visible.

Flagella

Bacterial flagella originate from basal granules inside the cell membrane and are hair-like structures about 0·02 μm thick and usually several times the total length of the bacterial body (Plate 2.1b, facing p. 13). They may be situated either at the bacterial poles or over most of the bacterial surface (peritrichate). The purpose of flagella is not known but presumably the motility which they impart enables bacteria to come into contact with high concentrations of nutrients, and may facilitate the dissemination of infection in the tissues. Motility can be readily observed microscopically in hanging-drop preparations (e.g. *Salmonella*, *Escherichia*) or from the characteristic spreading growth over the moist surface of solid media (e.g. *Proteus*, *Clostridium tetani*).

Bacterial flagella consist almost entirely of protein (flagellin). In the case of *Proteus* and *Bacillus subtilis* this protein consists of long thin molecules composed of at least fourteen amino acids which differ only slightly between these two bacterial species. The genus *Salmonella* contains a wide variety of antigenically distinct flagella which are made use of for distinguishing between the many hundreds of different serotypes. It is probable that these antigenic differences are determined by variations in the arrangements of amino acids constituting the protein molecules of flagella.

Fimbriae

These are small filaments which project from the surfaces of some bacterial species. They are markedly smaller than flagella, measuring up to a maximum of about 1·5 μm in length and only about 0·5–0·8 μm in width, and can be observed under the electron microscope as straight appendages occurring over the entire bacterial surface. They are composed of protein, produced by some of the bacterial species belonging to the family *Enterobacteriaceae*, and may occur on flagellate as well as non-flagellate organisms. The production of fimbriae may be enhanced or inhibited by conditions of laboratory culture. Special fimbriae or pili, known as sex-pili, are concerned with conjugation and the transference of DNA from one bacterium to another.

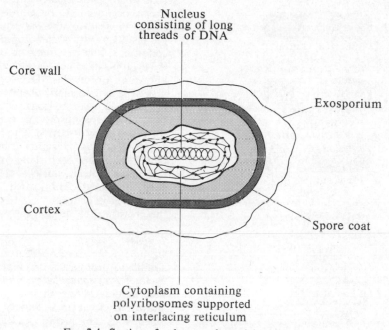

Nucleus
consisting of long
threads of DNA

Core wall

Exosporium

Cortex

Spore coat

Cytoplasm containing
polyribosomes supported
on interlacing reticulum

FIG. 2.4. Section of a dormant bacterial spore.

Most but not all fimbriate bacteria have the property of adhering to tissue cells, and perhaps in this way are able to remain in a nutritionally favourable environment in the host's tissues. Most of these strains also adhere to red blood cells, particularly those derived from the horse, pig, chicken and guinea-pig. A mixture of fimbriate bacteria with red blood cells results in the formation of easily visible haemagglutination.

Spores

When some species of bacteria are in an environment unfavourable for rapid multiplication they will develop into spores, which are dormant forms capable of survival for long periods of time under adverse conditions. Each bacterium develops into one spore, and during this process of sporulation part of the bacterial cytoplasm and nuclear material become incorporated within a thick cortex and an outer protective spore coat which is responsible for the characteristic resistance of the spore to adverse environments (Fig. 2.4). In *Bacillus cereus*, for example, part of the nuclear material becomes situated at one end of the bacillus, and this includes RNA and an amount of DNA equivalent to about half that which is present in an actively growing vegetative bacterium. A thin septum then develops from opposite sides of the cell, close to one end of

the bacillus and enclosing the nuclear material and some of the cytoplasm. This stage in sporulation may develop within about 35 minutes after the last cell division has taken place, and is followed by the development of a cortex, about 0·1 μm thick and then a protective spore coat, sometimes covered on the outside by an exosporium. Finally, the remaining part of the vegetative cell disintegrates. Although the exosporium, spore coat and cortex are antigenic it is probable that the antigens of the exosporium are primarily responsible for stimulation of spore antibody production.

Spores vary in situation and shape according to the bacterial species. They may develop centrally (*Bacillus anthracis*), subterminally (*Clostridium chauvoei*) or terminally as spherical (*Clostridium tetani*) or ovoid (*Clostridium tertium*) structures (Fig. 2.5). The size of the spore may be sufficiently large to bulge the walls of the cell during development in some bacterial species.

Compared with vegetative bacteria, spores are highly resistant to extremes of physical and chemical environments, including high temperatures, desiccation and disinfection. Some are not killed in a moist atmosphere unless heated to a temperature as high as 120°C for 10–15 minutes. Under dry conditions or in soil they may remain viable for many years, and at any time during this period they can develop into

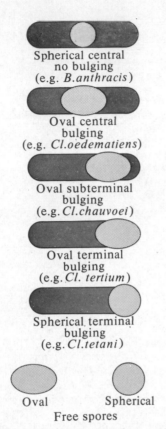

Spherical central
no bulging
(e.g. *B.anthracis*)

Oval central
bulging
(e.g. *Cl.oedematiens*)

Oval subterminal
bulging
(e.g. *Cl.chauvoei*)

Oval terminal
bulging
(e.g. *Cl. tertium*)

Spherical terminal
bulging
(e.g. *Cl.tetani*)

Oval   Spherical

Free spores

FIG. 2.5. The shape and disposition of spores developing in bacteria.

vegetative bacteria as soon as they are placed in a favourable environment with adequate nutrients. Under these conditions each spore will develop into one bacterium. During the initial stages of germination the cortex begins to disappear and the core wall increases in thickness. In the final stages the exosporium and spore coat are shed, leaving the core wall to form the cell wall of the new vegetative bacterium.

Most experiments to determine the nature of the substances required to initiate germination of spores have shown that simple sugars and amino acids are particularly important. For example, spores of *Bacillus mycoides*, *Clostridium welchii*, *Clostridium chauvoei* and *Clostridium sporogenes* will germinate in the presence of glucose; those of *Bacillus anthracis* in a medium containing adenosine plus tyrosine plus L-alanine; *Bacillus subtilis* in L-alanine plus glucose; and *Clostridium botulinum* in glucose and L-alanine plus L-arginine plus L-phenylalanine.

Protoplasts

Bacterial protoplasm is usually enclosed in a cell wall which gives rigidity and a characteristic shape to an organism. Damage to the wall commonly results in death of the bacterium consequent upon the disintegration of the protoplasm. Under defined conditions, however, removal of the wall may leave the protoplasm intact, usually in the form of a sphere known as a protoplast. Development of protoplasts may arise as an osmotic phenomenon after treatment of bacteria with various concentrations of salt solutions. It may also occur from the destruction of the cell wall by lysosyme. The properties of *Bacillus megaterium* protoplasts have been studied in some detail and it has been shown that they are able to synthesise proteins, nucleic acids and enzymes; that they are capable of growth, multiplication and production of endospores; and that they can support the growth of bacteriophages.

L phase

In 1935 Klieneberger-Nobel found that structures similar to protoplasts developed as part of the life cycle of *Streptobacillus moniliformis* and these have been designated as L phase. L phases have since been shown to occur in a variety of bacterial species when they are grown under adverse conditions (see Chapter 27).

Physiology

Bacteria require certain basic materials to provide energy for growth, multiplication and movement. These include carbon, nitrogen, potassium, sodium, calcium, magnesium, iron, hydrogen, oxygen and certain trace elements including manganese and cobalt. In addition, some bacteria require growth factors for the synthesis of essential metabolites. These substances are needed for the production of the main components of bacteria which include proteins, carbohydrates, fats, vitamins and enzymes.

Bacteria vary widely in their ability to synthesise these components, and on this basis can be divided into two main groups designated autotrophs and heterotrophs.

Autotrophs

Many bacterial species have developed an ability to synthesise complex organic molecules from simple inorganic substances. Thus, they require as food a source of carbon which is derived either from atmospheric CO_2 or from carbonates and various other inorganic substances. From these materials autotrophic bacteria are able to live and multiply, and most of them will grow in the absence of light. Some species, however, require sunlight as a source of energy and these organisms are mainly found in brackish and sewage contaminated water.

Heterotrophs

These bacteria cannot derive energy solely from simple inorganic substances but are dependent upon at least one organic compound for growth. This is usually supplied in the form of carbohydrates, amino acids, peptides or lipids. Parasitic bacteria are typically heterotrophic and many of those which cause disease in animals and man can only be grown in culture media containing various organic compounds. Among these bacteria, the development of their enzyme structure and cell protein is derived from amino acids incorporated in the media. The synthesis of nucleic acids depends upon the availability of purines and pyrimidines; and other growth factors are required for the formation of coenzymes and vitamins (e.g. thiamine, riboflavin, nicotinic acid, pyridoxine, p-amino-benzoic acid, folic acid, biotin, vitamin B_{12}, etc.)

Recent advances in knowledge on bacterial nutrition have shown that the original classification of bacteria into autotrophic and heterotrophic groups has become less precise because a number of examples have been observed which are exceptions to the general rule. These include certain intestinal bacilli which will grow inorganically with sodium citrate as a carbon source, and some soil bacteria which can adapt themselves to exist either autotrophically or heterotrophically.

Respiration

The process of bacterial respiration consists of oxidation by dehydrogenation in which hydrogen is enzymatically removed from a suitable nutrient, thus releasing energy which is absorbed into high-energy phosphate. The removal of hydrogen occurs through the action of dehydrogenases on the substrate nutrient, and the hydrogen is then passed on to other molecules (hydrogen acceptors) until finally released from the bacterium, leaving the dehydrogenase available to take up more hydrogen.

Aerobes

Many bacterial species are able to grow in the presence of atmospheric oxygen which is used as the final extracellular hydrogen acceptor. This process of transferring hydrogen from bacteria to atmospheric oxygen is carried out by the enzyme *cytochrome oxidase*, and those organisms which can only make use of free oxygen as the hydrogen acceptors are known as strict or obligate aerobes. Adaptation of enzymes in other bacteria enable them to use glucose and atmospheric oxygen from which carbon dioxide, water and energy are formed.

$$C_6H_{12}O_6 + 6O_2 \longrightarrow 6CO_2 + 6H_2O + energy.$$

With some bacterial species this process of oxidation may be incomplete, as in the production of acetic acid and water from alcohol.

$$C_2H_5OH + O_2 \longrightarrow CH_3COOH + H_2O + energy$$

Anaerobes

Among the bacterial species causing disease in animals and man, some are anaerobic and do not possess the necessary enzyme systems to utilise atmospheric oxygen as the final hydrogen acceptor. Moreover, some of these organisms are so sensitive to the presence of oxygen that the atmosphere may be toxic to them (e.g. *Sphaerophorus necrophorus*). These strict anaerobes must be grown in the absence of atmospheric oxygen and they have to make use of other substances as final hydrogen acceptors. A compound such as $NaNO_3$ can be used as a suitable hydrogen acceptor as it is reduced to $NaNO_2$, and the oxygen which is given up is used as a hydrogen acceptor. The reduction of nitrates to nitrites is a test frequently applied in the laboratory for identifying the properties of various bacterial species.

Growth

Multiplication

Bacterial multiplication occurs by **binary fission** and under appropriate conditions this is a continual process which is maintained so long as the environment of the organisms can supply the required nutrients and remove metabolic products which would otherwise interfere with development. For this to occur the synthesis and activity of suitable enzymes must be developed and maintained throughout the period of growth, and techniques for continual cell culture have been evolved which can sustain bacterial multiplication for long periods.

During the process of binary fission the bacterial cell becomes enlarged to approximately twice its length and a septum from the plasma membrane and cell wall develops, transversely, dividing the parent cell into two daughter cells. This division, followed by separation, may take place rapidly at an approximate rate of once every 30 minutes. Sometimes the process of division and separation is incomplete or delayed with the result that the two daughter cells do not separate from each other. Under these circumstances the multiplication process gives rise to bacterial formations characteristic for certain species, including pairs (*Diplococcus*), chains (*Streptococcus*), groups (*Staphylococcus*) or filaments (*Sphaerophorus*).

Growth environment

We have already noted the chemical requirements for the growth of autotrophic and heterotrophic bacteria, including carbon, nitrogen, inorganic salts, and the different atmospheric requirements for aerobic and anaerobic organisms. There are, in addition, certain other optimal conditions necessary for the cultivation of various species of pathogenic bacteria.

Carbon dioxide. Bacteria utilise the small amount of CO_2 which is in the atmosphere, but some species, particularly primary cultures of *Brucella abortus*, require a higher concentration of 5 per cent or more in the atmosphere for maximum growth rate.

Hydrogen-ion concentration. Most bacterial species associated with animal diseases require a pH range of 7·2–7·6 in the medium for optimal growth conditions. Environments which are either more acidic or more alkaline are rapidly lethal. Some species (e.g. *Mycobacterium tuberculosis*) are relatively resistant to the bactericidal effect of an acid pH, and this property is made use of for the isolation of this organism from contaminated material.

Temperature. Bacterial species which are parasitic in animals and man have become acclimatised to growing at body temperatures. The optimum temperature for their cultivation in the laboratory is about 37°C. Some species will grow more slowly at temperatures as high as 44°C or as low as 25°C, and a few will multiply at even lower temperatures in the range of 5–6°C.

Temperatures higher than 45°C are lethal to species of bacteria which naturally occur in the animal body, and the higher the temperature to which they are exposed under standard conditions the more rapid is the lethal effect. This lethal effect is greater in a moist atmosphere than it is in a dry one. In a moist atmosphere a temperature of about 60°C for 15–20 minutes is lethal to vegetative organisms because under these conditions the cell proteins become denatured. Most bacterial spores are more resistant and are killed in a moist atmosphere when the temperature is raised to about 120°C for 20 minutes. These conditions are provided by pressurised steam generated in an autoclave or pressure cooker. The lethal temperature for bacterial spores in a dry atmosphere requires to be at least 140–150°C. These conditions are produced in a hot air oven which is commonly used in laboratories for the sterilisation of laboratory glassware.

Moisture. Moisture is essential for bacterial growth and survival. This will be readily appreciated when it is realised that water accounts for approximately 80 per cent of the weight of bacteria. Conversely, desiccation under most conditions is lethal. It is important to emphasise, however, that frozen bacteria which are rapidly desiccated and then stored in a vacuum will remain viable for years. This method of preservation is known as **freeze drying** or **lyophilisation**.

Light. Pathogenic bacteria are susceptible to light and are killed rapidly when exposed to ultraviolet light derived from a u.v. lamp or from direct sunlight. They are killed more slowly by daylight passing through glass.

Rates of growth

Under customary laboratory conditions for bacterial cultivation, the growth of organisms occurs in a characteristic pattern which includes four stages. Immediately after inoculation of bacteria into a fixed volume of medium and subsequent incubation at a suitable temperature, there is an initial period of time before bacterial multiplication commences. This is known as the **lag phase**, and is followed by a period of **accelerating growth phase** leading to the **logarithmic phase** in which the rapid multiplication bears a linear relationship to time. This, in turn, is followed by a **declining growth phase** resulting from the increasing depletion of one or more of the nutrients in the media. Initially, the number of cells dying equals the number of cells dividing, and this is followed by an **accelerating** or **logarithmic death phase**, ultimately leading to the **stationary** or **dormant phase** in which bacteria remain viable but unable to multiply, and the low death rate almost balances the slow rate of multiplication.

The two important features to note are first, the initial delay in multiplication which occurs immediately after inoculation of the media; and second, the limited period of active growth which is controlled by the availability of all the nutrient requirements in a given volume of culture media (Fig. 2.6).

From the time when bacteriologists first grew organisms in the laboratory until the present day, the main purpose has been to provide suitable media, atmospheric conditions and temperatures which would allow multiplication to occur according to the order of events just described. It must be emphasised, however, that this cycle is unnatural, that it is controlled and limited by the artificial environment of laboratory techniques, and that it bears little relationship to the growth rates of bacteria in the tissues of the host. It is common practice for bacteriologists to examine some of the characteristic properties of bacteria when these are derived from pure cultures which have been incubated overnight or for longer periods. Under these conditions it is usual for the growth rate of cells to have passed the logarithmic phase and to be in the stage of declining growth phase or even the stationary phase.

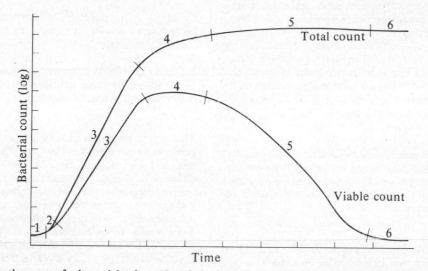

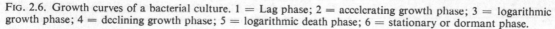

FIG. 2.6. Growth curves of a bacterial culture. 1 = Lag phase; 2 = accelerating growth phase; 3 = logarithmic growth phase; 4 = declining growth phase; 5 = logarithmic death phase; 6 = stationary or dormant phase.

Recently, it has been shown that bacteria vary in size and chemical constitution according to the time in the growth cycle at which they are examined. For example, cells multiplying rapidly in the logarithmic phase are larger than those which are in the stationary phase, and the former have a higher RNA content and a lower DNA content than similar bacteria in the stationary phase. We have seen that immediately after fresh culture media have been inoculated with resting bacteria there is a characteristic lag phase before multiplication occurs. During this lag phase considerable changes are going on within the bacteria in preparation for multiplication and these are apparent from the rapid increase in bacterial size and in RNA content, until the latter approaches the high concentration associated with rapidly multiplying bacteria.

Proteins and nucleic acids are essential components for the life of bacteria and it will be evident from the above discussion that the concentrations of these substances vary according to the external environment and the stage in the growth cycle of microorganisms in chemically defined media. When bacteria are dividing at a steady rate in a particular medium, there must be a dynamic equilibrium between all the molecular components associated with the production and maintenance of proteins and nucleic acids. There will also be an equilibrium between these components and the external environment. If these bacteria are then transferred to chemically different media, this will inevitably lead to an alteration in the internal components of the organisms. A consequent adaptation of the bacteria to the new environment must occur before equilibrium is re-established and multiplication can again take place. It is this period of adaptation which results in the characteristic lag phase occurring immediately after bacteria have been inoculated into different media.

Whereas proteins and nucleic acids are essential materials required for bacterial growth, polysaccharides and lipids are less important constituents which are stored by bacteria either intracellularly or extracellularly as capsules or slime. Little is known about the precise mechanisms which produce these accumulations except that they concern alterations in the production and activity of enzymes; and a shift of the enzyme equilibrium may result in either the synthesis or the breakdown of storage materials including polysaccharides and lipids. Polysaccharides can be synthesised when the external environment contains the necessary ingredients (e.g. glucose) and also in the presence of only minimal nitrogenous materials required for growth. Synthesis of polysaccharides can, therefore, take place independently of growth rate, and is not necessarily related to different phases in the growth cycle as is the case with proteins and nucleic acids.

Genetics

Present knowledge of bacterial genetics has been developed from studies carried out during little more than the last 20 years, and much of the current information is younger than this. The wider implications of these studies, particularly their importance in relation to the pathogenesis and control of bacterial diseases in man and animals, is now becoming apparent and will be of increasing significance in the future.

The study of genetics has necessarily included the development of a special terminology for the precise descriptions of the various processes involved, and the reader should have a clear understanding of the following terms which are used when discussing bacterial genetics.

Genes

These are inheritable units capable of independent segregation and rearrangement, which determine the inherited characters of bacteria; genes are intimately associated with parts of the DNA molecule in the nucleus of the cell.

Chromosomes

These consist of the entire double-helix DNA macromolecule occurring in the nucleus as a fine thread, and to which the genes are attached.

Genotype

This refers to all the heritable characteristics of a particular organism, some of which may not be observable under particular environmental conditions, although they may be potentially present within the organism.

Phenotype

This indicates the observable characteristic properties of a particular organism. These may be affected by both the genotype (i.e. heritable characteristics) and also by the environmental conditions.

Factors or episomes

These refer to genetic elements which may be added to a cell in which they then become autonomously replicating units in the bacterial cytoplasm or completely integrated with the chromosomes, in which case they replicate along with the chromosomes. Factors may or may not be lethal to bacteria, and are responsible for transferring properties to the organism which are additional to those controlled by the genes. There are three types of factors known as F or fertility factor, Cf or colicinogenic factor and R or resistance transfer factor.

F factor. Cells with F factors are designated F+ and those without as F−. The transfer of the F factor from an F+ cell to an F− cell renders the latter F+. The F factor confers on a bacterium the ability to conjugate ('maleness') with another bacterium through special fimbriae which form

tubes for the passage of the F factor from one cell to another.

Cf factor. Concerned with transferring from one bacterium to another the ability to produce colicins (i.e. bacteriocins).

R factor. This factor transfers to bacteria the quality of resistance to some antibiotics and occurs particularly among enteric organisms.

Mutation

This refers to bacterial multiplication in which a gene becomes altered or lost, so that the daughter cell and its progeny have a genetic constitution different to that of the parent cell.

Investigations into the relationships between genes and enzymes suggest that one gene has a controlling influence on one particular enzyme. However, this concept may be an over-simplification of a complex situation, because apart from the direct controlling effect which a gene may have on an enzyme, other genes may influence indirectly the activities of that enzyme by causing alterations in substrates, activators and inhibitors related to its activity. For these reasons it is difficult to establish beyond doubt that one gene is solely responsible for the activity of one particular enzyme in complex 'autosynthetic' bacteria, in which genes have not been chemically analysed and enzyme activity is determined by observable activities instead of chemical constitution. Nevertheless, experiments in this field do provide strong evidence for direct relationships existing between individual genes and enzyme activities.

Spontaneous mutations

During the process of reproduction it is normal for the genes to be exactly replicated. In this way, the daughter cells of each bacterial generation maintain the same properties as the parent cells. Occasionally a gene may become altered, either in its chemical structure or translocated with respect to the other genes in the bacterium. In either event the activity of the gene will be modified by an intrinsic cause resulting in the daughter cells becoming mutants. In other circumstances, some factor or factors in the bacterial environment may be responsible for a mutation occurring in which case the activity of a gene may be modified by an extrinsic cause. But these mutants will only be detected provided that they can survive in the environment in competition with parent cells; often this may not occur and the mutant strain will then die out. However, under various conditions survival of mutants with alterations in genetic constitution may give rise to important and easily detectable modifications to the properties of a particular species of bacterium (Fig. 2.7).

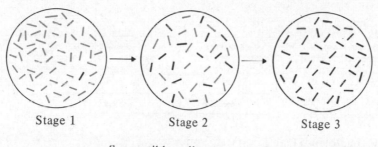

Stage 1   Stage 2   Stage 3

— = Susceptible cell   ▬ = Resistant cell

FIG. 2.7. The development of bacterial resistance to an antibacterial drug by spontaneous mutation. Stage 1 represents the initial growth of a susceptible culture in the presence of the drug, resulting in the selection of a resistant mutant. Stage 2 shows the rapid growth of this mutant. Stage 3 depicts the development of the resistant mutant of the culture which has finally developed from the original mutant cell.

One example of a mutation which is commonly observed in the laboratory is the delayed fermentation of lactose by cultures of certain bacteria (e.g. some strains of *Escherichia coli*) which may be incubated for as long as a week before fermentation is observed. Other examples include the development of drug resistance consequent upon the growth of bacteria in the presence of penicillin, streptomycin, etc.; the loss of somatic (O) antigens and the variation of smooth to rough forms (S → R): the loss of flagellar antigens; increased virulence as a result of passaging bacteria repeatedly from one animal to another in a particular species, leading to the development of a mutant capable of living in that animal species; or increased virulence resulting from growing the organism in media supplemented with blood, serum, ascitic fluid, etc.

Induced mutations

Mutations can be produced as a result of the controlled treatment of either dividing or resting bacteria with ultraviolet radiation, x-rays, nitrogen mustard and some other substances. There is no relationship between the nature of the inducing substance and the type of mutation which may occur.

Transformation

This refers to the transfer of DNA containing genes from one bacterium to another (Fig. 2.8). The DNA may be liberated spontaneously into the medium or extracted from the cells, and then taken up by the recipient, integrated into its chromosome, resulting in a change of phenotype. An example of transformation of this sort, which has been successfully carried out in the laboratory, is related to the ability of some strains of pneumococci to produce capsules. Thus, the DNA from encapsulated pneumococci has been isolated and successfully incorporated into the nuclei of non-encapsulated pneumococci, and as a result the latter organisms have developed the ability to form capsules (i.e. complex sugars).

Conjugation

This refers to the transference of chromosomal or episomal DNA from one bacterium to another as a result of direct contact, the development of a 'bridge' between the two organisms and a process which resembles mating. A bacterial population in which conjugation can take place includes donor and recipient cells. Donor cells which are also referred to as male or F+ cells, possess an F or sex factor which endows them with the property of developing special appendages called sex-pili on their surfaces, and it is via these pili that DNA passes from the

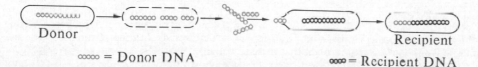

Donor   Recipient

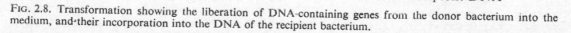

ᴏᴏᴏᴏᴏ = Donor DNA   ᴏᴏᴏᴏ = Recipient DNA

FIG. 2.8. Transformation showing the liberation of DNA-containing genes from the donor bacterium into the medium, and their incorporation into the DNA of the recipient bacterium.

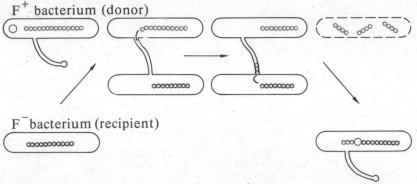

F$^+$ bacterium (donor)

F$^-$ bacterium (recipient)

○ = F (sex) factor

FIG. 2.9. Conjugation showing the transfer of genetic chromosomal material with F factor from an F⁺ (male) bacterium through a sex pilus to an F⁻ (female) bacterium as a result of contact. The reduction of DNA in the donor may cause death of the cell. The transfer of F factor to the recipient bacterium results in the cell acquiring the F⁺ (male) capacity to develop a sex pilus.

donors to the recipient cells. Recipient bacteria which are also known as female or F⁻ cells, possess neither the F factor nor sex-pili, but after conjugation has taken place the female cells become endowed with male properties, can develop sex-pili and are then capable of transferring DNA to another female cell.

In one type of conjugation the transfer of chromosomal DNA may occur in which it seems that genetic properties are transferred in a definite order, lending support to the theory that the genes, linearly organised on the chromosome, are transferred in the same lineal sequence to the receptor cell (Fig. 2.9).

In the other type of conjugation, episomal DNA is transferred from one cell to another and this process is concerned particularly with the transference of drug resistance. It is now known that the genes associated with drug resistance (R factors) are present in episomes which also contain resistance transfer factor (RTF), and it is the RTF portion of the episome which endows a bacterium with the property of developing a sex-pilus. When conjugation takes place the episome transfers from the donor to the recipient cell causing the latter to develop the property of drug resistance (Fig. 2.10).

Transduction
Under certain conditions bacteriophages may transfer genetic material from one bacterium to another (Fig. 2.11). To be able to demonstrate this process of transduction the donor strain of bacterium must differ genetically from the recipient strain; and the former must also be sensitive to a phage which is capable of transducing genetic material to the recipient strain. The first step is to produce a phage lysate from the donor bacteria by mixing the phage with bacteria under conditions which allow multiplication of the phage and subsequent bacterial lysis. The lysate so formed will contain some phages which have incorporated within themselves a small quantity of DNA from the lysed donor bacterium (about 1 in 10^6 of all phage particles), and these will have become temperate phages. If these temperate phages now infect recipient bacteria under conditions which allow the phages to develop in the living cells without causing lysis, a small proportion of the surviving recipient bacteria will acquire characters derived from the donor bacteria. In a typical experiment transduction can be observed only in about 1 in 10^4 bacteria. Usually only one character is carried from the donor to the recipient and this is not surprising in view of the relative sizes of bacteria and phages and the fact that only about 1/100 of total bacterial DNA can be carried by one phage particle to a recipient bacterium.

Classification
Bacteria belong to the Class Schizomycetes and their classification is based on the study of a variety of properties, including morphology and staining reactions, physiological properties and antigenic structures. An outline of the biological classification of bacteria which are of veterinary importance is shown on pages 26-28. For a more comprehensive classification the reader should consult Bergey's *Manual of Determinative Bacteriology*.

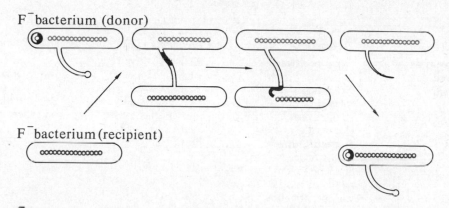

F⁻ bacterium (donor)

F⁻ bacterium (recipient)

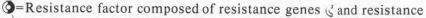

◐=Resistance factor composed of resistance genes ⚬ and resistance
transfer factor ❫

FIG. 2.10. Conjugation showing the transfer of a cytoplasmic resistance factor (episome) composed of resistance genes and resistance transfer factor (RTF) from an F⁺ (male) bacterium through a sex pilus to an F⁻ (female) bacterium. The transfer of RTF to the recipient bacterium results in the cell acquiring the F⁺ (male) capacity to develop a sex pilus. The loss of RTF by the donor bacterium causes the sex pilus to become useless.

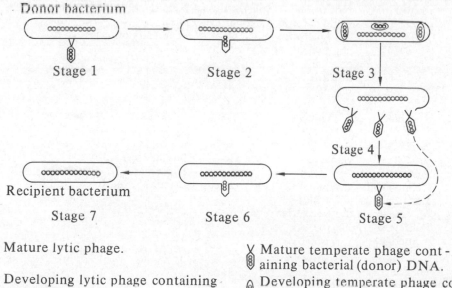

Donor bacterium

Stage 1   Stage 2   Stage 3

Stage 4

Recipient bacterium

Stage 7   Stage 6   Stage 5

⚟ Mature lytic phage.

⚟ Developing lytic phage containing no bacterial DNA.

⚟ Mature temperate phage containing bacterial (donor) DNA.

⚟ Developing temperate phage containing bacterial (donor) DNA.

FIG. 2.11. Transduction. Stages 1–4 show the life cycle of a lytic phage in which one phage unit incorporates some DNA from the donor bacterium and becomes a temperate phage. Stages 5–7 show the life cycle of the temperate phage in which the DNA it acquired from the donor bacterium becomes incorporated in the DNA of the recipient bacterium which can subsequently divide and produce genetically similar daughter cells. The transducing phage particle loses its own viral genetic material and cannot replicate in or lyse the recipient cell.

CLASS — SCHIZOMYCETES

ORDERS

Pseudomonadales
Gram-negative rods — straight, curved or spiral. Occur usually singly; motile with polar flagella.

Eubacteriales
Gram-positive or Gram-negative spheres or straight rods. Occur singly, in groups, in chains or in filaments. Non-motile or motile with peritrichous flagella. Some genera produce spores.

Actinomycetales
Gram-positive rods or filaments, also mycelia with conidia. Usually non-motile. Some genera are acid-fast.

Spirochaetales
Gram-negative slender spirals. No flagella but motile by body flexion.

ORDER — EUBACTERIALES

Family

Entero-bacteriaceae
Gram-negative rods; many are motile

Brucellaceae
Gram-negative rods or cocci

Bacteroidaceae
Gram-negative rods or filaments. Many are anaerobes and difficult to grow on nutrient media.

Micrococ-caceae
Gram-positive spheres; occur singly or in pairs, clumps or clusters

Lactobacil-laceae
Gram-positive cocci or rods. Occur singly or in pairs or chains

Corynebac-teriaceae
Gram-positive rods; some-times club-shaped

Bacillaceae
Gram-positive rods. Form endospores

Genera | Genera | Genera | Genera | Genera | Genera | Genera

Escherichia
Salmonella
Arizona
Klebsiella
Shigella
Citrobacter
Cloaca
Hafnia
Aerobacter
Enterobacter
Proteus
Morganella
Rettgerella
Providencia
Serratia
Yersinia

Brucella
Pasteurella
Actinobacillus
Haemophilus
Moraxella
Bordetella
Francisella

Sphaero-phorus
Strepto-bacillus
Fusobacterium
Bacteroides

Staphylo-coccus
Micrococcus

Streptococcus
Diplococcus
Lactobacillus

Coryne-bacterium
Erysipelothrix
Listeria

Bacillus
Clostridium

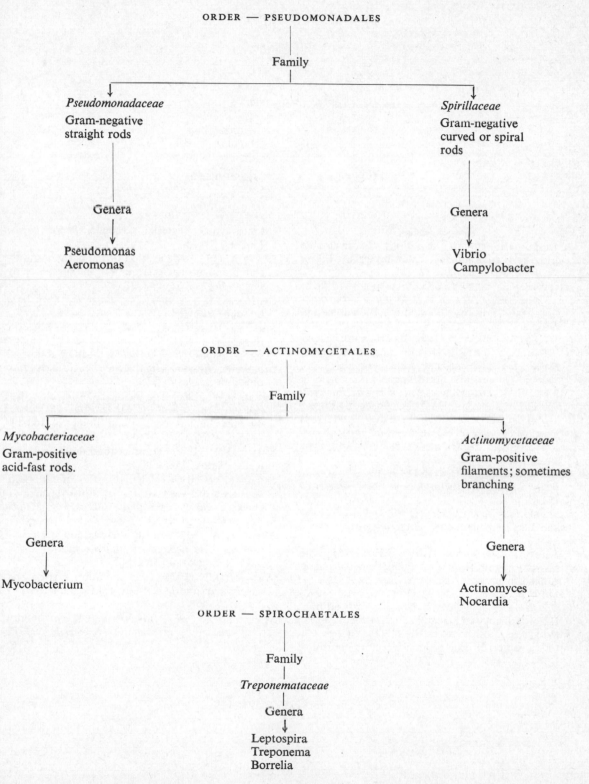

ORDER — PSEUDOMONADALES

Family

Pseudomonadaceae
Gram-negative
straight rods

Spirillaceae
Gram-negative
curved or spiral
rods

Genera

Genera

Pseudomonas
Aeromonas

Vibrio
Campylobacter

ORDER — ACTINOMYCETALES

Family

Mycobacteriaceae
Gram-positive
acid-fast rods.

Actinomycetaceae
Gram-positive
filaments; sometimes
branching

Genera

Genera

Mycobacterium

Actinomyces
Nocardia

ORDER — SPIROCHAETALES

Family

Treponemataceae

Genera

Leptospira
Treponema
Borrelia

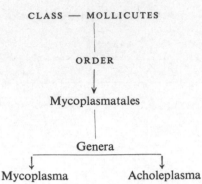

CLASS — MOLLICUTES

ORDER

Mycoplasmatales

Genera

Mycoplasma   Acholeplasma

Further reading

ANDERSON E.S. (1968) The ecology of transferable drug resistance in the Enterobacteria, *Annual Review of Microbiology*, **22**, 131.

BREED R.S., MURRAY E.G.D. AND SMITH N.R. (1974) *Bergey's Manual of Determinative Bacteriology*, 8th Edition. Baltimore: Williams and Wilkins.

COOKE, E.M., SHOOTER, R.A., BREADEN, A.L. AND O'FARRELL, S.M. (1971) Antibiotic sensitivity of *Escherichia coli* isolated from animals, food, hospital patients and normal people. *Lancet*, **2**, 8.

GOULD, G.W. AND HURST, A. (1969) *The Bacterial Spore*. London and New York: Academic Press.

FUHS G.W., ITERSON W.VAN, COLE R.M. AND SHOCKMAN G.D. (1965) Symposium on the fine structure and replication of bacteria and their parts. *Bacteriological Reviews*, **29**, 277.

GUNSALUS I.C. AND STANIER R.Y. (1960) *The Bacteria*, Vol. 1 (Structure), New York: Academic Press.

JONES D. AND SNEATH P.H.A. (1970) Genetic transfer and bacterial taxonomy. *Bacteriological Reviews* **34**, 40.

LAKHOTIA, R.L. AND STEPHENS, J.F. (1973) Drug resistance and R factors among enterobacteria isolated from eggs. *Poultry Science*, **52**, 1955.

MANDELSTAM, J. AND MCQUILLEN, K. (1973) *Biochemistry of Bacterial Growth*, 2nd Edition. Oxford: Blackwell Scientific Publication.

MEYNELL E. AND MEYNELL G.G. (1968) Phylogenetic relationships of drug resistance factors and other transmissible bacterial plasmids. *Bacteriological Reviews*, **32**, 55.

RYTER A. (1968) Association of the nucleus and the membrane of bacteria: a morphological study. *Bacteriological Reviews*, **32**, 39.

SALTON M.R.J. (1964) *The Bacterial Cell Wall*. London: Elsevier.

SHOOTER, R.A., COOKE, E.M., ROUSSEAU, S.A. AND BREADEN, A.L. (1970) Animal sources of common serotypes of *Escherichia coli* in the food of hospital patients. Possible significance in urinary tract infections. *Lancet*, **2**, 226.

SMITH, H.W. (1966) The incidence of infective drug resistance in strains of *Escherichia coli* isolated diseased human beings and domestic animals. *Journal of Hygiene*, **64**, 465.

SMITH, H.W. (1968) Antimicrobial drugs in animal feeds. *Nature*, **218**, 728.

SMITH H.W. (1970) The transfer of antibiotic resistance between strains of Enterobacteria in chicken, calves and pigs. *Journal of Medical Microbiology*, **3**, 165.

SMITH, H.W. (1974) Antibiotic-resistant bacteria in animals: the dangers to human health. *British Veterinary Journal*, **130**, 110.

WALTON, J.R. (1970) Contamination of meat carcases by antibiotic-resistant coliform bacteria. *Lancet*, **2**, 561.

WATANABE T. (1963) Infective heredity of multiple drug resistance in bacteria. *Bacteriological Reviews*, **27**, 87.

CHAPTER 3

IMMUNOLOGY

CHAPTER 3

Immunology

Immunology concerns the study of host responses to the introduction of foreign substances into the tissues, and the methods by which the body tries to eliminate these substances and protect itself against any further invasion by them. In more specific terms, microbes and their metabolic products stimulate the immunological mechanisms of the body: a process which is important to us in discussing methods for the control and prevention of infectious diseases in animals and man.

The relationship between an immune response and resistance to infection formed the main focus of attention for the earlier studies on immunology. It has long been known that some immunological responses are protective to the host and others can result in the development of hypersensitive reactions which may be the antithesis of defensive or protective mechanisms. Only during recent decades has the study of various aspects of hypersensitiveness developed into a new and important aspect of immunological research. To relate these two aspects of immunological protection and hypersensitivity within the context of microbes and infectious diseases, we can summarise by noting that as a result of an immunological response to a particular microbial infection, the host subsequently becomes less sensitive or more sensitive (hypersensitive) to that infection. The less sensitive individual will have developed a resistance which may protect it from similar infections in the future, whereas the more sensitive one may have become hypersensitive and react violently to further contact with the particular microbe or with some of its chemical components. It is important to realise that in both instances an immune response has taken place, and that in one it is beneficial but in the other it may be harmful.

Under modern conditions we see many examples of the beneficial effects of immunity in the control of infectious diseases. The expanding facilities for international travel and communication have increased the likelihood of infections, which hitherto have remained confined to certain countries or continents, now becoming distributed among human and animal populations on a world-wide basis. The practice of vaccination (i.e. immunization) is accepted as a valuable method for preventing the spread of infectious diseases among susceptible populations throughout the world; and many human diseases (e.g. typhoid fever, poliomyelitis, yellow fever, smallpox) are largely controlled by this method. Following the injection of killed or living microorganisms or their products, the individual develops an **active immunity** by producing specific antibodies against the microorganisms which enables him to withstand the natural disease for a period of time after the immunization course has been completed. Similarly, among domestic animals a number of infectious disease ares controlled by vaccination with varying degrees of success; some examples are contagious bovine pleuropneumonia (*M. mycoides*), the virus diseases of rinderpest, canine distemper, rabies, infectious laryngotracheitis, Newcastle disease, and the bacterial diseases caused by species of *Clostridium*, *Erysipelothrix*, *Brucella* and *Leptospira*. In each case the animal, which develops an active immunity against the microorganisms and their products contained in the vaccine, is able subsequently to resist natural infection for a period of time after immunization.

A cursory glance at scientific literature is sufficient to show us that the control of infectious diseases by vaccination is not always successful. The degree and duration of immunity developing as a result of this procedure may differ from one group of animals to another, according to age, breed, and methods of husbandry and hygiene. Microorganisms vary in their ability to produce clinical disease, so that an increase in their **virulence** results in relatively few organisms being sufficient to initiate disease in a susceptible animal, and only a highly immune individual can withstand such infection under natural conditions. Many animals which have been immunized against a particular microorganism and subsequently become infected with the same microbial species, may remain clinically normal but continue to harbour and excrete the infective agent, thus becoming sources of infection for other susceptible individuals in the flock or herd. Newly-born animals do not have the matured cellular organisation to develop their own immunity against infectious diseases to the same extent as adult animals, but they may obtain ready-made antibodies (**passive immunity**) transferred to them from their mothers either *in utero*, from ingestion of colostrum or via egg yolk. A passive immunity can also be conferred on an animal by injecting it with antiserum prepared in another individual who has already developed an immunity against the particular microorganism.

We have noted that an immune response may not always be beneficial to the host; on the contrary, it may be harmful and even fatal under particular circumstances. For example, an immune response may involve tissue cells, and sometimes results in their destruction and the release of toxic substances characteristic of hypersensitive reactions. Alternatively, an immune reaction may be associated with the malfunction of an organ, as occurs sometimes, in autoimmune reactions when the response is directed against the tissues of the host and more particularly against certain types of cells in organs or systems.

During the entire life of an individual, immune responses are biological processes which are constantly developing as a result of a variety of different and successive stimuli. More recent investigations have not only confirmed that the result may be to the advantage or to the disadvantage of the host, but that there may be more than one qualitatively different response by the host to a particular stimulus. One response may increase the resistance of the individual while another may cause the establishment of a hypersensitive state which can lead to pathological reactions and even to the death of the host.

In this chapter, we shall discuss immunology as it relates to the control and prevention of microbial diseases in animals; giving particular attention to the response of an animal to infection, to the development of an immune state, to the detection of immunity by various serological and other tests, and to the interpretation of these tests as a means of assessing the presence or absence of infection. In addition, we shall discuss the possible risks to the host of an immune response and how the response may be harmful and even fatal to some individuals.

Antigens

Definition

A good antigen is a substance of large molecular weight which has chemical groupings on its surface rendering it capable of stimulating an immune response by the host. In addition, a good antigen is one that is foreign to the host, being a substance with chemical groupings which are not normally present in host tissues. The introduction of antigen into the body causes a response to take place resulting in the production of substances called antibodies which are usually detectable in the serum, but may also stimulate a cellular immunity in the absence of serum antibodies. These will be described in the next section. It is sufficient for this discussion to state that antibodies are globulin molecules which can combine specifically with the antigen which stmulated their production.

Composition and specificity

Substances which readily stimulate an immune response in an animal are known as good antigens. Proteins are some of the best antigens and the larger their molecular weight the better are their antigenic properties. For example, ovalbumin (mol.wt 40 000) is a good antigen and foreign globulin (mol.wt 160 000–1 000 000) is a better antigen than either insulin (mol.wt 6000) or the enzyme ribonuclease (mol.wt 1400). These large molecules are composed of amino acids and peptide chains folded into a pattern characteristic for each protein. Provided that part or all of the exposed pattern of a protein is unlike the chemical groupings or antigenic determinants which the body tissues normally contain, the protein will be recognised by the tissues as foreign and will stimulate the production of antibodies. Thus, if the globulin fraction of rabbit serum is separated and inoculated back into the rabbit from which it was derived, that rabbit will not produce antibodies to the globulin. In contrast, bovine globulin is foreign to rabbits and will stimulate an immune response in that species because bovine globulin is antigenically distinct from rabbit globulin.

Polysaccharides consist of large complex molecules composed mainly of a variety of sugars, and we would expect that, like proteins, these large molecular substances would be good antigens. In fact, some of them are antigenic (e.g. pneumococcal capsular material; blood group polysaccharide) although the immune responses produced as a result of their injection into the body are not as marked as those stimulated by protein antigens, and the degree of response of the tissues also depends upon the animal species concerned. Complexes of protein and polysaccharide or of protein, polysaccharide and lipid constitute antigens. In these complex macromolecular substances the antigenic determinants may be derived from either the carbohydrate or peptide fractions. Antibodies to these complex antigens have reactive sites which combine with these determinants.

Haptens

These substances are of small molecular weight which do not stimulate antibody production when inoculated by themselves into animals; but after attachment to a large protein molecule (carrier molecule) they provide the antigenic specificity of the complex macromolecule and stimulate production of antibodies specific for themselves. The unattached hapten is also capable of reacting with these antibodies. An example of a hapten is penicillin which in an acid pH becomes degraded into compounds capable of combining with protein. This combination of a penicillin hapten with protein results in the formation of complex antigenic molecules capable of stimulating production of antibodies specific for penicillin.

Bacterial antigens

Although many bacterial structures are immunologically important, since they are known to be antigens and to stimulate the production of specific antibodies, our knowledge of the antigenic properties of bacteria is haphazard because the stimulus to investigate only some of them has been determined either by their potential importance in disease processes or by the ease with which they can be prepared in the laboratory. The following brief summary will give the reader some idea of the multiplicity of antigens which are associated with bacteria.

Somatic antigens

Among Gram-negative bacteria (e.g. *Salmonella, Escherichia, Brucella, Vibrio*) somatic antigens are composed of lipopolysaccharide–protein complexes which are good antigens and readily stimulate antibody production. Some of the purified polysaccharide fractions are haptens and when incorporated in complex antigenic molecules provide the specificities (determinant groups) of the antigens on which are based the serological typing procedures for *Salmonella, Escherichia* and other similar bacterial groups.

Gram-positive bacteria (e.g. *Streptococcus, Staphylococcus, Corynebacterium*) have somatic antigens composed of a protein layer which is on the surface of the bacterial body, and underneath this is a complex mucoantigen composed of carbohydrates and amino acids. The carbohydrate fraction provides the determinant groups of this inner antigen which forms the basis for Lancefield's grouping of streptococcal organisms. The mucoantigen of intact bacteria is partially masked by the protein layer so that to use the former in antigen-antibody reactions for streptococcal grouping, the organisms have to be disrupted in order to expose this antigen to the action of antibody.

Capsular antigens

Capsules are produced by a variety of bacterial species (e.g. *Pasteurella, Yersinia, Escherichia, Klebsiella, Bacillus*), and these substances are incorporated in the outer surfaces of bacterial bodies. Capsules commonly consist of polysaccharides but some are composed of polypeptides (e.g. *B. anthracis*). Well developed capsules may envelop the somatic antigens so effectively that the latter are prevented from reacting with their own specific antibodies until the capsular substances have been removed from the bacteria.

Flagellar antigens

Some bacterial genera of veterinary importance form flagella (e.g. *Salmonella, Escherichia, Proteus*). These flagella are composed of protein (flagellin) with a molecular weight of over 40 000, and they are good antigens. Among the salmonella group which possesses numerous antigenically distinct flagella, the antigenic varieties occur as a result of different arrangements of the amino acids constituting the protein molecules.

Fimbrial or piliate antigens

Under the electron microscope fimbriae (or pili) appear as short rod-like structures projecting from the surfaces of bacteria. They have been found in many genera of Gram-negative bacteria, including *Salmonella, Shigella, Escherichia* and *Proteus*. Fimbriae are antigenic and chemically distinct from flagella. Although fimbrial antigen-antibody reactions may sometimes interfere with and mask somatic antigen–antibody reactions and may also cause agglutination of erythrocytes, they do not appear to be of great importance in the prevention and control of disease. However, the modified form of fimbriae known as sex-pili form the interbacterial bridges which develop during the process of bacterial conjugation.

Spore antigens

Bacterial spores of importance in animal diseases are those which occur in the *Clostridium* and *Bacillus* groups. Recent research has shown that bacterial spores are complex structures with thick walls composed of chemically different layers. It is probable that spores contain a number of antigens, but so far, only the surfaces (exosporia) have been shown to be antigenic.

Soluble antigens

Animals are susceptible to infections with bacterial

species which produce soluble protein antigens known as toxins (e.g. *Clostridium, Corynebacterium, Staphylococcus*). These extracellular toxins are antigenic, and antibodies produced against them are known as antitoxins which are used in the control of some toxaemic infections. A difficulty in preparing antitoxins for therapeutic purposes is that injections of toxins into suitable animals may prove fatal. However, if toxins are mixed with formaldehyde they lose their toxic properties but maintain their antigenicities. The resulting non-toxic substances, known as **toxoids**, have the advantage that they are not only antigenic and can stimulate the production of antitoxins, but also that they can be injected into animals without causing severe toxaemia and death.

$$\text{toxin} + \text{formaldehyde} \longrightarrow \text{toxoid}$$

Blood group antigens

Most of these antigens are situated on the surfaces of erythrocytes but some also occur as soluble substances in the body fluids and on other cell types. Blood group systems have been well defined in horses, cattle, sheep, goats, pigs, dogs, cats, rabbits, chickens, mice and rats. From seven to more than thirty antigenic factors have been described in each of these species, except among cattle where more than 100 different antigens have been identified, compared with aproximately sixty antigens in man.

Viral antigens

Animal viruses vary in size and complexity of structure, but essentially they consist of nucleic acid surrounded by a protective coat of protein. During their life cycles, new viral particles are built up intracellularly from molecular components formed in tissue cells (See Chapter 39). Many components are of large mol. wt. and antigenic, so that under suitable conditions specific antibody production will be stimulated against the components as well as against the intact viral particle. During the final aggregation of these macromolecules into complete viral particles, some of the antigenic components will become buried beneath the outer surface of the virus and will not be available for antigen–antibody reactions. Antibodies against these masked antigens will, therefore, have no effect on intact, extracellular viral particles, and will be of little value to the host as a protective mechanism against infection. On the other hand, antibodies specific for the outer protein layer of viruses will have opportunities in the infected animal of reacting with this antigen and such antibodies may be of value to the host in controlling infection.

Heterophile antigens

These are immunologically related groups of antigens which occur in the cells of some bacterial species and also of some species of animals. **Forssman antigens** constitute an example of a group of related heterophile antigens. They occur on the surfaces of red blood cells of horses, sheep, dogs, cats and mice, and have also been detected in some bacteria including certain members of the genera *Clostridium, Streptococcus, Shigella* and *Salmonella*. The antigens are not present on red blood cells derived from man, monkeys, rabbits, guinea-pigs, rats and ducks, but these species often possess Forssman serum antibodies which have been produced as a result of contact with bacteria possessing this type of antigen. By contrast, animals possessing these antigens in their tissues do not develop the corresponding antibodies because the antigens are not recognised as foreign by the host and, therefore, do not stimulate the production of antibodies. Other examples of heterophile antigens are those shared by human blood group A and pneumococci and human blood group B and *E. coli*.

Antibodies

Definition

Antibodies or **immunoglobulins** are substances produced by the body in response to the presence of a foreign antigen, and they consist of globulins which combine specifically with the antigens that stimulated their production. This high degree of specificity of antibodies for their respective antigens is the most important characteristic property of these substances, and forms the basis for all antigen-antibody reactions, whether they occur *in vivo* as a defence mechanism of the host or *in vitro* in a serological test performed in the laboratory.

Composition and properties of antibodies

The heterogeneity of immunoglobulins

In recent years the development of newer methods for the study of the properties of immunoglobulins has yielded important information on the heterogeneity of these proteins. One of these methods is electrophoresis which consists of observing the migration of serum proteins in paper or gel under controlled conditions. The degree of migration of a protein fraction is a reflection of its size and charge; and by carrying out the tests in paper or gel it is possible to isolate and elute protein fractions having different migration characteristics.

Another method used for studying immunoglobulins is ion exchange chromatography which relies upon differences in the charges and sizes of globulin molecules for the separation of various fractions. The essential features of the method are first, to allow absorption of globulin molecules on to a resin, diethylaminoethyl cellulose (DEAE), and second, to elute with buffers of different molar strengths and pH values. In this way a complex immunoglobulin solution can be separated into fractions differing in their molecular charges.

A third technique is ultracentrifugation and the measurement of sedimentation constants. For example, in the case of the smaller molecules these constants are recorded as 7 Svedberg Units (or 7S), and the larger ones as 19 Svedberg Units (or 19S). The 7S fraction has a molecular weight of approximately 145 000 while that of the 19S fraction is about 900 000 and is sometimes referred to as a macroglobulin.

Immunoglobulins are themselves good antigens and it is possible to compare the antigenic structures of different preparations of these globulins. By using absorption techniques and agar gel diffusion methods, it has been shown that although there are common antigens there are also antigens specific for each fraction.

From all these tests it has been possible to characterise five different human immunoglobulins (abbreviated to Ig) which have been designated IgG, IgA, IgM, IgD and IgE. Table 3.1 summarises some of the properties of these human immunoglobulins and their relationships to various immunological reactions.

Similar studies in animals have not been developed to the same extent as those in man but present information may be summarised as follows. Fractions analogous to human IgG and IgM have been identified in many animals species, including horses, cows, sheep, goats, pigs, dogs, turkeys, ducks, chickens, rabbits, mice, rats, guinea-pigs and hamsters. It should be noted, however, that the IgG fractions in chickens, ducks and some other species have some characteristic properties which differ from those of human IgG. Sheep, cattle, goats, horses, pigs, dogs, cats, hedgehogs, rabbits and mice also possess an IgA fraction, and further investigations may show the existence of this fraction in additional species, particularly rats, guinea-pigs and chickens. A fraction similar to human IgE has been identified in pigs, cattle, dogs, rabbits and rats in relation to allergic reactions.

Structure of antibodies and their combining sites

The structure of immunoglobulin molecules has been studied by observing the results of splitting the molecules by the action of proteolytic enzymes (e.g. papain, pepsin) or separating the constituent peptide chains by dissolving the disulphide bonds. These studies have shown that IgG immunoglobulins are Y-shaped, possess a pair of 'heavy' and a pair of 'light' polypeptide chains, and also two combining sites each of which occurs on a different fraction after the molecule has been split by enzyme action (Fig. 3.1). The combining sites are situated on the

TABLE 3.1. Summarizing some of the properties of human immunoglobulins and their relationships to various immunological reactions.

Characteristic properties of immunoglobulins	IgG	IgA	IgM	IgE	IgD
Molecular weight	145 000	160 000	900 000	200 000	160 000
Sedimentation constant	7S	7–17S (mainly 7S)	19S	8S	7S
Concentration in normal serum (mg/100 ml)	800–1500	50–200	50–100	0·0001–0·0007	0·3–30
ASSOCIATION WITH ANTIBODIES					
Antibodies against Salmonella O antigens			++++		
" " E. coli O "			++++		
" " Salmonella H "	++++				
" " E. coli H "	++++				
" " clostridial toxins (i.e. antitoxins)	++++				antibody activity unknown
" " spirochaetes	+		+++		
" " viruses	++	+	+		
Complement-fixing antibodies	++		++		
Opsonins	++		++		
Bacteriocidins — lysins	++		++		
Natural isoantibodies (ABO blood group antigens)			++++		
Immune " (" " " ")	++++				
Antibodies in secretions (saliva, colostrum, digestive tract, respiratory tract)		+++			
Autoantibodies	++		++		
Reaginic antibodies (skin sensitizing)	+			+++	
Antibodies against Forssman antigen			++++		

++++, +++, ++, + = Decreasing degrees of association with immunoglobulin fractions.

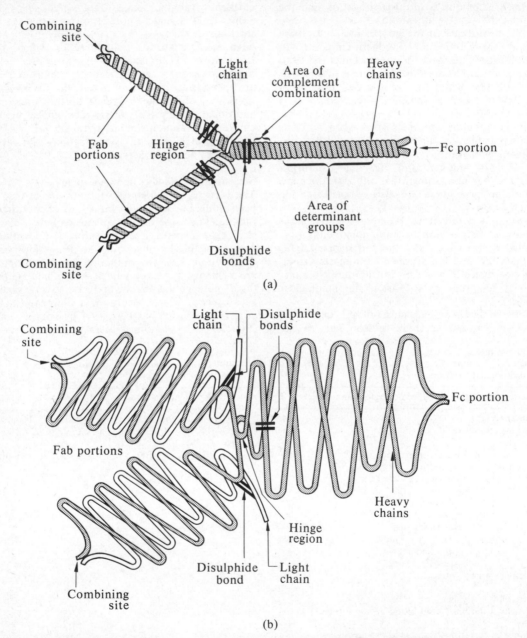

FIG. 3.1. An IgG molecule with the polypeptide chains folded (a) and partially unfolded (b).

The two fragments with antibody-combining activity (Fab portions) each consist of a large heavy (mol. wt. 53 000) polypeptide chain and a small light (mol. wt. 22 000) polypeptide chain folded on each other and held together by disulphide bonds. The two heavy chains constitute the hinge region and continue in a twisted formation, held together by disulphide bonds, to form the crystallizable fragment (Fc portion). This latter portion includes the areas where complement combines and the determinant groups are situated.

terminal parts of the heavy chain portions of the molecule, and although isolated light chains do not combine with antigen they do potentiate the combining activity of the heavy chains in the complete molecule. These peptide chains are of considerable length, twisted spirally around each other, and consist of large numbers of amino acids in sequences. There is evidence that the specificities of the combining sites are related to the sequence of these amino acids. Only a slight alteration in their sequence is probably sufficient to destroy the specificity of the combining site for a particular antigen. Since IgG immunoglobulins are composed of many hundreds of amino acid units, and because only a small proportion of these is concerned with the formation of each combining site, it is clear that potentially a great number of amino acid sequences can occur, enabling the development of combining sites on immunoglobulins (i.e. antibody production) to be modified to react with any one of a wide variety of antigens.

Studies on the structure of IgM immunoglobulins have shown that they are considerably larger and more complex than IgG molecules (Fig. 3.2a). They are stellate in shape when fully expanded and have five units radiating from hinged portions at the centre. Recent observations have shown that each unit may subdivide into two, giving a total of ten possible combining sites situated peripherally at the end of each subunit. However, a maximum of only five combining sites are usually involved in antigen antibody reactions, and this may be because of either steric interference with antigen which may combine with one site and block combination with the neighbouring one, or the IgM molecule may not be fully expanded at all the hinged areas.

IgA immunoglobulins occurring in sera are monomers and of similar configuration to IgG immunoglobulin. In other sites of the body, however, IgA is characterised by additional components known as secretory piece and 'j' (for joining) component which links together two monomers to form one dimer, thus conferring additional combining sites to the dimeric form (Fig. 3.2b). The secretory piece which is synthesised in epithelial cells and independently from the immunoglobulin, increases the resistance of IgA to the action of proteolytic enzymes and probably enhances the binding capacity of the immunoglobulin to epithelial surfaces. The dimeric form of IgA is secreted locally into the mucous surfaces of the intestinal and respiratory tracts, into saliva and colostrum, and it constitutes the most important immunoglobulin fraction in external secretions of most mammals. In addition, the concentration of IgA in milk from pigs, horses and rabbits remains substantially high throughout lactation, in contrast to bovine milk

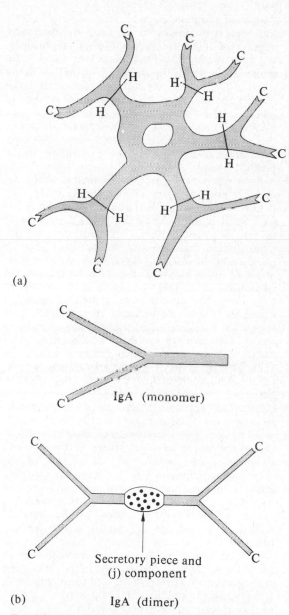

(a)

IgA (monomer)

Secretory piece and
(j) component

(b)   IgA (dimer)

FIG. 3.2.(a). An IgM molecule consisting of a central ring with five 'legs' of variable length and width. Each leg divides into two sections each of which terminates in an antigen-combining site (C). There is also a hinge region (H H) on each leg which enables the molecule to take up a variety of configurations when attached to antigen. (b) An IgA monomer with two combining sites (C) as it occurs in serum, and an IgA dimer with four combining sites as it occurs in external secretions.

in which the concentration decreases markedly after the initial secretion of colostrum has ceased.

Formation of antibodies

The processes involved in antibody formation constitute a focus for current research and theories. We have already noted that antibodies are globulin molecules in which the specificity of the combining site is related to the sequence of amino acids in the peptide chains. Thus, the formation of antibodies involves the constitution of the peptide chains, the folding of these chains to form protein molecules, and the circumstances in which these processes become modified by the presence of antigen in the host's tissues.

As a result of an antigenic stimulus, antibodies may be present in an animal for relatively long periods of time after the initial stimulus. Since the half-life of IgM molecules is about 3 days and that of IgG is about 3 weeks, the production of immunoglobulin must be a continuous process. Theories on globulin formation suggest that peptide chains are built up of amino acids under the influence of ribonucleic acids, and after completion, the chains fold into the characteristic shapes of globulin molecules. Under the influence of an antigen, it is suggested that the sequence of amino-acids is modified to give the specificity to the immunoglobulin combining sites. The question which has stimulated a great deal of experimentation and theory is how this process continues long after the antigenic stimulus has occurred. Moreover, is it essential for determinant groups of the antigen to be constantly present in cells which produce antibody, or does their initial presence result in modification of the cellular enzyme systems so that antibody production can continue in the absence of the determinant groups? We do not know the complete answers to these questions but successive theories have been proposed in an attempt to explain the process of antibody formation in the light of increasing knowledge of certain aspects of the problem.

In 1900 Ehrlich put forward a hypothesis that on the outer surfaces of certain cells in the body there were receptors which were adapted to combine with foreign proteins and toxins (i.e. antigens) when these gained access into the body. When these foreign substances came into contact with the receptors the two combined and both were then shed from the surface of the cell. As a result of this loss of receptors, the cells produced new ones at an increased rate and the excess became detached from the cells and distributed throughout the body. Ehrlich believed that these liberated receptors were the antibodies detectable by antigen–antibody reactions.

Some 30 years later, Haurowitz and his colleagues suggested that the essential first stage in antibody production was the entry of antigen into globulin-producing cells and the incorporation of the antigen in an intracellular template. The formation of such a template would then result in globulin produced by the cell becoming modified to possess specific receptors related to the antigen, and having the properties of antibody molecules. The presentation of this **instructive theory** stimulated considerable lively discussion among immunologists, and the critics were particularly concerned with two aspects. Firstly, it provided no satisfactory explanation of how the presence of antigen in a cell could suitably modify the template for globulin production into one for specific antibody (i.e. immunoglobulin) production. In 1952, Haurowitz suggested that the specificity of antibody did not originate at the time of peptide synthesis, but developed later, at a stage when the chain becomes folded. In this way the specificity of antibody resulted from the configuration of amino acids on the surfaces of globulin molecules as a result of the folding of the peptide chains.

The second criticism of Haurowitz's theory was in connection with the production of antibody over relatively long periods of time. The point of discussion was whether the antigen or part of the antigen had to remain in the cell in order to maintain the production of antibodies. If this was so, the question arose as to how antibody production could continue over a period of many months, since this would inevitably result in antibody being produced by cells which had not come into direct contact with antigen.

In 1955 Jerne put forward an entirely new hypothesis for antibody production. He believed that globulin molecules carry the receptors for any foreign antigen which enters the body but not for exposed tissue antigens belonging to the host. He then suggested that when foreign antigen enters the body it combines with those globulin molecules possessing related receptors and that this combination is then taken up by cells capable of forming antibody. These cells then produce replicas of the globulin molecule receptors which are liberated as antibodies.

More recent studies on globulin synthesis, using immunofluorescence techniques and other methods have provided evidence for the current theory on immunoglobulin formation. It is believed that in cells which produce globulin the sequence of amino acids constituting the peptide chains is controlled or coded by the ribonucleic acid in these cells. Consequently, the production of immunoglobulin in response to an antigenic stimulus develops from the alteration of the ribonucleic acid coding system within the cell which controls the development of the specific receptors on the immunoglobulin molecules.

Recognition of 'self'; immunological tolerance; autoimmunity

An important aspect of antibody production is the ability of the antibody-forming cells to recognise that antigens associated with the structure of the host's own healthy tissues are not foreign, and therefore, the body does not normally produce antibodies against its own tissue antigens. To understand the importance of this recognition by the host itself, it must be appreciated that the cells of the body contain multiple antigens and are potentially capable of stimulating antibody production when inoculated into a suitable host. For example, if lymphocytes or kidney cells from one animal species are inoculated into another species, the recipient will produce antibodies against these cells. It is essential for the normal functioning of healthy tissue cells in the host's body that they are not recognised as being antigenically foreign and that consequently, they will not stimulate the production of antibodies against themselves. It is known that provided these tissue antigens are exposed to the antibody-forming mechanism from embryonic life onwards (i.e. during the developmental stages of the antibody-forming mechanism), the body will not normally develop an immune reaction against them, although there is recent evidence to suggest that some modification to this view may have to be made. In other words, the antibody forming mechanism of the host is able to recognise the difference between 'self' and 'not self'.

To explain this phenomenon, Burnet and Fenner postulated a self-marker **selective theory** in which the body antigens have self-markers which are characteristic for each antigen. When the antibody-forming mechanism comes into contact with these self-marker units during fetal life, recognition units are formed so that in later life antibodies are not produced against the host antigens; in this way, the antibody-forming mechanism develops an **immunological tolerance** to the host's own tissue antigens. Another example of immunological tolerance can be demonstrated by inoculating foreign antigen into a developing embryo. This antigen will also become recognised by the antibody-forming mechanism so that during adult life the individual may fail to produce specific antibodies when further challenged with the same antigen.

Immunological tolerance was demonstrated particularly clearly by Medawar and his co-workers in a series of experiments on skin grafting, using two strains of inbred mice, one coloured white and the other brown. They found that skin grafts made from one adult to another within either group always took; whereas transference of a skin graft from an adult white mouse to an adult brown mouse (or *vice versa*) did not take and was rejected. It was then shown that if fresh spleen or bone marrow cells from a brown mouse were injected intravenously into white mice immediately after birth, those white mice when adults did not reject skin grafts derived from brown mice because of the immune tolerance which they had developed. The converse was also true. Additional tests showed that immune tolerance was a specific reaction limited to the cellular antigens employed, and that it developed only when the cells were inoculated into mice immediately after birth. Moreover, it was also shown by other related experiments that immune tolerance did not develop as the result of any interference with, or inhibition of antigen–antibody reactions, but was produced by failure of the tolerant recipient to develop an immune response against the particular antigens associated with the skin graft. Under the conditions of these experiments, tolerance to a skin graft is maintained only so long as the cells from the donor survive in the recipient.

The reader will recognise the similarity between the basic immunological processes which are involved in the experimental demonstration of immune tolerance related to skin grafting and the recognition of 'self' as a natural phenomenon in the adult. Both recognition of 'self' and immune tolerance develop as a consequence of cellular antigens being in contact with the developing lymphoid system during embryonic growth or immediately after birth.

There are circumstances under which the recognition of 'self' and the established state of immune tolerance in an adult may become destroyed or at least modified to the extent that an individual develops **autoantibodies** against his own tissue antigens. The circumstances under which this may occur and the precise function of autoantibodies in disease have not been fully determined. We have already noted in the discussion on the theory for the recognition of 'self', that the individual does not usually recognise his own tissues as foreign and does not, therefore, produce antibodies against them. There are various possible circumstances under which this state of self-recognition may become broken down and lead to the production of autoantibodies. For example, the body possesses a variety of hidden tissue antigens which do not usually come into direct contact with the immune mechanisms of the host (e.g. brain), and consequently a tolerance to these antigens is not developed. Under abnormal conditions, exposure of these antigens will result in the production of autoantibodies and in the case of the brain, this can result in the development of an allergic encephalomyelitis. Another example of the emergence of a hidden tissue antigen leading to autoantibody production, is the exposure of the determinant groups of complement after it has combined with an antigen–antibody reaction leading to the production of an antibody to complement known as **immunoconglutinin**. Damage to tissue cells by viruses, leading to the exposure of intracellular components and contact between these and the lymphoid system, may also give rise to auto-antibody production against these cellular components.

Other circumstances leading to the production of autoantibodies occur when heterologous antigens partially related to the tissue antigens of an individual, are capable of stimulating the production of antibodies which will cross-react with the host's tissues and are, therefore, autoantibodies. For example, haemolytic streptococci (Group A) have an antigen in common with human heart tissue, and heart autoantibodies have been demonstrated in sera from patients recovering from infection with these bacteria. Similarly, there is evidence to show that the presence of common antigens between some bacterial species belonging to the family *Enterobacteriaceae* and the tissues of rabbits and mice may lead to autoantibody production in these species consequent upon the establishment of enterobacterial infections.

There is some doubt concerning the relationship of autoantibodies to the development of disease, and whether these antibodies are produced as a result of a disease process or are involved in the aetiology of a condition. In some diseases, autoantibodies may be specific for certain tissues (e.g. human chronic thyroiditis, pernicious anaemia) while in others they may be non-specific for particular organs but directed against nuclear antigens, as occurs in human lupus erythematosus when the patient develops antibodies against constitutents of various cell types. It is interesting to note in this connection that there is recent evidence indicating that autoantibodies against certain tissue antigens can be detected in the sera of some apparently healthy animals, and that the production of these so-called cytotoxic antibodies is a normal function of the healthy animal, being associated with the removal of effete tissue cells and their destruction by macrophages. This process constitutes a cytotoxic hypersensitive response, classified by Coombs and Gell as a Type II hypersensitive reaction.

Since it is now recognised that autoantibody production may be a normal homeostatic mechanism, the question arises as to the circumstances which cause excessive autoimmune responses against particular tissues or cell constituents in an individual. There seems to be a variety of conditions which may give rise to these circumstances involving the sudden availability to the reticuloendothelial system of relatively large quantities of a particular type of tissue cell or tissue antigen. This may occur as the result of tissue damage (e.g. burns, wounds) or the alteration in the constituents of cells resulting in the formation and release of new and foreign antigenic components. These conditions may arise from infection with viruses; for example, glomerulonephritis in Aleutian disease of mink and in the NZB strain of mice infected with virus in the kidneys from birth, encephalomyelitis in dogs associated with nervous symptoms following canine distemper, and virus infections associated with tumour formation. Autoimmunity may also develop as a consequence of infection with species of bacteria having antigens in common with tissue cell components (e.g. common antigens of streptococci and the tissue cells of heart and kidney). Indications that a disease condition may be associated with an autoimmune reaction include the demonstration of the particular autoantibody, the presence of concentrations of lymphoid cells in the affected tissue, and an increase in the levels of serum gamma globulins.

Cellular origin of antibodies

The fact that antibodies are modified globulins and that the specific modifications to these protein molecules takes place intracellularly, means that the sources of antibody will be those cells which are responsible for the production of globulin. Although this basic concept has been realised for many years, there has been some doubt as to the relative significance of lymphocytes, plasma cells and macrophages in the process of antibody production.

Lymphocytes

These cells comprise the major cellular constituents of lymphoid tissue and are described as large, medium and small. Following a secondary antigenic stimulation, there is enlargement of germinal centres in the cortices of the lymph nodes and a marked increase in the numbers of lymphocytes of all sizes as well as of plasma cells in the red pulp of the spleen. These changes are characteristically far greater than those which take place after a primary antigenic stimulation, and it is believed that this is because of the development of so-called **memory cells** following the primary response to antigen. The rapid and intense production of humoral antibody by plasma cells following a secondary response is controlled by the preformed 'immunological memory' which was established after the primary response. The question arises, therefore, as to the cell types involved in the development of immunological memory.

Experiments designed to observe the respective functions of large, medium and small lymphocytes have demonstrated that when attempts are made to deplete rats of lymphocytes by cannulation of the thoracic duct, there is a marked decrease in small but not in medium or large lymphocytes. This is due to the rapid multiplication and replacement of medium and large lymphocytes only. It has been shown that small lymphocytes readily pass from the blood stream into various centres of lymphoid tissue throughout the body, and it has been postulated that these are in memory cells which respond to primary antigenic stimulation in any part of the lymphoid system of the body. This hypothesis is based on experiments which have shown that the response to antigenic stimuli in animals depleted of small lymphocytes was greatly reduced, and that the response could be enhanced when the number of small lymphocytes was again increased. Recent experiments also suggest that each cell produces only one type of antibody and that antibody production develops as the result of **clonal proliferation** of each antibody-producing cell.

The recognition of the immunological importance of small lymphocytes led to further investigations into the role of these cells in both humoral and cell-mediated immune responses. The fundamental difference between these two types of response is that a humoral immunity involves the synthesis and release of antibody into body fluids, whereas cell-mediated immunity refers to the synthesis of antibody which remains fixed to the surfaces of lymphocytes. These latter cells are then referred to as 'sensitized' lymphocytes. Humoral antibody is able to react directly with microbes, microbial toxins and to enhance phagocytosis, whereas cell-bound antibody is involved in delayed hypersensitivity reactions (e.g. tuberculin test) and rejection of tissue transplants. Thus, the small lymphocyte is involved in two different antibody-producing mechanisms which result in either the production and release of antibody from the cells into body fluids, or the production and maintenance of cell-bound antibody by 'sensitized' lymphocytes.

Interest has been centred on the possible differences between these two functional types of small lymphocyte, particularly in relation to the thymus and to the bursa of Fabricius in birds. Both functional types of lymphocyte are derived from similar stem cells in yolk sac, fetal liver and bone marrow, and these stem cells migrate via the circulation to the thymus and bursa of Fabricius where they proliferate and develop into lymphocytes. Removal of the thymus gland from mice at birth has the effect of causing a marked reduction in both the number of circulating small lymphocytes and in the ability of the host to reject tissue transplants. In contrast, the removal of the bursa from newly-hatched chicks causes a fall in the number of circulating small lymphocytes together with a reduction in humoral antibody response. From these and other experiments it has become clear that the two functions of

lymphocytes are associated with two distinct varieties of cell:

(1) Lymphocytes derived or dependent upon the thymus (T-lymphocytes) which develop into lymphoblasts and produce but do not secrete antibody.

(2) Lymphocytes derived or dependent upon the bursa (B-lymphocytes) which develop into plasma cells and are responsible for the production and secretion of humoral antibody.

Recent experiments also suggest that T-lymphocytes produce a substance which stimulates B-lymphocytes to develop into plasma cells producing humoral antibody, and that both types of lymphocyte are involved in enhancing the ability of macrophages to fix antigen and so to stimulate antibody production. Lymphocytes also produce a macrophage inhibition factor (MIF) which inhibits the migration of macrophages from the site of an immune reaction, thereby maintaining a high local concentration of cells which phagocytose bacteria already coated with specific antibody (opsonin). Consequently, these cellular interactions increase the overall bactericidal activity at the local site of an immune reaction.

Plasma cells
These are derived from small bursa-dependent lymphocytes (B-lymphocytes) as a result of antigen stimulation, and they actively synthesise and secrete humoral antibody.

Lymphoblasts
These are derived from the transformation of small thymus-dependent lymphocytes (T-lymphocytes) as a result of antigen stimulation, and they actively synthesise antibody which is not secreted but remains associated with the cell membrane.

Macrophages
The role of macrophages in the process of antibody production is not clearly defined but there is evidence from tissue culture experiments to suggest that the function of these cells is to take up and prepare antigen in such a way that it can stimulate the T-lymphocytes to produce antibody. No such effect has been observed with B-lymphocytes. Animal experiments have shown that mice can be subjected to a dose of x-rays which renders them unable to produce antibodies to bacterial antigens. If these animals are then injected with an adequate dose of normal mouse macrophages which had been previously incubated with bacteria and subsequently washed, these irradiated mice respond by producing antibodies. Another experimental approach has been made using phage as the antigen. Following ingestion of phage by macrophages a substance sensitive to ribonuclease was produced which could

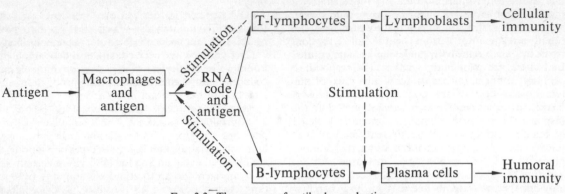

FIG. 3.3. The process of antibody production.

interact with lymph node cells, resulting in the production of antibody.

This relationship between macrophages and antibody production is also exemplified by many experiments which have demonstrated that either bacterial endotoxins or Freund's adjuvant, when mixed with antigen, may increase antibody production under controlled conditions. It is known that one effect is to increase the concentration of macrophages at the site of inoculation of the mixture of one of these agents and the antigen, thus giving rise to relatively extensive contact between macrophages and the antigen. It has been suggested that this contact results in the production of a specific RNA messenger code by the macrophages, and that subsequent contact between these cells and lymphocytes leads to antibody production under the control of the RNA code (Fig. 3.3).

Antibody production by different organs
In view of the importance of lymphocytes in the process of antibody production it is to be expected that the spleen and lymph nodes are the organs primarily concerned with this process. Nevertheless, experiments have shown that the development of antibodies by different organs depends upon a variety of factors, including the route by which the antigen enters the body, the nature of the antigen, the type of immunological response by the host (e.g. primary or secondary), the age of the host, and the physiological condition of the animal (i.e. pregnancy, lactation, egg-laying, etc.). The following is a summary of present knowledge of antibody production by various organs of the body and the conditions which determine the extent of these responses.

Spleen
This is the most important single organ concerned with antibody production. The extent to which it is involved depends largely on the route of antigen inoculation and the size and number of doses which the animal receives. Intravenous injections of antigen give rise to intense antibody production by the spleen and under these conditions the concentration of antibody in this organ is greater than that in the serum. Conversely, when antigen is inoculated subcutaneously, the eventual concentration of antibody in the serum will be greater than that in the spleen because antibody production will have occurred primarily in local sites in the body proximal to the area at which the antigen was inoculated. These results emphasise that the intensity of antibody production by the spleen is directly related to the facility with which the antigen comes into direct contact with that organ, and this applies to all tissues of the body which are potential antibody-producers.

Lymph nodes
The lymph nodes distributed throughout the body constitute important sites for antibody production. The level of response depends upon the proximity of the nodes to the site of antigen introduction. Thus, if antigen is inoculated into the hind foot, antibody production will occur first in the popliteal lymph nodes; similarly, injection of antigen into the ears stimulates antibody production initially in the cervical glands. The production of antibodies in lymphoid tissues related to the digestive tract, particularly the tonsils, Peyer's patches, mesenteric lymph nodes, lymphoid tissue in the appendix and caecum, follows the introduction of antigen into the digestive tract.

Thymus
The main cell types found in the thymus are lymphocytes and reticular cells which include macrophages. There is a constant, slow transfer of stem cells from bone marrow, fetal liver and yolk sac via the blood

stream to the thymus where they develop into T-lymphocytes.

These cells leave the thymus as immunologically competent T-lymphocytes to become distributed via the lymph stream to various lymphoid centres in the body. Thymectomy in the young animal results in a marked depletion in the numbers of lymphocytes and also in the immunological capacity of the individual to reject a homograft or develop a state of delayed hypersensitivity. Thymectomy in the adult leads to some reduction in the number of circulating lymphocytes. It has little immediate effect on the immunological capacity of the individual but may have a delayed effect, presumably due to the eventual depletion of immunologically competent cells whose development is controlled by the thymus. The functions of the thymus are not fully understood but it is clear that it is intimately associated with the development of the immune mechanism in the young and with the functioning of this mechanism during adult life particularly in relation to cell-mediated immunity.

Bursa of Fabricius
This organ consists largely of lymphoid follicles, and its function in birds seems to be concerned with the development of humoral immune responses in relation to B-lymphocytes, whereas the avian thymus has a controlling influence on cellular immune responses through the medium of T-lymphocytes. The inoculation of antigen into bursectomised birds results in a marked depletion of plasma cells and lower levels of antibody production compared to the responses of normal birds.

Mammary gland
Local antibody production confined to this organ can occur and has been demonstrated experimentally. For example, the inoculation of bacteria into one-quarter of a bovine udder results in the production of antibodies in that quarter before their appearance in other quarters. It is important to remember, however, that under conditions of natural disease, antibodies in milk are usually derived almost entirely from antibodies in blood serum originating from a generalised immune response of the body. Antibodies in colostrum which are of special importance for conferring a passive immunity on the newborn are composed mostly of IgA, and these immunoglobulins are also present in milk throughout lactation in pigs, horses and rabbits.

Vagina and uterus
Antibodies can be detected locally in the mucus from these organs. The extent to which these antibodies are either produced locally or are transferred from elsewhere has not been clearly defined.

Intestines
Antibodies occur in the intestines of animals, they are secreted locally and are known as **coproantibodies**. These intestinal antibodies belong mainly to the class of IgA immunoglobulins, they are resistant to digestion by trypsin or pepsin, and probably play an important role in the defence mechanisms of the body against enteric infections.

Complement

Definition
Complement is a substance present in fresh normal serum of animals and man which enhances the activity of antigen-antibody reactions. It does not, itself, have any effect on the combination of antigen with antibody — a process which can take place in its absence — but it may become involved in the reaction and be directly responsible for damage to cells. Thus, it is concerned with immunological reactions resulting in phagocytosis, bacteriolysis (disintegration of bacteria), haemolysis (disintegration of red blood cells) and the destruction of normal tissue cells and tumour cells. These reactions involve the incorporation of heat-labile components of complement which are destroyed by a temperature of 56°C for 30 minutes and by certain chemicals. The concentration of complement in sera of immunized animals remains fairly constant, and it does not combine with antigen or antibody but becomes bound up with an antigen–antibody reaction (e.g. lysis of red blood cells in immune haemolytic reactions).

Composition
The composition of complement has been studied since the beginning of this century and it is now known to be composed of at least four main components, all of which are associated with the globulin fractions of serum.

First component (C'_1) is a water-insoluble euglobulin fraction which is heat-labile.

Second component (C'_2) is a water-soluble globulin and is heat-labile.

Third component (C'_3) is a heat-stable euglobulin fraction destroyed by zymosan (yeast cell walls). It is a complex of six separate components all of which are required for immune haemolytic reactions.

Fourth component (C'_4) is a heat-stable pseudoglobulin fraction destroyed by ammonia or ether.

Although complement is present in the sera of man and most vertebrates, the proportion of each of the four main components varies from one species to another. Guinea-pig complement has been studied in particular detail, and is known to contain all the components but its activity is limited by the quantity of C'_3. Human complement is similar to that of guinea-pig. Complements derived from cow, sheep, horse, pig, dog and mouse contain no fraction C'_2. For this reason they fail to haemolyse red blood cells in an antigen–antibody system.

Antigen–antibody reactions

Bacterial agglutination reactions (Fig 3.4)

When a saline suspension of a particular bacterial

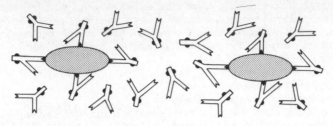

(a) Antibody excess

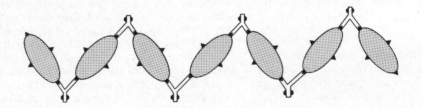

(b) Optimal proportions

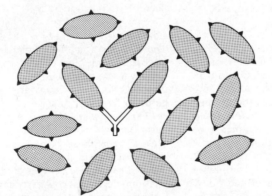

(c) Antigen excess

 IgG antibody molecule with two combining sites (C) and two determinant groups (D)

Antigen with four determinant groups (D)

FIG. 3.4. Bacterial antigen–antibody reactions occurring in (a) antibody excess (prozone effect) causing minimal or no agglutination, (b) optimal proportions causing complete agglutination with no excess of antigen or antibody, and (c) antigen excess causing minimal or no visible agglutination.

species is mixed with serum containing antibodies to these bacteria, the latter will become clumped or agglutinated. This is a specific antigen–antibody reaction which is widely used either for identifying the presence of serum antibodies against a known bacterial species, or for determining the antigenic structure of an unknown organism by using sera containing agglutinins against known bacterial antigens. The essential ingredients for an agglutination test are bacterial antigen, antibody (agglutinin) and an electrolyte (saline). The antigen may consist of a suspension of living or killed organisms, but for reasons of safety, killed suspensions are usually employed.

The principle of the test is that antibodies to bacterial antigen possess two receptor sites that will combine specifically with the antigens (determinant groups) on the surfaces of the bacteria. Under suitable conditions one antibody molecule will combine with the determinant groups on the surfaces of two bacteria, and in this way the bacteria become joined together or agglutinated. Agglutination can be observed microscopically or macroscopically, according to the technical methods employed.

The process of agglutination occurs in two stages. The first stage, consisting of the specific attachment of antibody to bacterial antigen, is known as **sensitization** and can occur rapidly within a few minutes of mixing antigen with antibody. The second stage may take several hours to develop completely, and will occur only in the presence of an electrolyte. The importance of an electrolyte in the second stage of agglutination can be demonstrated in the following way. When antigen and antibody are mixed together in distilled water, subsequent incubation of the mixture will result in sensitization of the bacteria. This can be confirmed by observing the absence of antibody in the supernatant fluid after centrifugation. Other tests can be used to detect antibody on the surfaces of the bacteria. In distilled water, however, the final stage of agglutination of the sensitized bacteria seldom occurs. It is probable that in the presence of an electrolyte the bacterial surfaces become more hydrophobic than hydrophilic.

The tube agglutination test
This is a relatively simple serological technique and is widely used for the detection of infectious diseases in animals (e.g. brucellosis, salmonellosis) and for the identification of unknown microorganisms. In the test the specific combination of bacterial antigen with antibody takes place following collisions between the two. It follows that any technique which increases the likelihood of collisions taking place will increase the speed and efficiency of the agglutination reaction. For this reason, tests are often incubated in waterbaths so that the level of water in the bath

is almost halfway up the columns of fluid in the agglutination tubes. Convection currents are set up in the tubes and this accelerates the sensitization and agglutination of the bacterial antigen. The agglutination reaction is also enhanced by carrying out the test at body temperature or above. The range of temperatures usually employed is from 37° to 52°C. At temperatures higher than 52°C there is a risk that sensitization may be followed by dissociation of the antigen–antibody complexes, giving rise to false negative reactions.

The tube agglutination test is commonly used to determine the presence and concentration of antibodies in sera to a particular bacterial antigen. The principle of the test is to make a series of increasing dilutions of serum in saline, to each of which is added a constant amount of bacterial antigen. After incubation the greatest dilution of serum which has caused macroscopic agglutination is recorded as the agglutinin **titre** of the serum. Alternatively, if the titre of the serum is 1/1000 and the volume of the reactants in the tube is 1·0 ml, the concentration of serum antibodies may be recorded as 1000 units/ ml. The titre of a serum will be affected by the concentration of antigen used in the test. A high concentration of antigen will require a correspondingly high concentration of antibody to produce visible agglutination and more than would be necessary to produce a similar result using less concentrated antigen. Thus, the greater the concentration of antigen the lower will be the apparent titre of the serum. To be able to compare the titres of a number of sera against a particular antigen, the latter must be standardized so that it contains approximately the same number of organisms per millilitre for each test in the series.

It may happen that when carrying out an agglutination test using a high titred serum, some of the strongest concentrations of sera fail to cause agglutination. This appears as a prozone in the early dilutions of a titration when the surfaces of the bacteria become saturated with antibody (Table 3.2). Under these conditions none of the antibody molecules can act as a bridge or linkage between two antigenic particles and agglutination fails to occur.

The rapid slide agglutinating test
This is a useful modification of the tube agglutination test and is used extensively as a laboratory procedure for the indentification of bacteria. Single drops or loopfuls of sera containing antibodies to known bacterial antigens are placed on a glass slide and, using a straight wire, part of a bacterial colony to be identified is transferred to the antiserum and evenly suspended in it. If the bacterial antigens are related to the agglutinins, agglutination will occur rapidly and this can be observed under a hand lens or

TABLE 3.2. Results of an agglutination test showing the prozone effect.

1/10	1/20	1/40	1/80	1/160	1/320	1/640	1/1280	1/2560	1/5120	1/10240
−	−	++	+++	++++	++++	++++	++++	++++	++	−

Prozone (under 1/10, 1/20). Titre (under 1/5120).

++++ = Complete agglutination. +++, ++ = Partial agglutination. — = No agglutination.

dissecting microscope. In this way, an unknown culture can be tested relatively quickly against a variety of known antisera, and the probable antigenic structure of the organism can be determined. However, the results of this rapid method may be affected by non-specific or minor antigen–antibody reactions and it is important that rapid slide tests are confirmed by the tube agglutination method before making a final diagnosis of the bacterial species under test.

The rapid plate test
This is another modification of the bacterial agglutination test which is often applied to the control of diseases in animals. One example is the rapid pullorum test for the control of pullorum disease in poultry, and another is the plate test for the control of brucellosis. For the former test the antigen consists of a heavy suspension of killed *S. pullorum* to which has been added crystal violet as a preservative and as a convenient colouring agent. One standard drop of this coloured antigen is placed on a white tile or glass plate and is mixed with a standard loopful of either whole blood or serum. If the serum contains agglutinins to *S. pullorum* the antigen is rapidly clumped and the violet colour facilitates the reading of the test. Similarly, the brucellosis plate test can be used for the control of brucellosis by mixing whole blood or serum with a heavy suspension of brucella organisms.

The Brucella milk ring test
This is a further modification of the agglutination test for the control of brucellosis in cattle. In this method one drop of a 4 per cent suspension of brucella antigen stained with haematoxylin is added to about 6 ml of milk, mixed and incubated at 37°C for 1 hour. If the milk contains agglutinins for *Br. abortus*, the agglutinated particles of antigen rise to the top with fat globules and form a visible ring near the surface in the layer of cream. In the absence of agglutinins the antigen remains evenly dispersed throughout the milk sample.

Haemagglutination reactions
Agglutination of red blood cells is often used as a basis for a variety of serological tests and many variations of the method have been developed including both tube and rapid plate tests. The results are read according to the pattern which the red cells form when they sediment in round-bottom tubes or wells.

The direct haemagglutination test
This is used for determining blood groups in man and animals. Red blood cells contain antigenic determinant groups on their surfaces (blood group antigens), and when a suspension of cells is mixed with an appropriate serum containing specific antibodies (isoantibodies) for these determinant groups, the cells will be agglutinated. Figs. 3.5 and 3.6a diagrammatically represent haemagglutination by IgM and IgG immunoglobulins, respectively.

The antiglobulin haemagglutination test (Coombs test)
This is a modification of the direct haemagglutination test and is employed in those cases when a serum may contain antibodies to a particular blood group antigen which sensitizes the cells but fails to cause haemagglutination. Antibodies of this sort were known as **partial**, **univalent** or **incomplete** antibodies because it was thought that one of the combining sites was masked and was not available to combine with antigen and link together or haemagglutinate two red blood cells. It is now known that sometimes the surface antigens on a cell may be situated at the bases of grooves on the surface structure and the shape of the immunoglobulin molecules and the disposition of their combining sites may render them physically incapable of combining with two particles of antigen (Fig. 3.6bi). Alternatively, haemagglutination may not occur when the Fab portion of IgG immunoglobulin does not fully expand to enable each receptor to combine with a separate red blood cell (Fig. 3.6ci).

Antibodies are immunoglobulin molecules which are themselves antigenic, and if they are derived from (say) chicken serum then they are composed of chicken globulin. Chicken globulin is a foreign antigen to rabbits and when inoculated into these animals, will stimulate the production of antibodies specific for chicken globulin. Thus, anti-chicken globulin serum can be prepared in rabbits, and if this antiserum is then added to washed red blood cells which had previously been sensitized but not agglutinated by antibodies derived from chicken

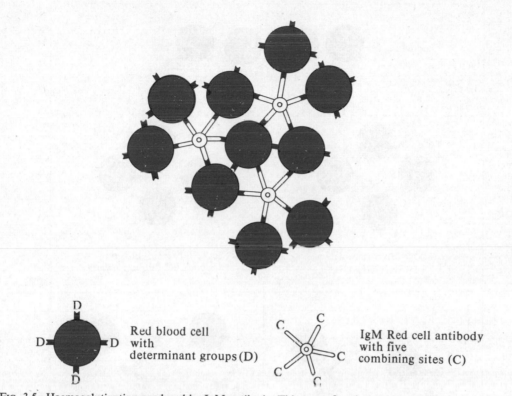

Red blood cell
with
determinant groups (D)

IgM Red cell antibody
with five
combining sites (C)

FIG. 3.5. Haemagglutination produced by IgM antibody. This type of agglutination is stronger and more efficient than a similar reaction with IgG antibody which has only two combining sites.

serum, the red blood cells will be agglutinated. The explanation is that the rabbit anti-chicken globulin serum contains divalent antibodies to chicken globulin. These combine with two molecules of antibody which are already attached to the surfaces of red blood cells and cause haemagglutination, (Figs. 3.6 bii and cii). Before use in the antiglobulin haemagglutination test it is important to absorb the antiglobulin serum with the species of red cells being used in the test to ensure that any normal antibody to the cells has been completely removed and will not cause false positive reactions in the antiglobulin haemagglutination test.

A modification of the Coombs test can be used for the diagnosis of brucellosis by detecting the presence in serum of non-agglutinating antibodies to *Br. abortus*. When these antibodies are mixed with the bacterial antigen they become attached to but fail to agglutinate the bacteria. If these sensitized cells are washed, resuspended in saline and an appropriate antiglobulin serum added, the antibodies in this serum cause agglutination of the sensitized bacteria. This test is particularly useful for detecting cases of chronic human brucellosis and has also been applied to infection in cattle.

The viral haemagglutination inhibition test
This is based on the property of some viruses being able to combine with the surfaces of red blood cells and cause haemagglutination. If, however, the virus is mixed with a serum containing specific viral antibodies before the addition of red cells, an antigen–antibody reaction occurs which subsequently inhibits the haemagglutinating property of the virus. This is the basis of the haemagglutination inhibition (HI) test which is used for detecting certain viral infections in animals (Fig. 3.7). Samples of sera are tested for the presence of specific antibody by observing their capacity to inhibit haemagglutination by the virus. The HI test can be used for detecting infection with poxviruses, togaviruses and myxoviruses. The last group includes Newcastle disease virus, for which the HI test is widely used for diagnosing infection in birds. (See Chapter 42)

The indirect haemagglutination test
This has been developed as a result of the demonstra-

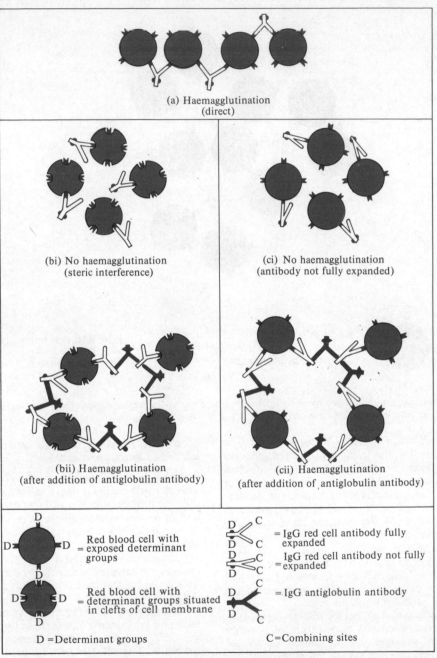

Fig. 3.6. Haemagglutination and antiglobulin haemagglutination produced by IgG antibody. (a) Shows direct haemagglutination between red blood cells with determinant groups exposed on their surfaces and fully expanded IgG antibody molecules. Haemagglutination may not occur when either the determinant groups of the blood cells are situated in clefts (bi) because of steric interference with antibody combination, or when the Fab portion of the IgG antibody molecule does not fully expand (ci). Under both conditions the red blood cells have become sensitized with antibody (i.e. globulin) and the subsequent addition of antiglobulin antibody causes haemagglutination (bii and cii).

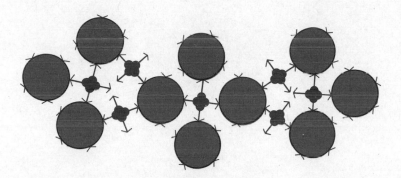

Viral haemagglutination

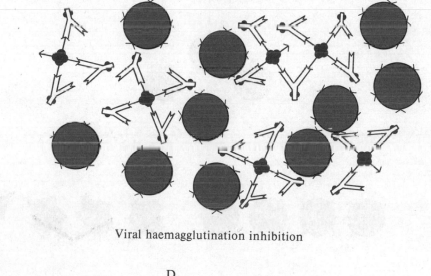

Viral haemagglutination inhibition

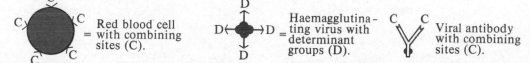

FIG. 3.7. Viral haemagglutination and haemagglutination-inhibition. Some viruses are able to attach themselves to red blood cells and cause haemagglutination. This reaction can be inhibited when viruses are mixed with specific anti-viral antibody before the addition of red blood cells.

tion that antigens and haptens from a variety of bacterial and fungal species can be extracted and, under suitable conditions, attached to the surfaces of normal, washed red blood cells. These modified cells which have become coated with microbial extracts will be agglutinable by antisera containing homologous antibodies to the organisms, and haemolysis will occur when complement is added to the system (Fig. 3.8). For example, preparations of O-antigen polysaccharides from *Salmonella* or *Escherichia* can be obtained by various extraction methods (e.g. trichloracetic acid, phenol or sodium hydroxide) and when these O-antigens are mixed with washed red cells, the latter become coated with the polysaccharides. In addition, red cells can adsorb, simultaneously, a number of serologically distinct

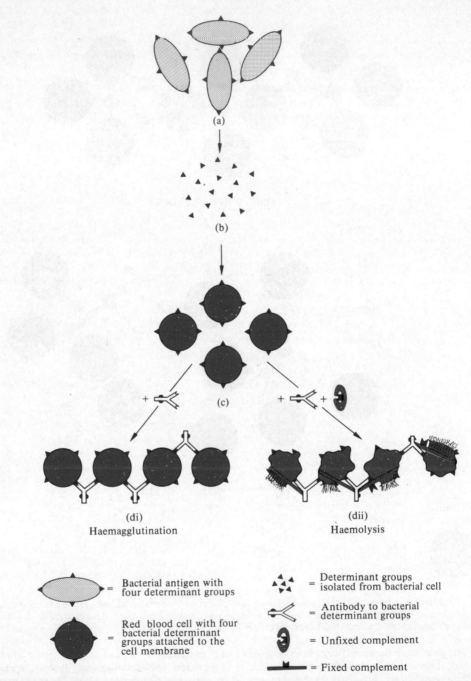

FIG. 3.8. Indirect haemagglutination and haemolytic reactions. Under *in vitro* and *in vivo* conditions microbial determinant groups on the surfaces of organisms (a) may become removed (b) and subsequently attached to the surfaces of normal red blood cells (c). In the presence of antibody specific for the microbial determinant groups, these modified red cells become haemagglutinated (di) or haemolysed when complement is also available (dii). In the laboratory this system can be used for *in vitro* tests to determine specific microbial antibodies in sera, and the process can also be responsible for the development of *in vivo* haemolytic anaemias in diseased animals.

polysaccharides from different bacterial species and these cells then become agglutinable by antisera to any of the O-antigens which have been adsorbed on to their surfaces. Bacterial extracts containing protein (e.g. protein derived from *Myco. tuberculosis*) will not adhere to the surfaces of red cells unless the latter have been pre-treated with tannic acid. These so-called tanned cells will adsorb tuberculo-protein and thereafter can be used for testing sera for antibodies to *Myco. tuberculosis*. Similarly, some viruses which do not adhere to the surfaces of normal red cells will combine with tanned cells and the latter are than agglutinable by appropriate viral antisera.

Red cells modified with bacterial extracts constitute a very sensitive antigen which can be used to detect antibodies which would not be observed by the classical bacterial agglutination test. This type of indirect haemagglutination reaction may demonstrate a tenfold increase in antibody titres compared with the bacterial agglutination test. In addition, the sensitivity of the test can be increased still further by using these modified red cells in an anti-globulin haemagglutination test.

Precipitation reactions

There are many circumstances in which antigen to be used in a serological reaction consists of a colour-less solution instead of a particulate suspension as in the agglutination test. Examples of antigens which consist of molecular solutions are bacterial poly-saccharides and proteins, serum proteins (globulins and albumens), and viruses. These substances can combine with their respective antibodies to form antigen–antibody complexes. Provided that these complexes are sufficiently large and numerous, they will be observable with the aid of a hand lens and in most cases will be seen with the naked eye as fine precipitations. The essential ingredients for precipita-tion tests are antigen (precipitinogen), antibody (precipitin) and an electrolyte (saline); and the reaction which takes place is fundamentally similar to the agglutination of a particulate antigen. A variety of techniques have been devised to adapt the method to suit different circumstances.

The precipitin ring test

This and recent modifications of the method are in common use for a variety of diagnostic and research purposes. The simplest technique consists of carefully layering antigen on to the surface of antiserum in a narrow tube so that the interface between the two fluids is relatively small compared with the total volumes of the reactants. An antigen–antibody reaction occurs at the interface and as this develops it can be observed macroscopically as a white ring which, in time, may break up and precipitate to the bottom of the tube. Both solutions of antigen and antibody should be water-clear in order to obtain the most accurate results.

When a precipitation test has been set up in a series of tubes containing a constant amount of antiserum in each tube and with decreasing amounts of antigen, it will be noticed that precipitation occurs more quickly in one tube of the series than in the others. The tube which shows this rapid reaction contains **optimal proportions** of antigen and antibody, which are the amounts combining together without any excess left over. This can be confirmed by examination of the supernatant fluid after the reaction is completed and by showing that there is no remaining detectable antigen or antibody.

When the precipitation reaction is a complex one involving more than one antigen–antibody system, two or more separate rings may be observed at the interface but usually the reactions become clouded and indefinite. To overcome this difficulty an agar diffusion technique (**Oudin's method**) can be used. In this method the serum is incorporated in an agar gel and allowed to set at the bottom of a tube. The antigen is then layered on to the surface and the tube allowed to stand for several hours or days. During this time antigens will diffuse into the agar at different rates, depending upon a number of factors including molecular size and concentration. Precipitin lines will form at different levels in the agar gel in the region of optimal proportions for each antigen–antibody system.

Another modification is **Ouchterlony's method** of double diffusion. Variations of this method have been developed but the basic technique consists of carrying out the precipitation test in an agar plate. A number of circular wells are cut out of the agar and into each of these is placed antigen or antiserum. Both antigen and antibody will diffuse towards each other from two adjacent wells and when they meet in optimal concentrations, a visible line of precipita-tion will be formed (Plate 3.1a, facing p. 58). One advantage of this technique is that two or more antigens can be tested simultaneously against a particular antiserum, and several antigen–antibody systems can be demonstrated simultaneously.

A number of modifications to this technique have been made to adapt it to particular uses. For example, the diagnosis of viral antigen in tissues from pigs infected with swine fever and from cattle infected with rinderpest can be made in a thin layer of agar gel on a glass slide. A central well containing known antiserum is surrounded by a number of wells containing tissue (i.e. suspected viral antigen) and one control well filled with an extract from known infected tissue. If the unknown tissue contains specific antigen, a characteristic precipitation line or lines are formed which can be observed macroscopically. Other modifications have included the incorporation of dyes to facilitate the observation of precipitin lines.

Immunoelectrophoresis is a further modification which is particularly useful for determining the globulin components in a sample of serum. Two wells are made in a suitable agar-buffer medium; one is filled with a known serum and the other with the serum sample to be examined. An electric current is then passed through the medium for an appropriate time (e.g. 1 hour). This causes the protein components to migrate at different rates characteristic for each component. Subsequently, a serum containing known antibodies to the various components is placed in a trough situated between the two wells and time allowed for antigen–antibody (precipitation) reactions to take place. The result is a series of precipitation arcs which occur along the edges of the trough, each one being representative of a particular protein component of the test serum which can be compared with those derived from the known serum sample in the other well (Plate 3.1b, facing p. 59).

Flocculation tests

These tests using bacterial toxins and antitoxins demonstrate clearly the significance of optimal proportions in the formation of visible precipitation. In this system, mixtures of antigen and antibody in either antigen excess or antibody excess give rise to soluble complexes, and it is only in the region of optimal proportions that visible precipitation occurs. This technique can be used to estimate the concentrations of bacterial toxins and antitoxins. The Lf dose of toxin is that amount which flocculates most rapidly with one unit of antitoxin.

Non-precipitating antibodies

These do not cause visible precipitation when mixed with an antigen and, under certain conditions, may not be revealed by a precipitation test. We have already referred to this type of antibody in connection with the antiglobulin haemagglutination test and discussed how they can be detected by adding an appropriate antiglobulin serum to the test. These antibodies are of particular significance during the early stages of an infectious disease when the precipitation test may be of little value for determining the early production of antibodies because the greater proportion of them may be of the non-precipitating variety. If antigen is mixed with these antibodies and subsequently added to a serum known to contain precipitating antibodies, the latter will not cause precipitation of the antigen because of the blocking effect of the non-precipitating antibody.

Lytic reactions and complement-fixation

The addition of bacteria to a fresh unheated sample of serum containing homologous antibodies will result in the organisms becoming disintegrated or lysed. Lysis takes place as the result of an antigen–antibody reaction in which complement has become involved. Conversely, if the activity of complement is prevented by heating the immune serum to 56°C for 30 minutes before adding it to the bacteria, no lysis will occur. We have already noted that guinea-pig serum is a rich source of all four main fractions of complement. If fresh guinea-pig serum which does not contain homologous antibodies is added to bacteria, no lysis will occur because complement alone cannot cause lysis. These experiments demonstrate two important features of lytic reactions, namely:

(1) Complement causes lysis of bacteria in the presence of homologous bacterial antibody.

(2) Complement does not cause lysis of bacteria in the absence of an antigen-antibody reaction.

The involvement of complement in an antigen-antibody system is referred to as **complement-fixation**.

The earliest studies on the role of complement in bacterial lysis were carried out by Bordet in 1909, who observed the lysis of vibrio organisms by complement in the presence of specific antibody. Later, he made similar experiments using red blood cells as antigen and observed lysis (haemolysis) of the cells in the presence of antibody and complement. Haemolysis can be readily observed in the laboratory and this type of reaction has formed the basis of an indicator system in the complement-fixation test, which can be applied to a variety of *in vitro* antigen-antibody reactions. The fixation of complement in a haemolytic system occurs in stages. First, C'_1 becomes attached to the antigen–antibody complex in the presence of Ca ions, and this is followed by C'_4 and C'_2 in the presence of Mg ions. Finally, C'_3 becomes incorporated and this is followed by haemolysis of the cells (Fig. 3.9).

Complement-fixation in an antigen–antibody reaction has been studied extensively using a haemolytic indicator system which includes red blood cells (usually from sheep), an antibody to red blood cells and complement. Antisera to red blood cells can be prepared by inoculating cells from one animal species into another. For example, the inoculation of sheep red blood cells into rabbits stimulates the production of antibodies specific for sheep cells. Complement is usually obtained from pooled serum samples derived from two or more guinea-pigs. To ensure that this is the only source of complement in the system, the antiserum to sheep cells should be heated to 56°C for 30 minutes beforehand, to destroy any haemolytic complement which it may contain. The haemolytic effect of complement on red blood

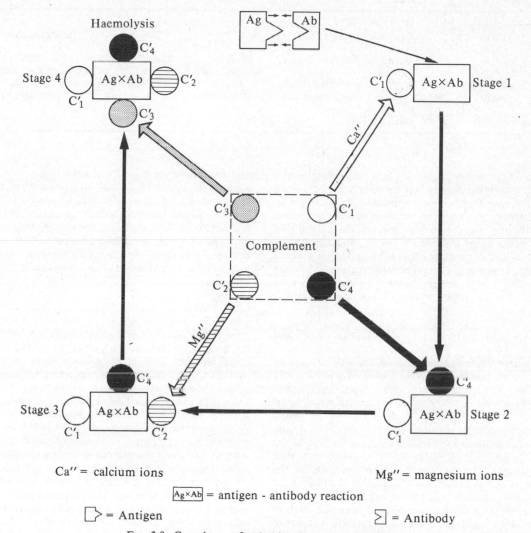

Ca″ = calcium ions   Mg″ = magnesium ions

Ag×Ab = antigen - antibody reaction

▷ = Antigen   ◁ = Antibody

Fig. 3.9. Complement-fixation in a haemolytic system.

cells in an antigen–antibody system can be summarised as follows:

Red blood cells + specific antibody (heated) ⟶ no haemolysis

Red blood cells + specific antibody (heated) + complement ⟶ haemolysis

The amount of complement (i.e. fresh guinea-pig serum) required to lyse a given volume of red blood cells can be found by mixing different concentrations of complement with constant amounts of red blood cells plus heated antiserum, and observing the least amount of complement which will cause complete lysis of all the red blood cells. This amount is known

as the **minimal haemolytic dose (MHD)** of complement. Under these standardized conditions all available complement will become combined with antibody on the red cell surfaces and cause lysis.

It has long been established that in immunological systems involving cellular antigens, antibody and complement, it is complement and not antibody which is responsible for the lytic reaction. Recent experiments have shown that under these conditions the action of complement is to produce holes in the surface membranes of the cells which consequently alters their osmotic stability and results in cellular lysis. This mode of action, which occurs in conjunc-

TABLE 3.3. Diagrammatic representation of the complement-fixation test.

STAGE 1	STAGE 2	STAGE 3	STAGE 4	STAGE 5	STAGE 6
Mix primary system		Add indicator system		Result	Interpretation
Antigen + unknown serum (heated) + complement	Incubate at 37°C for 30 minutes or at 4°C overnight	Red blood cells + antibody (heated) to red blood cells	Incubate at 37°C for 30 minutes	Haemolysis → or No haemolysis→	Negative (antibody not in unknown serum) Positive (antibody in unknown serum)

tion with either IgG or IgM immunoglobulin fractions, takes place when the cellular antigen is an erythrocyte (haemolysis), a tissue cell, a bacterium (bacteriolysis) or a virus, provided that the respective antibodies are directed to the surface antigens of erythrocytes or tissue cells, the somatic antigens of bacteria or the surface coats of viral particles. There is also evidence to show that under certain conditions clusters of holes are produced as a result of complement-fixation which may enhance and accelerate the lytic effect.

Complement-fixation test (CFT) (Fig. 3.10 and Table 3.3)
This test is used in a variety of immune systems to detect the presence of antibodies in sera, particularly against viruses and less comonly bacteria. The test is performed in two stages. In the first stage, serial dilutions of the heated serum under test are mixed with a constant amount of antigen (e.g. virus), and to each dilution mixture is added two to four MHD of guinea-pig complement. The tubes are then incubated. The purpose of the second stage of the test is to ascertain in which serum dilutions an antigen–antibody reaction has occurred by observing whether complement has become fixed. To each of the above mixtures is added a standard volume of sheep red blood cells and antiserum to sheep red blood cells. The mixtures are incubated and subsequently the presence or absence of haemolysis is determined. If haemolysis has occurred it means that complement was still available after incubation of the primary test, and that no antigen–antibody reaction had taken place in the primary system. Conversely, no haemolysis indicates that the complement present in the primary test had been fixed by an antigen–antibody reaction, that none remained available to cause lysis of the red blood cells, and that the serum under test contained antibodies against the particular antigen. (See also Appendix 1)

Immunoconglutinin test
Since the beginning of the century it has been known that bovine serum contains a substance which will agglutinate red blood cells, provided that these cells have already absorbed complement on to their surfaces. This haemagglutinating substance is a heat-stable serum globulin known as **conglutinin,** and one of its characteristic features is that it will combine with 'fixed' but not with 'unfixed' complement. This combination will only occur in the presence of fractions C'_1, C'_2 and C'_4 of complement.

Since the original description of bovine conglutinin, similar substances have been identified in the sera of other animal species, particularly after they have been inoculated with either an antigen–antibody complex or immunized with an antigen. Under both conditions the level of conglutinin rises and falls, and shows a typical antibody response. Conglutinin which appears under these conditions is an antibody known as **immunoconglutinin** because its presence is directly related to a known immunological reaction. After an antigen–antibody complex has been inoculated into an animal, complement becomes fixed, and it has been suggested that this involves an unfolding of the complement molecules and exposure of some previously hidden determinant groupings which stimulate antibody production against complement. Thus, immunoconglutinin is an example of an autoantibody. Similarly, if an animal is immunized with a bacterial antigen, antibodies will be produced which will combine with the antigen and fix complement. In this way the fixed complement then stimulates the production of immunoconglutinin. The exact function of immunoconglutinin in the disease process is not known but its presence appears to be associated with increased resistance to infection, and the immunoconglutination test is occasionally used to estimate the immune status of an animal. Fig. 3.11 shows diagrammatically the incorporation of immunoconglutinin in antigen–antibody reactions.

Fluorescent antigen–antibody reactions
The principle of these reactions is that antigens and antibodies can be labelled with fluorescent dyes and

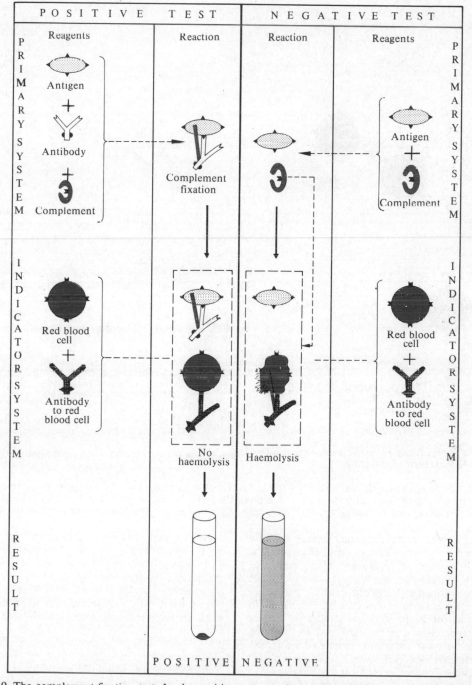

FIG. 3.10. The complement-fixation test. In the positive test, complement becomes fixed to the antigen–antibody reaction in the primary system and is not available in the indicator system which consequently shows no haemolysis. In the negative test no antigen–antibody reaction takes place in the primary system and the available complement becomes incorporated in the indicator system causing haemolysis.

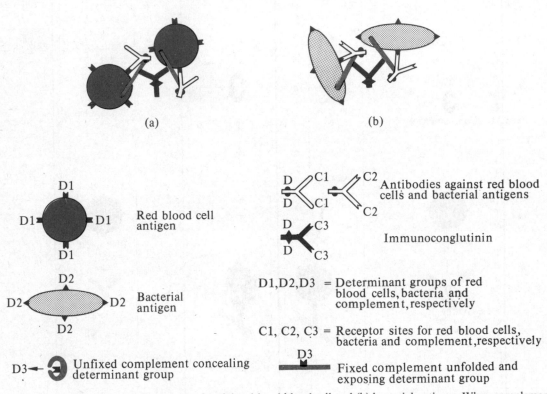

FIG. 3.11. Immunoconglutinin reactions involving (a) red blood cell and (b) bacterial antigens. When complement becomes fixed in an antigen–antibody reaction it exposes the determinant group to immunoconglutinin receptors. Immunoconglutinin may consist of IgG as well as IgM immunoglobulin. The former is depicted in the diagram.

that when subsequently examined microscopically by ultraviolet light the antigen–antibody reactions fluoresce. Since the combination of antigen with antibody is a highly specific reaction, this technique has been developed as a useful diagnostic procedure for the identification of microbial infections in animals and for immunological studies. A variety of fluorescent dyes can be used and for staining antibodies the most commonly employed are fluorescein isothiocyanate (FITC) which emits a green light and lissamine rhodamine B (RB 200) emitting an orange-yellow colour. The conjugation of antibody with fluorescein or RB 200 consists of precipitating immunoglobulin out of a serum sample with ammonium sulphate, dissolving the precipitate in

distilled water, removing excess ammonium sulphate by dialysis, adjusting to pH 9·2 with buffer solution and mixing with the dye at 4°C. Subsequently, excess dye is removed by dialysis and the final preparation can be stored frozen at −20°C or freeze dried. The two techniques used for routine work are the direct and indirect fluorescent antibody tests.

Direct test
This consists of adding a preparation of known antibody labelled with a dye to sections, cell cultures or fixed smears containing suspected microorganisms or antigens, allowing time for an antigen–antibody reaction to take place, washing off excess

of dyed antibody and examining the preparation under the microscope with u.v. illumination. When an antigen–antibody reaction has taken place this will be observed by an area of fluorescence resulting from the dyed antibody globulin having combined with the antigen (Fig. 3.12a).

been labelled with a fluorescent dye. Thus, if the serum containing unlabelled microbial antibodies was derived from (say) a chicken, the dyed anti-globulin serum must contain antibodies to chicken globulin. To carry out the test the specimen containing the suspected antigen is flooded with specific

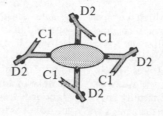

(a)   Direct test

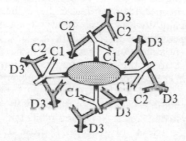

(b) Indirect test

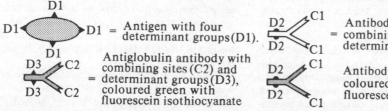

D1 = Antigen with four determinant groups(D1).

Antibody to antigen with = combining sites (C1) and determinant groups (D2)

Antiglobulin antibody with combining sites (C2) and = determinant groups(D3), coloured green with fluorescein isothiocyanate

Antibody to antigen coloured green with fluorescein isothiocyanate

FIG. 3.12. The direct and indirect fluorescent antibody tests using fluorescein isothiocyanate. In the direct test antigen is detected by adding specific antibody labelled with fluorescein and examining under u.v. illumination. The indirect test consists of adding unlabelled specific antibody which combines with the antigen. The preparation is then treated with appropriate antiglobulin antibody previously treated with fluorescein. This method is more sensitive than the direct test and gives a greater concentration of fluorescence around the particles of antigen.

Indirect (sandwich) test

This method is more sensitive than the direct test and incorporates an antiglobulin test in the reaction. The ingredients required are a known undyed antibody to the particular antigen to be identified, and an appropriate antiglobulin antibody which has

undyed antiserum to the antigen, time allowed for an antigen–antibody reaction to take place, and excess serum washed off. The preparation is then covered with an appropriate labelled antiglobulin antibody, time allowed for an antigen–antibody reaction to take place and excess washed off. If antigen was present this will be observed microscopically as areas of fluorescence. The method is more sensitive than the direct test because the greater amount of dyed antiglobulin antibody compared with undyed antibody to the antigen will give a larger and more intense area of fluorescence (Fig. 3.12b). (See also Chapter 42)

Neutralization reactions

Neutralization tests are procedures which consist essentially of observing the extent to which specific antibody will combine with and neutralize the toxic effect of an antigen in the animal body, the skin, the developing avian embryo or in cell cultures. These tests have been used for many years in the study of bacterial toxin–antitoxin reactions and latterly they have been applied extensively to observe the neutralizing capacity of antisera to viruses. It is probable that the IgG class of antibodies is particularly effective in neutralizing soluble toxins.

Bacterial neutralization tests

These are commonly applied to clostridial toxins as a measure of toxin or antitoxin concentration and also as one method for determining the specificity of an unknown toxin suspected of causing disease. The value of the tests is based on the ability of a toxin to combine specifically with homologous antitoxin and to have its characteristic toxic properties neutralized by this combination. The neutralizing power of a particular antitoxin can be determined by mixing it with a known toxin and observing any subsequent reduction in the systemic toxic reactions in an experimental animal. The activity of toxins can be determined by assaying under standard conditions the smallest dose or minimal lethal dose (MLD) which will cause the death of a particular animal species within a given time. Conversely, the standardisation of antitoxins can be carried out in animals by observing the amount of antitoxin which will neutralize a standard dose of toxin. Antitoxins can be preserved and stored without any deterioration in their biological activity, whereas toxins tend to develop into toxoids during prolonged storage. For this reason, international standards for antitoxins are available for reference so that all fresh batches of antitoxin can be prepared to the same standard. For example, one international unit of tetanus antitoxin is the activity contained in 0.3094 mg of dried standard antitoxin, and similarly, one international unit of *Cl. welchii* type A antitoxin is the activity contained in 0·1132 mg of dried standard antitoxin.

Fresh preparations of toxins can be assayed against standard antitoxins. The **Lo dose of toxin** is that amount which is just neutralized by one unit of antitoxin. The **L+ dose of toxin** is the smallest amount which, when mixed with 1 unit of antitoxin will produce a standard effect. This effect may be the death of a particular animal species (e.g. mouse, guinea-pig) of known weight in a given time.

An alternative method for estimating toxin-antitoxin reactions is to inoculate mixtures into the skin of rabbits. Small quantities of many clostridial toxins will cause necrosis at the site of intradermal inoculation. In the presence of adequate specific antitoxins the necrotizing activity of toxins will be neutralized and prevent the development of lesions. The test can be used for estimating the strength of an unknown toxin against a standard unit of antitoxin or *vice versa*. In this method, the **Lr dose of toxin** is the amount which will produce a standard lesion when inoculated with 1 unit of antitoxin. Mixtures of toxin and antitoxin are allowed to stand for $\frac{1}{2}$–1 hour before being inoculated so that maximum neutralization will have occurred beforehand. This intradermal method is very sensitive and a number of tests can be carried out on the shaved skin of one rabbit.

Viral neutralization tests

These have been increasingly used as antigen–antibody reactions to determine immunological specificities and the capacity of antisera to prevent virus infections. A common sequel to virus infection is the production of symptoms or lesions which can be easily observed. These effects can usually be inhibited by the presence of specific antibody which combines with viral particles and prevents their attachment and subsequent penetration into susceptible host cells. To inhibit viral growth in this way it is important that antibody combines with virus before the latter has become attached to the tissue cell. After attachment greatly increased quantities of antibodies are required to prevent penetration of virus into the cell and, if penetration has already occurred, the addition of high concentrations of antibody to the infected tissue cells will not prevent intracellular viral growth.

When virus and homologous antibody are mixed together an antigen–antibody reaction occurs. The extent to which subsequent viral growth in tissue culture will be prevented depends upon the amount of antibody fixed to each particle of virus. For example, only a few molecules of antibody attached to the tails of bacteriophages will prevent their fixation to the surfaces of bacteria. Animal viruses vary greatly in size and the larger the particle the greater is the amount of fixed antibody required to inhibit viral attachment, penetration and growth in tissue cells. Even under optimal conditions the prevention of viral growth is only an indirect effect of antibody, since the latter is specific for the outer antigenic protein coat of the viral particle and not for the nucleic acid which is the infective component and contained within the body of the virus.

The general procedure for carrying out a neutralization test is to mix a constant amount of virus with increasing dilutions of antiserum, allow to react for an appropriate time at a suitable temperature depending on the particular virus being used, and then to inoculate the mixtures into a susceptible host system which is then observed for signs of infection. (See Chapter 42)

Several variations of the test are possible using different hosts and indicator effects, e.g. counting deaths in groups of unweaned mice inoculated intracerebrally with Aujeszky's disease virus, counting of 'pocks' on the chorioallantoic membrane of eggs inoculated with fowl pox virus, observing infected cell culture monolayers for the development of specific cytopathic effects, haemagglutinins or haemadsorption, or counting 'plaques' of cell degeneration in petri-dish cell cultures overlaid with agar after inoculation.

The neutralization test is the most widely applicable, but not necessarily the most convenient serological test for investigational work since it is very expensive in both time and materials. It is very sensitive, however, and is usually highly specific and can be performed with viruses which neither haemagglutinate nor react in complement-fixation tests. It should be noted that combination of virus and antibody is often a loose one and the virus may not be inactivated in the process. Thus, the two components may be dissociated by simple dilution, filtration or change in pH, resulting in the release of infectious virus. The results of neutralization tests vary according to the lability of the virus, the type of cell used, etc., and for this reason comparative tests between acute and convalescent sera must always be made. Immunity is closely related to the persistence of neutralizing antibodies in the animal and a four-fold or greater rise in titre is diagnostic.

Phagocytosis and pinocytosis

The digestion and removal from the body of foreign material and effete or damaged tissue cells by phagocytes constitutes the processes of phagocytosis or pinocytosis which form an integral part of the defence mechanism. The cells involved are polymorphonuclear leucocytes (microphages) and mononuclear macrophages which are variously termed monocytes in the blood, histiocytes in connective tissue or Kupffer cells in the liver. Thus, phagocytosis refers to the absorption of particulate substances by leucocytes, which is facilitated by movement of wandering cells and the development of pseudopodia. Pinocytosis, on the other hand, is the term used to describe ingestion through cell membranes of fluids or colloids, and it is probable that some

animal viruses (e.g. pox viruses) are ingested by this process. Phagocytosis can occur in the absence of antibody but samples of normal sera often contain natural antibody, known as **opsonin**, which can prepare cells for phagocytosis by combining with them in an antigen–antibody reaction. This process of preparation involves the attachment of sufficient antibody protein to the surfaces of the cells to change their electrical potential and facilitate their adhesion to leucocytes.

This reaction process can be demonstrated in the laboratory by showing that when bacteria, which have been mixed with fresh serum containing antibodies are subsequently washed free from the serum, they become more susceptible to phagocytosis than similar untreated cells. Conversely, the mixing of leucocytes with normal serum followed by washing, does not enhance their phagocytic properties towards untreated cells.

Bacteria + antibody — wash — add leucocytes → marked phagocytosis

Leucocytes + antibody — wash — add bacteria → very slight phagocytosis

An antibacterial serum containing a relatively high concentration of specific thermostable antibody (**immune opsonin**) will have a far stronger opsonic activity than normal serum. The degree to which a serum is able to prepare bacteria for phagocytosis is known as the **opsonic index** and this will vary according to the concentration of antibody. By using a standard technique it is possible to compare the opsonic indices of a number of sera. A mixture consisting of the serum to be tested, a suspension of the particular bacterial species concerned and a suspension of leucocytes is incubated, a film prepared and stained, and the number of bacteria ingested by more than fifty leucocytes is counted. The calculated average number of bacteria ingested by one leucocyte is the **phagocytic index** for that serum. Similarly, the phagocytic index for a normal serum is obtained and the opsonic index calculated as follows:

$$\text{Opsonic index} = \frac{\text{phagocytic index of unknown serum}}{\text{phagocytic index of normal serum}}.$$

Phagocytosis includes not only the removal of foreign material from the body (e.g. bacteria) but also effete or damaged tissue cells. This raises the question of the processes which are involved in the recognition, preparation and finally the phagocytosis of particles, and how this process allows discrimination so that only those particles are phagocytosed which are required to be removed from the body to maintain the health of the host. Current information indicates that antibodies against specific cell types are responsible for the discrimination which apparently controls this cleansing mechanism. For example, the removal of effete red blood cells is an important cleansing process mediated by antibodies to these particular cells which enhance their phagocytosis. Similarly, recent investigations indicate that the phagocytosis of other types of effete tissue cells and of tumour cells is also controlled by antibodies specific for each cell type.

It is a well established fact that the phagocytosis of bacteria by leucocytes may or may not lead to the death and dissolution of these organisms. After the action of antibody, possibly enhanced by complement, has lead to the phagocytosis of bacteria, the ingested organisms are subjected intracellularly to the destructive actions of lysozyme, phagocytin (a bactericidal protein particularly active against Gram-negative bacteria), and to other substances. Some organisms are susceptible to the destructive actions of these intracellular substances and are destroyed, while others are resistant and will survive. There is additional evidence to indicate that the presence of immune opsonin on the surfaces of phagocytosed bacteria may increase the likelihood of their destruction by the leucocyte. However, there are circumstances under which phagocytosed bacteria may survive ingestion by leucocytes. This gives rise to a balanced situation in which the leucocyte acts as a protection for the bacteria against the action of antibodies and antibacterial drugs, and the host may become a carrier of that particular organism. Moreover, the ingested bacteria may be responsible for the destruction of the leucocytes containing them.

Hypersensitive reactions

In the preceding discussion on antigen–antibody reactions we have been concerned with the direct and specific combination of antigen with antibody, in which the latter was present in the serum and associated with an increased resistance or immunity of the host to a particular microbial infection. There are circumstances, however, in which antigen–antibody reactions occur *in vivo* and are related to an increased reactivity, or sensitivity of the body to a particular antigen involving damage to tissue cells. Such a state of increased reactivity, known as **hypersensitivity** or **allergy**, may not be beneficial to the host and may be the cause of profound reactions possibly terminating in death. The development of hypersensitive reactions in the tissues depends upon a variety of conditions and we still know little about how tissue cells become involved or the exact nature of the cell damage which may develop. One aspect of these reactions which assists their classification is that some may occur rapidly, within 2–3 minutes, when demonstrable circulating antibodies are present in the serum; while others may take several days or weeks to develop in the apparent absence of detectable humoral antibodies but associated with immunologically activated lymphoid cells (T-lymphocytes). It is, therefore, convenient for discussion to classify hypersensitivity into 'immediate reactions' and 'delayed reactions'. It should be noted that Coombs and Gell have proposed an alternative method for classifying hypersensitive responses which they have grouped into four types of allergic reactions.

Whether a hypersensitive state develops as an immediate or a delayed type of reaction depends upon a number of factors, including the nature of the antigen–antibody reaction, the class of immunoglobulin produced, the tissue cells involved, and the properties of the pharmacologically active substances which may be released as a result of the immune reaction. The five pharmacologically active substances which have been studied most closely in relation to hypersensitivity are histamine, serotonin, bradykinin, slow reacting substance of anaphylaxis (SRS-A) and lymph node permeability factor (LNPF). The following is a summary of the characteristic features of these substances.

Histamine

This substance is stored in the granules of mast cells and some is also produced continually outside these cells. As a result of a hypersensitive reaction, mast cells become destroyed or degranulated and the stored histamine is released. The ability to form new histamine is particularly high in tissues which are rapidly growing, as in the developing fetus and in inflammatory conditions. The action of histamine on the tissues is to cause rapid contraction of smooth muscle, vasodilatation and increased capillary permeability.

Serotonin (5-hydroxytryptamine)

Occurs in varying concentrations in platelets, particularly those from rabbits, and also has been reported in mast cells of rodents. As the result of an immunological reaction, serotonin is released from platelets and may then cause contraction of some smooth muscles and increased vasodilatation and permeability of small blood vessels.

Bradykinin

This substance is produced from kininogen, a globulin precursor in plasma, by the action of an enzyme released from tissues following an antigen–antibody reaction involving tissue cells, and it then becomes detectable in the blood stream. Since the half-life of bradykinin in blood is about 30 seconds it must be produced in high concentrations before becoming detectable. It is a slow reacting substance causing contraction of smooth muscles, vasodilatation and increased permeability of capillaries. Unlike histamine and SRS-A (see below) the

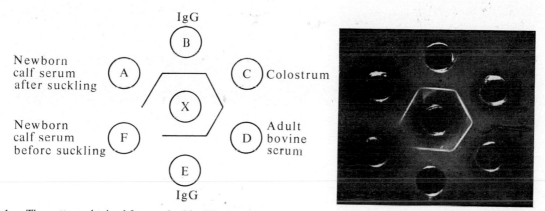

IgG

Newborn calf serum after suckling — A

B

C — Colostrum

X

Newborn calf serum before suckling — F

D — Adult bovine serum

E

IgG

3.1a   The pattern obtained from a double diffusion (Ouchterlony) test. The antigens have been placed in wells A–F and antibody to bovine IgG prepared in a rabbit was placed in the central well (X). Following diffusion of antigens and antibody through the agar, lines of precipitation formed opposite all wells except F. These lines also joined up with each other showing that a similar antigen-antibody reaction had taken place in each case. The test reveals that IgG is present in all samples except newborn calf serum obtained before suckling.

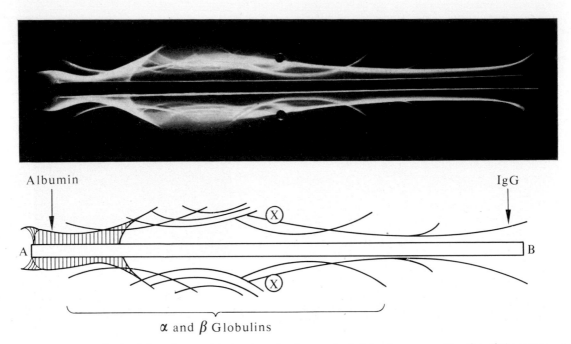

3.1b   The pattern obtained from immunoelectrophoresis of normal adult bovine serum. Samples of the serum were placed in each of the two wells (X) and subjected to electrophoresis resulting in the albumin fraction migrating to the left. Subsequently, an anti-whole bovine serum prepared in a rabbit was placed in the trough (AB). The preparation was left overnight and precipitation arcs developed representing the different antigenic components present in the bovine serum. The diagram simplifies the interpretation of the typical complex picture which developed.

production of bradykinin can be triggered off by immunological reactions involving complement.

Slow reacting substance of anaphylaxis (SRS-A)

There are difficulties in preparing and analysing a purified form of SRS-A and it is probable that there are a number of different SRS substances. This may be the reason for some confusion in the literature as to the exact nature and activity of SRS-A. Recently, it has been shown that under experimental conditions this substance can cause damage and severe congestion to blood vessels of the duodenum and small intestine in rats — lesions which have a strong resemblance to those associated with severe anaphylactic shock in that species. Present information suggests that SRS-A has an affinity for lipids which results in it being rapidly absorbed by cells in the locality of its formation; and this rapid attachment to cells may be related to a close association which has been demonstrated between SRS-A and lecithin. SRS-A causes contraction of smooth muscles, is slow in onset and has a prolonged action. Thus, following a hypersensitive reaction the release of SRS-A occurs later than that of histamine and lasts longer. The action of SRS-A is not inhibited by antihistaminic drugs.

Lymph node permeability factor (LNPF)

This material is derived from mononuclear leucocytes and can be prepared from cells of the spleen or lymph nodes. The constitution of LNPF has not been defined but it is not composed of protein or polypeptide. It is known to contain RNA but this does not appear to be involved in the biological activity of the substance. LNPF is associated with delayed types of hypersensitive reactions which are characterised by leucocytic infiltrations (e.g. tuberculin reaction). Intradermal inoculation of LNPF characteristically causes increased permeability of local blood vessels and a lymphocytic infiltration. It has only slight activity on smooth muscle.

Immediate hypersensitive reactions (Fig. 3.13)

General reaction (anaphylaxis)

This is also classified as a Type I allergic reaction by Coombs and Gell. It has been known for a long time that guinea-pigs may react violently to two injections of an antigen given under suitable conditions and that this reaction may be so severe as to cause death. The classical type of experiment consists of inoculating a normal guinea-pig with a dose of a harmless foreign antigen (e.g. egg albumin, serum from another species, etc.). If a second dose of the same antigen is then given intravenously about a fortnight later, the guinea-pig may show severe symptoms of distress and die from asphyxia within

a few minutes. This syndrome is known as anaphylactic shock. An explanation of the cause of such sudden and profound reactions has been the subject of very many experiments and it is important to note some of the features associated with this type of immunological response. First, it is necessary that sufficient time elapses between the inoculation of the first dose of antigen (**sensitizing dose**) and the second dose (**shocking dose**) to allow for the animal's tissues to produce specific antibodies before administration of the shocking dose. Second; although the sensitizing dose of antigen may be given by any route, so long as it is able to stimulate adequate antibody production, a general systemic reaction will only occur when the shocking dose of antigen is given intravenously. Third; the symptoms and lesions of anaphylactic shock vary according to the animal species concerned, but certain features are common to all species and include a sudden fall in blood pressure, contraction of smooth muscle and respiratory distress. Fourth; the immune reaction causing the shock is specific and will only take place when the same antigen has been inoculated on both occasions.

Consideration of these salient features of an anaphylactic shock indicate that they arise from an antigen–antibody reaction occurring throughout the body and that this reaction is closely associated with tissue cells. The early classical experiments of Schultze and Dale confirmed this when they showed that if the intestines or uterus were removed from a guinea-pig which had already received a sensitizing dose of antigen, and the organ was suspended in a bath of balanced salt solution, the smooth muscle of these tissues would contract when antigen (similar to that used for sensitization) was added to the fluid. This type of experiment is known as the Schultze–Dale reaction and clearly demonstrates the immunological specificity of the reaction and the involvement of tissue cells. The explanation of these results is that after inoculation of the sensitizing dose of antigen the animal produces specific antibodies some of which become attached to tissue cells (e.g. mast cells, macrophages). In the presence of a second dose of antigen (i.e. shocking dose) an antigen–antibody reaction occurs on cell surfaces and causes the release of some cellular constituents which are responsible for the reactions characteristic for anaphylactic shock. The exact nature of the releasing mechanism is unknown but probably occurs as the result of the action of an enzyme system in the cells. It is known, however, that one of these liberated substances is histamine and that it appears in the circulation within a few seconds of the antigen–antibody reaction having taken place. Moreover, symptoms closely resembling those of anaphylactic shock can be reproduced by inoculating histamine

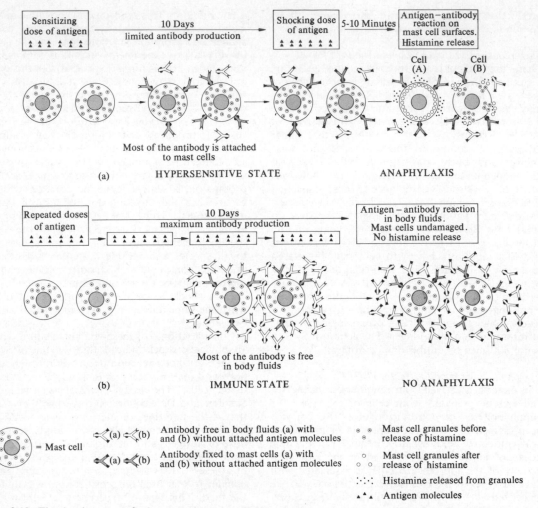

Sensitizing dose of antigen | 10 Days limited antibody production | Shocking dose of antigen | 5-10 Minutes | Antigen–antibody reaction on mast cell surfaces. Histamine release

Cell (A)   Cell (B)

Most of the antibody is attached to mast cells

(a)   HYPERSENSITIVE STATE   ANAPHYLAXIS

Repeated doses of antigen | 10 Days maximum antibody production | Antigen – antibody reaction in body fluids. Mast cells undamaged. No histamine release

Most of the antibody is free in body fluids

(b)   IMMUNE STATE   NO ANAPHYLAXIS

= Mast cell

(a) (b) Antibody free in body fluids (a) with and (b) without attached antigen molecules

(a) (b) Antibody fixed to mast cells (a) with and (b) without attached antigen molecules

Mast cell granules before release of histamine

Mast cell granules after release of histamine

Histamine released from granules

Antigen molecules

Fig. 3.13. The development of a hypersensitive state leading to anaphylaxis (a) and of an immune state (b).
Following the inoculation of a sensitizing dose of antigen the majority of antibody molecules become fixed to mast cells (a). After the intravenous inoculation of a second (shocking) dose of the same antigen 10 days later, the antigen molecules become attached to antibody already fixed to mast cells. The result is either the migration of granules to the periphery of the cell and the release of histamine through the cell membrane (cell a), or movement of granules through the ruptured mast cell membrane followed by release of histamine from these granules (cell b) causing anaphylaxis.
Following the inoculation of repeated doses of the same antigen (b), maximum antibody production occurs resulting in a high concentration of antibody molecules in tissue fluids which combine with all available antigen. Consequently, antibody molecules attached to mast cells are prevented from combining with antigen, the mast cells remain intact, histamine is not released and anaphylaxis does not develop.

into normal animals. It has also been noticed that eosinophils are associated with anaphylactic shock. The exact role of these cells is unknown but they are probably concerned with the host's response against the pharmacological action of histamine.

Other approaches to this problem confirm that tissue cells are actively concerned in anaphylactic reactions. For example, some gamma globulins, whether they are antibodies or not, can become absorbed on to tissue cells. By using this property it is possible to confirm experimentally by **reversed anaphylaxis** that the antigen–antibody reaction involves tissue cells. To demonstrate this a guinea-pig is inoculated with gamma globulin (antigen) which becomes absorbed on to tissue cells. Thereafter, if the animal is inoculated with an immune serum containing antibodies against the gamma globulin antigen, typical anaphylactic shock will develop.

Sensitization to an antigen may be transferred in serum from one animal to another. This can be shown as follows: the serum from a guinea-pig which has become sensitized after one injection of antigen is inoculated into a second normal guinea-pig. Subsequently, when this second animal is injected intravenously with an adequate dose of the same antigen a typical anaphylactic reaction develops. This is known as **passive anaphylaxis** because the shocked animal passively acquired the sensitizing antibody.

Many of these immediate types of hypersensitive reactions arise from artificial and experimental conditions, and they show that an individual who has become sensitized to a particular antigen may be in a critical state, since the introduction into the body of a shocking dose of that same antigen may precipitate a violent and sometimes fatal anaphylactic reaction. Similar situations can occur naturally, particularly in atopic individuals who are in a state of immediate hypersensitiveness (i.e. allergy) to various antigens (also termed **allergens**), including pollens, feathers, dust, etc., and in others who have developed a sensitivity to certain foodstuffs or drugs. The antibodies concerned in these hypersensitive reactions are known as **reagins** or **reaginic antibodies**. They have a particular affinity for tissues, especially skin and macrophages, and this characteristic property appears to be associated primarily with the IgE class of immunoglobulins. One method of treatment for atopic individuals is to de-sensitize them by giving a series of injections of the known allergen in small doses. This results in the production of **blocking antibodies** which are so-called because they combine with the allergen and prevent the development of a hypersensitive reaction by blocking the combination of allergen with reagin. These blocking antibodies belong to the IgG class of immunoglobulins and do not have the affinity for tissue cells characteristic of reagins. In many cases de-sensitization may have only a temporary effect, and in the course of some months the individual may again become hypersensitive to the particular antigen.

Local reaction (*Arthus*)

Immediate hypersensitive reactions may develop locally under suitable conditions. The classical demonstration of this type of response was made originally by Arthus who noticed that after repeatedly inoculating horse serum into rabbits, a further subcutaneous injection of serum produced a localised inflammatory response (Arthus reaction). This type of immune response has been studied in some detail and it is now established that an Arthus reaction develops only when antigen is inoculated into the skin of an animal that has already been immunized against that antigen and in which serum antibodies can be demonstrated by customary serological methods. Within a few minutes of inoculating the antigen a local reaction begins to develop. With the aid of fluorescent techniques it has been possible to observe antigen–antibody complexes which form in the linings of small blood vessels and in the tissues around the area of injection. Blood flow in these vessels is reduced or inhibited by accumulations of platelets and leucocytes. Oedema begins to develop and large numbers of polymorphs pass through the vessel walls into the tissues and ingest the antigen–antibody complexes. During the following 12–24 hours the lesion becomes infiltrated with lymphocytes and macrophages; polymorphs begin to degenerate and towards the end of this period eosinophils migrate to the site. In severe reactions a necrotic lesion of the skin may develop. This type of local response which can also occur in sites other than the skin is classified by Coombs and Gell as Type III allergic reaction.

Serum sickness is a Type III hypersensitive reaction which is a more generalised or systemic form of the Arthus reaction. Following the inoculation of a large therapeutic dose of hyperimmune serum, the recipient responds to the antigenic properties of the foreign proteins by developing antibodies which react with residual antigen remaining in the tissues, leading to the consequent formation of antigen–antibody complexes. These complexes can cause a variety of reactions including a raised body temperature, arteritis and glomerulonephritis.

The Shwartzman reaction is an artificially produced condition similar to the Arthus reaction but its aetiology is not properly understood. If a small dose of polysaccharide extract from a Gram-negative bacterium is inoculated into the skin of a rabbit, only a very slight and transitory inflammatory response develops. However, when a second dose of extract is given intravenously on the following day, the skin around the site of the first inoculation shows a rapid and severe inflammatory response. Some haemorrhages develop which coalesce. Microscopically, the lesion is similar to an Arthus reaction and shows a rapid accumulation of platelets and leucocytes followed by a deposition of polymorphs, destruction of the smaller blood vessels and sometimes necrosis. Although the lesion suggests a typical hypersensitive reaction there are certain features which are not wholly consistent with this type of immunological response. For example, the same bacterial polysaccharide does not have to be used for both injections and the reaction will develop after injection of extracts derived from a number of different Gram-negative bacteria. The fact that the reaction only develops when there is an interval of some 24 hours between the first and second injections is difficult to explain on present knowledge of immunological reactions because of the short time interval available for antibody production. It may be significant, however, that animals used in this type of experiment will have had a lifelong intestinal bacterial flora containing Gram-negative organisms, which will have provided favourable conditions for the development of an immune response to the O antigens and polysaccharides of these organisms before inoculation.

Delayed hypersensitive reactions or cellular immunity
Although it may be difficult in certain circumstances to draw a clear distinction between immediate and delayed hypersensitive reactions, the essential characters of the latter are that they take longer, sometimes 2 days or more to develop fully, that they can occur in the absence of circulating antibodies demonstrable by customary techniques, and that this delayed type of hypersensitivity can be passively transferred by cells but not by serum. Hence, this delayed-type hypersensitivity is also known as cellular or specific cell-mediated immunity. Delayed hypersensitive reactions occur in a variety of conditions, particularly some chronic bacterial and fungal diseases, in some skin lesions associated with chemical substances, and probably in association with some of the lesions related to autoimmune diseases. These conditions are classified by Coombs and Gell as Type IV allergic reactions. The tuberculin reaction is the best known example and although not typical of all delayed-type reactions, it will be described first as a basis for further discussion.

Reactions associated with the tubercle bacillus
The technique for the tuberculin test is based on the original observations of Robert Koch who compared the two distinct reactions which occurred in healthy and in tuberculous guinea-pigs. He noticed that if tubercle bacilli were inoculated into a healthy animal, no response occurred until 1–2 weeks later, when a nodule formed at the site of inoculation and developed into a persistent ulcer; local lymph glands became enlarged and these lesions persisted until the animal died. In contrast, the inoculation of tubercle bacilli into the skin of an infected guinea-pig gave rise to a response after a few days, when a necrotic lesion began to develop at the site of inoculation and thereafter, the underlying ulcer healed. Similar results can be elicited by inoculating either killed tubercle bacilli or tuberculin which is a purified protein derivative (PPD) extracted from the tubercle bacillus. When a small quantity of tuberculin is inoculated into the skin of a healthy guinea-pig no reaction develops, whereas a similar

dose inoculated into the skin of a tuberculous guinea-pig results in the slow development, during 2 days, of a cutaneous response. Initially, there is an accumulation of polymorphs but this and oedema are less marked than in the Arthus reaction. Within a few hours the polymorphs are superseded by a persistent concentration of macrophages and lymphocytes around the site of inoculation.

Reactions associated with other microorganisms
Delayed hypersensitive reactions in the skin similar to the tuberculin reaction, can be produced in animals infected with a variety of microorganisms, and in some instances advantage has been taken of this type of reaction to develop routine methods for diagnosing infection. For example, the johnin test is used for diagnosis of Johne's disease. The preparation of johnin from *Mycobacterium paratuberculosis* and the method of applying the test is similar to the tuberculin test. Glanders in horses, a bacterial disease caused by *Pseudomonas mallei*, can also be diagnosed by a skin test. A variety of other delayed-type skin reactions have been produced experimentally by inoculating appropriate microbial extracts into the skin of infected animals. Examples of these include bacterial extracts prepared from *Salmonella, Escherichia coli, Brucella abortus*, and fungal extracts derived from species of *Aspergillus, Coccidioides, Histoplasma* and *Trichophyton*.

Characteristics of delayed hypersensitive reactions
The experiments quoted above and others related to a variety of infections, suggest that a delayed-type hypersensitivity is an immunological response which commonly develops as a result of microbial infection and may be intimately concerned with the pathogenesis of infectious diseases. At present, we know little about the significance of this type of immune response but there are certain characteristic features of interest.

(1) A delayed hypersensitive state develops more intensely in chronic than acute infections.

(2) The presence of protein in microbial extracts appears to be advantageous for optimal development of skin reactions in chronically infected animals.

(3) This type of immune response cannot be passively transferred from one animal to another by serum antibodies but only by cells or extracts prepared from cells.

The fact that immunity can be transferred from one individual to another by cells or cellular extracts in the absence of serum antibodies is an important characteristic feature of a delayed hypersensitive reaction (i.e. cellular immunity) which distinguishes it from other types of immunological responses and is exemplified by the following type of experiment. When cells from the spleen or lymph nodes of a hypersensitive animal (donor) are injected into a normal animal (recipient) the latter will become hypersensitive to the particular antigen concerned. This transferred hypersensitivity will last only so long as the cells in the inoculum remain intact in the recipient, and the duration of their existence will be affected partly by the degree of genetic relationship between donor and recipient.

Transfer factor. The realisation that the condition of delayed hypersensitivity is one of cellular immunity has led to the development of a variety of experiments to investigate the nature of this type of immunological reaction and to identify the substance or substances responsible for the transfer of cellular immunity from one individual to another. In this respect, the following type of experiment is of particular interest. Human leucocytes derived from a patient who has developed delayed hypersensitivity to tuberculin are concentrated, washed and disrupted. An extract prepared from these cells (i.e. transfer factor) is then inoculated into the skin of a non-hypersensitive individual. When tuberculin is subsequently injected into the skin of the recipient on the following day a typical delayed hypersensitive reaction occurs. Similar experiments have shown that specific transfer factors are developed by individuals subjected to one or other of a variety of microbial antigens or to tissue antigens following organ transplantation.

Transfer factor can be liberated from leucocytes either mechanically (lysis or repeated freezing and thawing) or immunologically (antigen–antibody reactions). It has a molecular weight of < 10 000 and is dializable; it is neither an antigen nor an antibody but has biological properties indicating that it is a replicating informational molecule. The function of transfer factor may be to convey immunological information to a small number of lymphocytes (about 2–3 per cent), which consequently become antigen-responsive and undergo clonal proliferation, causing the host to develop a state of delayed hypersensitivity.

Immunological reactions related to abnormal tissues

Neoplasia

A great deal of interest has been focussed on the immunological aspects of neoplasia and recent studies during the last decade have been particularly significant in relation to virus-induced tumours in animals. The agents concerned include certain DNA viruses (e.g. polyoma, SV40, Shope papilloma and some adenoviruses) and the RNA leukoviruses (oncornaviruses). (See also Chapter 46)

Antigenic studies have shown that after a DNA virus has induced tumour formation the virus is no longer demonstrable as an infectious entity within the cells but can be detected immunologically in subsequent cell divisions of the tumour. Conversely, the continued presence of DNA infectious virus in tumour cells will result in the death of those cells. Tumour cells induced by RNA viruses, on the other hand, usually contain the complete infectious viral particles which continue to survive in subsequent cell divisions. In these cells it is often possible to detect specific viral envelope antigens on their surfaces as well as internal group specific (gs) structural viral antigens in the cellular cytoplasm. These observations emphasise the important feature that virus-induced tumours may possess specific antigens related to the viruses and foreign to the host, as well as 'self' antigens derived from the host's own tissues. In addition, virus-induced tumours develop new antigens, including transplantation antigens which occur on the surfaces of transformed cells and so-called T (tumour) antigens located within these cells as small, probably enzymatic particles associated with the nucleus. Both these antigens appear to be virus-coded because their production is controlled by the oncogenic viruses causing the tumours. In neoplasms caused by chemical carcinogens the specificities of antigens related to these abnormal tissues are dissimilar to those of virus-induced tumours, because the antigens are distinct in different animals although the carcinogen stimulating their development may be the same in all cases.

A variety of techniques have been used for the detection of tumour antigens and these usually involve reactions between specific antibodies to corresponding available antigens on the surfaces of cells. The tests have included complement-fixation and cell lysis observed by vital staining of test cells, fluorescent antibody techniques, observations on reduction in growth rates of tumour cells in tissue culture media containing specific antibodies, and a variety of other tests using sensitized lymphocytes to detect cellular immune responses. The use of these techniques has demonstrated the general principle that humoral immune responses as well as cell-mediated responses can be demonstrated against virus-induced tumour cells. Sometimes the results have been difficult to relate to the pathogenesis of tumour development for a variety of reasons, including the complexity of some of the tests, the fact that only the surface antigens of cells may be involved in some of the antigen–antibody reactions, and that these antigens are not strongly immunogenic and stimulate only weak humoral responses in the host. These studies have also shown that the total immune reaction against virus-induced tumours consists of both a delayed hypersensitive cell-mediated response as well as a humoral response, that the former is more effective at controlling the growth of the primary tumour, and that antibodies may prevent the spread of virus and subsequent development of secondary tumour formation. Recent observations suggest that under certain conditions the establishment of a myxovirus infection in a tumour may result in regression, possibly due to an increased immunogenicity of the tumour cells in relation to the presence of myxoviral antigens causing a stimulation of the host's immune response to the tumour.

The recognition that virus-induced tumours have specific antigens foreign to the host both on cell surfaces and within transformed cells, has led to the following observations on the immunological significance of these antigens in the development and possible control of these tumours.

(1) It is a feature of both DNA and RNA virus-induced tumours that their development is affected by the age of the host. In both animals and man the increased susceptibility of the young and the aged to the development of tumours corresponds with the times at which the immunological reactions of the host are least responsive; whereas mature animals which have highly responsive immune mechanisms are less susceptible than neonates to tumour formation following infection with oncogenic viruses. It is also known that in the newborn animal, the capacity to produce cell-mediated immune responses (delayed hypersensitive reactions) develops more slowly than the ability to produce humoral antibody responses.

(2) Resistance to some virus-induced tumours (e.g. polyoma) can be transferred passively from one animal to another by inoculation of sensitized lymphoid cells but not by immune serum.

(3) Various techniques are now available for suppressing immune responses in adults, including x-irradiation of the whole body, the use of antilymphocytic serum and thymectomy. When these methods of immune suppression are applied it has been shown that animals become significantly more susceptible to oncogenic virus infections. It is also known that in man there is an increased incidence of tumours among patients being treated with antilymphocytic serum.

(4) There is evidence to show that adult animals inoculated with oncogenic viruses develop a resistance to the subsequent inoculation of a related virus-induced transplantable tumour derived from a genetically similar donor.

(5) With certain oncogenic virus infections, including avian lymphomatosis and mouse leukaemia, the development of immune tolerance may have a significant effect on the susceptibility of the host. It has been noticed that when newborn animals become infected with virus they cannot be immunized during adult life by virus inoculation against a subsequent challenge with tumour cells. Whereas, animals which have not become infected neonatally can develop a resistance to challenge with tumour cells following inoculation of virus during adult life.

Although immune responses against virus-induced tumours are known to develop and include delayed hypersensitive reactions as well as humoral immunity, attempts to prevent and control tumour formation by immunological methods have been generally unsatisfactory. The experiments have usually been concerned with the development of humoral immunity and beneficial effects have only been demonstrated under defined conditions by actively immunizing animals against virus-induced tumours, employing oncogenic viral vaccines or passive immunization with antisera prepared against virus or tumour cells. The latter method, particularly, has shown the unexpected feature that tumour development may actually be increased in certain cases following the inoculation of antibodies specific for the tumour cells. This phenomenon is known as **immunological enhancement**, and one possible explanation is that the antibodies inhibit the development of a delayed hypersensitive reaction against the tumour, either by reducing the rate of production of sensitized lymphoid cells or by preventing them from coming into contact with the tumour.

Tissue transplantation

The advancement of surgical techniques enabling the satisfactory transplantation of organs (e.g. kidney, heart, lungs, liver) from donor to recipient have emphasised forcibly the immunological hazards culminating in grafted tissues subsequently being rejected by the recipient. These problems arise from the fact that tissue cells of the transplant are antigenic, that the antigens they possess are specific for the donor and foreign to the recipient, and that the degree to which they may be foreign depends upon the genetic relationship between donor and recipient.

It has long been recognised that skin can be grafted satisfactorily from one site to another on the same individual (**autograft**) because all the antigens of the graft correspond to those of the host. Similarly, grafts can be satisfactorily transferred between identical or monozygotic twins (**syngeneic homograft**) because of their antigenic identity; and success has also been achieved for the same reason when grafts are transferred between strains of mice which have been repeatedly inbred for several generations. The problems of graft rejection arise when a graft is transplanted from one individual to another of the same species but not genetically identical (**allogeneic homograft**) or from one species to an individual of another species (**xenograft**).

An important feature of transplant antigens is that they are also present on the blood leucocytes of the donor. Consequently, the antigenic structures of circulating cells, which can be readily obtained for laboratory tests, reflect the antigenic composition of the graft tissue. This has led to the development of laboratory serological tests which can be used to assess the degree of incompatibility between the potential donor of a graft and the recipient. Many antigens are involved, some are strong, others weak, and it has been shown that incompatibility of strong antigens is more likely to lead to early rejection of the graft by the recipient than incompatibility of weak antigens.

Antisera against transplant antigens can be obtained from individuals following transfusion of relatively large volumes of blood containing leucocytes, from the injection of lymphocytes or from recipients of skin grafts. The two methods which are most commonly used for detecting antibodies are the leucocyte agglutination and leucocyte cytotoxicity tests. The antigen for the agglutination test is prepared from blood which has been defibrinated either mechanically or by the addition of ethylene-diaminetetraacetate (EDTA) anticoagulant. The leucocytes are collected, washed and resuspended at the desired concentration. The antigen for the cytotoxic test consists of lymphocytes concentrated from a blood sample which are added to the serum under test followed by complement. If there is combination of antibody with lymphocytes in the presence of complement, the cell membranes are damaged and this is observed by the uptake of dyes (eosin, trypan blue) which penetrate the cell membranes damaged by the antigen–antibody reaction. An alternative procedure is to add fluorescein diacetate which causes undamaged cells to fluoresce but not damaged ones, because the dye can pass out of the latter through the damaged cell membranes. Thus, using dark ground illumination, dead cells (i.e. those which have combined with antibody and complement) appear dark while live undamaged cells fluoresce.

Graft rejection is a complex immunological and inflammatory process. Histologically, it has been shown that the immune response of the host is mainly cell-mediated, characterised by a marked infiltration of lymphocytes and by the fact that these cells can transfer the property of graft rejection from one host to another. Serum antibodies are also produced but under experimental conditions it has not been possible to show that they can transfer the property of graft rejection from one host to another. Nevertheless, there is evidence that antibodies are closely associated with the immunological rejection of grafts because they are cytotoxic for graft cells and are probably in high concentration in the immediate vicinity of the lymphocytes involved in the rejection process.

The overriding problem associated with successful transplantation operations is one of preventing the immunological reactions of the recipient from rejecting the graft, and at the present time no permanently satisfactory method has been developed. However, it is important to match as nearly as possible by serological techniques, the antigens of the donor with those of the recipient before undertaking a transplant operation, because the closer the antigenic relationship between the two the less likelihood there will be of a relatively rapid and severe rejection process developing after transplantation. Secondly, various methods have been used for suppressing the immune responses of the recipient. These have included whole-body x-irradiation, the use of immuno suppressive drugs, the administration of antilymphocytic serum (ALS) or of combined immunosuppressive drugs with ALS. All these methods are drastic because the recipient is unable to respond immunologically to subsequent microbial infections, and the risk of infectious diseases has become a more common cause of death than graft rejection and consequent malfunction of the transplanted organs. Possible future developments to overcome these serious problems might be the isolation of the tissue antigens concerned, followed by their inoculation into the recipient to produce a condition of immunological tolerance before transplantation is carried out. Alternatively, the condition of **immunological enhancement** might be developed in the recipient before transplantation occurs. This would involve the inoculation of tissue cells from the donor into the recipient and stimulating the production of antibodies which may subsequently protect the graft from immunological rejection.

Further reading
AITKEN, M.M., SANFORD, J. AND ZARKOWER, A. (1974) An investigation of the association between circulating antibody levels and systemic anaphylactic sensitivity in cattle. *Research in Veterinary Science*, **16**, 199.

BECKER E.L. (1971) Nature and classification of immediate-type allergic reactions. *Advances in Immunology*, **13**, 267.

BELL, R.B. (1974) Histology of the local cellular response of ducks to injections of antigenic material. *Journal of the Reticuloendothelial Society*, **15**, 213.

BIENENSTOCK, J., GAULDIE, J. AND PEREY, D.Y.E. (1973) Synthesis of IgG, IgA, IgM by chicken tissues: immunofluorescent and ^{14}C amino acid incorporation studies. *Journal of Immunology*, **111**, 1112.

BLOOM B.R. (1971) *In vitro* approaches to the mechanism of cell-mediated immune reactions. *Advances in Immunology*, **13**, 101.

BOURNE F.J., CURTIS, J., JOHNSON, R.H. AND COLLINGS, D.F. (1974) Antibody formation in porcine fetuses. *Research in Veterinary Science*, 16, 223.

BURNET SIR MACFARLANE (1969) *Cellular Immunity*, p. 726. Melbourne: Cambridge University Press.

CARR, I. (1973) The macrophage. A review of ultrastructure and function. New York and London: Academic Press.

CEBRA J.J. (1969) Immunoglobulins and immunocytes. *Bacteriological Reviews*, 33, 159.

COCHRANE, C.G. AND KOFFLER, D. (1973) Immune complex disease in experimental animals and man. *Advances in Immunology*, 16, 185.

COHEN S. AND MILSTEIN C. (1967) Structure and biological properties of immunoglobulins. *Advances in Immunology*, 7, 1.

COWAN K.M. (1973) Antibody response to viral antigens. *Advances in Immunology*, 17, 195.

CRUICKSHANK R. AND WEIR D.M., Eds. (1967) *Modern Trends in Immunology* 2, p. 342. Butterworth: London.

DRESSER, D.W. AND MITCHISON, N.A. (1968) The mechanism of immunological paralysis. *Advances in Immunology*, 8, 129.

GLYNN L.E. AND HOLBOROW E.J. (1965) *Autoimmunity and Disease*. Oxford: Blackwell Scientific Publications.

GRAPPEL, S.F., BISHOP, C.T. AND BLANK, F. (1974) Immunology of Dermatophytes and Dermatophytosis *Bacteriological Reviews*, 38, 222.

HELLSTROM, K.E. AND HELLSTROM, I. (1974) Lymphocyte-mediated cytotoxicity and blocking serum activity to tumor antigens. *Advances in Immunology*, 18, 209.

HERBERT W.J. (1970) *Veterinary Immunology*. Oxford: Blackwell Scientific Publications.

HOLBOROW E.J. (1968) *An ABC of Modern Immunology*. London: The Lancet, Ltd.

HUDSON, R.J., SABEN, H.S. AND EMSLIE, D. (1974) Physiological and environmental influences on immunity. *Veterinary Bulletin*, 44, 119.

HUMPHREY J.H. AND WHITE R.G. (1970) *Immunology for Students of Medicine*, 3rd Edition. Oxford: Blackwell Scientific Publications.

JEFFCOTT L.B. (1972) Passive immunity and its transfer with special reference to the horse. *Biological Reviews*, 47, 439.

KIRSTEN W.H. (1966) Malignant transformation by viruses. In *Recent Results in Cancer Research*. Berlin: Springer-Verlag.

LACHMANN P.J. (1967) Conglutinin and immunoconglutinin. *Advances in Immunology*, 6, 479.

LANCE E.M., MEDAWAR P.B. AND TAUB R.N. (1973) Antilymphocyte serum. *Advances in Immunology*, 17, 1.

LINDENMANN J. AND KLEIN P.A. (1967) Immunological aspects of viral oncolysis. In *Recent Results in Cancer Research*. Berlin: Springer-Verlag.

MULLER-EBERHARD, H.J. (1968) Chemistry, and reaction mechanisms of complement. *Advances in Immunology*, 8, 1.

MURRAY, M. (1973) Local immunity and its role in vaccination. *Veterinary Record*, 93, 500.

ROGERS BRAMBELL, F.W. (1970) *The transmission of passive immunity from mother to young*. Amsterdam: North Holland.

ROITT I.M. (1974) *Essential Immunology*, 2nd Edition. Oxford: Blackwell Scientific Publications.

SAMTER M. AND ALEXANDER H.L. (1965) *Immunological Diseases*. London: Churchill.

SCHULTZ, R.D. (1973) Developmental aspects of the fetal bovine immune response: a review. *Cornell Veterinarian*, 63, 507.

SCHULTZ, R.D., SCOTT, F.W., DUNCAN, J.R. AND GILLESPIE, J.H. (1974) Feline immunoglobulins. *Infection and Immunity*, 9, 391.

SKARNES R.C. AND WATSON D.W. (1957) Antimicrobial factors of normal tissues and fluids. *Bacteriological Reviews*, 21, 273.

SULITZEANU D. (1968) Affinity of antigen for white cells and its relation to the induction of antibody formation. *Bacteriological Reviews*, 32, 404.

SVENDSEN, J. AND BROWN, P. (1973) IgA immunoglobulin levels in porcine sera and mammary secretions. *Research in Veterinary Science*, 15, 65.

Symposium on Nonspecific Resistance to Infection (1960). *Bacteriological Reviews*, 24, 2.

TIZARD I.R. (1971) Macrophage-cytophilic antibodies and the functions of macrophage-bound immunoglobulins. *Bacteriological Reviews*, 35, 365.

TURK J.L. (1967) Cytology of the induction of hypersensitivity. *British Medical Bulletin*, 23, 3.

TURK J.L. (1972) *Immunology in Clinical Medicine*, 2nd Edition. London: Heinemann Medical.

UHR J.W. (1966) Delayed hypersensitivity. *Physiological Reviews*, 46, 359.

WATANABE, H. AND ISAYAMA, Y. (1973) Chicken immunoglobulins in serum and ascitic fluid. *Japanese Journal of Veterinary Research*, 21, 33.

WEIR D.M. (1973) *Immunology for Undergraduates*, 3rd Edition. Edinburgh: Churchill Livingstone.

WHEELOCK, E.F. AND TOY, S.T. (1973) Participation of lymphocytes in viral infections. *Advances in Immunology*, 16, 123.

CHAPTER 4

THE PATHOGENESIS OF
INFECTIOUS DISEASES

CHAPTER 4

The pathogenesis of infectious diseases

Throughout life man and animals are constantly subjected to the metabolic processes of microorganisms. Some of these organisms do not cause disease because they are unable to adapt themselves to living within the body tissues. Other species have modified their life cycles so that they are able to live on food available in the intestinal tract without interfering with the well-being of the host. This harmless relationship is known as **commensalism**. In other instances, organisms living in the intestinal tract metabolise some of the foodstuffs and break them down into substances more readily digestible by the host. This specialised and beneficial relationship is known as **symbiosis**. The final group of organisms with which we are particularly concerned are those which the host attempts to reject because they have acquired the ability to interfere with the normal metabolic processes of the body. This challenging relationship is known as **parasitism**. Because of their parasitic existence these organisms are the cause of pathological changes in the tissues of the host which responds in an attempt to rid itself of these **pathogenic** organisms.

Increasing knowledge and application of epidemiological, immunological and chemotherapeutic principles to the control of infectious diseases in man and animals, have helped to reduce but not to prevent the risks of world-wide epidemics. In addition to world plagues, man and animals are constantly subjected to infectious diseases spreading within a limited community and it is in the experience of all of us to have suffered and recovered from an infectious disease. One notable feature arising from this experience is that after recovery and return to normal health, the individual may have developed an increased resistance or immunity to that particular infection which may last for a few months or for a lifetime. By overcoming the clinical effects of an infectious disease the body does not only rid itself of the pathogenic organisms or at least succeed in reducing their numbers below the danger level, but it also builds up a specific immunity against them, thus

enabling it to withstand reinfection more effectively in the future. In this context, freedom from disease depends upon a fine balance between the ability of pathogenic organisms to penetrate the defences of the body and create a parasitic existence within the host to complete their life cycles, and the success of the host in preventing or at least curtailing the existence of pathogenic organisms within the body. In these circumstances a condition known as **premunity** often develops in which the organisms continue to exist in the tissues in small numbers which are insufficient to produce clinical disease but are capable of constantly stimulating antibody production, thus providing the host with long-term protection against reinfection.

In this chapter we shall discuss the salient features concerned with first, the routes by which animals become infected with pathogenic organisms; second, the general and special ways by which the body defends itself against infection; and third, the properties which pathogenic microorganisms have developed to enable them to overcome the body defences, organise themselves in the tissues, and give rise to consequent development of lesions which are the sites where host and parasite come into direct contact one with another.

The spread of infection among animals
The development of intensive methods for rearing domesticated animals for human food production means that the veterinarian is concerned on an increasing scale with the prevention and control of disease on a herd or flock basis and to a less extent with the individual animal. Intensive methods of animal production markedly affect the ecology of pathogenic organisms, particularly in relation to their natural habitats, mode of life and environment. Host–parasite relationships are not stable but always being modified by changing conditions of environment; and the introduction of intensive methods of animal production involving the crowding together of animals into groups, tends to increase the rate of

transfer of pathogenic organisms from one host to another and hence to increase the incidence of parasitism.

The maintenance of life-cycles of pathogenic microorganisms depends upon their ability to pass from one host to another, to penetrate the defences of susceptible hosts and to colonize in their tissues. Many of these organisms have developed highly specialised life-cycles which affect their routes of transfer from one host to another. The frequency with which this occurs is affected by the environment of the host species as well as the particular properties of the organisms. The following is a brief survey outlining the various routes by which some pathogenic microorganisms commonly pass from one host to another.

Ingestion

This is one of the commonest routes for the transfer of infection from one host to another. Outstanding examples are the *Salmonella, Arizona, Proteus, Shigella* and *Escherichia* groups, all of which have adapted themselves to live in the intestines. Consequently, they are organisms which are excreted in the faeces and thus contaminate the environment, including food, water, pastures and litter. In this way they are likely to be ingested by other susceptible hosts because they are able to remain viable for many weeks or months in humid atmospheres, and in addition, are able to colonise initially in the intestinal tract after ingestion. Close contact between susceptible animals kept intensively are ideal conditions for the rapid dissemination of these organisms from one individual to another. This is exemplified in salmonellosis of sheep where the spread of the disease occurs especially when these animals are brought together in confined spaces for lambing or transport. Cross-infection rarely occurs among sheep well dispersed on grazing lands except when a common source of infection, for example a water supply, becomes contaminated.

Bacillus anthracis the cause of anthrax, is another pathogenic species which can be disseminated by ingestion but in this case the life cycle shows an additional modification. These organisms are able to sporulate in the atmosphere and the spore coat is highly protective to the organism which is able to remain viable for many years in the soil under a variety of climatic conditions. After ingestion by susceptible animals the spores develop into vegetative forms and colonise initially in the walls of the intestines. The likelihood of colonisation taking place is probably increased by abrasions to the intestinal wall from sharp pieces of material passing through the intestines.

Several pathogenic species of *Clostridia* are spread from one animal to another by ingestion. For example, *Clostridium welchii* are normal inhabitants of sheeps' intestines and under favourable conditions become disseminated among groups of animals multiplying rapidly in the intestines and causing lamb dysentery and other enterotoxaemic infections. Similarly, *Clostridium septicum*, an inhabitant of the intestines, causes braxy in sheep as a result of rapid multiplication in the abomasum, and is also responsible for some cases of blackquarter in cattle and sheep in which the route of infection is considered more likely to be from ingestion than via surface wounds of the skin. *Clostridium chauvoei* a common cause of blackquarter, is another inhabitant of the intestines and ingestion is probably a more common route of infection than skin wounds. Although strains of *Clostridium oedematiens* causing Black disease, bacillary haemoglobinurea and localised gas gangrene lesions, usually develop primarily as a result of contamination of skin wounds, the organisms are frequently inhabitants of the intestines in certain districts, and may be spread by ingestion and cause intestinal infections. *Clostridium botulinum* is another toxigenic member of the clostridial group which is ingested by animals and is an inhabitant of the intestines of herbivores in certain areas. As a consequence, no disease is produced in the living animal but after death the environment of the putrefying carcase is suitable for toxin production by the organisms, and subsequent ingestion of the carcase meat containing preformed toxin by other animals may lead to a fatal toxaemia (e.g. Lamsiekte).

Leptospira comprise another group of bacteria which is commonly transmitted from one host to another by ingestion. These organisms have a predilection for the kidneys resulting in the excretion of infected urine, and susceptible animals usually contract leptospirosis from the ingestion of material contaminated with infected urine. *Leptospira* may also be spread by the ingestion of leptospires derived from infected fetuses, placentae and milk.

Other species of pathogenic bacteria which may be transmitted by ingestion and excreted in the faeces are *Erysipelothrix insidiosa* particularly in pigs, *Listeria monocytogenes* among a wide variety of animal hosts, *Yersinia pseudotuberculosis* infections among rodents, *Brucella* which may also be transmitted by other routes, ovine infections with *Campylobacter fetus* (*intestinalis*) and *Actinomyces bovis*, and equine infections with *Pseudomonas mallei* the cause of glanders which may also be transmitted by other routes.

The alimentary route of infection is not as commonly used by viruses as it is by bacteria, but there are many occasions when viruses are introduced by means of contaminated foodstuffs and fomites. Most animal viruses are readily inactivated by bile, acid and digestive enzymes in the alimentary tract but a few, such as enteroviruses, reoviruses and adeno-viruses are resistant and are capable of establishing enteric infections. The majority of enterovirus infections are symptomless but a small proportion give rise to febrile illness associated with viraemia and, in a few cases (e.g. poliomyelitis of man and Teschen disease of pigs), the virus spreads to the central nervous system and causes meningitis and paralysis.

Inhalation

This is a particularly common route of infection among animals kept under intensive methods of husbandry which facilitates the inhalation of air-borne droplet infection leading primarily to respiratory diseases. Examples include *Haemophilus, Klebsiella* and some species of *Pasteurella*. After inhalation of these bacteria they may remain viable in various sites of the respiratory tract or in local lymph glands. The subsequent development of clinical infection is often secondary to respiratory virus diseases which are also commonly disseminated by the same route of infection. The bacterial species involved are not particularly resistant to environments outside the animal body and cross-infection occurs most readily among calves, pigs and poultry under intensive methods of management. Similarly, *Pseudomonas mallei* the cause of glanders, may be spread by inhalation when susceptible animals are in close contact one with another; thus providing conditions for the rapid transfer of droplets containing viable organisms which rapidly lose their infectivity due to dessication when exposed to the atmosphere. There is also evidence to suggest that *Brucella abortus* infection in cattle may occasionally be transmitted by inhalation.

Virus commonly causing or associated with upper respiratory tract infections of animals include orthomyxoviruses (e.g. equine and avian influenza), paramyxoviruses (e.g. Newcastle disease in birds and parainfluenza 3 of 'transit fever' of cattle), reoviruses, coronaviruses and rhinoviruses. Moreover, in a number of severe generalized virus infections including rinderpest and sheep pox, the virus may also enter the host through the respiratory tract.

Coitus

Some bacterial infections are venereal and transmitted from male to female during coitus. A typical example is *Treponema cuniculi* the cause of rabbit syphilis. Other infections are *Campylobacter fetus (venerealis)* and *Brucella abortus* in cattle, and *Brucella suis* in pigs. These brucella infections may also be transmitted by ingestion and other routes. All these bacterial species and also *Corynebacterium renale* have adapted themselves to living in the urogenital tract; they are comparatively non-resistant to climatic conditions outside the host's body but may contaminate the local environment of diseased animals and in this way may indirectly infect healthy animals which come into contact with freshly contaminated bedding. The urogenital tract may be the site of primary lesions in a number of disease conditions in man and animals such as lymphogranuloma venereum (PLGV) and genital herpes in humans, and contagious pustular vulvovaginitis in cattle. There is also evidence that parainfluenza 3 virus, Bittner's mouse mammary tumour virus and the Marburg rhabdovirus may be present in the semen of the male and may be transmitted during coitus.

Infection of the fetus in utero

Vertical transmission of infection from mother to fetus *in utero* may occur during the course of a viraemic illness in the dam. In human medicine, the rubella virus of German measles is a notable example, while in veterinary medicine vertical transmission has been reported in swine fever, avian leukosis, lymphocytic choriomeningitis infection of mice, equine infectious anaemia, equine rhinopneumonitis, bluetongue of sheep and malignant catarrhal fever in wildebeest. Similarly, infection of the bovine fetus *in utero* can occur during bacterial and fungal illnesses, including *Br. abortus* and mycotic abortion associated with *Aspergillus fumigatus* and *Absidia ramosa*.

Skin wounds

These form common sites of entry for a wide variety of pathogenic organisms into the body. Examples are pyogenic bacteria including *Staphylococcus, Streptococcus, Corynebacterium* and *Sphaerophorus*. A number of toxigenic clostridial species may also produce infection of the host via skin wounds, including *Clostridium tetani* the cause of tetanus, *Clostridium oedematiens* and *Clostridium welchii* type A which produce lesions of gas gangrene following dermal inoculation, and *Clostridium septicum* associated with the development of malignant oedema. It has also been suggested that among cattle, skin wounds may be a less common site of entry into the tissues than the alimentary tract for *Clostridium chauvoei* which causes blackquarter. Although clear indications of skin wounds associated with this bovine disease are seldom observed, this route of infection is known to be common for *Clostridium chauvoei* infections in sheep, particularly in relation to contamination of wounds associated with lambing, docking, castration and shearing.

Other bacterial pathogens which may also gain entry into the tissues through damaged skin are *Actinobacillus ligniéresi, Actinomyces bovis* via skin wounds on the udders of pigs or in association with *Brucella abortus* in the aetiology of fistulous withers or poll-evil in horses, *Nocardia farcinica* the cause of farcy in cattle, and *Bacillus anthracis*. Although leptospiral infections are commonly transmitted from animal to animal by ingestion of material contaminated with infected urine, there are circumstances under which the organisms may gain entry into the body via the skin. This latter route of infection may occur via wounds among various species of animals or through the intact skin of pigs, particularly when the integument has become softened by repeated contact with water and mud.

Species of fungi (e.g. Dermatophytes) may also gain entry through the skin.

Small superficial abrasions of the skin may allow viruses to enter and infect susceptible cells in the epidermis or dermis. Papilloma, contagious pustular dermatitis (orf) and fowl pox viruses can penetrate in this way and give rise to localised lesions without systemic spread of infection. Notable examples of viruses which may gain entry through skin wounds and progress to severe systemic infections include rabies and herpes-B virus of monkeys which are usually transmitted by the bite of an infected animal.

Insect bites

A variety of pathogenic microorganisms are transmitted from one host to another through the intermediary of biting insects. The frequency with which this occurs depends upon a variety of factors including climatic conditions, the natural habitats and hosts for the insects as well as the incidence and life history of the pathogenic microorganisms. Some species of pathogenic bacteria which may be transmitted by this method are *Borrelia anserina* the cause of spirochaetosis in poultry, which is transmitted by the fowl tick (*Argas persicus*), the pigeon tick (*Argas reflexus*) and more rarely by the red mite (*Dermanyssus gallinarum*) or by mosquitoes (e.g. *Culex pipiens*). Bubonic plague in man is caused by *Yersinia pestis* and the disease is spread by the bite of the rat flea (*Xenopsilla cheopsis*) which becomes infected from rats in which the disease occurs as an epizootic. *Francisella tularensis*, the cause of tuleraemia in wild rodents in many countries, is disseminated by infected ticks, and the aetiology of tick pyaemia (lamb pyaemia) is also related to tick bites. When the sheep tick (*Ixodes ricinus*) bites the skin of lambs during the spring and early summer, *Staphylococcus pyogenes* already on the surface of the skin, becomes mechanically inoculated and causes the pyogenic infections characteristic for the disease.

It should also be remembered when considering the epidemiology of infectious diseases, that flies can mechanically transfer pathogenic organisms from contaminated areas to the surfaces of skin and mucous membranes. Some examples of this form of dissemination are streptococcal species causing bovine mastitis, *Bacillus anthracis* particularly in tropical countries, and *Moraxella bovis* the cause of infectious bovine keratoconjunctivitis.

Rickettsial infections (e.g. heartwater disease in cattle, sheep and goats, and tick-borne fever in sheep) and many virus diseases are transmitted from one host to another by insect bites. Inoculation may be by mechanical means (e.g. mouth parts of rabbit fleas contaminated with myxoma virus) or by arthropod vectors in which the virus undergoes a cycle of development in the arthropod which may remain infected for the rest of its life. Arthropod-borne virus diseases include African horse sickness and bluetongue of sheep (orbiviruses) as well as equine encephalomyelitis, Rift Valley fever, louping-ill of sheep, and numerous other togavirus infections.

General defence mechanisms of the body

Pathogenic organisms must penetrate the skin or enter the host by one of the natural orifices to complete their life cycles. The general defence mechanisms of the body constitute important barriers which help to protect the individual against these infections, and the following section summarizes the methods of defence associated with different parts of the body.

Skin

Hair, fur and feathers help to protect animal skins from traumatic damage. The intact skin, itself, is an efficient covering to the body and capable of disposing of large numbers of pathogens which come into direct contact with it. Although the mechanism by which this cleansing process functions is not clearly understood, experiments have shown the efficiency with which it operates. For example, under experimental conditions Gram-negative organisms including *Escherichia* and *Salmonella*, cannot survive for longer than 10–15 minutes on the surface of human skin. Gram-positive organisms, particularly *Streptococcus* and *Staphylococcus*, are similarly disposed of by the bactericidal activity of the skin although they may persist for longer than Gram-negative organisms. In addition to these potentially pathogenic bacteria which normally lead a temporary existence on the skin, there are other microbial species always present in this situation and they constitute the normal flora of the skin. These latter organisms are non-pathogenic and may include some aerobic spore-bearing bacilli, diphtheroid bacilli, sarcinae and some non-haemolytic streptococci. A question of special interest concerning the pathogenesis of infection is the nature of the mechanism which rids the skin of potential pathogens and still allows relatively harmless organisms to survive. This cleansing mechanism probably consists of a variety of processes which together produce the recognised effects. These include continual desquamation of epithelium which occurs from the surface of the skin and, to some extent, will assist in the removal of all types of microorganisms. More particularly, the acidity of the skin and the secretion of some fatty acids constitute a formidable barrier which pathogenic organisms must overcome before establishing themselves on the integument. The acidity of the skin may be as low as pH 4 or 3 due to lactic acid produced by sweat glands, and this bactericidal activity is enhanced by saturated and unsaturated fatty acids produced by sebaceous glands. It has also been suggested that bactericidal substances derived from the normal flora may also contribute to the bactericidal activity of the skin. Circumstances which alter these conditions will increase the risk of infective organisms penetrating beneath the outer surface of the skin and establishing themselves in the tissues. The most obvious of these conditions is trauma which involves damage to the continuity of the integument, consisting of cuts, abrasions and insect bites resulting in the inoculation of organisms already on the surface of the skin, or of other microbes which are carried and inoculated by biting insects. Another condition of some importance is the continual wetting of the skin's surface. This reduces the concentration of secretions and consistency of the epidermis to such an extent that some organisms (e.g. *Leptospira*) can penetrate the skin and infect the tissues.

Conjunctiva

The mucous membranes surrounding the eyes are constantly subjected to air-borne infections and without an efficient cleansing mechanism the conjunctiva could become a site of repeated infection. The important defence mechanism of this area of the body is the constant secretion of lachrymal fluid flowing from the upper eyelid to the inner canthus and then to the nasal cavity. A steady flow of this fluid which is ensured by repeated blinking, provides an efficient mechanical washing of the surface area. In addition, lachrymal fluid contains lysozyme which is able to lyse certain bacterial species.

Respiratory tract

Nasopharynx. The surface of the nasopharynx is subjected to contact with microorganisms inhaled from the atmosphere. The tortuous construction of the nasal cavity together with large quantities of mucus provide an efficient method of protection against the establishment of local infection. In addition to the mechanical washing of the mucous membranes the mucus, itself, probably contains some substance other than lysozyme which is capable of reducing the rate of multiplication of bacteria which become lodged in the area. There is also evidence to suggest that in man, at least, the mucus has an anti-viral action since it has been shown that it can neutralize influenza virus. In spite of this cleansing process a variety of bacteria, fungi and viruses are able to adapt themselves to this kind of environment and they constitute the normal microbial flora of the nasopharynx.

Trachea and bronchi. These structures are mainly protected by the mixture of ciliated epithelial and mucus secreting cells which line these organs. The surfaces are constantly washed by mucus which is moved by the cilia up the trachea and away from the lungs. Mucus which has reached the upper end of the trachea is removed from the respiratory tract by the coughing reflex.

Bronchioles and lungs. Under natural conditions some microorganisms may succeed in overcoming the cleansing mechanisms of the trachea and bronchi, pass through the bronchioles and be finally destroyed in the lungs. Experimentally, it has been shown that insufflated bacteria which reach the lungs are rapidly destroyed by histiocytes and lymphoid tissue.

Digestive tract

Mouth. The lining of the mouth is composed of a relatively thick and impenetrable layer of stratified squamous epithelium and connective tissue. The whole surface is constantly washed with saliva which flows backwards towards the larynx. In addition to this mechanical washing of the area, saliva has bacteriostatic and bactericidal properties against a variety of microorganisms. Nevertheless, some bacterial and fungal species have adapted themselves to the microenvironment of the mouth and constitute the normal mixed flora which is always present.

Stomach. The important defence mechanisms of the stomach consist of the vomiting reflex which enables the stomach to expel irritant substances, and also the acid pH of the contents due to the presence of hydrochloric acid. This latter mechanism varies greatly in its efficiency since the concentration of hydrochloric acid in the contents differs from one individual to another and at different times within the same individual. If microorganisms pass rapidly through the stomach the pH of the contents may be insufficiently acid to be lethal before the organisms have passed further down the alimentary canal. For example, *Escherichia coli* is relatively resistant to the acid pH of the stomach over a period of about 15 minutes, and salmonellae, streptococci and staphylococci may also survive rapid passage through the stomach.

Intestine. The two natural defence mechanisms of the small and large intestines are peristalsis and the normal bacterial flora. One of the effects of irritant and toxic substances is to increase peristaltic movements and speed up the expulsion of toxins and bacteria from the intestinal tract. For their normal functioning the intestines depend upon a resident bacterial flora which has adapted itself to this site. Potential pathogens commonly found in the intestines of healthy animals include *Escherichia, Proteus, Clostridium, Listeria, Streptococcus*, in addition to various species of viruses and fungi. The establishment of disease-producing organisms in this environment may be inhibited by other microbial species constituting the normal flora of the intestines. Constant microbial competition and antagonism has to be overcome by pathogenic organisms before they can establish themselves and produce clinical disease. Under certain conditions, however, some bacterial species normally present in the intestines (e.g. *Escherichia coli, Clostridium welchii*) may multiply rapidly and be associated with the development of gastro-enteric and enterotoxaemic infections.

Urogenital tract

Male. The male cleansing mechanism is provided by urine. The repeated expulsion of urine from the bladder helps to prevent the establishment of infection in the ureters and urethra, and any contaminating organisms in the external meatus are washed out. From time to time heavy contamination of the genital tract with organisms capable of surviving in this environment can take place and an ascending infection may develop (e.g. *Corynebacterium renale*).

Female. As in the male, the repeated expulsion of urine mechanically cleanses the urogenital tract of the female. In addition, the cervical plug in a pregnant animal also assists in preventing the establishment of pathogenic organisms.

Special defence mechanisms of the body

Lymphoreticular system
The foregoing discussion on natural defences of the body emphasises the importance of the intact skin and mucous membranes with their ancillary cleansing mechanisms as the initial defence barriers against infection. Mechanical injuries to the surface of the body which allow direct access of pathogenic organisms to underlying tissues require an immediate cellular response by the host if these organisms are to be contained and disposed of before they have had time to multiply extensively and produce their pathogenic effects. Such injuries to the continuity of the outer defences of the body can occur anywhere on the skin or in the digestive, respiratory or urogenital tracts. To protect the body against infection at any of these sites requires a cellular defence mechanism which can be mobilised quickly in any part of the body, and which must be composed of cells adapted to collecting and removing infective organisms. Such a specialised cellular mechanism is distributed throughout the tissues of the body and is collectively known as the lymphoreticular system.

The lymphoreticular system consists of phagocytic cells, some of them free and wandering, others fixed to tissues in various organs of the body. Collectively, they form a system of cells particularly adapted to the ingestion and disposal of foreign and effete material, including aged and dead erythrocytes, microorganisms, proteins, drugs, dyes, etc. The early classical studies of Metchnikoff revealed the extent and composition of this phagocytic system and subsequent studies have demonstrated the importance of these cells as a defence mechanism against microbial infection. The system is composed of mobile and sessile cells. The former include the actively mobile **microphages** (i.e. polymorphs or neutrophils) and the less actively mobile **macrophages** (i.e. monocytes or large mononuclear cells). Both these cell types are capable of actively phagocytosing foreign particles and the macrophages have a further characteristic property of fusing together to form giant cells. These multinucleated cellular masses are capable of phagocytosing larger particles, particularly some fungi. Other cells which may congregate in areas of infection are eosinophils. These are sluggishly amoeboid and accumulate in areas where antigen–antibody reactions are occurring. Their exact function is still unknown but they are particularly evident in the tissues surrounding some types of allergic reactions and parasitic diseases. Recent experiments have shown that they can be actively phagocytic and ingest foreign red cells in the presence of antibody.

Histiocytes comprise the fixed cells of the lymphoreticular system and are distributed as a framework in various organs of the body, particularly the Kupffer cells of the liver, cells lining the sinuses of the spleen and lymph nodes, the capillaries of the medullary sinusoids of the adrenals, the venous sinusoids of bone marrow and the capillaries of the pituitary. Histiocytes also occur in large numbers in the omentum ('milk spots') and in the alveolar wall of the lungs.

Thus, the lymphoreticular system comprises a formidable group of cells circulating in the blood stream and distributed in various organs of the body. Their ability to remove foreign particles from the blood stream can be assessed by inoculating carbon particles (India ink) intravenously and observing the rate at which they are ingested by phagocytes and removed from the blood after injection. Provided that the dose of carbon is not too great, the majority of particles (over 90 per cent) will be removed by the liver and spleen. With larger doses a good deal of the material will become collected in the lungs.

The destruction and removal of microorganisms from the body by phagocytosis can take place in the absence of serum antibodies specific for the particular organisms causing infection. However, the presence of antibodies greatly enhances this process and it is well known that the tissues of immune animals can respond to infection by showing an increased ability to remove and destroy pathogenic organisms. Thus, the developing reaction of the lymphoreticular system to microbial infection consists initially of cellular responses involving a limited degree of phagocytosis followed by the production of antibodies which enhance the intensity of both phagocytosis and lysis of the infecting organisms. The process of antibody production and involvement in host reactions to infection are discussed in Chapter 3.

The development of microbial infections

From earlier chapters the reader will appreciate that although man and animals exist in an atmosphere laden with microorganisms, only a small proportion of bacteria, fungi and viruses are adapted to life in or on the surface of the body. Some of these latter organisms have modified their way of life to such an extent that under suitable conditions they cause pathological changes in the body resulting in the development of disease. In this section we shall discuss the important characteristic properties of these disease-producing organisms which enable them to resist to varying degrees the defence mechanisms of the body. It is important to our discussion that we define what we mean by certain scientific terms, including pathogenicity, virulence and invasiveness, which at present are often loosely applied and may add confusion to any description of the characteristic features of disease-producing organisms.

Pathogenicity is a term which refers to the ability of organisms to produce disease in the host. To be able to determine that a particular organism is pathogenic for a given host species, we must ensure that the host is in a normal state of health beforehand and that the conditions of experiment (e.g. age, husbandry, route of inoculation, dosage, etc.) are clearly defined.

Only in this way can the pathogenicity of one organism be compared with that of another. Even under these conditions it soon becomes evident that different strains of the same species of microorganism differ in their ability to produce disease. For example, a comparison between the ability of strains of *Bacillus anthracis* to produce anthrax in (say) guinea-pigs shows that under similar conditions an acute and fatal disease is produced far more readily by some strains than by others. Nevertheless, the term pathogenicity should be applied to a genus or group of microorganisms and should describe the potential ability of that group to initiate a disease process.

Virulence, on the other hand, is the term applied to define the ability of a particular strain of microorganisms to produce disease under defined conditions. We have already noted that *Bacillus anthracis* organisms are pathogenic for guinea-pigs but that strains differ in their ability to produce acute and severe disease. We can, therefore, say that those strains which cause severe disease when inoculated in small doses are more virulent than strains which only produce mild forms of the disease even when inoculated in large doses. If comparative experiments of this nature are carried out under constant conditions the results show that differences in virulence are associated with differences in the characteristic properties of the organisms. In the case of *Bacillus anthracis* the presence of a well-developed capsule protects the organisms against the defence mechanisms of the host and enables the infection to develop more readily. Most capsulated strains are more virulent than non-capsulated strains. Similarly, some clostridial organisms produce potent toxins which damage tissue cells, and a comparison of the toxin-producing capacities of different strains of *Clostridium tetani* reveal that some strains are virulent since they produce more toxin than avirulent strains.

Invasiveness is a term which superficially describes the way in which a pathogenic organism attacks the host. For example, if a cow becomes infected with a virulent strain of *Bacillus anthracis*, the animal may die suddenly and examination of the blood and organs from the carcase would reveal *Bacillus anthracis* in large numbers distributed throughout the body. In other words, *Bacillus anthracis* is an invasive organism. In contrast, if a horse receives a wound in the foot which becomes contaminated with *Clostridium tetani*, the animal may die from the disease. Postmortem and bacteriological examination would show that *Clostridium tetani* had developed at the site of the wound but had not penetrated the body beyond this local area. The toxin, alone, would have diffused out from the site and become attached to neural tissue, giving rise to the characteristic symptoms of the disease. In this type of infection,

Clostridium tetani is an example of a non-invasive pathogenic organism.

Establishment of a primary lesion

The development of an inflammatory response following experimental inoculation of bacteria can be observed most easily in the skin. Within 10–15 minutes following inoculation, the blood vessels in the immediate vicinity begin to dilate and the blood flow increases. At the same time there appears to be a marked increase in the number of capillaries in the area because many which were not previously observable become dilated and filled with blood. This vasodilatation is probably induced by histamine released locally by mast cells, and the effect may be increased by small amounts of serotonin. This hyperaemic condition persists for about 1 hour and then becomes less severe. After a further 2–3 hours, hyperaemia again develops and may persist for a further 2–3 hours before declining.

The action of histamine in causing vasodilatation does not last for longer than 15 minutes under experimental conditions. The more prolonged inflammatory response may be associated with the local production of kinins (i.e. polypeptides) although, as yet, there is no conclusive evidence on the effect of these substances in an inflammatory response. Kinins are formed as the result of the action of enzymes on substrates which are present in the serum. Bradykinin, for example, is a slow acting substance which causes dilatation of small blood vessels and increased permeability of the vessel walls.

During the hyperaemic stage the walls of the capillaries develop an increased permeability to plasma proteins which pass through into the surrounding tissue spaces together with some erythrocytes. This abnormal permeability continues for about 4–5 hours and then returns to normal. During the early stages of the inflammatory response there is some infiltration of the tissues with leucocytes which increases in intensity as the hyperaemic stage terminates and the blood flow in the capillaries becomes sluggish. At the same time, tissue macrophages and endothelial cells lining the blood vessels become swollen. Circulating leucocytes begin to migrate to the margins of the blood vessels and become adherent to the swollen endothelial cells. They then begin to move along the walls of the blood vessels, apparently in search of some opening through which they can squeeze themselves and pass into the surrounding tissues. These cells are strongly attracted to the area and undergo extreme changes in shape in order to migrate through the vessel walls. They appear to push aside the endothelial cells, to squeeze through the intercellular gaps, and then to penetrate the basement membrane. In the early stages of leucocytic migration it is neutrophils which penetrate the walls and accumulate in the tissues. Later, these cells are replaced by monocytes and lymphocytes and as the lesion develops there will be a marked mononuclear infiltration in the area.

The migration of leucocytes into an area of inflammation is a most important initial response of the host to microbial infection, since the accumulation of these cells possessing phagocytic properties enables a rapidly mobilised cleansing mechanism to be concentrated in the area of infection. Although many studies have been made to determine the factors which control this sudden and differential migration of leucocytes into an inflammatory area, we still do not understand the chemotactic forces which are responsible for this reaction. Some living bacteria, including streptococci, salmonellae and *Mycobacterium tuberculosis* are chemotactic to polymorphs, whereas killed organisms fail to show this property. In other words, the extra activity shown by polymorphs migrating to within an inflammatory area appears to be excited by the presence of living organisms. Recent observations suggest that during the early stages of an inflammatory reaction the swelling of the endothelial cells coincides with a decrease in the repulsive forces between these cells and circulating polymorphs. In addition, it seems that one of the properties of inflammatory fluids is to excite the general activity and movement of polymorphs and so to increase the chances of contact between these phagocytic cells and infecting organisms.

The initial accumulation of polymorphs at the site of an inflammatory response is replaced by an infiltration of mononuclear cells, particularly macrophages and lymphocytes. The extent to which this transformation of cell types occurs varies with different infections. Lesions caused by pyogenic (i.e. pus producing) organisms always contain large numbers of polymorphs, whereas in lesions associated with *Escherichia coli* or salmonella infections these cells eventually become almost entirely replaced by mononuclear cells. With milder reactions, associated with viral infections, lymphocytes become the predominant cell type in the lesion.

Development of bacterial infections in the body

A brief consideration of the variety of symptoms associated with infectious diseases in man and animals is sufficient to show the different modes of infection which occur. Even within the field of bacteriology we have noted that individuals may die suddenly from an invasive (*Bacillus anthracis*) or a non-invasive (*Clostridium tetani*) infection. In other conditions the symptoms and lesions may be those of severe toxaemia (*Clostridium*), enteritis (*Salmonella*), arthritis (*Staphylococcus, Erysipelothrix* and other organisms), pyaemia and necrosis (*Staphylococcus, Streptococcus, Corynebacterium, Sphaerophorus*) and granulomata (*Mycobacterium tuberculosis*). Each type of lesion depends upon the characteristic properties of the different pathogenic organisms and the particular mechanisms that each has developed in order to establish itself in the host's body. In contrast to these examples, the most successful host-parasite relationship is that which occurs in the symptomless carrier animal which harbours a potential pathogen but continues to lead a normal life until such time as circumstances may upset this fine balance between host and parasite. In the following section we shall discuss some of the characteristic properties of pathogenic bacteria which enable them to withstand the body defences and develop their pathogenic capacities from the primary lesion.

Toxaemic infections

Toxins are substances produced by bacteria which have a toxic action on tissue cells. These substances are usually separable from the whole organism. One of the characteristic properties of pathogenic clostridia is their ability to produce a variety of toxins. Each organism has its own particular battery of toxins which interferes with the normal metabolism of tissue cells; and these toxic effects can be neutralized by specific antibodies (antitoxins) provided that they are available in adequate concentrations in the early stages of infection. The conditions under which these organisms produce their toxins and the subsequent pathogenesis of disease differ considerably from one species to another even within the clostridial group. We have already noted that the characteristic method of attack of *Clostridium tetani* is multiplication, locally, at the primary site of infection which is commonly a contaminated skin wound. The organism produces tetanospasmin, a neural toxin acting upon nerve cells in the cerebrospinal axis. Under experimental conditions two clinical forms of the disease can be produced in animals. Injection of toxin intravenously results in the development of the 'general' form which gives rise to rigidity of the facial muscles, jaw, neck and latterly the limbs and trunk. If the toxin is injected intramuscularly, however, a spasticity of the muscles near the site of inoculation develops first, and this is followed by a toxic action on the brain stem. Many experiments have been designed to investigate the exact sites and mode of action of this toxin. Present evidence indicates that strong concentrations of toxin accumulate in the region of the primary lesion and that some disperses from the site and acts on neuronal elements. It does not pass up the axons but travels by muscular pressure from the site of infection along the inter-neuronal tissue spaces to the spinal cord, where it passes into the interstitial tissue of the central nervous system. The other toxin produced by *Clostridium tetani* is tetanolysin which can lyse erythrocytes of many animal species.

Clostridium botulinum also produces extremely potent neurotoxins, but unlike tetanus, botulism does not arise from a direct infection with the causal organism. It develops as the result of the ingestion of preformed toxin which is then absorbed through the wall of the intestine. Unlike tetanospasmin which acts on nerve cells in the cerebrospinal axis only, botulinum toxin has a specific action on all parts of the peripheral somatic and autonomic nerve fibres which are cholinergic. A feature which is common to both tetanus and botulinum toxins is their extreme lethality.

An important lethal toxin of *Clostridium oedematiens* is the alpha toxin which is produced by both type A and type B strains of the organism. The characteristic reaction produced by this toxin is a gelatinous oedema and haemoconcentration. It has been suggested that this is due to an enzyme-like action on the walls of blood vessels directed against the intercellular cement substance. The other toxins produced by *Clostridium oedematiens* have a variety of activities including haemolytic, necrotizing, lecithinase and also tropomyosinase which attacks the muscle protein, tropomyosin.

The lethal effect of *Clostridium septicum* appears to be associated with the haemolytic and necrotizing alpha toxin. In addition, the beta toxin is a deoxyribonuclease, the gamma toxin a hyaluronidase and the delta toxin is haemolytic.

Strains of *Clostridium welchii* produce at least twelve different toxins, nine of which are lethal and five are necrotizing. The alpha toxin is a lecithinase as well as being lethal, necrotizing and haemolytic. It is probable that oedema, haemorrhage, necrosis and shock resulting from the injection of *Clostridium welchii* toxins into animals are produced by lecithinase activity which causes permeability of capillaries, damage to cells and possibly damage to cell mitochondria. Other *Clostridium welchii* toxins contain haemolysins, collagenase, proteinase, hyaluronidase and deoxyribonuclease.

The above examples show that toxins produced by clostridial organisms have a variety of actions on tissue cells which can be demonstrated experimentally. The increased permeability of blood vessels at the site where the primary lesion is developing will facilitate the passage of toxins into various tissues of the body. A sufficient concentration of specific antitoxins in the host during the early stages of infection can neutralize the effects of the toxins. In practice this means that to treat successfully a toxaemic infection of this sort, an adequate concentration of antitoxin (i.e. hyperimmune serum) must be given as early as possible after infection is known or suspected to have occurred. Active immunization by inoculation of vaccines is of value provided that there has been sufficient time for high concentrations of antibodies to be produced before infection and toxin production have taken place.

Pyaemic infections

A feature of infection with some pathogenic bacteria is the formation of pus at the site of infection. When these pyogenic organisms spread from the primary site of infection via the blood stream to other parts of the body the condition is known as pyaemia. This type of condition is sometimes associated with staphylococcal, streptococcal and coryne-bacterial infections. The toxins which these organisms produce not only attack and destroy leucocytes to form pus at local sites of infection but in severe cases become distributed in the body and cause a generalised toxaemic condition. The following summary emphasises the variety of toxins produced by these organisms.

Staphylococci are pyogenic organisms which produce toxins having a variety of activities. They include lethal toxin which may kill a mouse or rabbit within 30 minutes; a necrotoxin which experimentally may cause necrosis of rabbit or guinea-pig skin; three haemolysins, and other toxins including leucocidins which have lethal effects on leucocytes; an enterotoxin associated with cases of staphylococcal poisoning; a coagulase which coagulates plasma and may inhibit the destruction of phagocytosed staphylococci because of the production of a film of fibrin on the surfaces of the organisms; a fibrinolysin which is produced by some strains, and hyaluronidase or 'spreading factor' which promotes the dispersion of staphylococci in the tissues.

Streptococci comprise another group of pyogenic organisms which produce a variety of toxins including two haemolysins — streptolysin S and streptolysin O which is lethal for mice, rabbits and guinea-pigs, and is toxic for leucocytes and erythrocytes. Additional toxins are fibrinolysin (streptokinase) having an anti-inflammatory reaction, streptodornase causing liquefaction of purulent exudates, hyaluronidase (spreading factor), and an erythrogenic factor responsible for the skin rash in scarlet fever. All strains do not produce the whole range of toxins and enzymes at the same time, and the concentration and variety of their production depends upon the environment of the bacterial growth. As in the case of staphylococci, all the toxic substances produced by streptococci are not individually lethal to the host but collectively they facilitate the establishment of the organisms in the body by interfering with the cellular defence

mechanisms, resulting in the distribution of bacteria and toxins in the tissues.

In the immediate neighbourhood of a primary lesion, some organisms will infect blood clots in small blood vessels (i.e. infected thrombi). In these clots organisms will be temporarily protected from the action of antibodies and phagocytes. Pieces of these thrombi may break off, become carried away by the blood stream and finally lodge in small blood vessels in various organs, particularly in the liver, lungs, and kidneys where they produce suppurative lesions.

Corynebacterium pyogenes produces a toxin which haemolyses red blood cells, is lethal to rabbits and mice and causes necrosis when inoculated into the skin of guinea-pigs. The precise way in which these toxic reactions occur and interfere with the cellular defences of the host are not clearly understood. Experiments using toxoid or toxoid plus whole organisms to stimulate immunity in various species of animals have, so far, proved unsatisfactory; and it is clear that antibodies to the toxin do not protect. Demonstrable immunity develops only after infection and the establishment of a necrotic lesion.

Bacteraemic infections

At certain stages in the development of some bacterial infections, organisms gain entry to the blood stream and become rapidly distributed in various organs of the body. We have already noted that in pyaemic infections, infected thrombi may break off from blood clots and be transplanted to various sites in the body. In cases of severe trauma when a wound becomes contaminated with bacteria, some organisms are forced into small blood vessels at the site of injury and then become distributed to other regions of the body. A bacteraemia may also develop from organisms in the lymphatic system which are conveyed to the thoracic duct and thence into the blood stream.

An outstanding example of a bacteraemia is acute infection with *Bacillus anthracis*. This disease develops from a local lesion where the organisms multiply rapidly, the cellular defences of the site are unable to cope with the high rate of bacterial multiplication, and phagocytosis may be inhibited by well developed bacterial capsules. Bacteria then break out from the lesion and become disseminated throughout the blood stream where they continue to multiply so fast that they overwhelm the cellular defence mechanism. The pathogenesis of anthrax has been studied in some detail during the last decade and it is now known that three bacterial products are, together, responsible for the development of disease. Two of these substances associated with the bacterial bodies are polyglutamic acid in the capsule which inhibits phagocytosis, and an anticomplementary lipoprotein fraction occurring in the bacterial bodies. The third substance is a toxin separable from the bacterial bodies, consisting of three components which together cause the production of oedema and are lethal.

Salmonella and Escherichia organisms may also produce a marked bacteraemia during the acute stage of infection, particularly in young animals. After ingestion of these organisms, a few will penetrate the wall of the intestinal tract and be filtered off into the local lymph nodes, and some will enter the blood stream (primary bacteraemia) and become distributed in other organs of the body. During the development of an acute and generalised infection these organisms continue to multiply in various sites in the body, become released into the blood stream in increasing numbers and give rise to a secondary and more severe bacteraemia which may prove fatal. Bacteraemias may also develop typically in young animals during the acute stages of infection with *Erysipelothrix*, *Pasteurella*, *Yersinia* and other bacterial infections.

Granulomatous infections

After the establishment of a primary infection in the tissues and the initial and local inflammatory response has occurred, subsequent development of the lesion will depend upon the characteristics of the infecting microorganism and the tissues in which the lesion is situated. Many pathogenic organisms are not highly virulent and as the lesion develops relatively slowly, the tissues react not only defensively to contain and eliminate the pathogenic organisms but also to repair damaged tissues at the site of the infected focus. In lesions which develop slowly over several months the process of repair is so marked that this type of reaction is often referred to as an **infectious granuloma**. The word granuloma has arisen from the descriptive term 'granulation tissue' which has for many years been applied to the granular surface formed by the accumulation of leucocytes, fibroblasts and vascular endothelial cells which attempt to rebuild areas of damaged tissue. Infectious granulomata develop in animals in a variety of chronic infections including tuberculosis, actinomycosis, glanders, some cases of chronic staphylococcal mastitis in cattle and pigs, chronic forms of *E. coli* and *Salmonella pullorum* infections in poultry and in some fungal diseases. A variety of cell types can be seen as would be expected in a lesion which, simultaneously, is trying to eliminate a focus of infection and to repair tissue damage. The relative proportions of cell types will differ according to the tissue in which the lesion is developing and the characteristics of the infecting organisms. For example, when a tuberculous lesion begins to develop in the liver of a susceptible animal, neutrophils comprise the first cell type which accumulate in the area and attempt to ingest the bacteria. Within 24 hours these cells are outnumbered by a concentration of macrophages which ingest any bacteria still remaining free and also some of the neutrophils which have already concentrated at the site.

There is experimental evidence to show that living tubercle bacilli stimulate the phagocytic properties of macrophages and in the early stages of the development of the lesion, phagocytosis is not always fatal to ingested microorganisms which may survive and liberate themselves by destroying the cells. As the lesion continues to develop, a dense accumulation of macrophages occurs in the centre and many undergo peculiar morphological changes which result in the fusion of groups of cells to form **giant cells**. These giant cells appear as large multinucleated structures in which the nuclei occur in circular formation around the circumference of the cell. This central mass of macrophages and giant cells increases in area with the result that the cells become more remote from blood vessels, their oxygen supply diminishes and eventually they die from anoxia. In addition, the toxic action which infecting bacteria may have on these cells will add to the rate of cellular destruction and give rise to a central pocket of pus in the lesion. At the same time, viable organisms liberated by these dying cells can often exist long enough to migrate outwards and extend the infective process to the margins of the lesion. Provided that this extension is sufficiently slow, fibroblasts proliferate around the periphery of the lesion which becomes walled off by a layer of fibrous tissue. The slower the rate of development of the lesion the more likely it is to be contained within the area of primary infection. Following the initial non-specific cellular response, the tissues of an immune animal will be more efficient at curtailing the spread of infection than those of a highly susceptible individual. For example, the presence of **immune opsonin** in serum will enhance the process of phagocytosis, and high concentrations of lytic antibodies will increase the rate of microbial destruction. There is growing evidence to show, however, that the immune response which develops from chronic infections may not always be beneficial to the host. It has been known for many years that inoculation into normal animals of purified protein derivative (PPD) obtained from tubercle bacilli gives rise to only very slight and transient reactions. On the other hand, injection of this material into an infected animal can lead to the development of a severe inflammatory response including necrosis. Moreover, this type of reaction which can occur after inoculation of PPD into any part of the body far removed from the area of the infective lesion, demonstrates that the animal has become allergic to the bacteria and their products, that sensitizing antibodies are present in the tissues throughout the body, and that the host has developed a state of hypersensitivity.

In an animal which has developed a specific hypersensitivity against a chronic microbial infection, antibodies situated either in or on tissue cells will be distributed throughout many tissues of the body. If these cell-fixed antibodies come into contact with the homologous bacterial antigen, an antigen–antibody reaction will occur resulting in damage to the cell in a manner discussed under hypersensitivity (Chapter 3). This cellular reaction may take place even when the antigen involved is not, itself, toxic to tissue cells. The importance of recognising this feature is that in a chronic lesion in which microbial destruction of tissue cells is continuing over a relatively long period of time, the dissemination of microbes or their antigens liberated into tissues surrounding the lesion in a hypersensitive animal, may result in an immunological reaction involving cell damage and a consequent inflammatory reaction which may ultimately lead to necrosis. In this way, lesions increase in size and new ones will develop. Foci of hypersensitive reactions such as these are often characterised by marked infiltrations with lymphocytes, plasma cells and eosinophils.

Development of viral infections in the body

At certain stages in the growth cycles of a number of animal viruses, a viraemia develops when viral particles are distributed in the body via the blood stream. Experiments with distemper virus in ferrets have shown that the disease is similar to that in dogs, and after intranasal inoculation, the virus penetrates the mucosa and multiplies in the underlying lymphatic tissue. Virus then becomes released into the blood stream and distributed to various organs where further multiplication occurs, giving rise to a secondary and more severe viraemia. This latter stage marks the end of the incubation period and the beginning of the development of symptoms at a time when virus is also present in mucous membranes. Although the initial site of infection and viral multiplication is in the region of the nasal mucosa, the animal is not infective to others until the secondary and more severe viraemia has developed. In the same way, young chickens infected with Newcastle disease virus may not transmit the infection to other chickens until clinical signs of the disease have begun to develop. Experiments with mouse pox (ectromelia) and rabbit pox have shown that after initial infection viral multiplication occurs in the respiratory tract, but cross-infection to other susceptible animals does not take place until the end of the incubation period and the development of clinical signs of disease.

An important problem arising from these observations is where and under what conditions does virus multiply during the incubation period, and what is the cause of death in fatal infections? We have already noted that after experimental intranasal infection of ferrets with distemper, the virus develops initially in the lymphatic tissue of the region. At about 3–4 days after infection, small amounts of virus can be detected in the blood and spleen. It is probable that some virus from the site of primary infection has found its way into the blood stream and has become lodged in the spleen. From about the fourth to sixth day after infection the amount of virus increases in the blood and particularly in the spleen; and by the ninth to tenth day the viraemia continues to develop and virus can be detected in many tissues of the body, including spleen, bladder and skin.

Viruses can only carry out their life cycles within living, susceptible cells where they are shielded from circulating antiviral agents. Development of measures designed to interfere with these life cycles are most likely to be effective in the early stages of viraemia. At this time, viral particles are circulating in the blood and becoming attached to the outer surfaces of tissue cells prior to penetration and intracellular multiplication. The presence of virus in the blood stream is also associated with circulating leucocytes as has been shown with myxomatosis, vaccinia and pox infections in rabbits, when the early viraemic stages involve the presence of virus in circulating leucocytes. In this way, virus becomes distributed in various organs of the body and, at the same time, cells of the reticuloendothelial system are highly active in phagocytosing viral particles.

Recently, it has been shown by fluorescent antibody methods that the virus of mouse pox occurs in the Kupffer cells of the liver. Other sites where virus may be found are in the capillary endothelia of various tissues of the body. This is partially confirmed by the observation that there is considerable proliferation of these cells at the time when they would be expected to be harbouring virus. Following this period of viral multiplication in different tissues of the body, increasing numbers of viral particles become released from cells and a second and more severe viraemia may develop, giving rise to clinical signs of disease.

The stage of secondary viraemia is particularly important in the ecology of arthropod-borne diseases like louping-ill, bluetongue and Nairobi sheep disease, in which the spread of infection depends upon the transmission of virus from one host to another by mosquitoes, ticks or other arthropod vectors. In typical arthropod-borne infections the virus particles inoculated into the subcutaneous tissues are engulfed by macrophages and are transported to the lymphatics and lymphoid tissues. After multiplying therein, the progeny virions enter the blood stream and are conveyed in the circulation to establish secondary foci of infection in other tissues of the body such as the central nervous system. In some arthropod-borne diseases the development of a marked viraemia is not associated with the development of clinical signs of the disease. This type of symptomless viraemia occurs, for example, in chickens infected with Eastern equine encephalitis virus. Mosquitoes are able to transmit infection from chickens to other animals, although the infected chickens remain clinically normal and are probably the main vertebrate reservoir for this and similar viruses. It also seems that in man and the horse, which are susceptible species, the development of a viraemia frequently does not lead to the development of encephalitis.

The apparent marked variation in pathogenicity of different viruses raises the problem of why some acute viraemias result in severe symptoms of disease and others fail to cause any clinical response in the host animal. So far, no highly toxic substance has been isolated from viruses which, alone, could account for the development of symptoms and lesions. It seems probable that cellular damage arising from extensive viral multiplication in the tissues may cause the release in adequate quantities of intracellular products of viral growth which are sufficiently toxic to cause general symptoms of infection. Symptoms and lesions associated with particular organs like the lungs or liver, arise from intense multiplication of virus in these organs with consequent damage to cells together with secondary bacterial invasion, causing serious derangement of the normal functioning of the organs. The extent to which this occurs may depend upon the virulence of any particular strain of virus. For example, an avirulent strain of Newcastle disease virus will multiply in the chorioallantoic sac of the developing chicken embryo without causing severe cellular damage. On the other hand, the rapid multiplication of a virulent strain under similar conditions results in marked cellular damage leading to necrosis and rapid invasion of the embryo with virus.

Development of fungal infections in the body

The pathogenesis of fungal infections in animals is an aspect of mycology which, until recently, has received comparatively little attention. Growing interest in these diseases has already shown that it is only under particularly favourable conditions that these organisms are capable of causing clinical infection. The development of disease is relatively rare when one considers the high incidence of potentially pathogenic fungi which occur in or on the animal body. Recent research has established that soil is a reservoir for a variety of pathogenic fungi and there is little doubt that the proximity to the soil of farm animals, in particular, is one important predisposing factor related to the development of fungal diseases in animals.

Dermatophytes

During the last decade it has been confirmed that ringworm fungi can lead a saprophytic existence in the soil. From there it is not difficult to imagine the facility with which these organisms can come into contact with the skin of animals. Under unspecified favourable conditions, ringworm spores will germinate on the skin and form hyphae which penetrate into hair follicles and subsequently attack the hairs. These fungi appear to have a predilection for keratinized tissue and the hyphae penetrate the area where keratinization is taking place. In fact, the general nutritional requirements of ringworm fungi do not appear to be very exacting, and it may well be that their pathogenicity is directly related to their ability to produce an enzyme capable of digesting keratin.

The first stage in the establishment of a ringworm lesion is the development of hyphae which travel from the epidermis down the hair follicles as far as the bulb, penetrating the hair just above this region. The local tissue reaction is often mild, consisting of congestion, leucocytic infiltration and exudate which dries and forms scabs on the surface of the skin.

The responses of the tissues to infection are not confined solely to the immediate area of contact between fungus and skin. For more than 50 years it has been known that in some human ringworm infections an allergic type of skin response may develop on parts of the body far removed from the primary lesion. These lesions do not contain the fungus and they disappear spontaneously when the primary focus of infection begins to heal. This type of remote immunological reaction and the tissue responses in the primary lesion indicate that hypersensitive reactions may play an important part in the establishment and subsequent development of fungal lesions on the skin of animals. A great deal still needs to be investigated before we understand the pathogenesis of these infections.

Other mycotic infections

As in the case of dermatophytes, relatively little work has been done on the pathogenesis of systemic mycotic infections in animals, but it is now becoming apparent that only under particular conditions do these organisms exert their pathogenic effects on the host, and this is often associated with characteristic changes in microbial morphology. Species of *Aspergillus* are commonly present in the environment of domesticated animals and under experimental conditions, naturally saprophytic strains are as pathogenic as strains which have been isolated from lesions of diseased animals. Morphologically, the pathogenicity of *Aspergillus* is associated with the transition of spores into mycelia and the latter occur in large numbers in active lesions.

A variety of animal species suffer from infection with *Aspergillus fumigatus*, and rabbits are known to be susceptible to experimental inoculation of the fungus which produces a haemolytic, thermolabile toxin. A more recent example of toxin production by aspergillus species was revealed from investigations into deaths of turkeys which had eaten certain consignments of groundnuts. It was shown that toxicity arose from contamination of groundnuts with *Aspergillus flavus* and the production of a toxin by this fungus. Day-old ducklings are also highly susceptible to the toxin under experimental conditions.

Allergic skin reactions may develop during aspergillus infections and this is particularly noticeable in rabbits about a fortnight after the inoculation of spores and subsequent to the development of a lesion containing mycelia. Similarly, eruptions can occur on the skin of individuals infected with *Coccidiodes immitis*, an organism which is commonly present in the soil of certain areas where infection is endemic.

Moniliasis is another fungal disease of man and animals usually caused by *Candida albicans*. The pathogenesis of this type of infection is not clearly understood but the organism does produce a toxin under suitable conditions. *Candida albicans* occurs naturally in the yeast-like cell form in the intestinal tracts of animals, and when the organism exhibits pathogenic properties, these are usually associated with the development of mycelia which penetrate the tissues underlying the colonies of yeast-like cells.

Further reading

BANG F.B. AND LUTTRELL C.N. (1961) Factors in the pathogenesis of virus diseases. *Advances in Virus Research*, **8**, 199.

MIMS C.A. (1964) Aspects of the pathogenesis of virus diseases. *Bacteriological Reviews*, **28**, 30.

NOWOTNY A. (1969) Molecular aspects of endotoxic reactions. *Bacteriological Reviews*, **33**, 72.

PLATT H. (1967) Pathogenesis. In *Viral and Rickettsial Infections of Animals*, p. 167, eds. Betts A.O. and York C.J. London: Academic Press.

SMITH H. (1968) Biochemical challenge of microbial pathogenicity. *Bacteriological Reviews*, **32**, 164.

SMITH H. AND PEARCE J.H., eds. (1972) Microbial pathogenicity in man and animals. In *22nd Symposium of the Society of General Microbiology*. London: Cambridge University Press.

SPECTOR W.G. AND WILLOUGHBY D.A. (1963) The inflammatory response. *Bacteriological Reviews*, **27**, 117.

CHAPTER 5

CONTROL AND PREVENTION
OF INFECTIOUS DISEASES

Control and prevention of infectious diseases

Chemotherapeutic and antibiotic substances

The history of science reveals a number of examples of early discoveries which were to lie dormant until similar observations made several decades later, stimulated a general interest in their significance. The study of antimicrobial agents and chemotherapy is a typical example of a scientific field in which the early work was not followed up for nearly half a century. From approximately 1890 onwards, there are reports of microbial antagonisms in which the responsible antibiotic agents were derived from microorganisms. Examples of these, made before the beginning of this century, included the antibiotic action of a product developed from *Pseudomonas aeruginosa* on *Bacillus anthracis*, and the beneficial effects of a fungus named as *Penicillium glaucum* on bacterial infections in guinea-pigs. Later, it was Ehrlich who first developed the term 'chemotherapy' to describe the action of substances which would combine with and inhibit the growth of microbes but at the same time have no effect on host tissues. His work led to the development of Gram's staining method using the basic aniline dyes, especially crystal violet which combines with nucleic acids in those bacteria which stain Gram-positive. Combination of the dye with bacteria prevents multiplication, and media incorporating crystal violet can be used selectively for the isolation of certain bacterial species from a mixed population.

The next important stage in the development of chemotherapeutic agents was the study of sulphonamide drugs derived from sulphanilamide which, like the basic aniline dyes, are effective mainly against Gram-positive bacteria. This was followed by the study of antibiotics including penicillin and other substances, which tended to overshadow the development and use of the sulphonamides. There followed in quick succession the discovery of streptomycin which is active against the tubercle bacillus and a variety of other bacterial species, and then the tetracyclines and chloramphenicol all of which became known as the 'broad spectrum' antibiotics because of the variety of bacteria which are susceptible to these substances. Continued widespread interest in the value of antibiotics has resulted in the isolation and study of many substances, particularly the polymyxins, the erythromycin group and several others which have been shown to be of practical value in the treatment of diseases in animals and man.

Today, the search continues on an increasing scale for new antibiotics which will broaden the variety of bacterial and fungal infections susceptible to treatment by chemotherapy. In addition, attention has been turned particularly to the problem of overcoming resistance to these agents by the introduction of new substances or the development of combined thereapy using two or more antibiotics, simultaneously. The search also continues on a wider field for agents of value in the control of protozoal infections, virus diseases and in the treatment of tumours. At the present time, many hundreds of antibiotics have been isolated and tested, and it is possible only to summarise briefly the properties and activities of the few which are presently recognised to be of value in the control of animal diseases.

Sulphonamides

The important antibacterial action of sulphonamides is the release of sulphonilamide residue which resembles paraaminobenzoic acid (PABA). In fact, the relationship is so close that sulphanilamide can replace PABA in folic acid metabolism which is involved in the synthesis of amino acids and proteins, causing inhibition of these activities in the cell.

A great variety of drugs related to sulphanilamide have been developed and tested as antimicrobial agents, and as already noted, the majority are active against Gram-positive bacteria, particularly staphylococci and streptococci. One of the first of these substances to be used was Prontosil, and some of the others of current interest are those which are rapidly absorbed from the intestines, including **sulphadimi-**

TABLE 5.1. Summarizing the significant properties of some antimicrobial agents

Antimicrobial agents	Susceptible microbial species								Site of antimicrobial action				Result of antimicrobial action		Intestinal absorption after oral dosage
	Gram-positive bacteria	Gram-negative bacteria	Lepto-spira	Borrelia and treponema	Myco-plasma	Rickett-sia	Chla-my-dia	Fungi	Cell wall	Cell memb-rane	Cyto-plasm	Protein syn-thesis	Bacterio-static	Bacteri-cidal	
Sulphonamides	+	+					l				+		+		Yes (some exceptions)
Penicillins	+	Varies according to agent	+	+					+					+	Varies according to agent
Streptomycin group	+	+	+									+		+	No
Polypeptide group	Varies according to agent	+								+				+	No (toxic)
Tetracycline group	+	+	+		+	+	+					+	+		Yes
Chloramphenicol	+	+				+	+					+	+		Yes
Erythromycin group	+	l			+	+	+					+	+		Yes
Lincomycin	+	l			+	+	+					+	+		Yes
Novobiocin	+	l										+	+		Yes
Vancomycin	+								+					+	No
Rifamycin group	+													+	
Cephalosporin group	+	+							+					+	No
Nitrofurans	+	+									+			+	Varies according to agent
Nalidixic acid		+									+			+	Yes
Griseofulvin								+			DNA metabolism				Yes
Polyenes								+		+					No (some agents are toxic)

+ = antimicrobial action, l = only limited number of species susceptible.

dine, **sulphamethoxypiridazine** and **sulphamethyl-phenazol**. **Sulphadimidine** is particularly useful because it is active against both Gram-positive and Gram-negative bacteria. Some preparations are absorbed only slowly from the intestines and these include **succinylsulphathiazole** and **phthalylsulphathiazole** which are effective against bacteria within the intestines. Others, including **sulphanilamide, sulphacetamide** and **sulphathiazole** are of limited value because they are rapidly absorbed and rapidly excreted. Since they are bacteriostatic rather than bactericidal agents it is often difficult to maintain an effective concentration of these drugs in the tissues unless they are used in topical applications. It is also important to remember that when culturing material from animals which have been subjected to sulphonamide treatment, PABA should be incorporated in the medium (5 mg/100 ml) to overcome inhibition.

Penicillin

The interesting observations of Fleming in 1928 that the growth of staphylococci was inhibited by the mould *Penicillium notatum* and by culture filtrates (penicillin) prepared from it, have been thoroughly recorded elsewhere, and penicillin is now a household word used throughout the world in connection with the control of human and animal diseases. Nevertheless, it is of interest to recall that this world-wide revolution in chemotherapy took place firstly, because Fleming realised the significance of his original observations and investigated the phenomenon in more detail; and secondly, because the work of Chain and his colleagues at Oxford in 1940 resulted in the purification and concentration of the substance, penicillin. This, in turn, led to commercial production methods being developed. The consequent impact of penicillin on the incidence and epidemiology of microbial diseases in animals and man has had far-reaching effects on the methods for controlling infectious diseases and has been a stimulus to the development of other antibiotic substances.

For the production of penicillin on a commercial scale, *P. notatum* or *P. chrysogenum* is grown for 10–14 days in large containers of fluid medium. The purified end-product contains, in fact, six different penicillins, of which one is **benzylpenicillin** or **penicillin G**.

More recently it has been possible to modify the growth of *P. notatum* by adding to the cultures synthetic side-chains resulting in the production of unusual forms of the penicillin molecule. An example is **penicillin V** which is less susceptible to the acid pH of the stomach, and can be administered orally. Some of the other semisynthetic penicillins include **methicillin, cloxacillin, oxacillin, propicillin** and

nafcillin which are fairly resistant to gastric acidity, can be given orally and are resistant to penicillinase. **Ampicillin** can also be given orally and has a wider range of antibacterial activity — being active against both Gram-positive and some Gram-negative bacteria, including *Salmonella, Shigella, Pasteurella* and *Pseudomonas*, but it is not resistant to the action of penicillinase.

The antibacterial action of penicillin depends upon its ability to inhibit the enzymic incorporation of muramic acid into the mucopolysaccharide complex of the bacterial wall — a process which is associated with multiplication. Thus, penicillin is particularly active against young cultures growing in the log phase. The effect of penicillin on bacterial cell walls can be seen in the development of large bizarre forms and of protoplasts and L-phase by bacteria growing under certain conditions in media containing penicillin. These unusual bacterial forms which develop are devoid of cell walls.

Penicillinases are enzymes produced by some strains of staphylococci and by some other bacterial species which destroy penicillins. The importance of these enzymes is that those bacterial species which produce penicillinase are resistant to the antimicrobial action of penicillin.

Streptomycin group

Streptomycin is produced by *Streptomyces griseus* and together with its hydrogenated derivative (**dihydrostreptomycin**) has an antibacterial activity on a fairly wide range of organisms including at least some members of the following genera, *Staphylococcus, Streptococcus, Mycobacteria, Pasteurella, Yersinia, Salmonella, Brucella, Bacillus, Klebsiella, Escherichia, Pseudomonas, Proteus* and *Bordetella*.

Some other members of the streptomycin group are **neomycin, kanamycin, framycetin, streptothricin, paromomycin** and **viomycin**, and it seems that the antibacterial activity of these substances is mainly associated with inhibition of protein synthesis. **Streptomycin**-resistant strains of bacteria can develop in patients undergoing treatment.

Polypeptide group

A variety of polypeptide substances derived from species of *Bacillus* have been isolated and tested for their antimicrobial activities. The most important include **bacitracin** and **subtilin** derived from *B. subtilis*, **polymyxins (B** and **E)** from *B. polymyxa*, **gramicidin S** and **tyrocidin** from *B. brevis*, **circulin** from *B. circulans*, and **colistin** which is similar to but less toxic than **polymyxin B**. This group of substances is limited in its use because of toxic effects when taken orally, and for this reason they are commonly employed for local applications only. **Bacitracin** is active mainly against Gram-positive organisms and also *Haemophilus*, while **polymyxin** and **colistin** are active against some species of Gram-negative organisms, including *Salmonella, Escherichia, Brucella, Campylobacter Pasteurella* and *Haemophilus*.

The antibacterial activity of the polypeptide group of substances is concerned with surface activity and alterations in cell membrane permeability. Their effects on bacteria are characterised by a loss of amino acids, purines, pyrimidines and organic ions. Unlike the action of penicillin, the antibacterial activities of the polypeptide group of substances do not depend upon bacterial growth and multiplication taking place; and compared with penicillin their action on bacterial membranes is relatively immediate.

Tetracycline group

This includes **chlortetracycline** (aureomycin) obtained from *Streptomyces aureofaciens*, **oxytetracycline** (terramycin) obtained from *Streptomyces rimosus*, **tetracycline** derived from chlortetracycline, **methacycline** derived from oxytetracycline and **demethylchlortetracycline**.

These substances are active against a wide variety of bacteria including Gram-negative and Gram-positive species and also against *Mycoplasma* and *Rickettsia*. Their activities are related to interference with protein synthesis in rapidly dividing cells. The tetracyclines are not highly toxic and can be given by mouth. Oral dosage may alter the normal intestinal flora and in severe cases can result in the development of thrush and other fungal disorders of the digestive tract.

The growth rates of young animals (e.g. pigs and poultry) can be increased by incorporating **chlortetracycline** in the foodstuffs. This practice leads to the development of strains of bacteria which are usually resistant to all the tetracyclines and not only to the one incorporated in the food. **Methacycline** has a similar antibacterial activity to the other tetracyclines but in addition, is active against *Mycoplasma* and has been used in the treatment of avian chronic respiratory disease (CRD).

Chloramphenicol

This substance is derived from *Streptomyces venezuelae* but is now produced synthetically. It is relatively non-toxic and can be given by mouth or by injection. It is similar to the tetracyclines in having a wide spectrum of antibacterial activity against Gram-positive and Gram-negative bacteria and also against *Rickettsia*, and this activity seems to be associated with interference in the synthesis of proteins but not of nucleic acid.

Erythromycin group (macrolides)

This group of drugs is sometimes referred to as the macrolides because they possess large complex molecules (lactone rings). The group includes **erythromycin** derived from *Streptomyces erythreus*, and the related drugs **oleandomycin, tylosin, spiramycin** and **carbomycin**.

These substances attack many species of Gram-positive organisms, some Gram-negative bacteria and like chloramphenicol, their activity seems to be concerned with inhibition of protein synthesis. Strains of organisms resistant to these drugs often develop when treatment is prolonged, but the development of such mutants may be delayed if other drugs (e.g. chloramphenicol) are used concurrently with the erythromycin group. Members of this group are sometimes used as alternatives to penicillin when strains of bacteria resistant to the latter are the cause of disease.

Lincomycin is derived from *Streptomyces lincolnensis* and has an antimicrobial activity similar to erythromycin.

Novobiocin and vancomycin

These antibiotics are produced by *Streptomyces niveus* and *Streptomyces orientalis*, respectively. Both substances are active against Gram-positive cocci and novobiocin is also active against *Proteus* and some other Gram-negative bacilli. They are mainly used in the treatment of infections with penicillin-resistant staphylococci which are susceptible to these antibiotics.

Rifamycin group

These substances are derived from *Streptomyces mediterranei* and one of them, **Rifamycin SV** is particularly bactericidal against staphylococci, streptococci and mycobacteria, attacking these organisms when they are actively multiplying. Encouraging results have been obtained from the use of this antibiotic for the treatment of bovine streptococcal and staphylococcal mastitis, and it is also effective against strains of these organisms which are resistant to other antibiotics.

Cephalosporin group

These antibiotics were originally isolated from a cephalosporium mould. Two derivatives of the natural substances are **cephalothin** and **cephaloridine** which are less toxic and of greater therapeutic value than the original cephalosporins. These derivatives are active against both Gram-positive and Gram-negative bacteria and also against penicillinase-producing staphylococci. Like penicillin, their activity is related to interference with the synthesis of bacterial cell walls. They are not readily absorbed from the intestines and need to be injected parenterally when they become readily distributed in the tissues.

Nitrofurans
These consist of synthetic nitrofuraldehyde compounds which are bactericidal for several Gram-positive and Gram-negative bacteria. **Nitrofurazone** and **furazolidone** are used for the treatment of bacterial enteritis, particularly salmonella infections in poultry and farm animals, while **nitrofurantoin** which is active against Gram-positive and Gram-negative bacteria, is rapidly absorbed by the intestinal tract, excreted largely by the kidneys, and is of value for the treatment of urinary tract infections.

Nalidixic acid
A synthetic substance mainly active against certain genera in the family *Enterobacteriaceae* due to inhibition of DNA synthesis.

Griseofulvin
This substance is derived from *Penicillium Janczewskii* and its action is primarily against some of the fungi that affect the skin and hair of animals and man (e.g. ringworm) and also against some plant pathogens. The mode of action is not known but it has been suggested that it interferes with the development of the cell wall and also possibly with nucleic acid metabolism. It has been observed to cause excessive branching and swelling of the hyphal wall.

Polyenes
Some species of *Streptomyces* produce conjugated polyenes which are antifungal agents. These include **hystatin, amphotericin, candicidin** and **filipin**, which act on fungal cell walls causing the leakage of intracellular material.

Drug resistance
The most serious current problem in relation to the use of antimicrobial drugs in the control of infectious diseases is the increasing frequency with which bacterial resistance to some of these substances has developed. In practice, this means that the treatment of specific infections with an antibiotic agent known to be potentially active against a particular microbial species, may be ineffective when used for the treatment of certain outbreaks of that infection.

The first recorded observations of a major epidemiological problem of this nature were made in Japan during the years following the end of the World War II. At that time, various sulphonamide derivatives were introduced into that country for the control of human dysentery caused by bacteria belonging to the *Shigella* group. Initially, the incidence of the disease became reduced but after a few years of this treatment it was noticed that by 1949 the incidence

began to increase and reached a peak in 1952. As a result of this new and serious situation, additional drugs were used for the therapy of the disease, including streptomycin, chloramphenicol and tetracycline. Subsequently, the incidence of dysentery again declined temporarily, only to be followed by a further increase. By this time it was noted that many strains of *Shigella* had become resistant to this latter group of antibiotics which had been introduced, and a more striking feature was that the larger proportion of these strains had developed a multiple resistance to all three of these antibiotics.

Detailed investigations into the epidemiology of this problem revealed a number of interesting features, the most important of which was the suggestion, later to be confirmed, that the property of multiple drug resistance can be transferred from resistant strains of *Escherichia* to *Shigella* in the intestinal tracts of patients as well as *in vitro* under laboratory conditions. Further experiments showed that the transfer of multiple drug resistance can take place among the majority of genera comprising the family *Enterobacteriaceae* as well as in certain other genera. These observations have led to extensive world-wide investigations into the genetic as well as epidemiological aspects of this problem in relation to the control of infectious diseases in animals and man by antimicrobial drugs. It is now known that within the family *Enterobacteriaceae*, multiple drug resistance may be transferred by conjugation from one bacterium to another by means of episomes known as R (resistance) factors in association with resistance transfer factors (RTF) (See Chapter 2). These episomes which consist of DNA, occur in the cytoplasm of the donor bacterium and multiply independently of the chromosomal DNA. Thus, a bacterium with an R factor only, is a cell that is resistant to one or more antimicrobial drugs but is not able to transfer this resistance to another susceptible cell. On the other hand, a bacterium with both an R factor and RTF is both resistant and capable under suitable conditions of transferring the resistance to another susceptible cell. It is now known that this transfer of antibiotic resistance from one bacterium to another can take place not only in the normal bacterial flora of the intestines of animals (e.g. calves, pigs, chickens) but also in the absence of antibiotics in the environment; that the frequency with which *in vivo* transfers take place will be higher when colonisation of the bacteria occurs in the intestines; and that transfers can occur between bacteria belonging to the same genus (e.g. from *E. coli* to *E. coli*) or from one related genus to another (e.g. from *E. coli* to *S. typhimurium*).

This newly-acquired knowledge means the original assumption that drug resistance developed in a bacterial population by a natural process of selection over a relatively prolonged period of time and only in the presence of the particular antibiotic, is not the sole method by which resistance can occur. These recent investigations have shown that by means of R factors and RTF, microbial resistance to drugs may also develop relatively quickly, can be transferred from one bacterial species to another, and the process can continue in the absence of the antibiotic from the microbial environment.

The results of these studies on the mode of development of drug resistance among bacteria, emphasise the facility with which this can take place even under conditions where the use of antibiotic agents is restricted to the control of serious diseases which can only be treated in this manner. During recent years, the widespread use of antibiotics in the fields of human and veterinary medicine and their further use as additives in animal foodstuffs to promote the growth of intensively reared food-producing animals, have resulted in the development of increasing numbers of bacterial strains possessing resistance to many of the drugs in common use. This is becoming particularly evident among strains of *Salmonella* and *Escherichia*. Although it is possible for human intestinal bacterial pathogens to develop a drug resistance from bacterial strains derived from animals, present evidence would indicate that this may not be the most important mode of development of drug resistance presently observed in man, but that it may be more commonly the result of antimicrobial therapy in human medicine. Nevertheless, both the medical and veterinary aspects of drug resistance are serious problems for the veterinarian, and there is no doubt that the use of those drugs in veterinary medicine which are also applied to the treatment of human diseases, must be employed with discretion.

Sensitivity testing

In view of the frequency with which pathogenic bacteria develop a resistance to antibiotics, it is important to be able to determine whether a particular bacterial strain isolated from diseased animals shows this property, and to obtain evidence quickly, concerning the range of antibiotics to which the organisms are susceptible. The following is a brief description of some of the methods commonly employed in routine laboratories.

Disc or tablet method

Commercially prepared tablets or discs of absorbent paper impregnated with an antibiotic are available for sensitivity testing. The general procedure is to place these at intervals of approximately 2 cm over the surface of an agar or blood agar plate which has been evenly inoculated over its surface with the organisms under test. Some sets of paper discs are joined together with paper in readiness for them to be evenly distributed over the surface of the medium. After subsequent incubation the growth on the plate is examined for zones of inhibition around the discs or tablets. The results are not precise but sufficiently accurate for clinical purposes and enable advice to be given as to the antibiotics most likely to be of value in the subsequent treatment of the condition.

Cylinder plate method

The procedure is similar to the above method except that in place of the discs or tablets, a series of small sterile glass, metal or porcelain cylinders are placed on the surface of the inoculated medium. Into these are placed dilutions of the antibiotic to be tested which will diffuse into the medium during subsequent incubation, and will cause zones of inhibition in the growths of susceptible organisms. The results are subject to variations according to a number of factors including the strength of the agar, the solubility and rate of diffusion of the antibiotic, the pH, time and temperature under which the test is carried out.

Serial dilution method

This consists of adding a standard volume of broth suitable to support the growth of the organism to be tested, to each of a number of screw-capped containers. To the series is added doubling dilutions of the antibiotic in broth. An additional control tube containing no antibiotic should be included. A loopful of an actively growing broth culture of the organism is inoculated into each tube, the cultures incubated overnight and examined for inhibition of growth by the absence of turbidity. To confirm that the greatest dilution of antibiotic showing no turbidity, known as the minimal inhibitory concentration (MIC), is the result of either a bacteriostatic or bactericidal action, the fluid must be subcultured into fresh medium free from antibiotic and incubated. No growth indicates a bactericidal action.

Bacterial vaccines and hyperimmune sera

Since the earliest studies were made on diseases caused by microbes, it has been known that infection with a potentially pathogenic organism followed by survival of the host is associated with the development of an immune state which may protect the individual from subsequent disease caused by similar organisms. This was clearly demonstrated by the work of Jenner, recorded in 1798, in which he showed that inoculation of a person with cowpox protected that individual from smallpox. Later, Pasteur found that inoculation of chickens with a strain of *Pasteurella* of low virulence, protected the birds from subsequent infection with a virulent strain of that organism. It was he who introduced the term 'vaccination' in recognition of Jenner's work, to describe this procedure of artificial protection or immunization. The word vaccination is derived from the Latin: *vacca*, a cow, and although it should be restricted to describing the control of smallpox, the terms vaccine and vaccination have now become accepted as referring to a wide variety of immunizing agents and their administration.

Methods for controlling infectious diseases by the inoculation of vaccines which cause the production of an **active immunity**, or by injection of hyperimmune serum which confers a **passive immunity**, need to be modified for different diseases. These modifications have to take into account the nature of the infective agents, their life histories, and the pathogenesis of the diseases they produce in animals of different ages and species. For the control of many diseases no satisfactory immunological procedures have been developed, for others the results are of limited value, and for only a few is immunization a wholly efficient and reliable method for controlling infection. The following section outlines some of the more important problems related to the use of immunological procedures in the control of infectious bacterial diseases in animals, and summarises the methods presently in use.

Immunization and disease control

Infections with potentially pathogenic organisms may give rise to a variety of host parasite relationships. For example, they may develop as severe reactions resulting in the sudden death of the animal (e.g. anthrax), or of undetectable responses in which the organisms may or may not survive in the tissues of the apparently normal individual for relatively long periods of time before being eliminated by the host or eventually causing disease (e.g. *Clostridium chauvoei*, as a cause of blackquarter in cattle). Infection may also give rise to a variety of pathological responses varying in severity between these two extremes. The nature of the disease will be affected by a number of factors, including the age of the animal and the extent to which it can respond immunologically to antigenic stimuli, the tissues and organs affected, and the nature of the organisms' pathogenic properties which may be associated with either endotoxins (e.g. *Salmonella, Escherichia*) or exotoxins (e.g. *Staphylococcus, Clostridium*). For these reasons the procedures for artificial immunization have to be adapted to meet the conditions and characteristic features of the various infections which are encountered.

Active and passive immunity
There are two distinct methods for artificially immunizing animals against infectious diseases. One

is to use a vaccine containing antigens in the form of bacteria and/or their products to stimulate the production of an active immunity. The other method is to confer a passive immunity by inoculating hyperimmune serum containing a high concentration of specific antibodies against a particular infective agent or its products (i.e. toxins). The serum will have been prepared artificially in another animal, usually a horse, by injecting it with repeated doses of bacteria or bacterial products.

There are important differences between these two forms of artificial immunization which can be conferred by the injection of vaccines or hyperimmune sera. Following injection of one dose of vaccine there will be a period of time lasting for some 7–10 days before the antibody-producing mechanisms in the body will have responded sufficiently to produce a detectable concentration of antibodies in the serum (inductive phase). It is important to remember that during this inductive phase immediately following vaccination, the animal will remain susceptible to infection and this susceptibility will decrease as antibody production develops. Moreover, under most conditions the degree of resistance developed by the animal during the first productive phase after receiving one dose of vaccine will not be maximal; and it is common practice to give a second dose of the same vaccine, sometimes referred to as a booster dose, at an interval of about 2–3 weeks after the first dose. The degree of active immunity which develops following this second dose (second productive phase) will be markedly greater than the level reached after the first dose, and in most circumstances will remain at a substantial level for 9–12 months. The level of immunity may be re-stimulated by injecting another dose of vaccine after this period of time.

In contrast to the responses stimulated by vaccines, a passive immunity conferred on an animal by the injection of hyperimmune serum has an immediate effect because the animal receives the high concentration of antibodies contained in the serum. The other important feature of this method of protection is that the immunity it confers on the recipient is of short duration and may not protect the individual from developing the natural disease for more than approximately 2–3 weeks.

An alternative method for conferring a passive immunity on newborn animals is to vaccinate the dam who then develops an active immunity and transfers this to her offspring via the colostrum in cattle, sheep and pigs and via egg yolk in birds. An example of this method is the passive protection of newborn lambs against lamb dysentery by vaccination of the ewe shortly before lambing. The resulting immunity in the lamb is of short duration since the antibodies only pass through the wall of the intestines from ingested colostrum during the

TABLE 5.2. Summarizing the main features of bacterial vaccines and hyperimmune sera used for the control of animal diseases.

Causal organisms	Diseases	Animal species vaccinated	Nature of vaccines	Remarks	Use of hyperimmune sera
Bacillus anthracis	Anthrax	Horses, cattle, sheep, goats, pigs	Living; spores of avirulent strain		Yes
Brucella abortus	Brucellosis	Cattle, sheep	Living; avirulent strain 19	Used in calves up to 6 months of age	
		Cattle	Killed; strain 45/20	Used with water-in-oil adjuvant	
Borrelia gallinarum	Spirochaetosis	Poultry	Killed; bacteria in tissues	Tissue or haemolysed blood from infected geese, treated with phenol or formalin. Or, formalinized chick embryo cultures	
			Living; followed by treatment with arsenical preparation		
Clostridium botulinum	Botulism	Cattle, mink	Alum precipitated toxoid		
Clostridium chauvoei	Blackquarter	Cattle, sheep	Alum precipitated toxoid or toxoid plus killed bacteria	Mixed vaccines prepared incorporating several of these toxoids	Yes
Clostridium oedematiens	Black disease	Sheep	Alum precipitated toxoid		Yes
Clostridium septicum	Braxy	Sheep	Alum precipitated toxoid or toxoid plus killed bacteria		
Clostridium tetani	Tetanus	Horses, cattle, sheep, goats, pigs	Alum precipitated toxoid		Yes
Clostridium welchii type B	Lamb dysentery	Sheep	Alum precipitated toxoid		Yes
Clostridium welchii type C	Struck	Sheep	Alum precipitated toxoid		Yes
Clostridium welchii type D	Enterotoxaemia and pulpy kidney	Sheep	Alum precipitated toxoid or toxoid plus killed bacteria		Yes
Corynebacterium pyogenes	Mastitis	Cattle, sheep	Alum precipitated toxoid plus killed bacteria	Unreliable	Yes
Erysipelothrix insidiosa	Erysipelas	Pigs, turkeys	Killed; virulent strain Living; avirulent strain		Yes
Escherichia coli	Enteric infections in young animals	Cattle, pigs	Killed; mixed serotypes	Sows may be vaccinated to give passive immunity to piglets	Yes

Organism	Disease	Animal	Vaccine	Remarks	
Leptospira icterohaemorrhagiae *Leptospira canicola* *Leptospira pomona* and other serogroups	Leptospirosis and abortion	Cattle, pigs, dogs	Killed; bacteria	Unreliable; reduces incidence of abortion	Yes
Mycobacterium paratuberculosis	Johne's disease	Cattle	Living; attenuated strain	Used in liquid paraffin and olive oil adjuvant for calves up to 4 weeks of age	Yes (in cattle)
Mycoplasma mycoides	Contagious bovine pleuropneumonia	Cattle	Living; attenuated strain	Used in liquid paraffin and lanoline adjuvants	
Pasteurella multocida	Pasteurellosis	Cattle, sheep, pigs	Killed; mixed capsulated serotypes	Autogenous vaccines often used	
Pasteurella multocida	Fowl cholera	Turkeys	Killed; mixed capsulated serotypes	Autogenous vaccines often used: also mixed vaccines of *Past. multocida* and *Past. haemolytica*	
Pasteurella haemolytica	Pneumonia	Cattle, sheep, pigs	Killed; mixed formolised strains	Immunity only temporary	
Salmonella abortus equi	Abortion	Horses	Killed; bacteria		
Salmonella cholerae suis	Salmonellosis	Pigs	Living; avirulent strain	Also gives some immunity against *S. typhi-murium* infection	
Salmonella dublin	Salmonellosis	Cattle	Living; avirulent strain		
Salmonella gallinarum	Fowl typhoid	Poultry	Living; avirulent strain		
Staphylococcus pyogenes	Acute pyaemic infections	Cattle, sheep	Toxoid	Variable results. β-propiolactone better than formalin for inactivating the vaccine	
Streptococcus equi	Strangles	Horses	Killed; bacteria		

first 36–48 hours after birth, but this is often sufficient to protect the neonate from immediate post-natal disease.

Age of the animal

An important factor governing a decision on the most appropriate methods for conferring an artificial immunity is the age of the animal. Although there is evidence that young animals begin to develop the capacity to produce antibodies very soon after birth, and indeed to a limited extent *in utero*, for practical purposes of disease control the young animal is unable to protect itself from infectious diseases by means of its own immunological tissue responses. For this reason, artificial immunization of young animals must depend upon a passive immunity which may be conferred on them either by their mothers via colostrum following vaccination of the dam shortly before parturition, or by the injection of hyperimmune sera.

For the control of some diseases it is important to be able to protect a young animal from infection soon after birth and to ensure that this protection will last for a longer period of time than would normally follow passive immunization, alone. This means that it may be desirable to inoculate a vaccine into a young animal which already has a passive immunity against the disease, so that it will remain immune because its own active immunity will replace the relatively short-lasting passive immunity. The problem that has to be considered in these circumstances is that when a vaccine is inoculated into an animal which is already passively immunized against the infective agent, the antibodies in the tissues will combine with the microbial antigens in the vaccine and markedly reduce the stimulating effect the vaccine would otherwise have on the development of an active immunity. This is because combination of antibodies with the antigen will result in the removal of the latter from the body before adequate stimulation of antibody production has occurred. For these reasons, vaccination of young animals may have to be delayed until such time as any passive immunity will have waned sufficiently to prevent interference with the antigenic stimulus of the vaccine to cause the development of an active immunity.

The nature of vaccines

Living and killed vaccines

The essential property of a satisfactory vaccine is that it will be highly immunogenic (capable of stimulating a strong immune response) and at the same time unable to cause disease. These are the two features which are to a certain extent mutually exclusive. It is a general rule that a live vaccine will give a stronger immunity and of longer duration than a killed vaccine. This is because living organisms multiply and persist in the host's tissues for a longer period than killed organisms, and thereby cause a more prolonged immunological response. It is also possible that certain labile antigenic components of importance for stimulating the production of a solid immunity, may be destroyed during the preparation of a killed vaccine. However, a vaccine consisting of a suspension of living, virulent organisms is clearly unacceptable because of the risk of spreading disease. Conversely, a vaccine containing killed organisms stimulates less response over a shorter time than a living vaccine.

For these reasons, attempts have been made during recent years to reach a compromise by developing living bacterial vaccines prepared from attenuated or avirulent strains which will be both safe to use and stimulate a maximum immune response in the recipient. Examples of living vaccines of this kind are contagious bovine pleuropneumonia (*M. mycoides*), fowl typhoid vaccine prepared from the avirulent 9R strain of *S. gallinarum*, and similar vaccines prepared from *S. choleraesuis* for use in pigs and *S. dublin* for the control of bovine infections. Other examples are anthrax vaccine consisting of a suspension of spores derived from an avirulent strain of *B. anthracis*, brucella vaccine containing the avirulent strain S19 of *Br. abortus*, swine erysipelas vaccine prepared from an attenuated strain of *E. insidiosa*, and on a more limited scale a vaccine against Johne's disease consisting of an attenuated strain of *Myco. paratuberculosis*.

Many attempts have been made to prepare killed bacterial vaccines which are of value in the control of animal diseases. Only a small proportion of the wide variety of those tested experimentally, have been found to give a satisfactory level of immunity under practical farming conditions. These include a killed vaccine for the control of brucellosis (*Br. abortus* strain 45/20), a vaccine for pasteurellosis caused by *Past. multocida*, the control of scours in calves and young pigs for which the vaccines contain several serotypes of *E. coli*, the prevention of erysipelas in pigs with a vaccine containing killed virulent organisms of *E. insidiosa*, a leptospiral vaccine for dogs which includes a suspension of killed *L. icterohaemorrhagiae* and *L. canicola* organisms and a similar vaccine containing other serogroups for the prevention of abortion in cattle. In addition, a wide variety of vaccines and mixed vaccines are used for the control of clostridial infections in various animal species. Many other killed bacterial vaccines have been tested but are not widely used.

The use of antiviral vaccines is discussed in Chapter 41.

Mixed vaccine

Attempts to control simultaneously a number of infectious diseases by vaccination have resulted in trials using mixed vaccines which contain several species of organisms and their products. It has been found in practice that with few exceptions this is usually an unsatisfactory procedure because of a variety of reasons. There is, for example, a limit to the maximum response an animal can make to the presence of one type of microbial antigen. If two or more antigenically distinct organisms are included in one vaccine, the maximum response to each component will be reduced, and furthermore one component may be more immunogenic than another and stimulate a disproportionate amount of the total immunological response. Exceptions to the limited value of mixed vaccines are the satisfactory responses derived from using clostridial vaccines, particularly for the control of these diseases in sheep. The toxins obtained from clostridial cultures are purified and formolised, causing them to be altered into **toxoids** in which the antigenic properties of the toxins remain intact but the toxic properties are destroyed. Vaccines prepared from individual clostridial species may consist of toxoid alone, or a mixture of toxoid and killed bacteria. Several different mixed clostridial vaccines are now used and some of them contain more than two of the following components: *Cl. welchii* type B (lamb dysentery), type C (struck), type D (enterotoxaemia and pulpy kidney), *Cl. septicum* (braxy), *Cl. chauvoei* (blackquarter), *Cl. oedematiens* (black disease) and *Cl. tetani* (tetanus).

Autogenous vaccine

This is prepared from the specific bacterial strain causing an outbreak of disease and is used for the control of that particular infection. The organisms are isolated from the condition (e.g. pasteurellosis), grown in the laboratory, killed and standardised to an appropriate concentration. An autogenous vaccine will stimulate a stronger immunity against the particular serotype of microorganism causing disease than will a similar vaccine prepared from various closely related serotypes with or without the inclusion of the one responsible for the particular outbreak.

Adjuvants

It is a general feature of a killed vaccine that it is safe to use but the immunity it stimulates is relatively shorter in duration than that produced by a similar live vaccine. However, the immune responses to killed vaccines can be prolonged when the antigens in the vaccine are combined with certain substances known as adjuvants. One of the most widely used adjuvants is aluminium hydroxide (alum) which has the property of adsorbing on to and precipitating clostridial toxoids. When alum-precipitated toxoid is inoculated into the tissues, the toxoid is not all immediately available as antigen capable of stimulating the immune mechanisms of the body, but is released slowly from its combination with the insoluble adjuvant at the site of inoculation. Thus, it provides a more prolonged antigenic stimulus than a similar dose of pure toxoid because the latter is soluble, becomes quickly dispersed in the tissues, and produces a more rapid antigenic stimulus of shorter duration.

Various types of water-in-oil adjuvants are incorporated in some killed vaccines (e.g. *Br. abortus* (strain 45/20), *Myco. paratuberculosis*), and one preparation known as **Freunds's complete adjuvant** which consists of a water-in-oil emulsion containing heat-killed mycobacteria, has been used experimentally but tends to produce a severe local reaction at the site of inoculation. The important mycobacterial constituents of this adjuvant are the lipids present in the waxy surfaces of these organisms.

Hyperimmune sera

Horses are usually employed for the preparation of antisera to be used therapeutically for the prophylaxis (prevention) of disease because a relatively large volume of serum can be obtained from each individual horse. Occasionally other species (e.g. cattle, sheep, goats, dogs, rabbits) may be employed for the preparation of special antisera. The animals are subjected to a course of injections with a particular bacterial antigen or toxoid, and after completion of the course, the sera are tested for antibody titres. When these have reached satisfactory levels the animals are bled, sometimes on a number of occasions over a period of several days, and the sera collected and stored or the globulin fractions concentrated by ammonium sulphate precipitation. This latter procedure is used, for example, in the preparation of various clostridial antisera for the prevention of tetanus (*Cl. tetani*), lamb dysentery (*Cl. welchii* type B), enterotoxaemia and pulpy kidney disease (*Cl. welchii* type D), blackquarter (*Cl. chauvoei*) and black disease (*Cl. oedematiens*).

The characteristically short duration of a passive immunity conferred on an animal by the inoculation of hyperimmune serum has already been referred to, but it is important to appreciate the conditions under which this temporary immunity may vary in length and the risks attached to prolonging a passive immunity by repeated injections of hyperimmune sera.

When a hyperimmune serum is prepared in a horse and is then injected therapeutically into another horse to protect the latter from disease, that animal will be receiving **homologous** antiserum, i.e. a serum derived from the same species of animal. Whereas, if the antiserum is inoculated therapeutically into an animal of a different species, the recipient will be receiving **heterologous** antiserum. The antibodies in the antisera are associated with gamma-globulin, and when an animal is inoculated with homologous serum, the gamma-globulin will persist for a longer period of time in the recipient than comparable amounts of heterologous gamma-globulin. This is because heterologous gamma-globulin is recognised as foreign by the recipient and will be eliminated more quickly by the protective mechanisms of the body than homologous gamma-globulin which has been derived from an animal of the same species. In practice, this means that under controlled conditions a passive immunity derived from homologous antiserum may persist at an effective level for some 3–4 weeks, whereas one derived from heterologous antiserum may be effective for only about 1–3 weeks.

When it is desirable to prolong the protective effect of an artificially produced passive immunity, it would seem logical to subject the recipient to a series of injections of hyperimmune sera at intervals. However, this procedure is not without risk, particularly when using heterologous sera. Heterologous gamma-globulin is highly immunogenic in an adult recipient and after receiving one dose the animal will not only be protected passively by the antibodies contained in the serum but will also begin to produce its own antibodies against the foreign gamma-globulin. Thus, if the recipient is subjected to a further dose of the hyperimmune serum 2–6 weeks or longer after the first dose, it may develop a hypersensitive reaction which will take the form of either a generalised anaphylactic reaction or a localised (Arthus) reaction. Hypersensitive reactions are far less likely to occur after repeated injections of homologous hyperimmune serum.

Further reading

GABRIEL K.L. AND SCHEIDY S.F. (1965) Sulfonamides. *Advances in Veterinary Science*, **10**, 245.

GARROD L.P. AND O'GRADY F. (1971) *Antibiotics and Chemotherapy*, 3rd Edition. Edinburgh: Churchill Livingstone.

HASH J.H. (1972) Antibiotic mechanisms. *Annual Review of Pharmacology*, **12**, 35.

HOWELL D.G. (1965) Principles of immunization in animals and man. I. A review of some immunological problems associated with veterinary preventive medicine. *Veterinary Record*, **77**, 1391.

JAWETZ E. (1968) The use of combinations of antimicrobial drugs. *Annual Review of Pharmacology*, **8**, 151.

NEWTON B.A. (1965) Mechanisms of antibiotic action. *Annual Review of Microbiology*, **19**, 209.

ROLLO I.M. (1966) Antibacterial chemotherapy. *Annual Review of Pharmacology*, **6**, 209.

SCHEIDY S.F. AND GABRIEL K.L. (1965) Antibiotics. *Advances in Veterinary Science*, **10**, 253.

WEHRLI W. AND STAEHELIN M. (1971) Actions of the rifamycins. *Bacteriological Reviews*, **35**, 290.

WHITE R.G. (1968) Antigens and adjuvants. *Proceedings of the Royal Society of Medicine*, **61**, 1.

CHAPTER 6

ESCHERICHIA

Escherichia

The family *Enterobacteriaceae* is composed of non-sporing, Gram-negative rods which may be motile with peritrichous flagella or non-motile. They grow on ordinary media and reduce nitrates to nitrites.

The very large number of bacterial types which comprise the family are segregated into groups (or genera). These groups can best be described as dense centres of population composed of bacteria giving similar biochemical reactions and showing close

in attempting to divide so large a family of closely related bacteria and transitional forms into groups, since the characteristic properties of many organisms do not correspond exactly with the typical characters of a particular group, and there are several biochemical and antigenic interrelationships between the groups.

Table 6.2 compares some of the properties which help to differentiate between the groups comprising

TABLE 6.1. The bacterial tribes, groups and species comprising the family *Enterobacteriaceae*.

Tribe	Group	Type species	Other species
Escherichieae	Escherichia	*E. coli*	
	Shigella	*Sh. dysenteriae* (Shiga)	*Sh. flexneri, Sh. boydii, Sh. sonnei*
Salmonelleae	Salmonella	*S. choleraesuis*	*S. typhi, S. enteritidis* and many others (including
	Arizona	*A. arizonae*	Bethesda-Ballerup)
	Citrobacter	*C. freundii*	
Klebsielleae	Klebsiella	*K. pneumoniae*	*K. ozaenae, K. rhinoschleromatis*
	Enterobacter		
	Subgroup A	*Ent. cloacae* (*Aerobacter cloacae*)	
	Subgroup B	*Ent. aerogenes* (*Aerobacter aerogenes*)	Subspecies *hafniae*
	Subgroup C	*Ent. liquifaciens* (*Aerobacter liquifaciens*)	
Proteeae	Proteus	*Pr. vulgaris*	*Pr. mirabilis, Pr. morganii, Pr. rettgeri*
	Providencia	*P. providenciae*	

serological relationships. In addition, there are many transitional forms continually being identified which complicate the clear-cut division of these organisms into easily characterized groups. This requires periodic modifications to the internationally recognized criteria on which the classification is based. Table 6.1 shows the various groups and species of organisms comprising the family.

It is inevitable that there are inherent difficulties

the family *Enterobacteriaceae*. The members of each group are further divided into subgroups according to certain biochemical reactions, and classification into individual serotypes is based upon the combination of somatic (O), flagellar (H) and/or capsular (K) antigens possessed by each organism. Further differentiation between strains of a particular serotype may be made by colicin or bacteriophage typing.

TABLE 6.2. Comparing some properties of the bacterial groups comprising the family *Enterobacteriaceae*.

Test	Escherichia	Shigella	Salmonella	Arizona	Citrobacter	Klebsiella	Enterobacter	Proteus	Providencia
Motility	+	−	+²	+	+		+	+	+
Glucose	+	+¹	+	+	+	+	+	+	V
Lactose	+ or X	−	−	+ or X	+ or X	+	+	−	−
Sucrose	V	−	−	−	V	+	+	V	V
Mannitol	+	V	+	+	+	+	+	V	V
Indole	+	V	−	−	−		−	+³	+
Methyl red	+	+	+	+	+	−	−	+	+
Voges Proskauer	−	−	−	−	−	+	+	−	−
Citrate	−	−	+	+	+	+	+	V	+
H₂S	−	−	+	+	+	−	−	V	−
Urease	−	−	−	−	−	+	−	+	−

+ = positive reaction or fermentation	¹ = production of acid only (i.e. anaerogenic)
X = late fermentation	² = *S. pullorum* and *S. gallinarum* are non-motile
V = variable reaction	³ = *Pr. mirabilis* gives negative reaction

Escherichia coli

In 1885–86, Escherich described the properties of an organism he named *Bacterium coli commune* and which he had identified in the faeces of new-born babies. Later, this organism became known as *Bacterium coli* and more recently as *Escherichia coli*. The group *Escherichia* is composed of the many different serotypes of *E. coli*.

Distribution in nature

E. coli are normal inhabitants of the intestinal tracts of vertebrates, including man. Under certain conditions the number of these organisms in the intestines undergoes a marked and rapid increase, and this may be associated with definite signs of ill health and sometimes death.

Morphology and staining

E. coli is a bacillus measuring approximately 2–3 μm in length by 0·6 μm in width (Plate 6.1a, facing p. 100). It does not form spores. Many strains possess peritrichous flagella but may be only sluggishly motile. Some strains develop capsules and produce a mucoid type of growth on solid media.

The organisms stain Gram-negative.

Cultural characteristics

E. coli is aerobic and facultatively anaerobic. It is readily grown on ordinary laboratory media without the addition of blood, serum, ascitic fluid, glucose, etc. The optimum temperature for cultivation is 37°C but growth will occur over a temperature range of approximately 20–44°C. On agar media the colonies usually develop to a size of 2–3 mm diameter but there may be considerable variation in colony sizes of different strains. Organisms which form well-developed capsules give rise to relatively large opaque, mucoid colonies. Growth of a smooth strain in broth results in a rapidly developing turbidity during the initial 18 hours' incubation and a slight deposit which can be easily dispersed on shaking.

Biochemical tests for the differentiation of *E. coli* from other closely related bacterial groups must be based on the reactions which occur in a variety of media. All strains of *E. coli* ferment glucose and lactose with production of acid and gas. The majority of strains ferment mannitol, form indole but fail to produce H₂S and do not grow in citrate medium. Most strains do not develop urease, give a negative Voges-Proskauer reaction and are positive to the methyl red test.

Methods of isolation

When attempting to isolate *E. coli* from faeces or tissues of dead animals it should be remembered that these organisms are normal inhabitants of the intestinal tracts of healthy individuals. The isolation of *E. coli* may be meaningless unless other factors are considered, including the detailed history of the case, the symptoms and the lesions. The amount and purity of growth on primary culture, and the sites from which isolations have been made are additional aids in making a final diagnosis. The isolation of *E. coli* from various organs of a fresh carcase, in addition to the intestinal tract, is usually indicative of disease associated with these organisms.

A satisfactory medium to use is MacConkey's agar. The presence of lactose and an indicator in this medium enables lactose fermenting organisms (e.g. *E. coli*) to be differentiated from lactose non-fermenters (e.g. *Salmonella, Proteus*). Growth of *E. coli* will appear as pink coloured colonies due to the fermentation of lactose and the production of acid shown by the indicator, (neutral red) (Plate 6.1b, facing p. 100). Conversely, lactose non-fermenters appear as pale, yellowish colonies on MacConkey's agar.

Blood agar plates can be a useful additional medium for the diagnosis of *E. coli* diseases. Haemolytic strains of *E. coli* can be readily observed on 5 per cent sheep blood agar and the K antigens develop well on this medium. Since blood agar is non-inhibitory, the relative proportions of *E. coli* to other bacterial species can be assessed, particularly in samples of intestinal contents which may yield a pure culture of *E. coli* when derived from cases of colibacillosis in young animals.

The growth characteristics of colonies on MacConkey's agar and blood agar can be observed after 18 hours' incubation at 37°C. Suspected colonies of *E. coli* can be picked off and tested for their biochemical reactions. If these are characteristic for the group the serotype can be determined on the basis of the antigenic structure (*vide infra*).

Resistance to physical and chemical agents
E. coli is relatively susceptible to physical and chemical agents. In the majority of instances a temperature of 55°C for 1 hour or 60°C for 20 minutes is lethal to these organisms, and they are killed rapidly by autoclaving at 120°C. Under natural conditions *E. coli* may survive for weeks or months in water, faeces and dust in animal houses. They are highly susceptible to the lethal action of phenol and cresol, but the efficacy of these disinfectants is reduced in the presence of mucus and faeces.

Antigens and toxins
The complex O, H and K antigenic structures of *E. coli* have been studied in detail because they form the basis on which the serotypes can be differentiated one from another.

O antigens
These are the somatic antigens occurring as part of the bacterial body and are composed of a poly-saccharide–phospholipid–protein complex. These antigens are not destroyed by heating to 100°C nor to 120°C, but after the latter treatment their ability to combine with specific antisera is reduced. They are not destroyed by alcohol.

K antigens
These antigens which occur as envelopes or capsules on most strains of *E. coli*, are composed of poly-saccharides, and can prevent agglutination between O antigens and homologous antisera. The K antigens show different degrees of thermolability which form the basis for subdividing them into L, A and B varieties. Inhibition of O agglutination by K antigens can be overcome by heating the bacteria to 100°C for 1 hour. In the case of A antigens, cultures have to be heated to 120°C for $2\frac{1}{2}$ hours to enable O agglutination to take place. Recent immunoelectrophoretic studies suggest that the lipopolysaccharide of the B antigen may be very similar to, if not identical with that of the O antigen.

H antigens
These are the flagellar antigens which are composed of protein. Frequently, the H antigens are poorly developed on newly isolated strains and consequently agglutination with homologous H antiserum is weak. Passage of the strain through semi-solid medium often results in increased development of H antigen and of motility.

Fimbrial antigens
Fimbriae occur as small filaments situated over the whole surface of a bacterium. They are shorter and thinner than flagella and can be seen under the electron microscope but not under a light microscope. Fimbriae are antigenic and although they occur on some bacteria belonging to different groups of the family *Enterobacteriaceae* (including *Escherichia, Salmonella, Proteus, Klebsiella, Shigella* and *Cloaca*), their antigens are not specific for bacterial serotypes nor for groups. Repeated subculturing of fimbriate bacteria on solid media may result in the loss of fimbriae, and conversely, growth in fluid media encourages their development. Bacteria possessing fimbriae agglutinate red blood cells of various animal species and of man, and organisms without fimbriae fail to show this property. This form of haemagglutination reaction is due to the adherence of fimbriae to the surfaces of red blood cells.

Common antigen (CA)
Detailed examination of the antigenic structures of *Escherichia* and *Salmonella* has shown that some serotypes (e.g. *E. coli* O14 and *S. typhimurium*) develop another somatic antigen in addition to the O antigen referred to above. Since it appears to be common to many members of different bacterial groups, it is referred to as the common antigen. Common antigen is composed of polysaccharide, it is not destroyed by a temperature of 100°C and is soluble in 85 per cent ethanol. It may be that this antigen plays a significant role in the pathogenesis of disease, since the presence of common antigen derived from one bacterial serotype in the host may stimulate an immune response against the common

antigen of a second and different serotype which subsequently invades the host's tissues.

Enterotoxin

Many experiments have been designed to identify the substance or substances produced by *E. coli* which cause diarrhoea in animals. The so-called enteropathogenic property of these organisms was demonstrated by inoculating strains of either living or heat-killed *E. coli* into ligated loops of small intestine and observing distension and accumulation of fluid. The results showed that these reactions were not produced by all strains but only by those producing enterotoxin. Enterotoxin is composed of a heat-stable and a heat-labile fraction. The heat-stable fraction is unaffected by a temperature of 60°C for 30 minutes, it is inactivated by heating to 121°C and occurs extracellularly in a culture. The heat-labile fraction is inactivated by a temperature of 60°C for 30 minutes and occurs mainly within bacterial cells. It is also antigenic and can be neutralized by antiserum. The ability to produce enterotoxin can be transmitted by conjugation from some strains to other deficient strains of *E. coli* and also to some strains of *S. typhimurium* and *S. choleraesuis*.

Colicins

These belong to a class of bacterial products known as bacteriocins. They are composed of proteins and have bactericidal activities. The first group of bacteriocins to be studied was derived from *E. coli* and termed colicins. Characteristically, they become attached to specific receptors on the surfaces of susceptible bacteria, causing the death of these organisms. The specificity of this bactericidal effect is of epidemiological value and is used as a method for differentiating between strains of *E. coli*.

Serological typing

The complex antigenic structures of strains of *E. coli* are composed of O, K and H antigens. Comparison of these antigens by serological methods has shown that there are 146 different O antigens, 91 K antigens, 49 H·antigens, and their identification (especially O and K antigens) is used as the method of classifying strains of *E. coli* into serotypes. Each serotype can be expressed by a formula recording its characteristic antigenic structure. An important epidemiological feature is the considerable amount of host species specificity shown by these organisms.

E. coli infections in horses

Epidemiology and pathogenesis

New-born foals can suffer from a disease known as joint ill, navel ill or 'sleepy foal disease', which may be associated with a variety of bacteria including *E. coli*, *Actinobacillus equuli* (*Bacterium viscosum equi*), salmonellae and streptococci. A small proportion of equine abortions has been attributed to *E. coli* infection.

Symptoms

E. coli infection causes a rise in body temperature and general weakness in foals during the first 2–3 days after birth. Some animals suffer from severe diarrhoea and death may occur rapidly. In others the symptoms include lameness resulting from localised infection of the joints.

Lesions

These are characteristic of a septicaemia and are not specific for *E. coli* infection. Lesions include petechial haemorrhages in the intestinal mucosa, some engorgement of the liver and spleen, absence of food in the stomach and very fluid contents in the small and large intestines. There may be a purulent inflammation of the joints.

Diagnosis

E. coli can be isolated in pure culture from the visceral organs of fresh carcases and from affected joints.

Control and prevention

In those cases which develop acute symptoms within a few hours of birth, death may supervene before treatment can be commenced. Antibiotic treatment similar to that employed for *E. coli* infections in other animal species can be adopted. As a preventive measure on premises where this condition is known to recur, antibiotic therapy may be of value. Beneficial results have also been claimed from the transfusion of maternal blood to foals as a means of enhancing passive immunity in the young animal.

E. coli infections in cattle

Epidemiology and pathogenesis

This is a disease of economic importance, and for over half a century *E. coli* has been associated with the aetiology of this condition. It must also be emphasised that a similar clinical condition in calves may be associated with salmonella infections and nutritional problems.

E. coli are normal inhabitants of the intestinal tracts of healthy calves, and colibacillosis only arises as a result of the rapid multiplication of certain serotypes of *E. coli*. For example, it has been estimated that there may be more than a 24-fold increase in the number of *E. coli* excreted in the faeces of calves suffering from diarrhoea, compared with the number excreted by healthy calves. The predisposing conditions which provide a suitable environment for this rapid multiplication are not clearly understood.

Very soon after birth a calf ingests *E. coli* from its environment and the organisms become established as part of the normal intestinal bacterial flora. The importance of colostrum as a means of transferring passive immunity from cow to calf is well established; and since adult animals normally develop antibodies against *E. coli*, colostrum may inhibit the sudden and abnormal rate of multiplication of these organisms in the calf and thus the subsequent development of a colisepticaemia. For this reason, it is important that the calf ingests colostrum during the first 48 hours after birth, when antibody globulins are readily absorbed by the intestinal mucosa. If the antibodies present in colostrum are heterologous for the antigens of *E. coli* in the calf, the beneficial effect will be either greatly reduced or absent.

Certain serotypes of *E. coli* predominate on different farms. Thus, when an in-calf cow is moved from one premises to another shortly before calving, the antibodies available in her colostrum will be related to serotypes of *E. coli* indigenous on the original farm, which may be antigenically distinct from those the calf will ingest from the environment where it is born. Under these circumstances the colostrum which the calf ingests may be of little benefit, and when passive immunity derived from colostrum is ineffective, the animal may suffer from a severe and sometimes fatal *E. coli* infection. Young calves which are subjected to the stresses and strains of movement from one premises to another, including dealers' premises and markets, develop an increased susceptibility to clinical infection with *E. coli*. In addition, they may have been deprived of colostrum, and ingest pathogenic serotypes of the organism from contact with other calves during transit.

Symptoms

In acute cases the symptoms are those of scouring, weakness and prostration. Death may occur in a matter of hours after the initial onset of symptoms.

In less acute cases the calf becomes listless, fails to suck and develops diarrhoea. The faeces are greyish-white in colour (hence the term White Scour) and have an unpleasant fetid odour. In some animals, tenderness and swelling of the joints may occur and also signs of pneumonia. The calf becomes increasingly weak, lies on the ground and is unable to rise. At this stage the body temperature may be several degrees above normal, the animal will show signs of abdominal pain, and the faeces will be of a very loose consistency containing mucus which may be blood stained. As the disease progresses, signs of general weakness increase, the temperature falls to subnormal and the animal becomes comatose and dies.

Lesions

Significant lesions may be absent except in those animals which have died from a colisepticaemia and where localised multiplication of *E. coli* has occurred in the tissues. In cases of pneumonia the lungs may show areas of congestion and necrosis. The spleen and mesenteric lymph nodes are sometimes enlarged and congested, and joint infections develop as a synovitis.

Diagnosis

Final diagnosis depends upon the isolation of *E. coli* from various organs in cases of septicaemic infections, and on the isolation of *E. coli* in profuse numbers and almost pure culture from the intestinal tract using blood agar or similar non-inhibitory media. It is important that cultures are made from the carcase as soon after death as possible to avoid the presence of post-mortem invaders increasing the difficulty of interpreting the results of bacteriological examinations.

Control and prevention

The importance of feeding colostrum during the first 48 hours after birth has already been discussed. This can provide the calf with passively acquired antibodies homologous to the *E. coli* serotypes which it ingests during early life. To obtain the maximum benefit from this passive immunity, the parent cow should not be moved to a new environment shortly before calving.

The injection of antisera as a means of conferring a passive immunity on the calf has been resorted to on many occasions with variable results. Advantage has been taken of the fact that adult bovine sera contain antibodies to *E. coli*, and sera derived from either the dam or other cattle have been injected by various routes into newborn calves. Doses of serum must be relatively large to be effective; and the development of methods for the concentration of serum globulins into smaller volumes provides a more practical method for preventing this type of disease.

It is important to remember that colostrum is not only a source of passive immunity for the calf but also a food containing proteins and vitamin A. There is a good deal of evidence to show that young calves on a diet which includes vitamin A are not so susceptible to White Scour, and that suckling calves born to cows which have been on a diet rich in vitamin A, and consequently with a high vitamin A content in the colostrum, are less likely to contract White Scour.

Calves should be kept under hygienic conditions

with adequate draught-free ventilation and sunlight in buildings which are well insulated from sudden changes in temperature. Vaccination of calves against *E. coli* infections has generally proved to be of little benefit.

Antibiotics have been used in the prevention and treatment of colibacillosis, particularly oxytetracy-cline, chlortetracycline and streptomycin. The greatest value has been derived when these substances are given orally for several days beginning within 24 hours of birth. It has been the practice on some farms to feed antibiotics as a prophylactic measure but this has resulted in the development of resistant strains of *E. coli*.

Bovine mastitis

E. coli is associated with a proportion of cases of acute bovine mastitis. In the United Kingdom there is evidence that the incidence of this type of mastitis has increased during the last decade.

Usually the disease is acute and one or more quarters of the udder become swollen, hot and painful. Milk production falls rapidly and may cease. There may also be generalised systemic disturbances including a rise in temperature and loss of appetite.

Antibiotics should be given parenterally because of the acute nature of this form of mastitis. Oxytetra-cycline, chlortetracycline and streptomycin given intramuscularly have been effective in the treatment of this condition.

E. coli infections in sheep and goats

Enteritis in lambs and kids caused by *E. coli* and sometimes associated with a septicaemia has been described on a number of occasions and is a similar disease to that which occurs in calves. Lambs and kids are particularly vulnerable to this infection during the first two days of life. Symptoms include a rise in temperature, weakness and lack of appetite. This is soon followed by coma and death within a few hours. In older animals there is a tendency for infection to localise itself in the joints of survivors. Lesions include enlarged, haemorrhagic spleens, and the accumulation of synovial fluid and sometimes pus in affected joints. *E. coli* can be isolated from the sites of lesions.

E. coli infections in pigs

Pigs are particularly susceptible to diseases associated with *E. coli* during the first 12 weeks or so after birth. Various names have been given to these conditions according to the age, symptoms and lesions which develop. For the sake of clarity all these infections will be considered under two headings, namely, piglet diarrhoea and oedema disease.

Piglet diarrhoea (*piglet scours*)

Investigations from many countries have emphasised the economic importance of this disease which is associated with the rapid multiplication of particular serotypes of *E. coli*. Many of these strains are haemolytic.

Symptoms. Baby pigs are highly susceptible during the first 4 days after birth and again when about 3 weeks old. Newborn piglets appear healthy for the first 12 hours or so after birth and then become listless and show signs of diarrhoea. Death will occur during the following 12–18 hours. In some instances piglets collapse and die without showing any definite symptoms. Usually there are a few survivors in each affected litter.

In young pigs aged 2–3 weeks the symptoms are mainly of severe scouring with sudden onset. The mortality rate is usually low.

Lesions. In cases of piglet diarrhoea there may be no specific lesions, but frequently the intestines show areas of congestion and the stomach is filled with clotted milk.

Diagnosis. Cultures taken from the small and large intestines will give a heavy and almost pure growth of *E. coli*. Similar results may also be obtained from the stomach. In fresh carcases *E. coli* is not usually detectable in sites other than these, with the possible exception of the brain. *E. coli* serotypes isolated from pigs usually belong to the groups O8, O138, O141 and O147.

Control and prevention. Successful treatment of piglet diarrhoea has been reported following the administration of antibiotics, including chloramphenicol, chlortetracycline and oxytetracycline. To prevent newborn piglets becoming affected, antibiotics have been injected into sows a few days before farrowing to obtain a sufficient concentration of the drug in the colostrum and milk soon after the birth of the piglets.

Attempts to prevent piglet diarrhoea by vaccination of the sow during pregnancy, thus enhancing the degree of passive immunity transferred via the colostrum and milk, have not always proved successful. Similarly, the dosing of newborn piglets with hyperimmune serum has also proved unreliable.

It is important to remember that piglet diarrhoea is a disease which develops largely as a result of modern intensive methods of pig husbandry, and a great deal can be done to prevent the disease by giving particular attention to maintaining high standards of hygiene. Piglets must be kept warm and free from draughts. Farrowing pens should be thoroughly disinfected before each litter, and pregnant sows should receive a diet rich in vitamin A and iron.

Oedema disease

Oedema disease is the name given to *E. coli* infections occurring in pigs of good condition at about 1 week after weaning. The name is descriptive and refers to the oedematous lesions which occur in various parts of the body.

Epidemiology and pathogenesis. The disease is commonly associated with only a few serotypes of *E. coli*, particularly those belonging to groups O139, O138 and O141. Consequent upon weaning and a change in diet, the microenvironment in the intestines becomes favourable for the rapid multiplication of *E. coli* in the intestines. The problem which continues to be a subject for debate is the manner in which this sudden increased population of *E. coli* is responsible for disease. It is believed by some that the production of a toxin or toxins is responsible for the development of the characteristic symptoms and lesions. Others have suggested that as the bacteria may be normal inhabitants of the intestines before the onset of disease, the host will have developed antibodies against them. Subsequently, when the organisms multiply rapidly there is an increased absorption of bacterial antigen or hapten by the intestinal wall, followed by antigen–antibody combination in the tissues giving rise to a hypersensitive reaction.

Symptoms. Oedema disease usually occurs about 1 week after weaning when the animals are about 8–12 weeks of age. Characteristically, the pigs show varying degrees of inco-ordination and in some cases paralysis. Occasionally, deaths occur suddenly and unheralded by obvious symptoms. Many affected pigs will show twitching of the ears and trembling, a staggering gait, and emit a peculiar hoarse squeal. There may be marked oedema of the eyelids, ears and face. Severe constipation commonly occurs.

Lesions. In many instances, examination of the intact carcase shows oedematous areas of the eyelids, ears and face. The abdominal cavity may contain a quantity of clear fluid, containing strands of fibrin, and similar accumulations of fluid may have developed in the pleural and pericardial sacs. In pigs examined soon after death, there is a characteristic oedematous thickening of the wall of the stomach, commonly in the cardiac zone, but sometimes in other areas of the stomach wall (Plate 6.1c, facing p. 100). This oedema may vary in thickness from 1–2 mm to 1–2 cm. In some instances oedema

may be seen in mesenteric lymph nodes and in the mesentery adjacent to the colon.

The main features revealed by histological examination are infiltrations of lymphocytes, plasma cells, and eosinophils around blood vessels in the submucosa, bronchi and in the connective tissue of the portal tract. Frequently, there are areas of haemorrhage in the lungs.

Diagnosis. This includes a typical history of the disease affecting pigs in good condition soon after weaning. The sudden onset of the characteristic symptoms, and the typical lesions observed in a fresh carcase are, collectively, strongly suggestive of the disease. Confirmation is obtained from the isolation in almost pure culture on blood agar or other solid media of one of the serotypes of *E. coli* commonly associated with oedema disease.

Control and prevention. No reliable methods are known for the treatment and prevention of oedema disease. Various approaches to this problem have included the use of *E. coli* antisera, vaccines and antibiotics.

E. coli infections in poultry

Epidemiology and pathogenesis

In recent years, colibacillosis has become an important disease particularly of broiler chickens aged about 6–9 weeks, and less frequently of young chicks during the first fortnight after hatching. Similar conditions have also been reported in turkey poults. The incidence of the disease has increased with the introduction and development of intensive methods of rearing young birds, and there is no doubt that methods of husbandry constitute important predisposing conditions.

Colibacillosis takes the form of either an acute generalised infection with *E. coli* which may be fatal, or a chronic, debilitating condition. Relatively few serotypes are involved in this disease. Organisms belonging to group O2 are isolated most frequently, and a smaller proportion of cases are infected with group O78, O1 and other serotypes.

Modern methods of broiler husbandry, particularly in relation to inadequate ventilation and overcrowding, are suitable for the build-up of *E. coli* infection in the environment of poultry houses, and for the rapid transfer of these organisms from one bird to another. It is probable that although *E. coli* is a normal inhabitant of the intestinal tract, the onset of colibacillosis under these conditions of husbandry may result from the inhalation of these organisms from an unusually heavily contaminated atmosphere.

E. coli can be isolated without difficulty from

various organs of affected birds and typical lesions of the disease can be produced following intravenous inoculation of *E. coli*. However, there is still some doubt as to the significance of the organism as a primary cause of disease. A variety of predisposing factors other than intensive methods of husbandry, may be of importance in the pathogenesis of colibacillosis, particularly concurrent infections with organisms of the pleuropneumonia group and respiratory viruses (e.g. infectious bronchitis).

Symptoms

The disease occurs more particularly in the winter months in birds aged 6–9 weeks. Mortality is usually about 5 per cent but sometimes higher. Deaths of some birds may occur rapidly while in others there may be loss of appetite, respiratory distress, diarrhoea and weakness. Survivors show signs of unthriftiness.

Lesions

Characteristically there is a pericarditis, usually appearing as a thickened pericardial sac adherent to the myocardium and containing a quantity of purulent exudate. Other lesions include inflammation of air sacs which may contain caseous material, an enlarged, congested liver with gelatinous exudate over its surface, an engorged spleen, and in younger chicks the caeca may be filled with caseous material.

Diagnosis

The clinical history, symptoms and lesions are strongly suggestive of colibacillosis. Confirmation is obtained by the isolation of *E. coli* from the visceral organs. The resultant growths derived from fresh carcases will be profuse and often consist of pure cultures of a particular serotype of *E. coli*.

Control and prevention

Good husbandry methods can do a great deal to reduce the factors which predispose to this disease. Particular attention should be given to maintaining high standards of cleanliness and disinfection of premises and equipment between each batch of chicks. Excessive overcrowding should be avoided, and adequate ventilation, particularly in cold weather, is essential to reduce the risks of inhalation of *E. coli* and other predisposing microorganisms, including mycoplasmas and respiratory viruses.

The use of antibiotics may be of limited value for financial reasons and also because of the increasing problem of the development of drug resistant strains of *E. coli*.

E. coli infections in dogs

E. coli, particularly haemolytic strains of serotype O42, have been associated with acute generalised infections in puppies and with either intestinal or urogenital infections in older animals, including pyometra and occasionally cystitis.

Symptoms

In newborn puppies the disease may be so acute that the only symptoms before death are weakness and a lack of appetite. Whole litters may be affected and this form of the disease has been referred to as 'fading puppy disease'. In older dogs the symptoms may be those of acute enteritis, a raised body temperature which may become subnormal during the terminal stages of the disease, excessive thirst, a persistent diarrhoea and general weakness. *E. coli* is also associated with some cases of pyometra in the bitch, causing distension of the uterus and a uterine discharge. In some cases the condition becomes acute and in others chronic over a period of a few years.

Lesions

The post-mortem examination of newborn puppies which have died from a generalised infection with *E. coli*, usually reveals petechial haemorrhages throughout the carcase, congested lungs and haemorrhagic gastroenteritis. Examinations of older dogs which have suffered from enteritis show congested livers, spleens and mesenteric lymph nodes, and acute gastroenteritis. In cases of pyometra the uterus is grossly distended and contains a brownish fluid.

Diagnosis

E. coli can be readily isolated from the fresh carcases of young puppies which have died from this infection. The organism often belongs to group O42. Bacteriological examination of older animals which have died from acute enteritis will show the presence of *E. coli* in some organs, including the spleen, mesenteric lymph nodes and intestines. *E. coli* can be isolated from the uterine contents in cases of pyometra.

Control and prevention

Some success has been claimed from the use of autogenous vaccines for the treatment and prevention of *E. coli* infections. Antibiotics are also of value provided that prompt treatment is instituted.

E. coli infections in laboratory animals

Disease associated with *E. coli* has been reported in various species of laboratory animals, including guinea-pigs, rats, mice and rabbits. A severe mucoid enteritis is a disease of rabbits which is of commercial importance since the mortality rate may be as high as 10–15 per cent. *E. coli* can be readily isolated from various sections of the gastrointestinal tract.

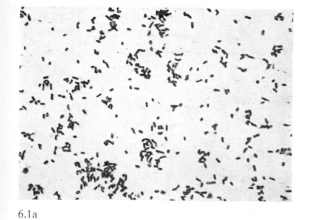

6.1a

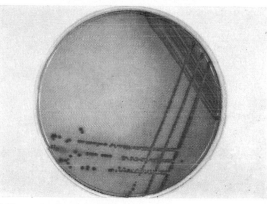

6.1b

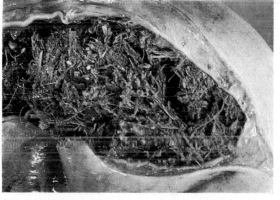

6.1c

6.1a Gram-stained film of culture of *Escherichia coli*, ×930.

6.1b Colonies of *Escherichia coli* on MacConkey's agar plate showing fermentation of lactose (pink colouration).

6.1c Oedematous thickening of the wall of a pig's stomach from a case of oedema disease.

However, although there is evidence to show that *E. coli* multiplies rapidly in affected animals, its role as a primary cause of disease is still in doubt. Ligated loops of rabbit intestine have been employed experimentally to assess the ability of different serotypes of *E. coli* derived from various animal species and from man, to cause dilatation of the gut.

Further reading

ALWIS, M.C.L. DE AND THOMLINSON, J.R. (1973) The incidence and distribution of colicinogenic and colicin-sensitive *Escherichia coli* in the gastro-intestinal tract of the pig. *Journal of General Microbiology*, **74**, 45.

BRANDENBURG, A.C. (1974) Immunity to *Escherichia coli* in pigs. IgG and blood clearance. *Research in Veterinary Science*, **16**, 171.

BUXTON A. AND THOMLINSON J.R. (1961) The detection of tissue-sensitizing antibodies to *Escherichia coli* in oedema disease, haemorrhagic gastro-enteritis and in normal pigs. *Research in Veterinary Science*, **2**, 73.

CLUGSTON, R.E. AND NIELSEN, N.O. (1974) Experimental edema disease of swine [*E. coli* enterotoxaemia] I. Detection and preparation of an active principle. *Canadian Journal of Comparative Medicine*, **38**, 22.

CLUGSTON, R.E., NIELSEN, N.O. AND ROE, W.E. (1974) Experimental edema disease of swine [*E. coli* enterotoxaemia] II. The development of hypertension after the intravenous administration of edema disease principle. *Canadian Journal of Comparative Medicine*, **38**, 29.

CLUGSTON, R.E., NIELSEN, N.O. AND SMITH, D.L.T. (1974) Experimental edema disease of swine [*E. coli* enterotoxaemia] III. Pathology and pathogenesis. *Canadian Journal of Comparative Medicine*, **38**, 34.

GAY C.C. (1965) *Escherichia coli* and neonatal disease in calves. *Bacteriological Reviews*, **29**, 75.

GRINDLAY, M., RENTON, J.P. AND RAMSAY, D.H. (1973) O-groups of *Escherichia coli* associated with canine pyometra. *Research in Veterinary Science*, **14**, 75.

HELLER, E.D. AND SMITH, H.W. (1973) The incidence of antibiotic resistance and other characteristics amongst *Escherichia coli* strains causing fatal infection in chickens: the utilisation of these characteristics to study the epidemiology of the infection. *Journal of Hygiene*, **71**, 771.

KENWORTHY, R. (1974) Digestibility and balance studies of gnotobiotic pigs undergoing acute intestinal infection with *Escherichia coli*. *Research in Veterinary Science*, **16**, 208.

LARIVIERE, S., GYLES, C.L. AND BARNUM, D.A. (1973) Preliminary characterisation of the heat-labile enterotoxin of *Escherichia coli* F11 [P155]. *Journal of Infectious Diseases*, **128**, 312.

LOGAN, E.F., STENHOUSE, A., ORMROD, D., PENHALE, W.J. AND ARMISHAER, M. (1974) Studies on the immunity of the calf to colibacillosis. VI. The prophylactic use of a pooled serum IgM-rich fraction under field conditions. *Veterinary Record*, **94**, 386.

PARISH W.E. (1972) Host damage resulting from hypersensitivity to bacteria. *Society for General Microbiology*, Symposium 22, p. 157.

PENHALE, W.J., LOGAN, E.F., SELMAN, I.E., FISHER, E.W. AND McEWAN, A.D. (1973) Observations on the absorption of colostral immunoglobulins by the neonatal calf and their significance in colibacillosis. *Annales de Recherches Vétérinaires*, **4**, 223.

PORTER, K., KENWORTHY, R., HOLME, D.W. AND HORSFIELD, S. (1973) *Escherichia coli* antigens as dietary additives for oral immunisation of pigs: trials with pig creep feeds. *Veterinary Record*, **92**, 630.

RUTTER, J.M. (1975) *Escherichia coli* infections in piglets: Pathogenesis, virulence and vaccination. *Veterinary Record*, **96**, 171.

RUTTER, J.M. AND LUTHER, P.D. (1973) Cytopathic factors in bacteria-free lysates of *Escherichia coli*. *Journal of Medical Microbiology*, **6**, 565.

SHREEVE, B.J. AND THOMLINSON, J.R. (1971) Hypersensitivity of young piglets to *Escherichia coli* endotoxin. *Journal of Medical Microbiology*, **4**, 307.

SOJKA W.J. (1965) *Escherichia coli* in domestic animals and poultry. Farnham Royal Commonwealth Agricultural Bureaux.

SOJKA W.J. (1971) Enteric diseases in new-born piglets, calves and lambs due to *Escherichia coli* infection. *Veterinary Bulletin*, **41**, 509.

STEVENS, J.B., GYLES, C.L. AND BARNUM, D.A. (1972) Production of diarrhoea in pigs in response to *Escherichia coli* enterotoxin. *American Journal of Veterinary Research*, **33**, 2511.

TENNANT, B. [Editor] (1971) Neonatal enteric infections caused by *Escherichia coli*. *Annals of the New York Academy of Sciences*, **176**, pp. 405.

TRUSCOTT, R.B. (1973) Studies on the chick-lethal toxin of *Escherichia coli*. *Canadian Journal of Comparative Medicine*, **37**, 375.

TRUSCOTT, R.B. LOPEZ-ALVAREZ, J. AND PETTIT, J.R. (1974) Studies on *Escherichia coli* infection in chickens. *Canadian Journal of Comparative Medicine*, **38**, 160.

WILKINSON, G.T. (1974) O-groups of *E. coli* in the vagina and alimentary tract of the dog. *Veterinary Record*, **94**, 105.

WRAY, C. AND THOMLINSON, J.R. (1972) The effects

of *Escherichia coli* endotoxin in calves. *Research in Veterinary Science*, **13**, 546.

WRAY, C. AND THOMLINSON, J.R. (1972) Dermal reactions to endotoxins in calves: their significance in the pathogenesis of Colibacillosis. *Research in Veterinary Science*, **13**, 554.

WRAY, C. AND THOMLINSON, J.R. (1972) Anaphylactic shock to *Escherichia coli* endotoxin in calves. *Research in Veterinary Science*, **13**, 563.

WRAY, C. AND THOMLINSON, J.R. (1974) Lesions and bacteriological findings in colibacillosis of calves. *British Veterinary Journal*, **130**, 189.

CHAPTER 7

SALMONELLA

Salmonella

Distribution in nature

The first member of this group to be studied was the typhoid bacillus, originally observed in human tissues by Eberth in 1880 and cultured by Gaffkey in 1884. Soon afterwards, Salmon and Smith reported on an organism (*Bacillus cholerae suis*) which they isolated from diseased pigs, and similar isolations were made in the following years from a wide variety of human and animal sources. The name *Salmonella* is in memory of Salmon and his early work on these organisms which now comprise a large group of more than 1000 different serotypes having a world-wide distribution.

A striking feature about the natural distribution of salmonellae is the relative host species specificity of a few serotypes and the ubiquitous habits of the majority. *S. typhi*, *S. paratyphi A* and *S. paratyphi C* are serotypes common to man, and it is only under unusual and rare conditions that these organisms are responsible for disease in animals. Similarly, among animals there are some organisms which show a particular specificity for certain species, including *S. abortus equi* for horses, *S. dublin* for cattle, *S. abortus ovis* for sheep, *S. choleraesuis* for pigs, and *S. pullorum* and *S. gallinarum* for poultry. The remaining members of the group are ubiquitous and potentially pathogenic for animals and man, alike. The most outstanding example is *S. typhimurium* which is frequently the cause of disease throughout the world in a variety of animal species as well as in man.

Since the majority of these organisms are potentially pathogenic for both man and animals, an important aspect of the epidemiology of salmonellosis is the risk of human infection arising from animal sources, and less frequently the occurrence of animal infections derived from man. Salmonellae are typically intestinal pathogens, and infected individuals may excrete the organisms intermittently in the faeces, contaminate the environment, and transfer infection to others. It is common for some infected individuals who excrete the organisms to remain clinically normal, and this 'carrier' condition may persist for months or years in several species of domesticated animals, and is particularly common among reptiles.

Morphology and staining

These organisms usually occur as short rods, measuring 2–4 μm in length and 0·5 μm in width (Plate 7.1a, facing p. 114). Occasionally, they develop into longer pleomorphic forms or very short coccobacilli after prolonged culture on laboratory media. With the exception of *S. pullorum* and *S. gallinarum*, all strains normally possess peritrichous flagella and are actively motile. Many serotypes are also known to develop fimbriae. Capsule formation has sometimes been observed and is associated more particularly with mucoid strains. Spore formation does not occur.

The organisms stain Gram-negative.

Cultural characteristics

Salmonellae are aerobic and facultatively anaerobic. They grow well on laboratory media at 37°C without the addition of blood, serum, ascitic fluid, glucose, etc., and after overnight incubation in broth a smooth strain will have produced an even turbidity, usually with no pellicle formation. With the majority of serotypes, growth on agar gives rise to round, smooth colonies of 2–3 mm in diameter (Plate 7.1b, facing p. 114). However, a few serotypes, including *S. pullorum*, *S. choleraesuis* and *S. abortus ovis*, grow less abundantly on solid media and develop characteristically as small dew-drop like colonies after 18 hours' and even 48 hours' incubation.

The fact that salmonellae commonly exist in the intestines where other related bacterial species are also present, means that reliable methods for isolation require the use of media which encourage the growth of salmonellae and inhibit that of other enteric organisms. A great variety of fluid and solid enrichment and selective media have been devised. Selenite broth is a useful fluid medium which allows the growth of salmonellae but inhibits other enteric organisms. Tetrathionate broth has similar properties. A number of different solid selective media have been developed and those most widely used are desoxycholate citrate agar (DCA), MacConkey's agar and brilliant green agar. Under most conditions, preliminary cultivation in fluid media followed by the use of selective media has proved more reliable than direct plating on selective media alone. One method is to inoculate material into selenite broth, incubate overnight and then plate on to desoxycholate citrate agar. After overnight incubation on this solid medium, salmonellae appear as pale coloured, lactose non-fermenting colonies. A more reliable modification of this method consists of inoculating material into selenite broth, incubating in a water-bath for 18–24 hours at 43°C, subculturing on to Difco brilliant green agar and incubating this mildly selective medium at 37°C. Meanwhile, the selenite broth is re-incubated for a further period of 18–24 hours at 43°C and then subcultured on to a second Difco brilliant green agar plate. Particular care should be taken when isolating *S. pullorum* and *S. abortus ovis*, since these organisms grow sparsely and may only appear as extremely small colonies on desoxycholate citrate agar plates after prolonged incubation. When isolating *S. choleraesuis* from contaminated material it is advisable to omit using enrichment media and to plate the material direct on to solid differential media. This direct method gives a higher isolation rate than the indirect method.

Detailed examination of cultural characteristics is required to distinguish between salmonellae and other closely related groups in the family Enterobacteriaceae (see Table 6.2, p.94). There are few exceptions to the rule that salmonellae do not ferment lactose, sucrose or salicin, and that they do ferment glucose, maltose, mannitol, dulcitol and dextrin with production of acid and gas. They are also characterised by their ability to reduce nitrates to nitrites and to produce H_2S. They do not decompose urea, liquefy gelatin or produce indole.

Resistance to physical and chemical agents
Salmonellae are relatively susceptible to chemical and physical agents. A temperature of 55°C for 1 hour or 60°C for 20 minutes is lethal to these organisms, and they are killed rapidly by autoclaving at 120°C. They are highly susceptible to phenol and cresol, although the lethal action of these disinfectants may be reduced in the presence of mucus or faeces. Similarly, the bactericidal effect of quaternary ammonium compounds is greatly reduced in the presence of protein. Formaldehyde vapour, which is used to fumigate egg incubators and other equipment on poultry farms, is effective as a disinfectant but its efficiency is reduced in the presence of colloidal or organic matter. The lethal effect of heat on salmonellae in human foods varies according to the serotypes involved and the materials which are contaminated. As a general rule, milk should be heated to 65·6°C for 1–2 seconds, egg yolk to 60°C for 30 seconds, whole egg to 55°C for 10 minutes and meat to 65°C for 10–15 minutes.

Antigens and toxins
The surface of the bacterial cell is composed of lipopolysaccharide–protein complexes which constitute the somatic (O) antigens. In addition, most salmonella serotypes possess flagella and are motile. These flagella are composed of protein (flagellin) and constitute the flagellar (H) antigen. A detailed study of these antigens has shown that there is a very large number of different O and H antigens and their identification is used as the basis for the serological classification of these organisms into serotypes. This method of classification, started by White and Kauffmann in 1929, has been continued and developed until now there are more than one thousand serotypes which can be distinguished, one from another, by their antigenic structures.

O antigens
There is a large number of different O antigens occurring in the salmonella group and the majority of organisms possess more than one of these on their surfaces. Each antigen has been designated by a number and in the case of *S. typhimurium*, for example, the O antigen complex is represented by the numbers 1, 4, 5, 12. This means that the surface of the organism is composed of four distinct antigenic groupings. Similarly, the O antigens of *S.dublin* are represented by the numbers 1, 9, 12 and those of *S. choleraesuis* by 6, 7.

The development of this classification has shown that numbers of organisms possess similar O antigens and they have been allocated into groups, accordingly. For example, group B consists of all those serotypes possessing O antigens 4, 12, group C1 organisms possess antigens 6, 7, group C2 includes antigens 6, 8, and group D1 includes 9, 12.

H antigens
The variety of flagellar antigens distributed among organisms belonging to any particular O group is used as a basis for distinguishing between individual serotypes within each group. For example, *S. abortus equi* and *S. abortus ovis* both possess the O antigens 4 and 12, and they can be distinguished one from the other by their different flagellar antigens. Detailed serological examination of flagellar antigens has shown that many organisms are capable of producing either one or two serologically distinct flagellar antigens. For example, the flagellar antigens of *S. typhimurium* are represented by either i or 1, 2,

the organism is called diphasic and the antigens are classified as either phase 1 (antigen i) or phase 2 (antigen 1, 2). Phase 1 antigens are identified by letters of the alphabet and latterly, as the number of these antigens has exceeded 26, the remainder have been given the letter Z and a number (e.g. Z_{10}, Z_{29}, etc.). Phase 2 antigens are signified by numbers (e.g. 1, 2, etc.). It should be emphasised that an individual organism of a diphasic serotype develops flagella belonging to only one phase and not to a mixture of both phases. Thus, a culture of *S. typhimurium* in phase 1 consists of a majority of organisms with i flagella and a minority with 1, 2 flagella. Conversely, a similar culture in phase 2 would consist of a majority of organisms with 1, 2 flagella.

Vi antigen

This is a somatic antigen additional to those already described above, and is associated with the virulence of *S. typhi* for mice and occurs on a few other serotypes. It is present on the surfaces of newly isolated virulent strains of *S. typhi* but is lost after repeated subcultivation when the organisms also lose their virulence for mice. Vi antigen is of little significance in relation to salmonellosis in animals but is of importance for the Vi phage typing of newly isolated strains of *S. typhi* in the study of the epidemiology of typhoid fever.

Smooth——→Transient——→Rough variation

The growths on solid media of newly isolated strains of salmonellae are characterised by the development of smooth colonies which are circular in outline with a convex, smooth, glistening surface. After repeated subcultivation, rough colonies may develop which have a roughened, crenated outline and a dull wrinkled appearance. This variation from smooth to rough (S——→R) may be associated with other changes, including the loss of O antigen and exposure of a serologically distinct and non-specific rough (R) antigen, the loss of virulence and the autoagglutination of rough bacteria when suspended in physiological saline or in a solution of acriflavine. Some strains develop T (transient) mutants which have properties intermediate between those of smooth and rough variants. These T mutants develop as smooth colonies on solid media although they are devoid of demonstrable O antigen, and have a strong tendency to mutate to the rough form.

Identification of serotypes

Preliminary rapid slide tests can be carried out using standard polyvalent O and polyvalent H (phase 1 and phase 2) antisera which are composite sera containing antibodies to all the respective O and H antigens. One drop of serum mixed with a small quantity of bacterial growth from solid medium will give rapid agglutination when the serum contains antibodies homologous for the antigens of the bacteria under test. Subsequently, a number of O group antisera, each one containing antibodies to the major O antigens in a group, should be used in slide tests to determine the group to which the unknown culture belongs. Thereafter, the culture should be similarly tested against antisera for particular flagellar (phase 1 and phase 2) antigens appropriate for individual serotypes comprising the suspected group to which the organism belongs. All rapid slide tests must be confirmed by tube agglutination tests. To obtain antigens for these latter tests it is customary to use alcohol for the preparation of O antigens and formalin for H antigens. In each case the density of antigen must be standardised before carrying out agglutination tests.

To type a diphasic organism it is necessary to identify both phases of flagellar antigen. The technique consists of growing the organism in semi-solid agar containing antibodies against the antigens to be suppressed. For example, cultures of *S. typhimurium* can be changed from phase 1 (antigen i) to phase 2 (antigen 1, 2.) by growing the organism in medium containing i antiserum. The organisms in phase 1 will be immobilised because their flagella become agglutinated by the antibodies in the serum; meanwhile, organisms in phase 2 will remain actively motile. Separation of the two phases is facilitated by the use of a Craigie tube (Fig. 7.1)

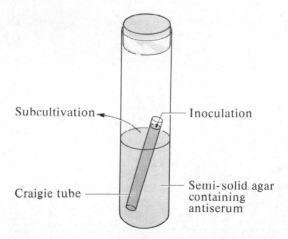

Fig. 7.1. Showing the use of a Craigie tube for changing the phase of salmonellae. Appropriate antiserum for the phase to be suppressed is mixed with the semi-solid agar. The culture is inoculated into the top of the Craigie tube and after the minimum period of incubation, the organisms are subcultured from the surface of the medium outside the Craigie tube.

TABLE 7.1. Classification of salmonellae showing representative serotypes (Kauffmann-White Scheme).

Group	Serotype	Somatic antigens	Flagellar antigens Phase 1	Phase 2
A	S. paratyphi A	1, 2, 12	a	—
B	S. paratyphi B	1, 4, 5, 12	b	1, 2
	S. typhimurium	1, 4, 5, 12	i	1, 2
	S. abortus equi	4, 12	—	e, n, x
	S. abortus ovis	4, 12	c	1, 6
	S. abortus bovis	1, 4, 12, 27	b	e, n, x
C1	S. paratyphi C	6, 7, Vi	c	1, 5
	S. choleraesuis	6, 7	c	1, 5
	S. thompson	6, 7	k	1, 5
C2	S. muenchen	6, 8	d	1, 2
	S. newport	6, 8	e, h	1, 2
	S. bovis morbificans	6, 8	r	1, 5
C3	S. kentucky	(8), 20	i	z_6
C4	S. kaduna	6, (7), (14)	c	e, n, z_{15}
D1	S. typhi	9, 12, Vi	d	—
	S. eneritidis	1, 9, 12	g, m	—
	S. dublin	1, 9, 12	g, p	—
	S. pullorum ⎱ S. gallinarum ⎰	1, 9, 12	—	—
D2	S. plymouth	(9), 46	d	z_6
E1	S. anatum	3, 10	e, h	1, 6
	S. meleagridis	3, 10	e, h	l, w
	S. london	3, 10	l, v	1, 6
E2	S. newington	3, 15	e, h	1, 6
	S. new brunswick	3, 15	l, v	1, 7
E3	S. canoga	(3), (15), 34	g, s, t	—
	S. thomasville	(3), (15), 34	y	1, 5
E4	S. niloese	1, 3, 19	d	z_6
	S. senftenberg	1, 3, 19	g, s, t	—
F	S. aberdeen	11	i	1, 2
	S. senegal	11	r	1, 5
G1	S. ibadan	13, 22	b	1, 5
	S. tanger	1, 13, 22	y	1, 6
G2	S. bracknell	13, 23	b	1, 6
	S. worthington	1, 13, 23	z	l, w
H	S. horsham	1, 6, 14, 25	l, v	e, n, x
I	S. weston	16	e, h	z_6
J	S. kirkee	17	b	1, 2
K	S. memphis	18	k	1, 5
L	S. minnesota	21	b	e, n, x
M	S. patience	28	d	e, n, z_{15}
N	S. urbana	30	b	e, n, x
O	S. adelaide	35	f, g	—
P	S. inverness	38	k	1, 6
Q	S. wandsworth	39	b	1, 2
R	S. tilene	1, 40	e, h	1, 2
S	S. waycross	41	z_4, z_{23}	—
T	S. weslaco	42	z_{36}	—
U	S. berkeley	43	a	1, 5
V	S. gamaba	44	g, m, s	—
W	S. karachi	45	d	e, n, x
X	S. bootle	47	k	1, 5
Y	S. hisingen	48	a	1, 5, 7
Z	S. greenside	50	z	e, n, x
51	S. meskin	51	e, h	1, 2

Also groups 52–60 with their respective O antigens (e.g. group 55 has O antigen 55).

which is open at both ends and inserted into the medium so that the upper end of the tube is well above the level of the medium. After heating and before the medium has solidified, the appropriate antiserum is added and mixed with the semi-solid agar. After inoculation of the culture into the top of the Craigie tube, the medium is incubated for the minimum time necessary for motile organisms, unaffected by the flagellar antibodies, to multiply and move to the surface of the medium outside the Craigie tube from where they are subcultured.

Bacteriophage typing

Phage typing of salmonellae was first applied to *S. typhi*. It has since been adapted to a number of other serotypes and has proved to be particularly useful for epidemiological studies on *S. typhimurium* in animals and man. By means of this technique it is often possible to determine whether the likely origin of *S. typhimurium* infection in a group of animals was derived from a particular source of domesticated or wild animals. In addition, phage typing is often of value in tracing the probable origins of human infections with *S. typhimurium* when these are derived from direct contact with diseased animals, from human foods of animal origin or from another human source.

Salmonellosis in horses

Epidemiology and pathogenesis

The serotypes commonly affecting horses are *S. abortus equi* and *S. typhimurium*.

Animals become infected with *S. abortus equi* usually from ingestion of pasture, food and water which have become contaminated with infected fetal fluids and fetal membranes expelled at the time of an abortion or from infected faeces. Animals of all ages and both sexes may be infected in this way, and subsequently many of them will develop into symptomless carriers and possibly rid themselves of infection during the course of a few months. Infected pregnant mares may abort towards the end of the gestation period or give birth to a dead foal at full term. *S. abortus equi* is occasionally associated with other conditions, including pneumonia, fistulous withers, testicular infections, joint infections and enteritis.

S. typhimurium causes disease in horses in association with predisposing factors, giving rise to gastroenteritis, bronchitis and pneumonia. Infection to young foals at birth may result in acute septicaemia and polyarthritis.

Symptoms

Abortions caused by *S. abortus equi* usually occur during the last two months of pregnancy or at full term, and the mare may show few premonitory symptoms other than mild diarrhoea, slight rise in temperature and inappetence. Newborn foals are susceptible to infection with *S. abortus equi* and the resulting septicaemia gives rise to weakness, diarrhoea, pyrexia, laboured breathing and death within 2–3 days. In some cases infection localises in the navel and joints, particularly the knee, hock and stifle which become hot, swollen and painful.

Lesions

Petechial haemorrhages occur in the heart, spleen and lungs of aborted fetuses and frequently there is excessive fluid in the abdominal cavity and pericardial sac. Fetal membranes are usually oedematous, haemorrhagic and show well-defined areas of necrosis.

Diagnosis

S. abortus equi can be readily isolated in pure culture from a freshly aborted fetus and from fetal membranes. Similar isolations can be made from the visceral organs of young foals which have died from acute septicaemic infections with *S. abortus equi* or with other serotypes. The diagnosis of enteritis in living animals caused by salmonellae depends upon the isolation of these organisms from faeces.

The agglutination test is used for the detection of infected animals. It is important to remember that healthy adults may have a low level of normal agglutinins to the O antigen of *S. abortus equi*, and this level can vary from one country or one district to another within a range of 1/20 to approximately 1/250. For diagnostic purposes positive agglutinin titres must be higher than the average for the district, and are usually in the range of 1/1000 or more. Shortly before an infected mare aborts, her serum agglutinin titre may fall to about 1/50 and increase again during the subsequent 2–3 weeks. Since agglutinins against the H antigen of *S. abortus equi* cannot usually be detected in healthy animals, the presence of these antibodies is strongly indicative of active infection.

Control and prevention

Horses infected with *S. abortus equi* develop an immunity and may become carriers of the organism. Because of this developing immunity, it is unusual for an infected mare to abort more than once. Many attempts have been made to immunize horses against *S. abortus equi* infection. Live vaccines give rise to a solid immunity but the animal may remain a carrier and a source of infection for other horses. Killed vaccines are safer to use but stimulate only a temporary resistance to natural infection.

Salmonellosis in cattle

Epidemiology and pathogenesis

S. dublin and *S. typhimurium* are the most common causes of bovine salmonellosis which affect cattle of all ages, and the disease may be acute or chronic. Calves are more susceptible to infection than adults.

S. dublin infections are known to occur in many countries, particularly throughout Europe, the United Kingdom and in parts of the U.S.A. Infected adults may act as symptomless carriers excreting the organisms intermittently in the faeces, and the incidence of such animals may vary from 0·4 per cent to as high as 10 per cent in some districts. *S. dublin* can survive in faeces for some 2–4 months depending upon the atmospheric conditions. Pastures, food and water may become contaminated from the faeces of carrier animals or from aborted fetuses and fetal membranes, and infection will spread to other cattle by ingestion. This can result in the development of acute and fatal infection, complete recovery, or the development of carrier animals which may continue to excrete the organisms intermittently in the faeces for several years. It is usual for only a few cattle in each infected herd to develop clinical signs of disease and a proportion of the remainder become subclinically infected. Among adult cattle, factors predisposing to the development of clinical infection include intercurrent diseases (e.g. parasitic infestations), poor nutrition and the stresses of transport and movement from one premises to another.

S. dublin infection of calves is usually acute and spreads rapidly from one calf to another. The disease commonly arises from the ingestion of infected faeces contaminating food, milk, water, bedding and pastures. Long distance transportation associated with stress and irregular feeding, increases the susceptibility of calves and the risk of contracting infection.

S. typhimurium is ubiquitous among different animal species and it is possible for this bovine infection to originate from disease in another animal species as well as from cattle. The epidemiology and pathogenesis of this disease is similar to infection with *S. dublin* except that the development of chronic carriers over a period of several years does not occur so frequently.

Symptoms

In adult cattle the signs of acute infection are a rise in temperature (40–41°C), inappetence, a sudden drop in milk yield and diarrhoea. During the following 24 hours the diarrhoea may develop into dysentery and the body temperature becomes subnormal. Pregnant animals may abort and death may occur during the following 2–3 days. More protracted cases rapidly become emaciated, dehydrated and show signs of abdominal pain. Complete recovery takes several months and some animals infected with *S. dublin* may remain carriers for years. Others may show little or no symptoms of infection but excrete salmonellae intermittently in the faeces for a period of several weeks or months.

Infection in young calves during the first 2 weeks of life causes a sudden loss of appetite, weakness, diarrhoea and death in a few days. In acute cases the faeces may be blood-stained and mucoid.

Lesions

In adult cattle there are areas of haemorrhagic inflammation and necrosis of the large intestine and similar areas of haemorrhage in the small intestine. The intestinal contents may be blood-stained. Mesenteric lymph glands are often oedematous and haemorrhagic. The wall of the gall bladder may be oedematous, areas of necrosis occur in the liver, and the spleen is often enlarged and congested. In less acute cases the lesions are not so severe but the lungs may show pneumonic areas.

In calves there are often haemorrhages in the myocardium and peritoneum. The mesenteric lymph glands and spleen may be enlarged and hyperaemic. As in adult cattle there may be areas of necrosis in the liver and pneumonic areas in the lungs.

Diagnosis

The symptoms can be only suggestive of salmonellosis and a final diagnosis must depend upon bacteriological examination. During the early febrile stage of the disease in adults, salmonellae will be present in the blood, sometimes in the milk and in faeces. Faecal samples from animals suffering from enteritis should be cultured in sodium selenite broth and desoxycholate citrate agar. There will usually be little difficulty in isolating *S. dublin* or *S. typhimurium* in this manner. At a later stage in the disease when obvious clinical symptoms have subsided, cattle may be excreting salmonellae intermittently in the faeces for periods of weeks or months, and in these cases it may be necessary to examine bacteriologically two or more faecal samples before being able to diagnose infection. At post-mortem examination it may be difficult to isolate the organisms from chronic carriers of *S. dublin* unless relatively large quantities of tissues (e.g. 10–20g) are examined bacteriologically.

Bacterial agglutination tests can be of diagnostic value when used in conjunction with bacteriological examination of faeces. For the interpretation of the agglutination test it is important to remember that one negative result from a suspected case does not necessarily mean that infection is absent because there may be a considerable delay between the initial development of infection and the first appearance of significant antibody titres in the serum. In addition, some chronic carriers of *S. dublin* fail to develop diagnostic agglutinin titres for periods of several months at a time. Many healthy adult cattle possess low levels of serum agglutinins to O and H antigens and it is generally considered that for diagnostic purposes serum titres should be at least 1/40 against the O and 1/320 against the H antigens. Young calves infected with *S. dublin* or *S. typhimurium* sometimes produce H agglutinins more rapidly than O agglutinins. It is important, therefore, to use phase 1 flagellar antigens as well as O antigens when testing calf sera for salmonellosis.

Control and prevention
Many attempts to vaccinate cattle against salmonellosis have had differing results. The problem is that a killed vaccine is safe to use but does not stimulate a high degree of protection. A stronger immunity develops after the use of a live vaccine and the immunogenic properties of live vaccines are related to the virulence of strains used in their production. Attenuated live cultures of *S. dublin* have been developed and are being assessed for safety as well as for protective capacity. To prevent disease in calves the dams have sometimes been vaccinated in an attempt to raise the concentration of antibodies transferred to their calves through the colostrum. The usefulness of this method is doubtful since it may reduce the mortality rate but not the incidence of infection under modern conditions of husbandry. Moreover, disease in calves can develop when they are some weeks old and after a passive immunity derived from colostrum is no longer present. Vaccination of young calves has also been attempted as a preventive measure but has proved unreliable.

Various chemotherapeutic agents have been used to treat salmonellosis, including chloromycetin, terramycin, neomycin, furazolidone, and other substances which may curtail clinical disease when applied promptly but do not always eliminate infection.

In addition to the measures already discussed it is most important to detect and remove all possible sources of infection from a known infected premises, including carrier animals and wild rodents which may harbour the organisms. It is also necessary to ensure that there is no contamination of food or water supplies, and to maintain a high level of farm hygiene.

Salmonellosis in sheep and goats

Epidemiology and pathogenesis
The common serotypes causing disease in these animals are *S. abortus ovis* and *S. typhimurium*.

Other serotypes including *S. dublin*, have been recorded less frequently.

Outbreaks of abortion caused by *S. abortus ovis* have been reported from several countries, particularly in Europe and in areas of south-west England. The common route of infection is by ingestion, and adult animals may be carriers of the organism. Other serotypes, particularly *S. typhimurium* and *S. dublin*, are responsible for enteric infections and occasionally abortions. Lambs are more susceptible than adults and the incidence of clinical disease can be affected by a variety of predisposing factors, including severe weather conditions, the collection of sheep into confined areas (e.g. lambing, shearing), the stresses of transport over long distances, and the presence of concurrent diseases.

Symptoms
Abortion is the classical symptom of infection with *S. abortus ovis* in pregnant animals, and usually occurs during the last two months of pregnancy. It is often preceded by a blood-stained or purulent vaginal discharge. The mortality rate among ewes is normally low. Deaths in lambs from *S. abortus ovis* infection may occur during the first day after birth in those individuals which are born weak, or during the first 10 days of life in strong lambs which suddenly become acutely ill with diarrhoea and dysentery. Other salmonella infections occur as enteric diseases of varying severity. Surviving lambs remain debilitated for many weeks. In adults the symptoms are usually less acute, consisting of intermittent diarrhoea, loss of weight, and areas of the fleece may fall out.

Infected goats show symptoms similar to those in sheep.

Lesions
These include areas of congestion and haemorrhage in the abomasum and small intestine, small haemorrhages in the myocardium and kidney cortex, congestion of the spleen and oedema of the mesenteric lymph nodes. The carcases of lambs which have died from *S. abortus ovis* infection often show lesions of lobar pneumonia.

Diagnosis
In outbreaks of abortion caused by *S. abortus ovis*, the organisms can be isolated in almost pure culture from newly aborted fetuses, fetal membranes and from infected uteri. In cases of acute enteric infection a septicaemia may have developed during the terminal stages of the disease, and salmonellae can be isolated from the visceral organs and blood as well as from the intestines. In less acute outbreaks the organisms are present in the intestines and mesenteric lymph nodes. *S. abortus ovis* can be isolated most

frequently by direct plating on to 5 per cent sheep blood agar or into selenite broth. Growths obtained in the latter may be subcultured on to 5 per cent sheep blood agar. It should be remembered that *S. abortus ovis* grows slowly on laboratory media and cultures may have to be incubated for as long as 72 hours before satisfactory growths are obtained for further examination.

Symptomless carrier animals can be detected by bacterial agglutination tests. Healthy sheep may have normal serum agglutinin titres against the O and H antigens of *S. abortus ovis* and *S. typhimurium*, and average flock titres will vary from district to district. A positive diagnosis of infection can only be made when agglutinin titres are higher than the average titres for the district.

Control and prevention

Vaccination with either killed or live attenuated cultures of *S. abortus ovis* have not proved to be reliable methods for the prevention of abortions. Chemotherapy is of limited value for the treatment of salmonellosis in small groups of animals but is not usually an economic proposition when applied on a large scale. It is of little practical value for the treatment of severe outbreaks of abortion caused by *S. abortus ovis*.

The incidence of disease can be reduced by giving attention to environmental and husbandry factors. Animals showing symptoms of enteritis should be isolated immediately. The crowding of sheep into pens or small areas of pasture for lambing, shearing or transport, should be avoided as much as possible, particularly when there is a history of subclinical infection in a flock.

Salmonellosis in pigs

Epidemiology and pathogenesis

Among domesticated animals, pigs constitute one of the most important reservoirs of salmonellae and are susceptible to disease caused by a wide variety of serotypes. Most important of these is *S. cholerae-suis* which is relatively species specific for pigs, and is the cause of pig paratyphoid. This organism is disseminated by symptomless carriers and infection occurs from ingestion of contaminated material. The most susceptible age is approximately 4–8 weeks after weaning, but the disease can occur in pigs of any age.

S. typhimurium is also an important cause of disease in pigs and less frequently a wide variety of other serotypes have been isolated from both diseased animals and from the mesenteric lymph glands, intestinal tracts and other sites in the carcases of apparently healthy animals at slaughter.

Symptoms

Pig paratyphoid can occur as an acute, subacute or chronic disease. The acute form is rapid in onset with discolouration of the skin which develops bright pink or purple areas, a rise in body temperature and lack of appetite. Death usually occurs in 1–4 days after the onset of symptoms. Less acute cases suffer from a profuse, yellowish diarrhoea, poor appetite and loss of condition, leading to general weakness and ultimately death of some animals. Survivors remain unthrifty and some may become symptomless carriers.

Lesions

Post-mortem examination of acute cases usually reveals haemorrhages in the mucosa of the stomach, intestines, kidney cortex and myocardium. The mesenteric lymph glands and spleen are usually enlarged and hyperaemic. Lesions are not constant in less acute and chronic cases but usually include inflammation and sloughing of areas of the gastric mucosa, and similar areas of ulceration may be seen in the small and large intestines. Mesenteric lymph nodes are enlarged. Occasionally the skin may show areas of discolouration, dermatitis and ulceration. The lungs may be pneumonic.

Diagnosis

As a result of the bacteraemia which develops in acute cases of pig paratyphoid, *S. choleraesuis* can be isolated from the visceral organs as well as from the intestinal tract and mesenteric lymph nodes. From cases of chronic pig paratyphoid and from other salmonella infections, the organisms may be identified in the intestinal contents and mesenteric lymph nodes. It should be recalled that *S. choleraesuis* is more difficult to isolate than most serotypes, and that sodium selenite or tetrathionate broth are unsuitable enrichment media. Direct inoculation on to desoxycholate citrate agar or Difco brilliant green agar is a more satisfactory method.

Control and prevention

When infection has been diagnosed in a group of pigs, apparently healthy animals should be isolated in clean accommodation and rigid disinfection procedures instituted. Some success has been claimed from the treatment of infected animals with sulphaguanidine, sulphasuxidine and sulphathalidine. More recently, nitrofurazone has proved to be of value in the treatment of infection with *S. choleraesuis*. Attempts to immunize pigs by vaccination with various preparations of killed or live attenuated cultures have not been uniformly satisfactory.

Salmonellosis in poultry

Epidemiology and pathogenesis

Poultry constitute an important animal reservoir for salmonellae, and a very wide variety of serotypes have been isolated from chickens, turkeys and to a lesser extent from ducks, geese and other species of domestic poultry. Diseases in poultry include infection with *S. pullorum* (pullorum disease; bacillary white diarrhoea), *S. gallinarum* (fowl typhoid), and other serotypes (avian paratyphoid).

Pullorum disease. This disease is almost world-wide in its distribution and is of particular importance in countries where intensive poultry farming forms an integral part of the agricultural industry. National schemes for control and prevention of the disease have reduced the incidence in some countries to less than 2 per cent and, in a few, the disease has been practically eliminated.

The dissemination of infection can occur in a number of ways according to the methods of poultry husbandry and the age of birds. Adults may be symptomless carriers of the disease and the ovaries are the organs where infection commonly persists. A proportion of eggs laid by adults with infected ovaries contain *S. pullorum* in the yolks, and the hatching of chicks from only a few infected eggs constitutes a serious source of infection for all the remaining chicks in an incubator and hatcher. Dried spicules of fluff contaminated with *S. pullorum* from infected chicks break off and become distributed by air currents throughout the hatching chamber and are a source of infection for all chicks in the hatch. The faeces of infected chicks contaminate the environment, including water, food and litter, thus spreading infection to other chicks. In acute outbreaks, the lungs of some chicks may be infected and cause *S. pullorum* to be exhaled, distributed in the atmosphere, and thus spread the disease from one bird to another by inhalation of infected droplets. In addition, pullorum disease can be disseminated indirectly by other means, including chick boxes and litter, chick sexers, clothing of attendants and utensils. Some young chicks which survive an epidemic may become symptomless carriers of *S. pullorum*, excreting the organisms intermittently in the faeces, and, in the case of female birds, harbouring infection in the ovaries. Contamination of the environment with infected faeces can lead to the spread of infection by ingestion among a flock of adult birds. The organisms can survive in litter for several months.

Fowl typhoid. The cycle of infection from the hen to the chick, as occurs in pullorum disease, can also take place with *S. gallinarum* infections. It is more usual, however, for fowl typhoid to develop as a disease of varying severity among growing birds and adult stock. The common route of infection is by ingestion, and it has also been shown that under experimental conditions the conjunctiva can act as a portal of entry. The severity of outbreaks can vary from acute with high mortality rates to chronic infections with low death rates and high proportions of carriers which excrete *S. gallinarum* intermittently in the faeces. The organisms can survive in litter for several months. There is no doubt that some strains of chickens are more susceptible to infection than others, and also that the virulence of *S. gallinarum* is enhanced by passage from one host to another, and markedly reduced following subcultivation in the laboratory.

Avian paratyphoid. A wide variety of serotypes have been isolated from domestic poultry, either from adults which sometimes appear to be clinically normal or from chicks and growing stock suffering from infection clinically indistinguishable from pullorum disease. Although many salmonella serotypes have been associated with severe disease in different countries, *S. typhimurium* is the most ubiquitous among different species of poultry, including chickens, turkeys, pheasants, ducks, geese, pigeons and other avian species. Among ducks, geese and turkeys, *S. typhimurium* may occur in the ovary as well as in the intestinal tract, and consequent infection of the egg may take place either via the ovary and yolk or from contaminated faeces infecting the outside of the egg shell as it passes through the cloaca or after it has been laid. When the outside of the eggshell becomes contaminated with these motile organisms, the latter are able to penetrate the shell and, under suitable conditions of storage and incubation, to multiply in the contents of the egg. Infection can also be spread by ingestion or inhalation of salmonellae from contaminated environments, especially hatchers, brooders, infected foodstuffs, litter, soil and utensils.

Symptoms

Pullorum disease. Young chicks are highly susceptible to this disease during the first fortnight after hatching. Deaths may occur suddenly and amount to some 95 per cent of the total hatch in severe outbreaks. In most instances, however, the disease is less acute and chicks appear sleepy, cold and huddle close to the source of heat. Some show nervous symptoms, including staggering and incoordination of the limbs, and others will suffer from inappetance, increased thirst, and signs of respiratory distress. The vents of chicks which survive for a few days at least, may be covered by an adherent mass of faeces. Growing stock are sometimes affected by a less acute form of the disease which causes slow growth rate, late feathering, intermittent diarrhoea and a low mortality rate. The majority of infected adults show no symptoms other than a lowered egg production, and in rare cases when the disease is severe, the symptoms are similar to those of fowl typhoid.

Fowl typhoid. When the disease occurs in young chicks the symptoms are indistinguishable from pullorum disease. The disease occurs more commonly among growing stock and adults, causing a mortality rate of 50 per cent or more in acute outbreaks. Most birds show signs of listlessness, diarrhoea with greenish coloured faeces, purple discolouration of the comb and wattles, collapse and death. Survivors show a marked loss of weight, a severe anaemia and intermittent diarrhoea.

Avian paratyphoid. Newly hatched birds are particularly susceptible to infection and the symptoms are indistinguishable from pullorum disease.

Lesions

Pullorum disease. In chicks which have died a few days after hatching, the spleen is congested and the surface of the yellowish coloured liver is streaked with haemorrhages. In dead chicks aged 7–10 days the most striking lesions are a hyperaemic liver with necrotic foci, congestion of the spleen and kidneys with distension of ureters with urates, pale areas in the myocardium and sometimes in the gizzard musculature. The caeca may be distended with caseous material. In birds of a few weeks of age the most striking lesions are pale areas of degeneration in the myocardium and a pericarditis.

Chronically infected adult hens often show characteristic lesions in the ovary consisting of pedunculate and misshapen ovules which are occasionally found detached in the abdominal cavity. A pericarditis and peritonitis may also be present. In adult birds which have died from acute infection the livers are congested and contain multiple small areas of necrosis. Spleens and kidneys are also enlarged and congested.

Fowl typhoid. In adult birds the most obvious lesions include enlarged, congested livers which are characteristically coloured dark red or reddish brown after exposure to the atmosphere (Plate 7.1c, facing p. 114). There may also be multiple necrotic areas throughout the substance of the livers. Spleens are similarly enlarged and necrotic, and areas of degeneration sometimes occur in the myocardia. The small

intestine may show catarrhal inflammation and petechial haemorrhages.

Avian paratyphoid. The lesions, alone, are not diagnostic. There may be congestion and necrosis of livers and spleens and a catarrhal enteritis.

Diagnosis

Pullorum disease. Although the history of disease on a premises, the symptoms of ailing chicks and the lesions may together be suggestive of pullorum disease, a final diagnosis must depend upon the isolation and identification of the causal organisms. In young chicks which have died from infection the organism can be readily isolated from the visceral organs and heart blood using the enrichment and selective media already described. It should be remembered, however, that *S. pullorum* grows poorly and small colonies on solid media develop only after incubation for 48–72 hours at 37°C. Similarly, *S. pullorum* can be isolated from the visceral organs and heart blood of adult birds which have succumbed to acute infection. In chronically infected birds the organisms can be isolated most frequently from the ovules of a laying bird and less readily from the inactive ovaries and from other organs in non-laying birds.

Various modifications of the bacterial agglutination test are used for the diagnosis of infection in carrier birds, including the tube agglutination test and the rapid whole blood test. The first of these methods consists of a straightforward bacterial agglutination test and it is generally accepted that a serum agglutinin titre of 1/50 and sometimes 1/25 is indicative of infection. The rapid whole blood test consists of mixing a given volume (one standard loopful) of fresh whole blood with one standard drop of antigen on a white tile. For this test the antigen consists of a heavy suspension in saline of killed *S. pullorum* to which crystal violet has been added to stain the bacteria and also to act as a preservative. A sample of whole blood containing a diagnostic titre of serum agglutinins will cause visible clumping of the antigen. The violet clumps which form can be easily observed against the white background of the tile, and a positive reaction will occur within two minutes of mixing the blood and antigen. This test has the advantage that it is carried out rapidly on the farm and that infected birds can be identified immediately and removed from the flock.

Fowl typhoid. The diagnostic procedures are similar to those used for pullorum disease. Among acutely infected birds, infection is generalised and the causal organisms can be isolated from the visceral organs and heart blood. The tube agglutination test and the rapid whole blood test for pullorum disease can be used for detecting fowl typhoid in living birds because the antigens of *S. pullorum* and *S. gallinarum* are similar (viz. 1, 9, 12). The methods for carrying out and interpreting the tests are similar for both diseases.

Avian paratyphoid. A conclusive diagnosis of salmonellosis in young birds caused by serotypes other than *S. pullorum* and *S. gallinarum* must depend upon the isolation and identification of the causal organisms. *S. typhimurium* and other motile serotypes can be isolated from the visceral organs of chicks, poults, ducklings and other young birds which have died from infection. Birds which survive an outbreak of disease may excrete the causal organism intermittently in their faeces for periods of several weeks or a few months, and it may be necessary to examine several faecal samples from individuals before being able to identify a carrier bird. A persistent infection with *S. typhimurium* may develop in the ovaries of turkeys, ducks, geese, pigeons and occasionally chickens. In these instances the organisms can be isolated from these organs in slaughtered birds.

The bacterial tube agglutination test can be used for detecting adult carrier birds. In the first instance it is essential to know which serotype is likely to be involved and to use the appropriate antigens for the test. It is also necessary to use both O and H (phase 1) antigens since a significant agglutinin titre against only one of these antigens may be present in a serum sample at any particular time. A titre of about 1/25 against an O antigen is indicative of infection, but it is not unusual for the serum of recently infected birds to have a titre of 1/50 or more against the H antigen and no demonstrable O agglutinins.

Control and prevention

Pullorum disease. This disease can spread so rapidly among a flock of birds that prompt control measures must take account of both the cycle of infection from one generation to another and the readiness with which the disease, arising from contamination of the environment and farm equipment, can spread through a group of birds. Survivors of an outbreak should be slaughtered, infected litter burned and all equipment and utensils disinfected. Incubators and hatchers should be fumigated with formaldehyde vapour and all movable parts disinfected. Eggs may be fumigated with formaldehyde or dipped in suitable bactericidal agents before being incubated to ensure the absence of infection on egg shells prior to incubation.

The rapid whole blood test is used widely for the detection of adult carrier birds. Reactors should be removed and the flock retested at intervals of 3–4 weeks until no further reactors are detected.

Fowl typhoid. Measures for controlling this disease are similar to those used for pullorum disease. In addition, the active immunization of adult birds with either killed or live attenuated cultures is practised. The immunity which develops from the use of a killed vaccine is usually inadequate to give solid protection. A live attenuated vaccine stimulates the development of a stronger immune response and does not cause clinical disease.

Avian paratyphoid. Methods of disinfection and fumigation used for the control of pullorum disease and fowl typhoid can be similarly applied to the control of disease caused by other serotypes. The detection of adult carriers may be a problem because some birds excrete salmonellae in their faeces and contaminate the environment at a time when bacterial agglutinins against the O and H antigens of infecting organisms cannot be detected in the sera. *S. typhimurium*, and less frequently other serotypes, may be carried by various species of domesticated animals and by rats and mice. Their infected faeces can contaminate food, water and poultry premises. It is important, therefore, to ensure that the risk of infection being derived from these other sources is reduced to a minimum.

Salmonellosis in dogs and cats

Epidemiology and pathogenesis

Many serotypes have been isolated from dogs and cats and, as in other species, the young are more susceptible than adults. The common route of infection is ingestion and this occurs most frequently from infected foodstuffs including meat, milk, eggs and wild rodents. Some infected individuals become symptomless carriers, excrete salmonellae intermittently in the faeces, and are potential sources of infection for other animals and man.

Symptoms

Young animals suffering from acute infection show signs of abdominal pain, vomiting, diarrhoea, dysentery and death. Milder cases develop less severe symptoms and sometimes only slight intermittent diarrhoea.

Lesions

Acute cases show petechial haemorrhages throughout the mucous and serous surfaces, congestion of the visceral organs and small necrotic areas in the liver and spleen. There is also a marked enteritis and congestion of the mesenteric lymph nodes.

Diagnosis
Isolation of salmonellae can be made from the visceral organs and heart blood in acute cases, and also from the intestinal tract.

Control and prevention
Severe infection can be controlled by the prompt use of antibiotics but the faeces of treated animals may be infected intermittently with salmonellae for several weeks afterwards.

Salmonellosis in wild rodents

Epidemiology and pathogenesis
Salmonellosis in wild rats and mice is a common disease of world-wide importance. *S. typhimurium* and *S. enteritidis* are the serotypes most commonly encountered. An increased incidence of a particular serotype among domesticated animals in a district may result in the wild rodents of that area becoming infected with the predominant serotype. For example, following an outbreak of *S. dublin* infection in cattle, the rats and mice on the farm may become infected with that organism for a period of time, and contaminate water supplies and food.

Rodents become infected by ingestion of contaminated material and, as in other animal species, a proportion of those infected become faecal excretors and contaminate both animal foods and the general environment of the farm on which they live. The incidence of salmonellosis in rodents is affected by the incidence of the disease in other animals species, and also by changes in climatic and environmental conditions which control the movement and density of rodent populations in the area.

Symptoms
Acute infection causes severe diarrhoea, listlessness and a harsh coat. Death may occur within a few hours from the onset of symptoms or after 2–3 days. Chronic infection may produce no definite symptoms.

Lesions
The lesions are characteristic of an acute generalised infection, including hyperaemia of the visceral organs and mesenteric lymph nodes, areas of necrosis in the liver and spleen, and severe enteritis.

Diagnosis
This must depend upon bacteriological examination. Salmonellae can be isolated from the liver, spleen, heart blood and intestines of animals which have died from acute infection, and from faecal samples and intestinal contents of chronically infected individuals.

Control and prevention
To reduce the incidence of salmonellosis in both man and domesticated animals, it is essential to control the population of wild rats and mice, and to attempt to eliminate faecal excretors, since these animals can act as reservoirs of infection on farm premises.

Public health aspects of animal salmonellosis
The majority of serotypes are potential pathogens for both man and animals. For this reason there is always the risk that disease in one animal may be the source of an epidemic among a group of animals or the origin of human infection.

The most important route for transference of salmonellosis from animals to man is via animal food products. Meat, milk and eggs are three of the commonest human foods of animal origin which may be contaminated at source and cause infection in man. The prevention of outbreaks of this type of human food poisoning constitute a world problem which emphasises that the responsibility of the veterinarian is to control and prevent animal salmonellosis not only from an economic and humane point of view, but also as an essential task in reducing the incidence of similar human infections. There is also considerable risk of human infection in a household being derived from close contact with diseased domestic pets, particularly dogs, cats, pigeons and tortoises. Farmers, animal attendants, veterinarians and others who come into contact with infected animals and carry out post-mortem examinations on diseased carcases are exposed to special risks of infection unless adequate precautions are taken.

Further reading

BASKERVILLE, A. AND DOW, C. (1973) Pathology of experimental pneumonia in pigs produced by *Salmonella cholerae suis. Journal of Comparative Pathology*, **83**, 207.

BROWN, D.D., DUFF, R.H., WILSON, J.E. AND ROSS, J.G. (1973) A survey of the incidence of infection with salmonellae in broilers and broiler breeders in Scotland. *British Veterinary Journal*, **129**, 493.

CLARK, G.McC., KAUFMANN, A.F., GANGAROSA, E.J. AND THOMPSON, M.A. (1973) Epidemiology of an international outbreak of *Salmonella agona*. *Lancet*, **2**, 490.

GHOSH, A.C. (1972) An epidemiological study of the incidence of salmonellas in pigs. *Journal of Hygiene*, **70**, 151.

GORDON R.F. (1971) Avian salmonellosis. *Veterinary Annual*, **12**, 95.

GRONSTOL, H., OSBORNE, A.D. AND PETHIYAGODA, S. (1974) Experimental salmonella infection in

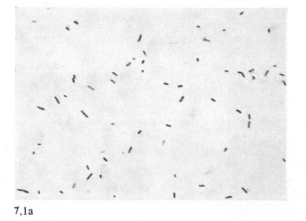

7,1a

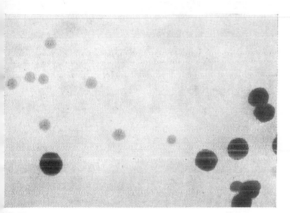

7.1b

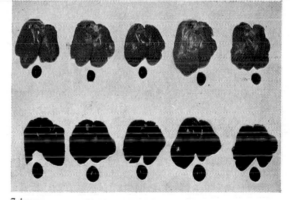

7.1c

7.1a Gram-stained film of culture of *Salmonella dublin*, ×930.

7.1b Colonies of *Salmonella dublin* (pale) and *Escherichia coli* (pink) on MacConkey's agar plate.

7.1c Livers and spleens from normal chickens (top) and chickens dead from fowl typhoid (below). Note discolouration and enlargement of the latter.

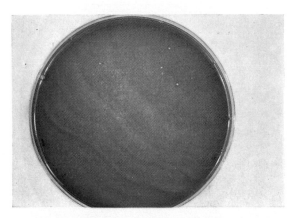

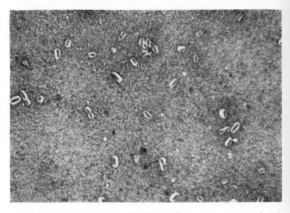

8.1a Growth of *Proteus vulgaris* on moist blood agar showing swarming. Culture sown top right.

8.1b India ink film of *Klebsiella aerogenes* stained methyl violet, showing capsules (colourless), × 930.

calves. I. The effect of stress factors on the carrier state. *Journal of Hygiene*, **72**, 155.

GRONSTOL, H., OSBORNE, A.D. AND PETHIYAGODA, S. (1974) Experimental salmonella infection in calves. II. Virulence and the spread of infection. *Journal of Hygiene*, **72**, 163.

HARVEY, R.W.S. AND PRICE, T.H. (1967) The examination of samples infected with multiple salmonella serotypes. *Journal of Hygiene*, **65**, 423.

HEARD, T.W., JENNETT, N.E. AND LINTON, A.H. (1969) The incidence of salmonella excretion in various pig populations from 1966 to 1968. *British Veterinary Journal*, **125**, 635.

HEARD, T.W., JENNETT N.E. AND LINTON, A.H. (1972) Changing patterns of salmonella excretion in various cattle populations. *Veterinary Record*, **90**, 359.

HINTON, M.H. (1973) *Salmonella dublin* abortion in cattle. I. Observations on the serum agglutination test. *Journal of Hygiene*, **71**, 459.

HINTON, M.H. (1973) *Salmonella dublin* abortion in cattle. II. Observations on the whey agglutination test and the milk ring test. *Journal of Hygiene*, **71**, 471.

JACK E.J. (1971) Salmonella abortion in sheep. *Veterinary Annual*, **12**, 57.

KATSUBE, Y., TANAKA, Y., IMAIZUMI, K. AND MASUDA, K. (1973) Salmonella carriers in swine. *Japanese Journal of Veterinary Science*, **35**, 25.

PROST E. and RIEMANN H. (1967) Food-borne salmonellosis. *Annual Review of Microbiology*, **21**, 495.

RICHARDSON, A. (1973) The transmission of *Salmonella dublin* to calves from adult carrier cows. *Veterinary Record*, **92**, 112.

ROBINSON R.A. (1970) Salmonella infection: diagnosis and control. *New Zealand Veterinary Journal*, **18**, 259.

ROWANTREE R.J. (1967) Salmonella O antigens and virulence. *Annual Review of Microbiology*, **21**, 443.

SMITH, H.W. (1960) The effect of feeding pigs on food naturally contaminated with salmonellae. *Journal of Hygiene*, **58**, 381.

SMITH H.W. (1967) Salmonellosis: The present position in man and animals. I Laboratory aspects with particular reference to chemotherapy and control. *Veterinary Record*, **80**, 142.

SOJKA W.J. and FIELD H.I. (1970) Salmonellosis in England and Wales 1958–1967. *Veterinary Bulletin*, **40**, 515.

SOJKA W.J. and GITTER M. (1961) Salmonellosis in pigs with reference to its public health significance. *Veterinary Reviews and Annotations*, **7**, 11.

SOJKA, W.J. SLAVIN, G., BRAND, T.F. AND DAVIES, G. (1972) A survey of drug resistance in salmonellae isolated from animals in England and Wales. *British Veterinary Journal*, **128**, 189.

STEVENS, A.J., GIBSON, E.A. AND HUGHES, L.E. (1967) Salmonellosis: The present position in man and animals. III Recent observations on field aspects. *Veterinary Record*, **80**, 154.

TAYLOR J. (1967) Salmonellosis: The present position in man and animals. II Public health aspects. *Veterinary Record*, **80**, 147.

THOMAS, G.W. AND HARBOURNE, J.F. (1974) Experimental *Salmonella dublin* infection in housed sheep. *Veterinary Record*, **94**, 414.

VAN OYE E. (1964) *The World Problem of Salmonellosis*. The Hague: W. Junk.

VENNEMAN, M.R. AND BERRY, L.J. (1971) Serum-mediated resistance induced with immunogenic preparations of *Salmonella typhimurium*. *Infection and Immunity*, **4**, 374.

VENNEMAN, M.R. AND BERRY, L.J. (1971) Cell-mediated resistance induced with immunogenic preparations of *Salmonella typhimurium*. *Infection and Immunity*, **4**, 381.

WENKOFF, M.S. (1973) *Salmonella typhimurium* septicaemia in foals. *Canadian Veterinary Journal*, **14**, 284.

WILLIAMS, L.P. AND NEWELL, K.W. (1968) Sources of salmonellas in market swine. *Journal of Hygiene*, **66**, 281.

CHAPTER 8

ARIZONA, PROTEUS, KLEBSIELLA
AND SHIGELLA

ARIZONA

PROTEUS

KLEBSIELLA

SHIGELLA

CHAPTER 8

Arizona, Proteus, Klebsiella and Shigella

ARIZONA

Synonyms
Paracolon arizonae; Paracolobactrum arizonae; Arizona paracolon.

Distribution in nature
This group of organisms is closely related to the salmonellae and commonly occurs in reptiles which constitute the main host reservoir. The name of the group is derived from the Tucson area of Arizona where the original isolations were made from lizards, gila monsters and other species of wild animals. The organisms are known to be pathogens for some species of domesticated animals, particularly turkeys, and for man.

Morphology and staining
Motile organisms similar to salmonellae.

Cultural characteristics
The general cultural characteristics are similar to those of salmonellae but in addition there are some properties which distinguish the arizona group. The great majority of strains ferment lactose with production of acid and gas, and in most cases this fermentation may be delayed (see Table 6.2). They do not ferment dulcitol but liquefy gelatin slowly.

Resistance to physical and chemical agents
Similar to salmonellae.

Antigens and toxins
The arizona group of organisms possess somatic (O) and flagella (H) antigens and the latter often occur in two and occasionally in three phases. These antigens are used for the serological identification of individual members of the group which now consists of nearly 200 different serotypes classified into more than thirty sub-groups on the basis of their O antigens. The close relationship between arizona organisms and salmonellae is emphasised by the fact that many O and H antigens are common to both groups. Arizona serotypes commonly isolated from diseased turkey poults are 7: 1, 2, 6 and 7: 1, 7, 8. No soluble toxins have been identified.

Epidemiology and pathogenesis
Arizona organisms occur most commonly in reptiles, turkeys and man, less frequently in chickens and rarely as a cause of disease in other animal species. The organisms are important pathogens for turkeys, poults being more susceptible than adults. Infection is spread from the ovaries of carrier birds via the yolks of eggs (cf. pullorum disease), by faecal contamination of the shell and subsequent penetration, or by ingestion from contaminated environments. Poults which survive infection may continue to excrete the organisms intermittently in the faeces and chronically infected female birds may harbour the organisms in the ovaries. It is probable that infected turkeys constitute an important source of infection for chickens, other animal species and for man.

Symptoms and lesions
Arizona organisms cause an enteric disease in turkey poults and chicks which is often clinically indistinguishable from salmonellosis. Birds which survive may develop nervous symptoms and an opacity of the iris with subsequent blindness. Arizona infections have occasionally been associated with enteritis in captive monkeys, in the young of other animal species and rarely with abortion in sheep.

Diagnosis
A final diagnosis cannot be made without isolating and identifying the causal organisms. The methods used are similar to those for the isolation of salmonellae and some workers claim that the most reliable technique is to inoculate suspected material into selenite broth and incubate the culture for 48 hours at 43°C before plating on to solid media.

117

Control and prevention

For the control of avian diseases, furazolidone medication in the drinking water reduces mortality rates but does not eliminate infection. Formaldehyde fumigation of eggs and the dipping of eggs in disinfectants prior to incubation have been used as control measures in hatcheries but are of limited value because of yolk infected eggs which remain unaffected by these procedures. Vaccination has also proved unreliable for the prevention of arizona infections in poultry flocks.

Public health aspects

Arizona organisms can cause human enteritis, and infection is probably derived most frequently from turkeys and from foods including ice cream, which may become contaminated from human sources.

PROTEUS

Distribution in nature

These organisms occur naturally in the environment of animals and man and particularly in the intestines, animal manures, human sewage, soil and water. In addition to this saprophytic type of existence, *Proteus* bacilli may be found in association with abortion and diseases of the newborn animal, otitis, peritonitis, dysentery and nervous disorders in dogs, enteritis in mice and in cases of dysentery in pigs. Infections due to *Proteus* are not uncommon in birds, reptiles and mammals in zoological collections. The organisms also constitute part of the bacterial flora of decomposing meat and eggs. The species most usually encountered are *Proteus vulgaris, Pr. morganii, Pr. rettgeri* and *Pr. mirabilis*.

Morphology and staining

Proteus are rod-shaped organisms commonly measuring 1–3 μm in length and 0·5 μm in width, but often showing considerable pleomorphism, occurring sometimes in coccal forms or as filaments measuring 10–20 μm in length. All strains are normally motile with peritrichous flagella and the majority produce fimbriae. Spores and capsules are not produced.

The organisms stain Gram-negative.

Cultural characteristics

These organisms are aerobic and facultatively anaerobic. They grow within a temperature range of approximately 20–40°C and optimally at 37°C, producing a characteristic smell. Growth on solid media shows the feature of 'swarming' when organisms spread rapidly as a thin film over the surface of the media (Plate 8.1a, facing p. 115). During the phase of rapid growth the bacilli are actively motile and tend to be longer than usual. The swarming phenomenon occurs in waves so that after inoculation of a culture on to an agar plate the resultant growth will develop as a series of rings. Swarming is inhibited when cultures are grown on solid media containing 6 per cent agar, on selective media or on media containing sodium azide.

None of the species ferment lactose but they all ferment glucose with the production of acid and gas, except most strains of *Pr. rettgeri* which are anaerogenic and produce acid only (Table 8.1). All species produce urease and this property enables them to be differentiated from salmonellae.

All species are positive to the phenylpyruvic acid (PPA) reaction since they are able to produce this substance from phenylalanine. This property is not possessed by any other groups in the family *Enterobacteriaceae*.

Resistance to physical and chemical agents

Similar to salmonellae.

Antigens and toxins

Serological studies of the somatic and flagellar antigens of these organisms has resulted in the development of an antigenic schema for their identification, leading to the recognition of numerous serotypes of *Pr. morganii, Pr. rettgeri, Pr. vulgaris* and *Pr. mirabilis*. Virulent strains inoculated into susceptible laboratory animals cause death in a few hours which may be due to a toxic substance produced by the bacteria.

TABLE 8.1.   Comparing the properties of some species of *Proteus*.

Species	Maltose	Mannitol	Indole	Gelatin	H$_2$S	Citrate
Pr. vulgaris	+	—	+	+	+	—
Pr. mirabilis	—	—	—	+	+	—
Pr. morganii	—	—	+	—	+	—
Pr. rettgeri	—	(+)	+	—	—	+

+ = fermentation   (+) = some strains do not ferment mannitol
                  — = no fermentation.

Epidemiology and pathogenesis

Proteus species are commonly present in the intestinal tracts of normal animals and frequently have to be differentiated from salmonellae and *E. coli* in cultures derived from intestinal contents. Under exceptional conditions the population of *Proteus* in the intestines increases markedly and may be associated with symptoms of severe diarrhoea and dysentery in young animals and less commonly in adults. Animal species in which this type of condition has been most frequently observed are cattle, sheep, goats, dogs and mink. *Proteus* organisms are also associated with otitis in dogs. Strains of the organism isolated from clinical cases of infection have an increased virulence which can be demonstrated by inoculation into mice or other susceptible species of laboratory animals. Under natural conditions proteus organisms are present in soil, water and decaying material, and the method of spread from animal to animal is similar to that for *E. coli*.

Symptoms and lesions

These are not characteristic for proteus infections.

Diagnosis

This depends upon isolation and identification of the causal organisms, enabling a differentiation to be made between these and other enteric infections.

KLEBSIELLA

Distribution in nature

These organisms are commonly found as saprophytes in water and soil, and also in the respiratory and intestinal tracts of healthy animals. *Kl. aerogenes* (syn: *Aerobacter aerogenes*) and *Kl. pneumoniae* (Friedländer's bacillus) are the most important members of the group associated with animal diseases.

Morphology and staining

These organisms are thick rod-shaped bacilli, often slightly oval in outline, varying in size from 1–3 μm in length and 0·5–1·0 μm in width. A characteristic feature is the production, both in laboratory cultures and in the hosts' tissues, of polysaccharide capsular material which gives rise to mucoid, slimy colonies. The bacilli usually occur singly but sometimes in pairs surrounded by capsular polysaccharide. They are non-motile and do not produce spores. Many strains develop fimbriae.

Klebsiellae stain Gram-negative, and well-developed capsules can also be seen by this staining method. Special staining techniques can be used for demonstrating capsules more clearly, and the India ink method is particularly suitable because it demonstrates extracellular slime undistorted by heat treatment (Plate 8.1b, facing p. 115).

Cultural characteristics

On solid media incubated at 37°C, capsulated strains develop as amorphous, opaque, mucoid colonies varying in diameter from 1–4 mm. After repeated subculturing there is a tendency for mucoid capsules to be lost and the cultures then develop as smaller colonies, less mucoid in consistency and similar to *Escherichia coli*. Colonies on MacConkey's agar are coloured pink resulting from the fermentation of lactose in the presence of an indicator. There is no haemolysis on blood agar.

Klebsiellae produce acid and gas in several carbohydrates, including lactose, glucose, sucrose and salicin. The majority of strains are Voges-Proskauer positive, methyl red negative, catalase positive, and they hydrolyse urea slowly.

Resistance to physical and chemical agents

These organisms are killed at a temperature of 60°C for 20 minutes and are susceptible to disinfectants. Like *E. coli*, they can survive for weeks or months at room temperature.

Antigens and toxins

The antigenic structure of these organisms is complex and consists of smooth (O), rough (R) and capsular (K) or mucoid antigens. Capsular antisera are used for typing these organisms because the K antigens mask the presence of O antigens and complicate serological techniques used for identification of the latter. There is a large number of serotypes comprising the group.

Epidemiology and pathogenesis

Klebsiellae develop in a variety of pathological conditions in animals as secondary infections, as well as primary causes of suppurative lesions or of generalised infections. They have been isolated from inflammatory and suppurative processes in foals, especially pneumonia, and from cases of metritis in mares and sows. In cattle and less frequently in pigs they may be associated with either acute or chronic forms of mastitis. The organisms have also been isolated from pigs affected with atrophic rhinitis, from air-sac infections in poultry, from the lungs of chicks affected with pullorum disease, and occasionally from the livers and intestines of diseased ducks. Klebsiellae can cause outbreaks of pneumonia in mouse colonies.

Symptoms and lesions

These are not characteristic and vary according to the site and severity of infection.

Diagnosis

A final diagnosis must depend upon the isolation and identification of the causal organisms.

SHIGELLA

Distribution in nature

This group of organisms is named after Shiga who, in 1898, was the first to isolate and identify these bacteria. Their natural habitat is the intestinal tract of man and they are the cause of human bacillary dysentery. Shigellae rarely affect lower animals but sometimes cause disease in primates. This group of organisms is divided into four subgroups, referred to as *Sh. dysenteriae* or Shiga bacillus (subgroup A), *Sh. flexneri* (subgroup B), *Sh. boydii* (subgroup C) and *Sh. sonnei* (subgroup D).

Morphology and staining

Shigellae occur as small rods measuring approximately 2–3 μm in length and 0.5 μm in width. They do not develop flagella, capsules or spores.

Shigellae stain Gram-negative.

Cultural characteristics

These are similar in many respects to the cultural characteristics of salmonellae (see Table 6.2). With the exception of a few strains of *Sh. flexneri* (subgroup B), shigellae are anaerogenic, failing to produce gas when fermenting carbohydrates. Glucose is fermented by all subgroups and mannitol by subgroups C, D and the majority of strains of subgroup B. Indole production is variable with strains of subgroups A, B and C, but is never produced by subgroup D.

Resistance to physical and chemical agents

Similar to salmonellae.

Antigens and toxins

On the basis of somatic antigenic structure, shigellae are divided into ten serotypes of *Sh. dysenteriae* (subgroup A), six of *Sh. flexneri* (subgroup B), fifteen of *Sh. boydii* (subgroup C) and one of *Sh. sonnei* (subgroup D).

Sh. dysenteriae serotype 1 produces a potent, diffusible exotoxin which consists of protein. The endotoxins derived from other members of the shigella group are associated with the somatic antigens.

Epidemiology and pathogenesis

Shigellae are of major importance as the causal organisms of human bacillary dysentery, a disease which is world-wide in distribution. Similar infections sometimes occur among captive apes and monkeys, usually associated with *Sh. flexneri* or *Sh. sonnei* infections. The disease can vary in severity from either an acute dysentery to a symptomless carrier state. In all cases the disease is an enteric infection, the causal organisms being excreted in the faeces where they can be isolated by methods similar to those employed for the isolation of salmonellae.

Other species of animals are very rarely affected but individual cases have been reported among dogs, rabbits and calves associated with *Sh. flexneri, Sh. boydii* and *Sh. sonnei*. Experimentally, *Sh. dysenteriae* is the most toxic member of the group and after intravenous inoculation into rabbits may cause haemorrhagic enteritis followed by paralysis. Oral dosage of live cultures seldom produces symptoms unless given in exceptionally large quantities.

Further reading

BRAMAN, S.K., EBERHART, R.J., ASBURY, M.A. AND HERMANN, G.J. (1973) Capsular types of *Klebsiella pneumoniae* associated with bovine mastitis. *Journal of the American Veterinary Medical Association*, **162**, 109.

COETZEE J.N. (1972) Genetics of the Proteus group. *Annual Review of Microbiology*, **26**, 23.

COWAN, S.T., STEEL, K.J., SHAW, C. AND DUGUID, J.P. (1960) A classification of the Klebsiella group. *Journal of General Microbiology*, **23**, 601.

EDWARDS, P.R., FIFE, M.A. AND RAMSEY, C.H. (1959) Studies on the Arizona Group of *Enterobacteriaceae*. *Bacteriological Reviews*, **23**, 155.

FRASER, G. (1963) Studies on *Proteus* organisms of canine origin. *Journal of Comparative Pathology*, **73**, 9.

GREENFIELD J., BIGLAND C.H. AND DUKES T.W. (1971). The genus Arizona with special reference to Arizona disease in turkeys. *Veterinary Bulletin*, **41**, 605.

GREENFIELD, J., GREENWAY, J.A. AND BIGLAND, C.H. (1973) Arizona infections in sheep associated with gastroenteritis and abortion. *Veterinary Record*, **92**, 400.

HARVEY, R.W.S., PRICE, T.H. AND DIXON, J.M.S. (1966) Salmonellas of subgenus III [Arizona] isolated from abattoirs in England and Wales. *Journal of Hygiene*, **64**, 271.

HARVEY, R.W.S., PRICE, T.H. AND HALL, M.L.M. (1973) Isolation of subgenus III salmonellas [arizonas] in Cardiff, 1959–1971. *Journal of Hygiene*, **71**, 481.

KOWALSKI, L.M. AND STEPHENS, J.F. (1968) *Arizona*, 7:1, 7, 8 infection in young turkeys. *Avian Diseases*, **12**, 317.

LAMONT, P.H. AND TIMMS, L. (1972) Experimental infection of turkey poults with *Arizona* serotype 7:1, 7, 8. *British Veterinary Journal*, **128**, 129.

TIMMS, L. (1972) Comparison of serological tests for detection of *Arizona* infection in adult turkeys. British Veterinary Journal, **128**, 412.

WEST, J.L. AND MOHANTY, G.C. (1973) *Arizona hinshawii* infection in turkey poults: pathologic changes. *Avian Diseases*, **17**, 314.

CHAPTER 9

PASTEURELLA, YERSINIA AND
FRANCISELLA

CHAPTER 9

Pasteurella, Yersinia and Francisella

PASTEURELLA

The name *Pasteurella* was introduced for this genus in recognition of the work carried out by Pasteur on fowl cholera, a disease of poultry caused by *Pasteurella multocida*. The most widely recognised species included in this group are *Past. multocida* and *Past. haemolytica*. Other species which have been recognised include *Past. anatipestifer* causing disease in ducklings, and *Past. pneumotropica* associated with pneumonia in laboratory rodents. Additional members of the genus which have now been re-grouped into other genera include *Yersinia pseudotuberculosis* (Syn: *Pasteurella pseudotuberculosis*), *Yersinia pestis* (Syn: *Pasteurella pestis*) and *Francisella tularensis* (Syn: *Pasteurella tularensis*).

Pasteurella multocida

Synonyms
Pasteurella septica; *Pasteurella boviseptica*; *Pasteurella suiseptica*; *Pasteurella aviseptica*, etc. according to the species of animal affected.

Distribution in nature
Past. multocida has been identified with disease in animals since the inception of bacteriology. During the last century Pasteur and his colleagues investigated epidemics of disease among poultry and isolated bacteria possessing the characteristic properties of *Pasteurella*. From their observations they formed the opinion that the symptoms of this poultry disease were so similar to those of human cholera, that they named it fowl cholera. Thereafter, there was some confusion in the literature between fowl cholera and fowl typhoid, a disease of poultry caused by *Salmonella gallinarum*, which was probably more widespread at that time than fowl cholera.

Similarly, pasteurellosis in cattle and pigs, sheep and horses was also studied extensively at the end of the last century, and *Past. multocida* was identified in these animals as the cause of some serious outbreaks of disease, variously named haemorrhagic septicaemia or cornstalk disease in cattle and barbone in buffaloes. It is now known that these organisms infect practically all domesticated and many wild species of animals and birds; that they can cause disease which may be chronic or acute; and that they are present throughout the world as commensals in the respiratory tracts of animals which are clinically normal.

Morphology and staining
Strains of *Past. multocida* newly isolated from the carcases of animals which have died from infection usually appear as short ovoid rods, measuring approximately 1·0 μm in length and 0·5–0·8 μm in width. However, the morphology of these organisms is variable, particularly when isolated from the upper respiratory tracts of clinically normal animals, and after repeated cultivation on laboratory media. They may then appear as relatively long rods measuring as much as 5 μm in length and 1·0 μm in width. The organisms are non-sporing and non-motile.

Past. multocida stain Gram-negative with a tendency to bipolar staining, which is clearly observed with newly isolated strains or with organisms in tissues when they are stained with methylene blue or Leishman's stain (Plate 9.1a, facing p. 126). After repeated subcultivation in the laboratory this characteristic property of bipolar staining may be lost. When observed in diseased tissues or in primary cultures from cases of acute infection, they have capsules which do not stain readily and may be difficult to observe. The amount of capsular material, which varies between different strains, is composed of complex polysaccharide and hyaluronic acid. The latter component is present in mucoid strains and may render the organisms inagglutinable. Agglutinability can be restored by heating the bacteria in a boiling waterbath for 10 minutes.

Cultural characteristics (Table 9.1)
Past. multocida will grow aerobically or anaero-

TABLE 9.1. Comparing some characteristic properties of *Pasteurella*, *Yersinia* and *Francisella* species.

Species of organism	Motility at 22°C	Growth on MacConkey agar	Haemolysis on blood agar	Production of indole	Production of urease	Production of H_2S
Past. multocida	—	—	—	+	—	+
Past. haemolytica	—	+	+	—	—	—
Past. haemolytica var. *ureae*	—	—	+	—	+	—
Past. anatipestifer	—	—	—	—	—	—
Past. pneumotropica	—	—	—	+	+	±
Yersinia pseudotuberculosis	+	+	—	—	+	+
Yersinia pestis	—	+	—	—	—	—
Francisella tularensis	—	—	—	—	—	+

± = strains vary in ability to produce H_2S

bically in an atmosphere with low oxygen tension, at an optimum temperature of 37°C. Growth takes place on ordinary laboratory media but is enhanced in the presence of serum or blood. Overnight incubation on nutrient agar of freshly isolated strains, particularly from cases of acute infection in cattle, results in the development of round, flat colonies of sticky, mucoid consistency, about 2–3 mm in diameter, containing well capsulated organisms. These smooth, mucoid strains are often derived from less acute cases of pasteurellosis. Other strains produce smaller round, smooth, iridescent colonies about 1 mm in diameter, and also colonies of circular shape which are non-iridescent. The organisms in these colonies possess smaller quantities of capsular substance. Some strains, especially those which have been repeatedly subcultured in the laboratory, may produce small colonies of about 1 mm in diameter which are of a drier consistency and difficult to suspend in fluid. These are rough cultures. Thus, colonial morphology of *Past. multocida* may be classified as mucoid, smooth (iridescent), smooth (non-iridescent) and rough variants.

Growth on blood agar is more profuse and the medium becomes characteristically darkened. This change in colour is particularly noticeable on plates which have been heavily inoculated. There is no haemolysis. Growth in broth of newly isolated and smooth strains results in an even turbidity which develops in 6–8 hours, and the rate of growth is increased when 10 per cent serum is added to the broth medium. Older strains tend to give a fine granular type of growth in broth which is visible as a deposit after 36–48 hours' incubation at 37°C.

Past. multocida produces indole and H_2S, and reduces nitrates. These organisms will not grow on MacConkey's bile salt medium and do not produce liquefaction of gelatin or inspissated serum. The great majority of strains do not produce urease.

Biochemical reactions of most strains include the production of acid, without gas, in glucose, sucrose, galactose, sorbitol, fructose, xylose, arabinose and mannitol. Dulcitol is fermented by some strains derived from poultry. No reaction occurs in lactose, maltose dextrin, raffinose, rhamnose or inulin. However, it should be remembered that variations to these biochemical reactions are shown by some strains isolated from different animal species and relate particularly to the reactions occurring in xylose, arabinose, dulcitol and lactose.

Resistance to physical and chemical agents
Past. multocida is readily killed by chemical and physical agents. Exposure on solid media to sunlight for 3–4 hours and also heating of suspensions to 55°C for 15 minutes are both lethal to these organisms. They are also killed by 0·5 per cent phenol in 15 minutes.

Antigens and toxins
Immunological studies of strains of *Past. multocida* isolated from a variety of host species, employing precipitin tests, capsular swelling tests, indirect haemagglutination tests and protection tests in mice, have shown that the antigenic structures of these bacteria differ. These differences formed the basis for earlier classification of the organisms into four distinct types which have been labelled Roberts types I–IV, based on protection tests in mice, and Carter types A–E related to capsular antigens.

Studies by Namioka and Murata have revealed the complex nature of the somatic antigens and the presence of shared antigens among strains derived from a variety of sources. A total of eleven different somatic antigens have been identified, and the antigenic structure of each serotype of *Past. multocida* can now be expressed by a number, referring to the somatic antigen, followed by a letter representing the capsular antigen. Table 9.2 shows the serotypes which are most frequently encountered in animals.

TABLE 9.2. Summarising the serotypes of *Past. multocida* most commonly encountered in animals. (Modified from Namioka and Bruner (1963) and Carter (1967)).

Serotype	Host species	Disease	Serotype	Host species	Disease
1:A	Pigs Mice	Pneumonia Sepsis	6:B	Cattle	Haemorrhagic septicaemia
3:A	Pigs	Pneumonia	1:D	Pigs Sheep	Pneumonia Pneumonia
5:A	Chickens Turkeys Ducks Pigs	Fowl cholera Fowl cholera Fowl cholera Pneumonia	2:D	Pigs	Pneumonia
			3:D	Cats	Pneumonia
7:A	Cattle	Sepsis	4:D	Pigs Sheep	Pneumonia Pneumonia
8:A	Chickens	Fowl cholera	10:D	Pigs	Pneumonia
9:A	Turkeys	Fowl cholera	6:E	Cattle	Haemorrhagic septicaemia

In addition to these serotypes it should be remembered that there are also a number of sub-types which have been described. There is little doubt that continued investigation of the antigenic structures of these organisms will lead to the recognition of further serotypes and sub-types in the future, and subsequently to information of practical value on the association of different serotypes with various host species, disease and immunity.

A toxin composed of protein has been described in relation to type B strains of *Past. multocida* in addition to lipopolysaccharide which may be derived from organisms in tissues and broth cultures.

Epidemiology and pathogenesis

The foregoing description of the properties of *Past. multocida* emphasises that these organisms are potential pathogens for many species of domesticated and wild animals, and that the diseases they cause have a world-wide distribution. The increased interest in these bacteria, particularly in relation to studies on epidemiology, has emphasised some important and poorly understood aspects of host-parasite relationships. The serological classification of these organisms shows some relationship to the diseases occurring in different host species, although there is a good deal of overlap between the varieties of animal species which are susceptible to infection with each serotype. For example, serotypes 5:A and 8:A are common causes of fowl cholera, and serotype 9:A usually infects turkeys. Similarly, serotypes 6:B and 6:E are the principal causes of epizootic haemorrhagic septicaemia in African cattle and buffaloes.

An important aspect of the epidemiology of pasteurellosis in animals is that the bacteria can be carried by individuals which show no signs of clinical infection. Since the organisms are relatively susceptible to chemical and physical agents, the carrier animal would seem to play an essential role in the life history of these bacteria and in their distribution from one host to another. *Past. multocida* has been identified frequently in the respiratory tracts and sometimes the intestines of apparently healthy domesticated and wild animals. There is evidence to indicate that among bovine animals, *Past. multocida* may be carried by clinically normal individuals and that under certain predisposing conditions, the organisms increase their rates of growth in these individuals until a severe and perhaps fatal infection has developed. This hypothesis has been put forward to explain outbreaks of disease which occur rapidly and simultaneously in groups of animals when these are subjected to certain stresses and environments, particularly among working animals during the rainy season in tropical countries, confinement of cattle for vaccination against other diseases or for transport, and concurrent virus infections. The rapid multiplication of *Past. multocida* in the respiratory tract can give rise to infected droplets which are exhaled into the atmosphere and become a source of infection for other individuals. Severely affected animals may also contaminate the environment by excreting large numbers of *Past. multocida* in the faeces.

Similarly, *Past. multocida* probably exists as a latent infection in a high proportion of healthy pigs and only becomes apparent under certain predisposing conditions. These include swine fever, swine influenza, swine pneumonia and other diseases which affect the respiratory tract. In these instances it seems that *Past. multocida* develops as a secondary infection and there is little evidence to show that these organisms are commonly a primary cause of disease in pigs.

Other animal species including poultry, sheep, rabbits, dogs and cats also act as carriers of *Past. multocida* which has been isolated from the throats and respiratory tracts of these species. In these animals, also, the development of disease is related to predisposing conditions concerned with climate, methods of husbandry and intercurrent diseases, particularly respiratory virus infections.

An attempt to summarise factual information on the epidemiology of *Past. multocida* infections in animals inevitably emphasises the lack of knowledge at the present time on this subject. We know that *Past. multocida* exists as a commensal in the respiratory tracts and sometimes the digestive tracts of animals, and that certain predisposing conditions alter this balance between host and parasite, which results in the development of disease. When this occurs, the virulence of the organism becomes enhanced and in cases of acute and fatal infection the degree of virulence is extremely high. In other instances chronic infections may develop, particularly in the respiratory tracts, causing the host to suffer a protracted form of pasteurellosis which may exist concurrently, as in acute cases, with some other microbial infection. Further research needs to be done on the biological activities of the toxic antigens of *Past. multocida* in relation to the conditions necessary for their development and into the reactions these antigens have on tissue cells.

Symptoms

Cattle
In acute cases of epizootic haemorrhagic septicaemia in the tropics the symptoms include a rise in body temperature, a sudden drop in milk yield, signs of abdominal pain, severe diarrhoea and dysentery. Respirations become rapid and shortly before death the mucous membranes appear cyanotic. In less acute cases there is a rise in body temperature and oedema develops subcutaneously in the region of the head, neck and brisket. Most animals suffer from severe diarrhoea and sometimes dysentery, and some show signs of respiratory distress and a nasal discharge which may be blood-stained or purulent. Death occurs within 2–4 days. In countries other than the tropics, *Past. multocida* infection may be associated with *Past. haemolytica* and give rise to symptoms of bronchopneumonia and the condition sometimes referred to as transit or shipping fever.

Sheep
The role of *Past. multocida* as a primary cause of infection has not been clearly established. In most cases when *Pasteurella* have been associated with disease the symptoms have been of pneumonia or occasionally mastitis.

Pigs
The role of pasteurellae as a primary cause of disease has not been definitely established. It is usual to isolate *Past. multocida* from the lungs of pigs which have shown symptoms of respiratory infection and pneumonia associated with virus infections, or from the upper respiratory tracts in cases of rhinitis.

Poultry
The acute form of fowl cholera can affect many species of wild and domesticated birds, including chickens, turkeys, ducks and geese, causing a high mortality rate. Death may occur suddenly without the development of any premonitory characteristic symptoms. Less acute cases show symptoms similar to fowl typhoid (i.e. infection with *Salmonella gallinarum*). Breathing is rapid through the open beak, the feathers are ruffled, and the comb and wattles become cyanotic. There may also be a yellowish diarrhoea. Chronic infection often results in the development of swollen wattles and comb, and sometimes the joints become hot and painful.

Dogs and cats
These animals are known to be symptomless carriers of *Past. multocida* which can give rise to septic bite wounds.

Rabbits
Outbreaks of acute infection can occur in colonies of rabbits. Deaths take place suddenly without any premonitory symptoms, and the mortality rate may be high among rabbits of all ages. Chronic infection sometimes develops and this is associated with respiratory symptoms of coryza.

Lesions

Cattle
Post-mortem examination of acute cases of haemorrhagic septicaemia show multiple haemorrhages on the serous membranes and organs together with blood-stained exudate in the thorax and abdomen. There will also be a severe gastroenteritis, the intestinal contents may be markedly blood-stained and the mesenteric lymph nodes enlarged and haemorrhagic.

The oedematous form of the disease includes those sub-acute cases in which the most striking lesion is oedema occurring in the subcutaneous tissues and sometimes in the region of the throat, including the tongue and the neck. There may be other lesions similar to but less marked than those associated with the acute form of the disease.

The pectoral form refers to sub-acute cases in which the lesions are mainly confined to the lungs and pleural cavity. Exudates may be present in the pleural cavity and also in the pericardial sac. The lungs have a marbled appearance due to thickened, yellowish septa distended with exudate and dividing the darker areas of pneumonia. The bronchial and mediastinal lymph glands will be enlarged. In addition, there may be lesions similar to but less severe than those associated with the acute form of the disease.

Sheep
A number of cases have been described in which the post-mortem appearances are of acute or subacute pneumonia. In acute cases there may be exudate in the pleural cavity and pericardial sac. More frequently, pasteurellosis occurs as a secondary infection and the lesions are related mainly to the primary infection. There have been some reports of acute mastitis caused by pasteurellae.

Pigs
Lesions related to a primary infection with *Past. multocida* are rare, the disease usually occurring as a secondary infection. In these latter cases the organisms occur as secondary invaders in pneumonic lesions associated with virus infections, and in the upper respiratory tract in cases of rhinitis.

Poultry
The liver and spleen are enlarged, hyperaemic and dark red in colour. The liver may become reddish brown on exposure to the atmosphere. There is a peritonitis, fluid in the pericardial sac and petechial haemorrhages on the serous surfaces.

The lesions of chronic infections include swelling of the comb and wattles. Sometimes infection which has localised in the joints causes the accumulation of sero-fibrinous fluid in these areas.

Rabbits
Lesions of the acute form of the disease are typical of a septicaemia, including multiple haemorrhages throughout the serous surfaces, in the myocardium, liver and sometimes the lungs. There may be a tracheitis. Subacute cases show multiple necrotic lesions in the liver and spleen and these organs are hyperaemic.

Diagnosis
The identification of pasteurella infection in any species of animal depends upon the isolation and identification of the causal organism. Leishman's stain applied to smears from heart blood, liver, spleen, lung or exudate from acute cases will usually show the organisms as bipolar staining, short ovoid rods. The site chosen for preparing these smears will depend upon the lesions present, but in acute cases there is usually little difficulty in identifying organisms from various sites. It is important to remember that some other bacterial species can show varying degrees of bipolar staining.

The organisms can be readily isolated in almost pure culture from the blood and organs of fresh carcases. The isolates should then be further examined to confirm that they possess the cultural characteristics of *Past. multocida*. A positive diagnosis of pasteurella infection in chronic cases of the disease is more difficult. Direct smears from any site suspected of being infected will not usually show typical pasteurella organisms because few may be present. Diagnosis depends upon the isolation and identification of *Past. multocida* by cultural and serological methods. As a general rule, strains isolated from cattle are pathogenic for mice and rabbits but not for ducks or chickens. Avian strains are pathogenic for different species of birds as well as for mice and rabbits.

Control and prevention

Immunization
The grave economic losses which can occur from haemorrhagic septicaemia in cattle have stimulated research into methods of protection which are both reliable and practical. A variety of immunizing agents have been prepared from filtrates of material derived from lesions in bovine animals and from living and killed bacteria with and without adjuvants. Some satisfactory results have been obtained from the use of a formolised vaccine prepared from iridescent cultures emulsified with lanolin and liquid paraffin. Similarly, alum precipitated vaccines have also proved useful. The protection derived from these vaccines which is measured in the laboratory by mouse protection tests may last for almost one year. To obtain the optimum results it is necessary to use vaccines prepared from capsulated strains of the same serotypes of *Past. multocida* as those which are responsible for the disease in the area or country concerned. Aerated cultures have been used for preparing vaccines since this technique for growth results in a greater density of bacteria in the fluid medium. The final density is appropriate for maximum stimulation of protection without having to concentrate the organisms as an additional step in vaccine production. There have been several reports of an anaphylactic type of reaction develop-

ing soon after the administration of vaccine to individual animals.

Attempts to control fowl cholera by vaccination were initiated by Pasteur who used live attenuated cultures. Subsequent investigations have shown that to produce the maximum degree of protection it is important to use capsulated strains antigenically related to the serotype responsible for disease. Formolised vaccines in oil emulsions have been used with variable results.

Hyperimmune serum has been used for the control of haemorrhagic septicaemia when immediate protection of cattle is required to contain an outbreak or prevent disease developing during transport or other conditions of sudden stress. In practice, the injection of hyperimmune serum confers immediate protection, although the passive immunity is of short duration and of limited value.

Chemotherapy

It is essential that treatment is initiated in the early stages of the disease if it is to be of value. For this reason the treatment of animals suffering from acute disease will be commenced too late to be effective. In less acute cases repeated high dosage rates are necessary and this may be economically practical for individuals or small groups of animals. Promising results in laboratory experiments have been obtained with penicillin G, carbomycin, chloramphenicol, chlortetracycline, and oxytetracycline. It should be noted that *Past. multocida* is one of the few Gram-negative bacterial species which is sensitive to penicillin.

Past. multocida does not develop resistance to chemotherapeutic agents as readily as other bacterial species but it has occurred as a consequence of administering streptomycin and bacitracin.

Public health aspects

Past. multocida has been isolated from the respiratory tracts of humans, particularly from those who have close contact with infected animals. Human infection can also develop from infected dog and cat bite wounds.

Pasteurella haemolytica

Synonyms

Pasteurella mastiditis

Distribution in nature

This organism has been isolated from cattle, buffaloes, sheep and goats. It is associated with pneumonic lesions in these animals but its role as a primary cause of disease has not been clearly established. *Past. haemolytica* has been identified as the causal agent of an acute septicaemic infection in lambs.

Morphology and staining

These organisms are sometimes morphologically similar to *Past. multocida*. They may appear as oval-shaped coccobacilli or show pleomorphism and develop into rods measuring about 2·5 μm or more in length and 0·5 μm in width. They are non-sporing, non-motile and stain Gram-negative. Bipolar staining is not a constant feature of these organisms. Smears prepared from infected lungs will contain a proportion of bacteria which fail to show this property.

Cultural characteristics

Past. haemolytica grows readily on most laboratory media. On nutrient agar the colonies are moist and translucent. Growth in broth results in an even turbidity. The organism is weakly haemolytic when grown on ox or sheep blood agar. The area of haemolysis is immediately beneath the bacterial growth and may not extend beyond the edges of the colonies. It can best be seen after 48 hours' incubation and when the colony has been removed from the surface of the blood agar medium. It has also been noted that when grown on bovine blood an extracellular substance is developed which increases the haemolytic effect of staphylococcal β toxin. On lamb-blood agar the narrow zone of complete haemolysis which occurs almost entirely underneath bacterial colonies of strains isolated from sheep is surrounded by a wider zone of partial haemolysis.

Past. haemolytica grows on MacConkey's bile salt medium but not usually on desoxycholate citrate agar. Acid, without gas, is produced by most strains in glucose, laevulose, maltose, saccharose, mannitol, sorbitol, fructose, galactose and xylose. Nitrates are reduced to nitrites. Gelatin and inspissated serum are not liquefied, indole and urease are not produced. Some strains produce H_2S.

Variant strains isolated from human respiratory tracts, have been named *Past. haemolytica* var. *ureae* because of their ability to produce urease. These variants do not grow on MacConkey's agar.

Strains of *Past. haemolytica* isolated from sheep have been divided into two types. Type T strains ferment trehalose but do not ferment arabinose; conversely, Type A strains ferment arabinose but not trehalose. Type T strains have been isolated more frequently from cases of septicaemia than from pneumonia, and Type A strains have been associated mainly with pneumonia.

Resistance to physical and chemical agents

The properties of *Past. haemolytica* are similar to those of *Past. multocida*.

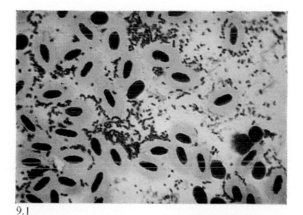

9.1

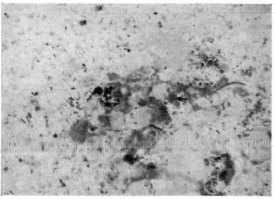

10.1a

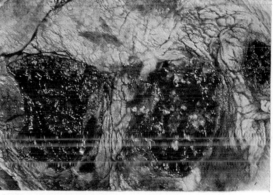

10.1b

9.1 Blood film from chicken infected with *Pasteurella multocida* showing coccobacillary organisms stained with Leishman's method, ×930.

10.1a Differential staining method applied to film from bovine cotyledon showing *Brucella abortus* organisms coloured pink, ×930.

10.1b Bovine placenta infected with *Brucella abortus*, showing hyperaemia of cotyledons and characteristic leathery appearance of intercotyledonary spaces.

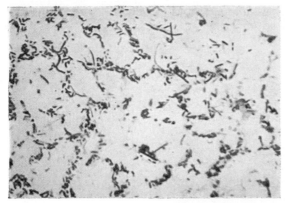

11.1a

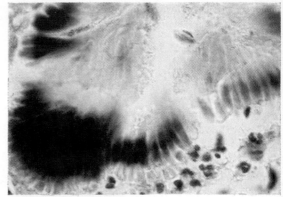

11.1b

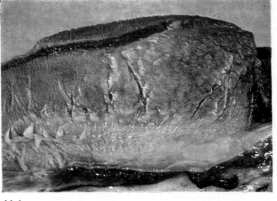

11.1c

11.1a Gram-stained film of culture of *Actinobacillus lignièresi*, ×930.

11.1b Film of pus stained by Ziehl-Neelsen method showing the characteristic ring of pink coloured clubs associated with *Actinobacillus lignièresi* organisms, ×930.

11.1c Cross-section of bovine tongue showing typical lesion of 'wooden tongue'.

Antigens and toxins

Strains of *Past. haemolytica* have been classified into eleven distinct serological types. The differentiation of these types has been based on diffusible surface antigens, which adsorb on to erythrocytes. Indirect haemagglutination tests against various antisera can then be carried out using these modified erythrocytes as antigen.

Epidemiology and pathogenesis

It is generally considered that the natural habitats for *Past. haemolytica* to occur as commensals are the respiratory tracts of sheep, goats, cattle, pigs, chickens and probably other species. The organisms have been isolated from the upper respiratory tracts of apparently normal animals, and predisposing factors include exposure to cold weather, the stresses of transport resulting in shipping fever (which may also be associated with concurrent *Past. multocida* infection), and other intercurrent infections (e.g. parainfluenza virus type 3). These conditions provide suitable environments for *Past. haemolytica* to invade lung tissue and cause pneumonia. *Past. haemolytica* also causes mastitis in ewes. Lambs are highly susceptible to septicaemic infections when a few weeks old, and develop an increasing resistance during the first year of life.

Symptoms

In cases of pneumonia (e.g. transport fever) there is a rise in temperature, respirations become increased and the animal collapses and dies within 12–48 hours after the symptoms have first been observed. In less acute cases there is spasmodic coughing and signs of general debility and dejection before death occurs in 2–3 days or later. Recovery is uncommon. In young lambs the symptoms are of an acute septicaemia and death occurs suddenly a few hours after the symptoms have first been observed.

Lesions

In adult animals the lesions are associated mainly with the respiratory tract. There are extensive areas of consolidation in the lungs. The alveoli are filled with mononuclear cells and erythrocytes. Interlobular septa are thickened by oedematous fluid containing polymorphs. The local lymph glands are enlarged and oedematous. In lambs there is congestion and oedema of the lungs, fluid in the peritoneal and pleural cavities and petechial haemorrhages throughout these areas.

Diagnosis

This depends upon the isolation and identification of the organism. *Past. haemolytica* can be isolated readily from the respiratory tract, particularly the lungs and oedematous fluid from fresh carcases of acute cases.

Control and prevention

Autogenous vaccines have been claimed to give protection against this infection in adult sheep. Mixed formolised alum-treated cultures of *Past. multocida* and *Past. haemolytica* have also been used to prevent clinical infections in sheep, cattle and pigs. The sensitivity of *Past. haemolytica* to antibiotics is similar to that shown by *Past. multocida*.

Public health aspects

Past. haemolytica does not cause disease in man although *Past. haemolytica* var. *ureae*, the urease-producing variant of the organism, has been isolated from human sputa and respiratory tracts.

Pasteurella anatipestifer

Synonyms

Pfeifferella anatipestifer; Moraxella anatipestifer.

This organism has been isolated from Canadian wild geese and is the cause of disease in ducklings known as Long Island duck disease or new duck disease.

The growth of *Past. anatipestifer* on medium is enhanced in the presence of serum and primary cultures may grow more satisfactorily in an atmosphere of increased CO_2. Carbohydrates are not fermented and neither indole nor H_2S is produced. The organism is catalase positive and liquefies gelatin.

The disease primarily affects young ducklings which show symptoms of depression, oculonasal discharge, incoordination of the limbs and greenish diarrhoea. The birds may also develop abnormal turning of the head and lie on their backs before death occurs 6–48 hours after the initial development of symptoms. Survivors are emaciated and often lame due to swollen hock joints. Post mortem examination may show enlarged congested liver and spleen, fibrous peritonitis and haemorrhagic enteritis.

Pasteurella pneumotropica

This organism causes pneumonia in mice and occurs only in the lungs and respiratory tracts. It exists as a latent infection in mouse colonies and has also been recovered as a latent infection from guinea-pigs, hamsters and rats which have been in contact with infected mice. The organism has also been isolated from the throats of cats.

Past. pneumotropica will not grow on MacConkey agar, is non-haemolytic, reduces nitrates to nitrites and produces indole. It ferments with acid production, maltose, sucrose, lactose, glucose and inositol, and does not ferment xylose. It is antigenically distinct from *Past. multocida, Yersinia pseudotuberculosis* and *Yersinia pestis.*

YERSINIA

The species *Pasteurella pseudotuberculosis* has recently been renamed *Yersinia pseudotuberculosis* and the genus *Yersinia* included in the family Enterobacteriaceae. However, for the convenience of the reader wishing to compare the genera *Pasteurella* and *Yersinia*, the latter is discussed in this chapter.

Yersinia pseudotuberculosis

Synonym
Pasteurella pseudotuberculosis.

Distribution in nature
This organism has a world-wide distribution and is particularly associated with a disease known as pseudotuberculosis in guinea-pigs and to a less extent in turkeys, pigeons, rats, rabbits and hares. It has occasionally been isolated from sheep, goats, pigs, cattle, cats, mice and man. It is known to be carried and disseminated by wild rodents and pigeons, and has been isolated from animal food-stuffs, soil and water.

Morphology and staining
Yersinia pseudotuberculosis sometimes occurs as short, ovoid rods, measuring about 1·5 μm in length and 0·7 μm in width, particularly when newly isolated from tissues, and these organisms then show bipolar staining with Leishman's stain. Pleomorphism may develop on subculture and the bacteria may appear as long rods or filaments. The organisms stain Gram-negative and do not form spores. *Yersinia pseudotuberculosis* is non-motile at 37°C but is motile. when cultures in broth medium are maintained at 22°C. This is a useful characteristic property for differentiating between *Yersinia pseudotuberculosis* and pasteurella organisms.

Cultural characteristics
Yersinia pseudotuberculosis grows on ordinary laboratory media including MacConkey's bile salt medium, which is a point of differentiation between this organism and *Past. multocida.*

Acid, without gas, is produced in glucose, maltose, arabinose, fructose, mannitol, salicin, galactose and rhamnose. Indole is not produced, nitrates are reduced to nitrites and the org; .ism is non-haemolytic.

Resistance to physical and chemical agents
The properties are similar to those of *Past. multocida.*

Antigens and toxins
Strains of *Yersinia pseudotuberculosis* possess a common flagellar antigen, a common somatic antigen which is similar to a somatic antigen of *Yersinia pestis*, and type specific antigens which have enabled strains of the organism to be subdivided into five distinct serological types.

Epidemiology and pathogenesis
Yersinia pseudotuberculosis has a wide distribution. Outbreaks of disease have been reported most frequently in guinea-pigs and rabbits as well as in turkeys, chickens, pigeons, cats, hares and very occasionally in other animal species including pigs, sheep and horses. The organism is known to occur in wild rodents and wood pigeons. It is probable that animals which suffer from clinical infection with *Yersinia pseudotuberculosis* contract the disease from ingestion of food which has become contaminated with infected faeces and urine of wild rodents or excreta from pigeons. It is also probable that cats can become infected from catching infected wild rodents.

Symptoms
The acute form of the disease develops as a sudden and fatal septicaemia. Deaths may be sudden and mortality rate high in a group of susceptible animals, particularly guinea-pigs and less commonly in poultry and rabbits. The more chronic form of infection is manifest by intermittent attacks of diarrhoea and emaciation which develop over a period of 2–5 weeks before death occurs. Some chronically infected animals will survive for longer periods particularly when infection remains localised in lymphatic glands and lymphoid tissue in the intestinal tract.

Lesions
In the acute form of the disease there is a severe enteritis. The spleen and mesenteric lymph nodes are enlarged and congested. In chronic cases there are numerous necrotic and caseous lesions, each about 1 mm in diameter but often coalescing to produce larger lesions in the spleen, liver and mesenteric lymph nodes. These lesions consist of necrotic and caseous foci surrounded by polymorphs, and there is no calcification. It is the appearance of the lesions which has given rise to the term pseudotuberculosis.

Diagnosis
The type of lesion and the animal species involved may be suggestive of infection with *Yersinia*

pseudotuberculosis. Confirmation must depend upon the isolation and identification of the causal organism from tissues, particularly the liver, spleen and sometimes from heart blood and bone marrow.

Control and prevention

Various chemotherapeutic agents can be used since the organism is susceptible to chloramphenicol, streptomycin and other antibiotics. When outbreaks of disease occur in guinea-pigs, poultry, or rabbits, it is advisable to destroy the survivors in the group and to thoroughly disinfect the cages and equipment. There is no reliable immunizing agent.

Public health aspects

Yersinia pseudotuberculosis in man can produce a chronic infection of the mesenteric lymph nodes and produce symptoms which are suggestive of an appendicitis. An acute septicaemic type of infection is rare.

Yersinia pestis

Synonym

Pasteurella pestis.

Distribution in nature

This organism is the cause of plague in man which has been one of the most serious diseases of the past. It is still present in areas of Asia, Africa and America, and depending upon the type of disease it causes, it is variously termed Bubonic Plague or Pneumonic Plague. The organism is carried by rats and infection is transferred to man by fleas, although man can become infected from rat bites. *Yersinia pestis* has also been identified in a wide variety of other rodents.

Morphology and staining

The organism is similar in appearance to *Past. multocida*, being a short, oval coccobacillus measuring about 1·5 μm in length and 0·7 μm in width. It shows considerable pleomorphism when subcultured on laboratory media and may appear as long rods which degenerate into variously shaped irregular forms. *Yersinia pestis* is non-motile, non-sporing and stains Gram-negative. In smears prepared from infected tissue the coccobacillary form shows well marked bipolar staining with methylene blue or Leishman's stain. This characteristic feature is less easily seen on subculture and is absent from pleomorphic forms. Tissue smears of the organism and newly isolated strains possess a capsule which becomes less obvious on subculturing.

Cultural characteristics

Yersinia pestis grows aerobically and anaerobically on ordinary laboratory media, but growth is enhanced in the presence of serum or blood. The organism does not produce haemolysis on blood agar. The optimum temperature for growth, particularly of primary isolations is about 27°C, but the organism will develop within a temperature range of 14–37°C. Capsule formation is optimal at 37°C.

Yersinia pestis grows on MacConkey's bile salt medium, does not produce indole or H_2S, and reduces nitrates to nitrites. Acid, without gas, is produced in glucose, galactose, fructose, maltose, mannitol, arabinose and xylose.

Resistance to physical and chemical agents

Yersinia pestis is relatively susceptible to chemical and physical agents and is similar in this respect to *Past. multocida*.

Antigens and toxins

The complex antigenic structure of *Yersinia pestis* includes a capsular antigen which is heat-labile at 100°C, and a heat-stable somatic antigen similar to the somatic antigen of *Yersinia pseudotuberculosis*. The capsular antigen will immunize mice but not guinea-pigs against experimental infection, and this property is enhanced when the vaccine has been prepared from cultures incubated at 37°C instead of 27°C to ensure maximal capsule formation. Bacterial products derived from *in vivo* cultivation of *Yersinia pestis* in guinea-pigs include a soluble and an insoluble fraction. The former is a toxin which is lethal to both mice and guinea-pigs, and the latter, which probably contains cell wall material is relatively non-toxic for mice and guinea-pigs but it immunizes both these species. This latter fraction can be produced by special *in vitro* culture of *Yersinia pestis*.

Epidemiology and pathogenesis

Infection in man can develop in two forms, either as bubonic plague arising from the bite of an infected rat flea, or as pneumonic plague which is a respiratory infection derived from inhaling infected droplets from another person with pneumonic lesions.

Plague occurs as an epizootic in rats and has also been identified in a variety of other rodents in which the disease does not occur as an epizootic. The common cycle for the spread of the disease involves infection of the rat flea (*Xenopsylla cheopis*) from the blood of an infected rat. The organisms multiply in the flea and are then inoculated into man when bitten by the flea.

Lesions

Yersinia pestis can cause the death of susceptible rats within a week following inoculation. On post-mortem examination there is an area of necrosis surrounded by oedema at the point of inoculation. The lymphatic glands and spleen will be swollen and haemorrhagic. In rats which have survived infection for more than a week, multiple necrotic areas will have developed in the spleen and liver. The post-mortem picture in guinea-pigs is similar to that seen in rats.

Diagnosis
Rats and guinea-pigs are used for the diagnosis of human infection, which is confirmed by observing the post-mortem lesions described above and by isolating and identifying the organism. The diagnosis of *Yersinia pestis* in rats which have died from natural infection may be difficult if the carcase is decomposing. In these circumstances material from a lesion in the carcase can be applied to the nasal mucous membrane of a guinea-pig or white rat which will develop infection, and *Yersinia pestis* can then be readily isolated and identified from the carcase.

Control and prevention
Cases of plague should be treated promptly with antibiotics and preferably tetracycline in large doses. Both live and killed vaccines are used for prevention but the degree and duration of immunity are limited, and repeated vaccination is required to maintain prolonged protection. Control of wild rodents is also necessary.

FRANCISELLA

Francisella tularensis

Synonym
Pasteurella tularensis

Distribution in nature
The organism derives its name from the district of Tulare, California, where it was first isolated from ground squirrels. *Francisella tularensis* occurs primarily among wild rodents in many areas of the world, including Asia, the Far East, some Western States of the U.S.A. and in some European countries. The species most commonly affected are rabbits, hares, squirrels and other wild rodents.

Morphology and staining
Francisella tularensis is a small coccobacillus measuring approximately 0·7 μm in length and 0·2 μm in width. It produces capsular material and shows bipolar staining. Pleomorphic forms develop after subcultivation on laboratory media. It is non-motile and does not produce spores. The organism stains Gram-negative.

Cultural characteristics
Francisella tularensis develops poorly on laboratory media and satisfactory growth only occurs in the presence of blood or serum to which has been added 0·1 per cent cystine. Growth will also occur on media containing egg yolk. Cultures develop as small mucoid colonies on primary culture after several days' incubation in an atmosphere of reduced oxygen tension.

Resistance to physical and chemical agents
The organism can survive for several months in infected carcases and in water. Its resistance to chemical and physical agents is similar to pasteurellae.

Antigens and toxins
Francisella tularensis possesses an antigenic relationship to *Brucella abortus* and *Brucella melitensis*.

Epidemiology and pathogenesis
As stated above the organism occurs naturally in wild rodents, and infection can be spread either by contact with infected animals or carcases, or from infected ticks. Domesticated animals show a considerable degree of resistance to infection.

Symptoms and lesions
Generally similar to those associated with *Yersinia pseudotuberculosis* infections in rodents.

Diagnosis
It is necessary to carry out bacteriological examinations of suspected material employing egg yolk or blood media containing cystine, using a heavy inoculum, and incubating the cultures in an atmosphere of reduced oxygen tension for 7–10 days. Hamsters or guinea-pigs may be inoculated with suspected material as these animals are susceptible to experimental infection.

Agglutination tests can be employed for the detection of carrier animals.

Public health aspects
Francisella tularensis is pathogenic to man and infection may be contracted from handling infected carcases, from tick bites or from laboratory cultures.

Further reading
BAIN R.V.S. (1963) *Haemorrhagic Septicaemia.* F.A.O. Agric. Stud. No. 62. Rome: FAO.
BIBERSTEIN, E.L., SHREEVE, B.J. AND THOMPSON, D.A. (1970) Variation in carrier rates of *Pasteurella haemolytica* in sheep. I. Normal sheep. *Journal of Comparative Pathology*, **80**, 499.
BRUNER D.W., ANGSTROM C.I. AND PRICE J.I. (1970) *Pasteurella anatipestifer* infection in pheasants. *Cornell Veterinarian*, **60**, 491.

CARTER G.R. (1955) Studies on *Pasteurella multocida*. I. A haemagglutination test for the identification of serological types. *American Journal of Veterinary Research*, **16**, 481.

CARTER G.R. (1957) Studies on *Pasteurella multocida*. III. A serological survey of bovine and porcine strains from various parts of the world. *American Journal of Veterinary Research*, **18**, 437.

CARTER G.R. (1967) Pasteurellosis: *Pasteurella multocida* and *Pasteurella hemolytica*. Advances in Veterinary Science, **11**, 321.

CARTER G.R. AND BAIN R.V.S. (1960) Pasteurellosis (*Pasteurella multocida*): A review stressing recent developments. *Veterinary Reviews and Annotations*, **6**, 105.

HUBBERT, W.T. (1972) Yersiniosis in mammals and birds in the United States. Case Reports and Review. *American Journal of Tropical Medicine and Hygiene*, **21**, 458.

JELLISON W.L., OWEN C.R., BELL J.F. AND KOHLS G.M. (1961) Tularaemia and animal populations: Ecology and Epizootiology. *Wildlife Disease*, **17**, 1.

MAIR, N.S. (1965) Sources and serological classification of 177 strains of *Pasteurella pseudotuberculosis* isolated in Great Britain. *Journal of Pathology and Bacteriology*, **90**, 275.

MARSHALL, J.D., HARRISON, D.N., MURR, J.A. AND CAVANAUGH, D.C. (1972) The role of domestic animals in the epidemiology of plague. III. Experimental infection of swine. *Journal of Infectious Diseases*, **125**, 336.

MOLLARET, H.H. [Secretary], KNAPP, W. [Chairman] (1971) Report [1966–1970] of the Subcommittee on Pasteurella, Yersinia and Francisella to the International Committee on Nomenclature of Bacteria. *International Journal of Systematic Bacteriology*, **21**, 157.

MOORE, T.D., ALLEN, A.M. AND GANAWAY, J.R. (1973) Latent *Pasteurella pneumotropica* infection of the gnotobiotic and barrier-held rats. *Laboratory Animal Science*, **23**, 657.

NAMIOKA S. AND BRUNER D.W. (1963) Serological studies on *Pasteurella multocida*. IV. Type distribution of the organisms on the basis of their capsule and O groups. *Cornell Veterinarian*, **53**, 41.

NAMIOKA S. AND MURATA M. (1961) Serological studies on *Pasteurella multocida*. I. A simplified method for capsule typing of the organism. II. Characteristics of somatic(O) antigen of the organism. III. O antigenic analysis of cultures isolated from various animals. *Cornell Veterinarian*, **51**, 498, 507 and 522.

PENN, C.W. AND NAGY, L.K. (1974) Capsular and somatic antigens of *Pasteurella multocida* types B and E. *Research in Veterinary Science*, **16**, 251

PRODJOHARJONO, S., CARTER, G.R. AND CONNER, G.H. (1974) Serological study of bovine strains of *Pasteurella multocida*. *American Journal of Veterinary Research*, **35**, 111.

REILLY J.R. (1971) Tularaemia, In *Infectious Diseases of Wild Mammals*, ed. J.W. Davis, p. 175. Ames: Iowa State University Press.

REPORT (1968) Symposium on Immunity to the bovine respiratory disease complex. *Journal of the American Veterinary Medical Association*, **152**, 713.

ROBERTS R.S. (1947) An immunological study of *Pasteurella septica*. *Journal of Comparative Pathology*, **57**, 261.

RUST, J.H. CAVANAUGH, D.C., O'SHITA, R. AND MARSHALL, J.D. (1971) The role of domestic animals in the epidemiology of Plague. I. Experimental infection of dogs and cats. *Journal of Infectious Diseases*, **124**, 522.

RUST, J.H., MILLER, B.E., BAHMANYAR, M., MARSHALL, J.D., PURNAVEJA, S., CAVANAUGH, D.C. AND U SAW TIN HLA (1971) The role of domestic animals in the epidemiology of Plague. II Antibody to *Yersinia pestis* in sera of dogs and cats. *Journal of Infectious Diseases*, **124**, 527.

SHREEVE, B.J., BIBERSTEIN, E.L. AND THOMPSON, D.A. (1972) Variation in carrier rates of *Pasteurella haemolytica* in sheep. II. Diseased sheep. *Journal of Comparative Pathology*, **82**, 111.

CHAPTER 10

BRUCELLA

Brucella

Distribution in nature

This group of organisms which includes *Brucella abortus, Br. melitensis, Br. suis, Br. ovis, Br. canis* and *Br. neotomae*, is an important cause of disease in animals and man throughout the world.

Animal species most frequently infected with brucellae are cattle, pigs, goats and sheep in which a common manifestation of the disease is infection of the reproductive tract and abortion. Similar infections occur less frequently in dogs. Horses are occasionally infected and develop a suppurative bursitis. Other animal species which may be associated with the disease and the transmission of infection are a variety of free-living animal species, including hares, deer, rats and other rodents, flies, mosquitoes and ticks. In man, brucellosis (i.e. undulant fever; Malta fever) is characterised by an acute septicaemic phase followed by a chronic stage which may extend over many years. The symptoms include a typically intermittent fever with muscle and joint pains, and hypersensitive reactions particularly among those who repeatedly come into contact with infective materials.

Morphology and staining

Brucellae are small bacilli or coccobacilli which show some variation in size, measuring from $0.6-2.0$ μm in length and about $0.3-0.5$ μm in width. In tissues the organisms often occur in groups as well as singly, and in laboratory cultures they sometimes develop as short chains. They are non-motile and do not form spores. Poorly developed capsules have been described in freshly isolated strains.

The organisms stain Gram-negative and although they are not acid-fast they can resist decolourisation by weak acids, including 0.5 per cent acetic acid, and this feature is incorporated in the brucella differential staining technique which is used for diagnosis. Films are stained with dilute carbol fuchsin for 15 minutes, washed and decolourised with 0.5 per cent acetic acid for 15 seconds, washed and counterstained with methylene blue for 1

minute, washed, dried and examined. The organisms appear pink against a blue background (Plate 10.1a, facing p. 126). An alternative is a modification of Köster's method which consists of staining for 1 minute in 2 parts of saturated aqueous solution of safranin and 5 parts of N KOH solution, wash in water, differentiate in 0.1 per cent H_2SO_4 for 10 seconds, wash in water, and counterstain with 1.0 per cent methylene blue for 3 seconds. The organisms are stained orange-red against a blue background.

Cultural characteristics (Table 10.1)

Growth on laboratory media is slow and often not visible until after 48 hours' incubation at 37°C. Primary cultures of *Br. abortus* and *Br. ovis* grow particularly poorly and require an atmosphere containing 5–10 per cent CO_2, whereas the other species grow under normal atmospheric conditions. On nutrient agar, colonies of smooth strains are about 0.5 mm diameter after 48 hours' incubation, and appear round, convex and translucent with a smooth glistening surface. The colonies become bigger during the following 2–3 days' incubation. Dissociation often occurs on agar media and colonies of rough cultures are larger, flatter, pale yellow in colour and have a granular appearance.

For optimum growth rate and for primary cultures a variety of solid media have been recommended, including serum agar, liver infusion serum agar, tryptose agar, dextrose potato or glycerol potato, and special media incorporating antibiotics. It is necessary to test new batches of medium with known cultures because some liver infusions are inhibitory, and it is also important to ensure that serum samples incorporated in the medium do not contain antibodies to brucellae. In broth cultures turbidity develops slowly with a fine granular deposit which becomes viscous after prolonged incubation. There is a tendency for some strains to dissociate more readily in broth cultures than on agar medium.

Although the organisms utilise various carbohydrates the amounts of acid and gas produced are

TABLE 10.1. Comparing some characteristic properties of *Brucella* species.

Species of *Brucella*	CO$_2$ required for growth	H$_2$S production	Urease production (time in hr.)	Growth in the presence of		
				Thionin		Fuchsin
				1:25 000	1:100 000	1:100 000
Br. abortus	Yes	Moderate	2 or more	—	±	+
Br. suis (American)	No	High	$\frac{1}{2}$	+	+	—
Br. suis (Danish)	No	None	$\frac{1}{2}$	+	+	—
Br. melitensis	No	None or trace	Variable	—	+	+
Br. canis	No	None	$\frac{1}{2}$	+	+	+
Br. ovis	Yes		None			
Br. neotomae	No	Moderate	None	—	+	—

+ = growth   ± = variable   — = no growth.

too small to be of practical use for identifying individual species, but this feature is of value in the identification of the brucella group.

Production of H$_2$S by American strains of *Br. suis* is vigorous but is less marked with strains of *Br. abortus*. Danish strains of *Br. suis* do not produce H$_2$S and *Br. melitensis* is usually negative but some strains may produce a trace reaction. In conjunction with other criteria the test for H$_2$S production is useful for the differentiation of brucella species. One method is to grow the organisms on a serum dextrose agar slope, having inserted a strip of filter paper previously impregnated with a 10 per cent lead acetate solution, and to observe any blackening of the paper during the subsequent days of incubation.

Urease activity is high with both the American and Danish strains of *Br. suis* but low with *Br. abortus*. *Br. melitensis* gives variable results. The tests can be made by inoculating one loopful of a 48 hour culture into 1·0 ml of a buffered 5·0 per cent urea solution (pH 4) with phenol red as indicator. The tubes are then examined after 30 minutes in a waterbath at 37°C, and subsequently at 1 hour and at hourly intervals, thereafter. A pink colour denotes a positive reaction and is due to the organisms' ability to produce NH$_3$ by the hydrolysis of urea. *Br. suis* will give a pink colouration within $\frac{1}{2}$–1 hour but *Br. abortus* will only give a positive reaction after 2 or more hours' incubation.

The sensitivity of brucellae to various dyes was first investigated by Huddleson and the technique is now used for differentiating various species of the organism. The dyes used are thionin, basic fuchsin, methyl violet and pyronin incorporated in serum dextrose agar plates. A loopful of culture is streaked over the surface of one-quarter of each dye plate and incubated for 5 days in an atmosphere of 10 per cent CO$_2$ before being examined. Thus, three unknown cultures can be tested on each plate and the fourth strain should be a known control for comparison. A modification to the technique consists of embedding sterilised dye-impregnated strips of filter paper in liver infusion agar on which is streaked at right angles the culture under examination. If the organism resists the dye it grows across the strip, whereas the growth of a sensitive strain is inhibited at some distance from the strip. For this test it is usual to use filter papers impregnated with thionin (1:800) or basic fuchsin (1:200), and sometimes with methyl violet (1:400) or pyronin (1:800). Cultures are incubated for 3 days in 10 per cent CO$_2$ before being examined. A method using dye tablets which are embedded in the medium has also been developed.

Most strains of *Br. abortus* are inhibited by thionin but not by basic fuchsin, and *Br. suis* is inhibited by basic fuchsin but not by thionin. Table 10.1 summarises these properties but does not include a number of variant strains of *Br. abortus* and *Br. melitensis* which have been described.

Resistance to physical and chemical agents

Brucellae are killed by heating to 60°C for 10 minutes and in milk by pasteurisation. They are susceptible to an acid pH, to disinfectants and to direct sunlight, but are known to survive several months in a fetus not exposed to sunlight. The organisms remain viable for long periods at low temperatures and will survive for a year or more in faeces at 8°C and can be stored at a temperature of –40°C for a great deal longer.

Antigens and toxins

Smooth strains of *Br. abortus*, *Br. suis* and *Br. melitensis* each possess two antigens which are labelled A and M. There is a quantitative difference between these antigens in *Br. abortus* and *Br. suis* on the one hand, and in *Br. melitensis*, on the other. The A and M antigens of *Br. abortus* occur in a ratio of 20:1 and in a slightly narrower proportion

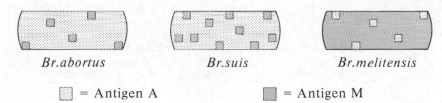

Br.abortus   *Br.suis*   *Br.melitensis*

▨ = Antigen A   ▩ = Antigen M

FIG. 10.1. The approximate proportions of A and M antigens in smooth strains of *Br. abortus*, *Br. suis* and *Br. melitensis*.

in *Br. suis*, whereas in *Br. melitensis* the proportion is 1:20 (Fig. 10.1). This means that *Br. melitensis* cannot be differentiated from the other two species by straightforward agglutination tests but only by agglutinin–absorption techniques using specific A or M. antisera. Because of the occurrence of these antigens in different proportions, it is possible to absorb A antibodies from a *Br. melitensis* antiserum and conversely, M antibodies from a *Br. abortus* or *Br. suis* antiserum. The resultant absorbed antisera will contain mono-specific M and A antibodies, respectively, which will agglutinate only those organisms possessing the predominant corresponding antigen. Thus, an absorbed antiserum containing only A antibodies will agglutinate *Br. abortus* and *Br. suis* but not *Br. melitensis*. This is because the A antigen of *Br. melitensis* constitutes only 5 per cent of the total antigenic complex and is insufficient to cause macroscopic agglutination. However, these absorbed sera should be used routinely in conjunction with biochemical and other tests for the identification of unknown cultures because some variant strains are known which may have the serological properties of one species but the biochemical, cultural and pathogenic properties of another. More recent studies on the antigenic structures of brucellae, using agar gel precipitation methods, have shown the presence of a number of other minor antigens in these organisms.

The surface antigen of *Br. canis* appears to be similar to the rough antigens of *Br. abortus*, *Br. suis* and *Br. ovis*.

No extracellular toxins have been identified.

Bacteriophage typing

Phages specific for *Br. abortus* have been isolated, and a standardised method of phage typing has been developed. This consists essentially of using a dilution of phage known as the routine test dilution (RTD) which is the highest dilution giving complete lysis. When the RTD is used against smooth cultures, only strains of *Br. abortus* are lysed; whereas a higher concentration of phage (e.g. 10 000 RTD) will also lyse strains of *Br. suis* but not *Br. melitensis*.

Application of the test on a wide scale is facilitated by the fact that diluted phage remains stable for a number of years when stored at 4°C.

Epidemiology and pathogenesis

Cattle

Br. abortus infection occurs in most parts of the world and the incidence may vary from 1 to 20 per cent or more in certain areas or in groups of animals exposed to particular sources of infection. A herd becomes diseased usually from the introduction of infected cattle and the disease subsequently spreads within the herd from aborted fetuses, placentae and genital discharges which contaminate the environment. The infection may also be transmitted via colostrum or milk which in some cases may be intermittently infected for several months after calving. Infected bulls used for artificial insemination can also be the cause of introducing widespread infection into a clean herd.

Under natural and experimental conditions it has been shown that cattle can become infected by various routes, particularly by ingestion, via the vagina during coitus with diseased bulls or artificial insemination with infected semen, through the conjunctiva and the skin, and possibly by inhalation.

Calves are relatively insusceptible to the disease but may excrete the organism during the period when they are fed infected milk and, consequently, may be responsible for the spread of infection on a farm during that time. In newly infected non-pregnant, yearling animals a temporary bacteraemia occurs and infection commonly develops in the udder and supramammary lymphatic glands.

In pregnant animals the organism has a predilection for the gravid uterus causing varying degrees of placentitis, resulting in abortion in suceptible animals or premature births of weak calves in herds where the disease is endemic. It is well known that *Br. abortus* has a predilection for fetal rather than adult tissues and it has now been shown that this is due to erythritol, a saccharide alcohol, which is present in the placenta of cattle, sheep, goats and pigs, and in the testicular tissues of these species. Experiments have also revealed that erythritol is a growth stimulant for *Br. abortus, Br. melitensis* and for *Br. suis*, and that it is a source of energy for avirulent strains of *Br. abortus*. These findings show clearly the close interrelationship between the occurrence of erythritol in the tissues and the pathogenesis of brucella infections in cattle, sheep, goats and pigs.

The introduction of *Br. abortus* infection into a clean herd may lead to acute and widespread disease giving rise to 50 per cent or more of abortions. Usually the initial abortion rate may not be greater than 30–40 per cent and this declines during subsequent years as the infection becomes more chronic in the herd. The introduction of susceptible animals into the herd will result in the recurrence of the acute form of the disease. The majority of infected animals excrete *Br. abortus* in the colostrum and milk following parturition, and excretion continues intermittently in many animals for several months and in some for 2 years or more.

The common sites for infection in bulls are the testicles, seminal vesicles and epididymis. Acute infection results initially in large numbers of organisms in the semen which becomes less heavily infected over a period of several months as the disease develops into a more chronic form.

Br. melitensis can cause disease in cattle and infection is usually derived from contact with infected goats or sheep. The organisms establish themselves in the udder and give rise to infected milk. Abortions may occur but less frequently than with *Br. abortus* infections. Cattle are also susceptible to infection with *Br. suis*.

Sheep

Br. melitensis is a major cause of disease in many countries and sheep of all ages are susceptible. Infection can take place by a variety of routes including the vagina, alimentary tract, conjunctiva, skin and possibly by inhalation. As in cattle, infection results in a transient bacteraemia and the organisms subsequently settle in the genital organs, mammary glands and lymph nodes. Infection is spread by diseased animals via aborted fetuses, milk and from vaginal discharges and urine which may be infected intermittently for several weeks and contaminate the environment.

Br. ovis causes epididymitis in rams and has been reported from New Zealand, Australia, Czechoslovakia and other countries. The tail of the epididymis and, to a less extent, the interstitial tissues of the seminal vesicles are the commonest sites for primary infection to occur. The semen from such animals may be infected. A bacteraemia develops later and subsequently the organisms settle in

additional sites, especially the kidneys, giving rise to intermittent infection of urine and, less frequently, the liver and spleen. Semen from infected rams may transfer the disease to ewes and cause inflammation of the uterus and cervix. Abortion may also occur.

Br. abortus has been reported as causing sporadic outbreaks of disease in sheep in some countries, including the United Kingdom.

Goats

Br. melitensis is a serious cause of disease, particularly in the area of the Mediterranean and in parts of the American continent. As with sheep, infection can occur by various routes, leading to a bacteraemia and the development of infection in the spleen and lymphatic glands in the majority of cases, and also in the uterus and udder in pregnant animals. Spread of infection arises from contamination of the environment with aborted fetuses, vaginal discharges, urine and faeces, which may be heavily contaminated for several months after an animal has aborted. In addition, *Br. melitensis* will also be excreted in the milk for several weeks or months.

Br. abortus has rarely been reported as causing disease in goats which appear to be relatively resistant to this infection.

Pigs

Br. suis is a widespread cause of disease among pigs in many countries, and animals of all ages are susceptible although the young do not develop symptoms as severe as those in adults. Infection can occur by a variety of routes, the most common being via the vagina during coitus. The organisms become localised primarily in the lymphatic glands draining the site of inoculation. Subsequently, a transient bacteraemia develops and, thereafter, the common sites for the establishment of infection are the genital organs, mammary glands, bladder, spleen and joints. Following infection of the male genital organs, the semen may be infected over long periods. In sows the gravid uterus is a predilection site for the organism and abortion may occur. Vaginal discharges at the time of parturition are heavily infected and constitute a serious source of contamination of the environment. The introduction of infection into a herd usually results initially in an acute form of the disease which later becomes more chronic and sometimes unrecognisable, until the re-introduction of fresh susceptible animals which results in the reappearance of the acute form of the disease.

It is noteworthy that hares are susceptible to infection with *Br. suis* as well as with other species of brucellae. Strains of organisms isolated from these animals are pathogenic for pigs and it is known that infected hares can be the sources of disease in swine herds.

Br. abortus has been isolated occasionally from pigs but it is not an important cause of disease in these animals.

Horses
Br. abortus is associated with chronic inflammatory conditions including fistulous withers, poll evil and also joint infections. The routes of infection have not been clearly established but the most usual are probably ingestion and contact. Predisposing factors related to the development of fistulous withers and poll evil may arise from other concurrent infections.

Dogs
Br. canis is host specific for dogs and causes abortion particularly among beagles. The disease has been reported from the U.S.A. but its existence may be considerably more widespread than previously realised.

Br. abortus is an uncommon cause of clinical disease and dogs show a marked resistance to this infection under natural conditions. However, there is serological evidence to indicate that dogs may acquire infection and be responsible for spreading the organism on farms.

Other species
A wide variety of animal species are susceptible in varying degrees to natural infection, particularly hares, deer and various wild rodents. Under natural conditions, cats and poultry show a strong degree of resistance but can be infected experimentally. In many countries it is evident that brucellosis can be spread by flies, mosquitoes and ticks. Recent work on the incidence of brucellae in free-living animals has shown that a very wide variety of species are susceptible, and that in some countries at least, the success or otherwise of an eradication programme may depend to a considerable extent on the incidence of infection in wild animals and the dissemination of organisms by arthropod vectors.

Symptoms
Among cattle, abortion is the characteristic symptom in the majority of animals infected with Br. abortus. In highly susceptible individuals abortion occurs usually at the seventh or eighth month of pregnancy and occasionally earlier as a result of heavy exposure to infection. In herds suffering from endemic infections, abortions are less common but placentae may be retained following parturitions at full term. Most animals abort only once although infection may be continually present in various body tissues. On a herd basis the introduction of infection into a group of healthy animals may result in abortions occurring in 30–40 per cent of individuals in 1 year, and then the abortion rate will decrease during subsequent years as the disease becomes endemic. However, the introduction into the herd of additional susceptible animals may cause a further rise in the rate of abortions.

Among sheep, the characteristic symptom of Br. melitensis infection is abortion which occurs most usually at the third or fourth month of pregnancy, and sometimes at almost full term. Other signs of infection are lameness and mastitis, recognised by discolouration of the milk which contains clots. In addition, animals infected with the acute form of the disease develop a rapid loss of condition, pyrexia and diarrhoea. Similar symptoms occur in goats infected with Br. melitensis. Br. ovis infection in sheep may be the cause of a low fertility rate and sometimes abortion.

Br. suis infections in pigs give rise to abortions or the birth of weak piglets, lameness and sometimes paralysis arising from the development of lesions in the spinal column. As a result of infection there is an increased infertility rate in both male and female animals.

Br. canis infection in dogs is characterised by early undetectable embryonic deaths or by abortions occurring at about the fiftieth day of gestation followed by a prolonged vaginal discharge. Male dogs may suffer from dermatitis of the scrotum and unilateral testicular atrophy, but many infected animals may remain symptomless.

Lesions
The gravid bovine uterus infected with Br. abortus develops a necrotic placentitis. Some of the cotyledons become swollen, hyperaemic and surrounded by a brownish exudate. The intercotyledonary spaces are thickened and have a characteristic, leathery appearance (Plate 10.1b, facing p. 126). The fetus shows no obvious lesions, and macroscopically the infected udder will usually appear normal but microscopically the parenchyma may show either heavy cellular infiltration or degeneration and necrosis. Infected bulls may develop an orchitis resulting in abscess formation or areas of necrosis in the testicle surrounded by fibrous tissue.

The lesions of Br. melitensis infection in sheep and goats are similar to those associated with Br. abortus infection in cattle. Br. ovis infection in sheep gives rise to lesions in the epithelium of the tail of the epididymis and in the interstitial tissue of the seminal vesicles.

Br. suis infection in pigs causes a placentitis and metritis in the pregnant animal, and an epididymitis and orchitis in boars causing necrosis and purulent lesions in the grossly enlarged testicles. Abscesses may also occur in various sites in the body including the spinal column and limb joints.

Lesions which may be associated with *Br. abortus* infection in horses are fistulous withers — a chronic inflammatory condition of the supraspinous bursa, and poll evil which is a similar type of lesion in the atlantal bursa.

Abortion in dogs caused by *Br. canis* gives rise to pathological changes similar to those described for cattle, sheep and pigs.

Diagnosis

A wide variety of methods have been used for the diagnosis of brucellosis in different animal species in various countries, and the following is a summary of the more widely accepted and reliable procedures.

Direct smear

In cases of abortion, brucella organisms can be seen in large numbers in films prepared from fresh samples of chorionic tissue, fetal stomach contents and uterine discharges. Films should be stained by the brucella differential staining technique (see p. 343). The organisms occur characteristically in clumps intracellularly as well as extracellularly. Smears prepared from abscesses in various animal species, and from fistulous withers in horses may not be of value for diagnostic purposes.

Bacteriological examination

Some suitable media for the routine isolation of brucellae are serum dextrose agar incorporating the antibiotics bacitracin, polymyxin B and actidione, trypticase soya agar or Albimi medium. All primary cultures of *Br. abortus* and *Br. canis* should be incubated in an atmosphere of 10 per cent CO_2 for at least 10 days before discarding as negative. Fetal membranes are usually grossly contaminated and a piece of cotyledon should be washed in saline several times, sliced into small pieces and rubbed over the surface of a solid medium. Pieces of lung or spleen from an aborted fetus should be similarly treated. Fetal stomach contents and meconium, often heavily infected with *Br. abortus*, should also be examined by spreading a few drops of material over the surface of solid medium. For the cultural examination of milk, Albimi medium has been used with actidione, polymyxin, bacitracin, circulin and ethyl violet instead of crystal violet.

Br. ovis can be isolated from various sites in diseased sheep, including semen, epididymis, spleen, placenta, mammary gland and aborted fetuses.

Guinea-pig inoculation

Guinea-pigs are susceptible to infection with brucellae and are used for diagnostic purposes. Material to be tested can be inoculated subcutaneously, intramuscularly in the case of milk samples, and by a variety of other routes, including the conjunctiva. Two animals are used for each test, one being killed at 3 weeks and the other at 6 weeks after inoculation. They are examined for brucellae and the sera tested for agglutinins. Typical lesions include miliary necrotic foci in the spleen, liver, lymphatic glands and an orchitis in male guinea-pigs after intraperitoneal inoculation of infective material. When necessary, the spleen can be inoculated on to serum dextrose agar.

Serological tests

A variety of serological tests are used for the control of bovine brucellosis because no single method is wholly satisfactory under all conditions. For example, none of the tests is reliable for detecting animals which are incubating the disease, and this period of incubation, when significant levels of antibodies are not produced, may last for several months in some cases. When antibodies are produced their presence may be detected more readily by one serological test than by another, and the antibody levels in sera from chronically infected animals show wide variations in concentration. An additional important problem is the difficulty of distinguishing between antibody production in healthy animals as a result of vaccination and that which arises from natural infection.

The serum agglutination test (SAT) is widely used as one of the more reliable methods for the diagnosis of *Br. abortus* infection in cattle, and is particularly valuable for use in unvaccinated cattle or on farms where calfhood vaccination is practised. Using standard antigen prepared at the Central Veterinary Laboratory, Weybridge, a titre of at least 50 per cent agglutination at 1:40 or more is indicative of infection. A titre of 1:20 is doubtful and the animal should be retested a few weeks later. The serum agglutinin titres developed by infected cattle show wide variation and positive titres may not develop in some individuals for a period of 1–4 or 5 months after infection, and others may never develop a positive titre although the infection causes abortion. In some cases the titre shows a sharp rise to a high level shortly before or soon after abortion. Young calves which become infected develop agglutinin titres which usually become negative by 6 months of age. However, infection contracted at about 6 months of age or later, results in a more persistent and clearly diagnostic titre.

The Rose Bengal plate test (RBPT) is a modification of the serum agglutination test and is used extensively for the routine testing of cattle in some countries. The antigen consists of a suspension of brucella organisms stained with Rose Bengal and adjusted to pH 3·6. It is claimed that the acid pH reduces the incidence of reactions caused by non-specific agglutinins sometimes present in bovine sera. The test is carried out by adding 0·3 ml serum to 0·3 ml stained antigen on a plate or tile, mixing and examining for agglutination after four minutes. The test has the advantages that it is cheap and convenient to carry out, it tends to give a positive reaction earlier than the SAT when testing sera from recently infected animals, and it gives results similar to the complement-fixation test (CFT) when used for the detection of chronically infected animals. In addition, the RBPT begins to give negative reactions sooner than the SAT with sera from calves which have been recently vaccinated.

The complement-fixation test is being used on an increasing scale for the control of brucellosis in cattle. It is particularly useful for the detection of chronically infected animals in which complement fixing antibodies fade less rapidly than agglutinins.

The milk ring test (MRT) is widely used as a general screening method. The test is based on detecting specific agglutinins in the milk which agglutinate stained antigen added to the composite milk sample derived from a number of cows. After incubation, the presence of agglutinins is determined by agglutination of the stained antigen which rises with the cream layer. For this test the antigen consists of killed *Br. abortus* organisms stained with haematoxylin (blue) or tetrazolium (red).

The whey agglutination test is of value for detecting animals which are excreting *Br. abortus* provided that they have not been vaccinated for a period of at least 3 months, beforehand. The higher the titre the more likely it is that excretion of the organism is persistent and not intermittent. The test consists of removal of cream from a milk sample by centrifugation, the addition of rennet followed by incubation, and separation of the whey which is then tested by the same method as the serum agglutination test.

The antiglobulin (Coombs) test has been introduced as an additional technique, mainly for detecting antibodies to *Br. abortus* in man and experimentally in animals. The method detects the presence of IgG antibodies and has been applied to the diagnosis of chronic human infections when antibodies associated with IgM immunoglobulins have disappeared.

Sheep infected with *Br. ovis* develop high serum titres detectable by the complement-fixation test, which may persist for at least 9 months after lambing.

Br. canis infection of dogs may be diagnosed by a bacterial agglutinin titre of 1:100 or more. In some cases this may be the only method of diagnosis but in others the infection may be suspected when abortion occurs at about 2 weeks before term or when bitches fail to whelp after apparently successful matings.

Control and prevention

The general basis for the control and prevention of brucellosis in cattle is the identification and elimination of infected animals from herds together with vaccination programmes designed to increase the resistance of animals to natural infection. Since the beginning of this century many attempts have been made to develop a vaccine which is both safe to use and sufficiently immunogenic to control the natural disease. It was eventually realised that virulent strains do not satisfy both these criteria and studies were made to find avirulent strains which were sufficiently immunogenic to be of practical value and yet remained stable and did not revert to the virulent form in the animal body. Two strains have been studied in particular detail. The first, known as *Br. abortus* strain 19, was originally isolated from milk and shown to be a smooth, non-virulent but immunogenic strain which, over several years' study did not appear to have changed its virulence. Strain 19 is now used extensively as a live vaccine which has the advantage when inoculated into calves aged 91–180 days, that it stimulates the development of a high level of immunity and only the transient production of agglutinins which disappear by the time of the first calving. One dose will give an immunity which remains high for as long as at least the fifth pregnancy. With the concurrent use of diagnostic tests for the detection and removal of infected animals from herds, this vaccine has enabled the incidence of bovine abortions to be greatly reduced in several countries. However, infection of milk still remains a serious public health problem.

The second vaccine which received wide attention was prepared from an avirulent strain known as 45/20. This was a rough strain which had the advantage that it did not stimulate agglutinin production against smooth antigens of *Br. abortus* and thus did not interfere with the serological detection of natural infection. Unfortunately, it was found that the strain was not stable and that it could give rise to both smooth and virulent mutants. On this account a killed 45/20 vaccine with adjuvant has been developed and used for the control of the disease. Following vaccination, the RBPT gives negative results sooner than the CFT in a non-infected animal and the titre of the SAT will not rise significantly and soon becomes negative.

Any reference to the control and prevention of brucellosis in cattle would not be complete without stressing the importance of ensuring that infection is not transmitted by a veterinarian from one farm to another. When handling animals, protective clothing should always be worn and thoroughly cleaned and disinfected after use. Material which is suspected of being infected (e.g. placentae, aborted fetuses) should not be handled unless the operator is wearing disposable gloves, and all equipment should be sterilised before and after use.

Attempts to control brucellosis in sheep have been based largely on the serological identification and slaughter of reactors. A variety of vaccines including strain 19 have been used in conjunction with sanitary measures to effect a considerable reduction of infection in diseased flocks.

It is important from the public health point of view in particular, that *Br. melitensis* infection in sheep and goats is adequately controlled. The agglutination test for the detection and elimination of infected animals should be carried out on a herd basis and used in conjunction with adequate standards of hygiene and disinfection. The development of a reliable vaccine is still awaited.

Public health aspects

Man is susceptible to infection with brucellae and the incidence of human infections and the species of organisms involved depend upon the environmental conditions in various countries which enable cross-infection between animals and man to take place. Human infections arise primarily from ingestion and contact but also probably via mucous membranes and inhalation. Infected milk and milk products, meat and meat products and sometimes other foodstuffs, constitute important sources of disease for man. The risk of infection is particularly severe for veterinarians, farmers and others concerned with the handling of infected animals, fetuses, afterbirths, discharges and laboratory cultures which are heavily infected with brucellae. It is a wise precaution for laboratory workers to manipulate infective material and cultures with great caution under protective hoods of proved efficiency.

Brucella neotomae

A new species of *Brucella* has been isolated from the desert wood rat, *Neotoma lepida*. This organism does not require CO_2 for primary isolation, it is sensitive to both thionin and basic fuchsin, and is antigenically related to *Br. abortus* and *Br. suis*. Under experimental conditions *Br. neotomae* can infect pigs with the production of agglutinins but without the development of clinical signs of infection. Experimental vaccines have been prepared from this organism.

Further reading

ALTON G.G. AND ELBERG S.S. (1967) Rev. 1 Brucella melitensis vaccine — a review. *Veterinary Bulletin*, **37**, 793.

ALTON G.G. AND JONES L.M. (1967) *Laboratory Techniques in Brucellosis*. W.H.O. Monograph No. 55, p. 92. Geneva: WHO.

BEH, K.J. AND LASCELLES, A.K. (1973) The use of the antiglobulin test in the diagnosis of bovine brucellosis. *Research in Veterinary Science*, **14**, 239.

BIBERSTEIN E.L. AND CAMERON H.S. (1961) The family Brucellaceae in veterinary research. *Annual Review of Microbiology*, **15**, 93.

BROWN, G.M., LOVE, E.L., PIETZ, D.E. AND RANGER, C.R. (1972) Characterisation of *Brucella abortus* strain 19. *American Journal of Veterinary Research*, **33**, 759.

CARMICHAEL L.E. AND KENNEY R.M. (1968) Canine abortion caused by *Brucella canis*. Journal of the American Veterinary Medical Association, **152**, 605.

CORBEL, M.J. (1972) Characterisation of antibodies active in the Rose Bengal plate test. *Veterinary Record*, **90**, 484.

CORBEL, M.J. (1973) Studies on the mechanism of the Rose Bengal plate test for bovine brucellosis. *British Veterinary Journal*, **129**, 157.

CORBEL, M.J. AND DAY, C.A. (1973) Assessment of indirect haemagglution procedures for the serological diagnosis of bovine brucellosis. *British Veterinary Journal*, **129**, 480.

HUNTER, D. AND ALLEN, J. (1972) An evaluation of milk and blood tests used to diagnose brucellosis. *Veterinary Record*, **91**, 310.

JONES, L.M. AND BERMAN, D.T. (1971) Antibody response, delayed hypersensitivity, and immunity in guinea-pigs induced by smooth and rough strains of *Brucella abortus*. *Journal of Infectious Diseases*, **124**, 47.

MCLAREN, A.P.C. AND BRINLEY MORGAN, W.J. (1973) The incidence of the various biotypes of *Brucella abortus* in cattle in the south-west of Scotland. *Veterinary Record*, **93**, 392.

MYLREA, P.J. (1972) The diagnosis of brucellosis in dairy herds. *Australian Veterinary Journal*, **48**, 369.

RENOUX, G. RENOUX, M. AND TINELLI, R. (1973) Phenol-water fraction from smooth *Brucella abortus* and *Brucella melitensis*: immunological analysis and biologic behavior. *Journal of Infectious Diseases*, **127**, 139.

STERNE, M., TRIM, G. AND BROUGHTON, E.S. (1971) Immunisation of laboratory animals and cattle with non-agglutinogenic extracts of *Brucella abortus* strain 45/20. *Journal of Medical Microbiology*, **4**, 185.

Symposium on brucellosis (1960). *Veterinary Record*, **72**, 917.

Symposium on the control and eradication of brucellosis (1968) *Veterinary Record*, **82**, 7.

THORNTON, D.H. AND MUSKETT, J.C. (1972) The use of laboratory animals in the potency test of *Brucella abortus* S19 vaccine. Response of guinea-pigs to graduated doses of vaccine and challenge. *Journal of Comparative Pathology*, **82**, 201.

CHAPTER 11

ACTINOBACILLUS

CHAPTER 11

Actinobacillus

These organisms are usually in the form of short rods but occasionally occur in longer forms or filaments. They are non-motile and stain Gram-negative. Organisms in this group which are pathogenic for animals include *Actinobacillus lignièresi* the cause of granulomatous lesions in cattle and sheep, and *Actinobacillus equuli* associated with disease in foals and occasionally pigs.

Actinobacillus lignièresi

Distribution in nature

This organism is named after Lignière who together with Spitz first described it at the turn of the century. They associated the organism with cases of subcutaneous granulomatous abscesses occurring among cattle in the Argentine. Since that time *Actinobacillus lignièresi* has been shown to have a world-wide distribution.

Morphology and staining

The organisms occur in tissues and in primary cultures as small rods measuring about 1.5 μm in length and 0.4 μm in width (Plate 11.1a, facing p. 127). After growth on laboratory media the organism shows considerable pleomorphism and may develop as coccobacilli, diplococci or as filamentous forms.

The organisms stain Gram-negative and are not acid-alcohol-fast.

Cultural characteristics

Primary cultures sown on to nutrient agar develop slowly when incubated aerobically at the optimal temperature of 37°C. After 24 hours, growth appears as small translucent colonies about $1-1.5$ mm in diameter. There is little improvement in growth rate of primary cultures when blood or serum is incorporated in the agar. However, the growth rate does improve after primary cultures have been subcultured several times on artificial media; colony sizes increase to 4–5 mm diameter and heavy inoculation

may give confluent growth over the surface of the medium.

Growth of newly isolated strains in nutrient broth is poor and granular. After subcultivation the organism grows more profusely producing a uniform turbidity and pellicle formation.

Cultures do not survive for more than a few days on laboratory media and should be subcultivated at frequent intervals to maintain viability. Acid without gas is produced in a number of carbohydrates including glucose, saccharose, maltose, laevulose, galactose and mannitol. Lactose is fermented after several days' incubation.

Resistance to physical and chemical agents

The organism is killed by a temperature of 60°C for 15 minutes, and is relatively susceptible to disinfectants.

Antigens and toxins

Common heat-labile antigens occur among all strains of *Actinobacillus lignièresi*, including those isolated from sheep as well as cattle. In addition, there are type-specific heat-stable antigens which enable the grouping of *Actinobacillus lignièresi* strains into six distinct types. Most cattle strains belong to type 1 and sheep strains to types 2, 3 and 4. An antigenic relationship has also been demonstrated between strains of *Actinobacillus lignièresi*, *Pseudomonas mallei* and *Pseudomonas pseudomallei*.

Epidemiology and pathogenesis

Under natural conditions, *Actinobacillus lignièresi* can cause disease in both cattle and sheep which is characterised by the development of infectious granulomatous lesions containing pus. The pathogenesis of the disease in cattle has become more clearly understood since the demonstration of the organism in the rumenal contents and tongues of apparently normal cattle, and also the presence of specific antibodies in their sera. This provides strong evidence that the disease is endogenous in origin

141

and may arise as the result of abrasions to the mucous surfaces of the tongue, pharynx and stomach. In sheep, the common sites of infection are in the region of the head, face and mouth, and arise from superficial skin wounds in these areas which become infected with the causal organism. Occasionally, the organism may be a cause of ovine mastitis.

Symptoms

These depend upon the mechanical interference resulting from the development of lesions in various parts of the body, especially in the region of the mouth, tongue and pharynx.

Lesions

The granulomatous infected lesions in cattle can occur in a wide variety of sites, particularly the tongue (hence the term 'wooden tongue'), cheeks, lips, gums, pharyngeal region, rumen, reticulum and omasum. In addition, lesions may develop on the skin, in the liver and sometimes in skeletal muscle. The lymph glands proximal to the areas of the lesions will also be affected. Similarly, in sheep the lesions occur on the skin and mucous surfaces.

The lesions commence as areas of chronic suppuration which become thick walled with the formation of granulomatous tissue. The pus characteristically includes very small granules which contain the causal organism in the centre surrounded by a ring of pear-shaped or club-shaped bodies (Plate 11.1b, facing p. 127). The precise function of these bodies is not known but they have been variously described as part of the defensive reaction of the tissues in the chronic inflammatory response.

Diagnosis

In cattle advanced cases of "wooden tongue" are characterised by extensive lesions of the tongue which becomes hardened and nodular (Plate 11.1c, facing p. 127). Gram-stained smears of the small greyish granules occurring in the pus from lesions in any part of the body, reveal zones of club-shaped bodies surrounding a central mass of *Actinobacillus lignièresi*. Material can be cultured by the methods already described either from the pus or from local lymphatic glands using serum or blood agar, or Phillips' medium containing oleandomycin and nystatin.

It may be necessary to carry out a differential diagnosis of these lesions from infections caused by *Actinomyces bovis*. The main points of difference are that *Actinomyces bovis* occurs in the tissues as Gram-positive organisms either in the form of filaments, short rods or cocci; pus from actinomycotic lesions contains particularly hard granules which after crushing and staining by Gram's method,

give the appearance of a number of Gram-negative staining club-shaped bodies surrounding a mass of Gram-positive organisms which often occur in filaments; there is a tendency for *Actinomyces bovis* to attack the bony structures of the body instead of soft tissues, particularly the jaw bones of cattle.

Control and prevention

Since it is now apparent that infections with *Actinobacillus lignièresi* are endogenous in origin, it is important to ensure as far as practicable that abrasions of the skin and mucous membranes occur infrequently. Iodine in the form of potassium iodide and Lugol's solution have long been used for the treatment of actinobacillosis. Considerable success has been claimed although it has been shown *in vitro* that potassium iodide is not exceptionally lethal to *Actinobacillus lignièresi*. Other methods of treatment include sodium iodide intravenously, streptomycin intramuscularly and sulphadimidine intravenously supplemented by additional oral dosage. No satisfactory vaccine is available.

Actinobacillus equuli

Synonyms

Bacterium viscosum equi, Bacillus nephritidis equi, Bacillus equirulis, Shigella viscosa, Shigella equirulis, Shigella equuli.

Distribution in nature

This organism occurs in the intestines of the equine species in many countries without causing disease. In foals, however, it may be associated with septicaemic infections, nephritis and joint ill. It has also been isolated from diseased pigs and calves.

Morphology and staining

In tissues and in primary cultures the organism occurs usually as oval-shaped rods measuring 1·5 μm in length and 0·8 μm in width. There is a tendency, particularly after subcultivation, for pleomorphic forms to develop as chains or filaments. Characteristically, the organisms produce material of mucoid consistency but whether they are really capsulated still remains doubtful. Spores are not formed and the organism is non-motile.

Actinobacillus equuli stains Gram-negative.

Cultural characteristics

Actinobacillus equuli grows well on ordinary laboratory media. On nutrient agar the colonies of newly isolated strains appear shiny and grey in colour. They have a characteristic mucoid consistency. Growth in broth develops as a slimy sediment.

Acid but no gas is produced in lactose, glucose,

maltose, sucrose and mannitol. Nitrates are reduced to nitrites, H_2S is produced and the Voges-Proskauer, methyl red and indole tests are negative.

Resistance to physical and chemical agents
This organism is relatively susceptible to the lethal actions of heat and disinfectants.

Antigens and toxins
There is considerable antigenic heterogeneity amongst strains of *Actinobacillus equuli* which limits the use of the bacterial agglutination test as a diagnostic procedure. In addition, there are antigens which are common to both *Actinobacillus equuli* and *Actinobacillus lignièresi*.

Epidemiology and pathogenesis
Actinobacillus equuli is known to occur in the intestines of healthy horses and predisposing factors, including overwork, exposure to the cold and parasitism, increase the susceptibility of individuals to clinical infection. The spread of the organism occurs commonly by ingestion, and infection of aborted fetuses may develop. It is difficult to set up experimental infection unless the organisms are inoculated intravenously when a fatal septicaemia may develop, causing acute arthritis and suppurative nephritis in foals. Subcutaneous inoculation results in the temporary development of a localised abscess. Although the organism has been isolated from young pigs, it is difficult to set up experimental infection in these animals.

Symptoms and lesions
Adult horses may be affected by an acute form of the disease and show signs of fever, difficulty in swallowing and salivation. Convalescence is usually protracted. In young foals the symptoms of infection are weakness and prostration. In acute infections, death occurs rapidly but in more protracted cases arthritis develops with consequent painful joints and lameness. Similar symptoms of acute infection have been described in young pigs, and in calves the signs of disease are diarrhoea, dehydration and nervous symptoms.

Lesions in foals include enteritis, arthritis, and an acute nephritis. Sometimes localised areas of necrosis are seen in the kidneys. In calves, areas of focal necrosis will be seen in many sites, including the lungs, spleen, rumen, small and large intestines.

Diagnosis
The symptoms and lesions may be suggestive of infection with *Actinobacillus equuli* but a conclusive diagnosis must be based on the isolation and identification of the organism from the tissues.

Control and prevention
Attempts have been made to use the bacterial agglutination test for detecting diseased individuals and vaccination as a method for preventing infection. Satisfactory results have been obtained from the treatment of infected foals with antibiotics, particularly streptomycin and the tetracyclines.

Actinobacillus suis
During recent years there have been several reports associating actinobacilli with disease in pigs. More recent studies on the characteristic properties of these organisms have shown that they constitute a species distinct from *Actinobacillus lignièresi* and *Actinobacillus equuli* and have been named *Actinobacillus suis*.

Strains of *Actinobacillus suis* are characterised by producing narrow but distinct zones of a-haemolysis on horse blood agar and wide zones of β-haemolysis on sheep blood agar. In addition, they differ from strains of *Actinobacillus lignièresi* and *Actinobacillus equuli* by their ability to hydrolyse aesculin and produce acid when grown in arabinose, cellobiose and salacin. *Actinobacillus suis* is also pathogenic for mice.

Actinobacillus suis can cause a fatal septicaemia in pigs 1–6 weeks of age. In older animals, infection manifests itself as an arthritis, polyarthritis, pneumonia or as a series of subcutaneous abscesses in the neck, shoulder and flank.

Further reading
CUTLIP, R.C., AMTOWER, W.C. AND ZINOBER, M.R. (1972) Septic embolic Actinobacillosis of swine: a case report and laboratory reproduction of the disease. *American Journal of Veterinary Research*, **33**, 1621.

FREDERIKSEN, W. (1971) A taxonomic study of *Pasteurella* and *Actinobacillus* strains. Journal of General Microbiology, **69**, viii.

MAIR, N.S. RANDALL, C.J., THOMAS, G.W., HARBOURNE, J.F., McCREA, C.T. AND COWL, K.P. (1974) *Actinobacillus suis* infection in pigs: a report of four outbreaks and two sporadic cases. *Journal of Comparative Pathology*, **84**, 113.

OSBALDISTON, G.W. AND WALKER, R.D. (1972) Enteric actinobacillosis in calves. *Cornell Veterinarian*, **62**, 364.

PHILLIPS J.E. (1960) The characterisation of *Actinobacillus lignièresi*. *Journal of Pathology and Bacteriology*, **79**, 331.

PHILLIPS J.E. (1961) The commensal role of *Actinobacillus lignièresi*. *Journal of Pathology and Bacteriology*, **82**, 205.

PHILLIPS J.E. (1964) Commensal actinobacilli from the bovine tongue. *Journal of Pathology and Bacteriology*, **87**, 442.

PHILLIPS J.E. (1965/66) Actinobacillosis. *Veterinary Annual*, 7, 42.

TILL D.H. AND PALMER F.P. (1960) A review of Actinobacillosis with a study of the casual organism. *Veterinary Record*, 72, 527.

WINDSOR, R.S. (1973) *Actinobacillus equuli* infection in a litter of pigs and a review of previous reports on similar infections. *Veterinary Record*, 92, 178.

CHAPTER 12

HAEMOPHILUS, MORAXELLA AND BORDETELLA

Haemophilus, Moraxella and Bordetella

HAEMOPHILUS

In 1892, Pfeiffer isolated and described for the first time the characteristic properties of an organism closely associated with human influenza. The most outstanding feature noted was that the organism would not grow on laboratory media except in the presence of two growth factors, both of which were present in whole blood. This dependence for growth on whole blood has given rise to the term *Haemophilus* as the descriptive generic name for these organisms. Some bacterial species closely related to this genus and which were at one time included in it are now classified separately in the genera *Moraxella* and *Bordetella*.

Distribution in nature

Animal pathogens of the genus *Haemophilus* are associated with infections of the respiratory tract, and include *Haemophilus suis* (Syn.: *H. influenzae suis*), *H. parasuis* and *H. pleuropneumoniae* (Syn.: *H. parahaemolyticus*) occurring in pigs; *H. agni* infects mainly sheep, and *H. gallinarum* is associated with chronic respiratory disease in poultry. A non-pathogenic species (*H. canis*) has been isolated from the prepuce of dogs.

Other species related to human infections include *H. influenzae* and *H. parainfluenzae* which occur in the respiratory tract, *H. aegyptius* the cause of conjunctivitis, and *H. ducreyi* which is associated with dermal lesions described as soft sore or chancroid.

Morphology and staining

These organisms are very small rods or coccobacilli measuring about 0·5–1·5 μm in length and 0·3 μm in width, occurring singly or in pairs. After repeated subcultivation, pleomorphic filamentous forms may develop. Capsules are produced by some strains after growth *in vivo* or after primary isolation but are absent from filamentous forms. Spores are not produced and the organisms are non-motile.

Haemophilus organisms stain Gram-negative but with some strains the depth of counterstaining may be improved by applying dilute carbol fuchsin for 10–15 minutes.

Cultural characteristics (Table 12.1)

The organisms are aerobes and many species will also grow anaerobically. Propagation of newly isolated strains on laboratory media will only take place when one or both of two growth factors (designated X and V) are present in the media. After repeated subcultivation some strains become less fastidious and will grow on media in the absence of these growth factors.

Growth factor X. This substance is haemin and is not destroyed by a temperature of 120°C.

Growth factor V. This is a co-dehydrogenase, diphosphopyridine nucleotide (DPN). It is present in yeast extract as well as in whole blood and is synthesised by staphylococci, giving rise to the phenomenon of satellitism.

Satellitism. This is the name given to an unusual feature of the growth characteristics which develop on solid media in a mixed culture of haemophilus organisms requiring factor V for growth and staphylococci. Colonies of the former grow more luxuriantly when they are adjacent to staphlococcal colonies and this is known as satellitism. It occurs because staphylococci synthesise V factor which becomes diffused into the medium in the immediate vicinity of the colonies.

On blood agar growth at the optimum of 37°C is poor and develops as very small discrete, transparent colonies.

On chocolate agar in which the contents of the red blood cells, including the X and V factors, have been liberated into the medium by heat, growth is more luxuriant than on blood agar. Similarly, relatively good growth occurs on Levinthal's medium

TABLE 12.1. Comparing the growth requirements and pathogenicity of different species of *Haemophilus*.

| Species of Haemophilus | Factors required for growth | | Pathogenicity | |
	X Haemin	V DPN	Host species	Nature of infection
H. suis (*H. influenzae suis*)	+	+	Pigs	Pneumonia associated with virus infections; Glasser's disease.
H. parasuis	−	+		
H. pleuropneumoniae (*H. parahaemolyticus*)	−	+	Pigs	Contagious pleuropneumonia.
H. agni	+*	−	Sheep Lambs Cattle	Bronchopneumonia Septicaemia Meningoencephalitis.
H. gallinarum (*H. paragallinarum*)	±	+	Chickens	Chronic respiratory
H. canis	+	−	Dogs	Infection of prepuce (non-pathogenic).
H. influenzae (*H. haemolyticus*)	+	+	Man	Respiratory infections laryngotracheitis; meningitis.
H. parainfluenzae	−	+	Man	Nasopharynx (non-pathogenic)
H. ducreyi	+	−	Man	Soft sore or chancroid
H. aegyptius (Koch-Weeks Bacillus)	+	+	Man	Conjunctivitis

+ = required for growth.
− = not required for growth.
± = strains differ in their requirement of X factor for growth.
DPN = diphosphopyridine nucleotide.
* = *H. agni* requires blood or tissue in the medium for growth. It does not show satellitism.
H. paragallinarum = strains of *H. gallinarum* not requiring X factor for growth.
H. haemolyticus = haemolytic strains of *H. influenzae*.

and Fildes' medium in which the red blood cells have been disrupted by heat or peptic digestion, respectively. Capsulated strains produce larger mucoid colonies than non-capsulated organisms.

Resistance to physical and chemical agents
These organisms are killed when subjected to a temperature of 55°C for 30 minutes.

Antigens and toxins
Studies on the antigenic structures of haemophilus organisms has shown that at least four distinct types of *H. suis* can be distinguished and that these are antigenically distinct from *H. pleuropneumoniae*.

Epidemiology and pathogenesis
The life histories of haemophilus organisms affecting animals are characterised by their natural habitats being commonly the respiratory tract and also by their apparent symbiotic relationships with respiratory viruses. An outstanding exception is *H. canis* which occurs on the prepuce of dogs and is generally considered to be non-pathogenic.

Those species associated with respiratory infections tend to spread rapidly from one individual to another either by droplet infection or indirectly from contact with infected equipment when animals are kept intensively.

H. suis is a cause of a condition in pigs known as Glasser's disease which develops as a serofibrinous pleuritis, pericarditis, peritonitis and arthritis in these animals. It should be noted that a clinically similar disease in pigs can be produced by *Mycoplasma hyorhinis*.

H. suis occurs in the respiratory tracts of normal pigs and is also associated with atrophic rhinitis and pneumonic infections when predisposing conditions favour the multiplication of these bacteria in the respiratory tract. Inflammatory reactions developing in response to infection with swine fever virus or swine influenza virus can provide a suitable environment for the rapid multiplication of *H. suis* in the lungs. Under experimental conditions, some strains of *H. suis* will not cause disease when introduced into apparently healthy susceptible pigs, but a mixture of *H. suis* and swine influenza virus will result in the development of severe pneumonia and pleurisy. In contrast, *H. pleuropneumoniae* has a greater degree of pathogenicity for pigs and will cause pneumonia when inoculated without virus into susceptible animals.

In chickens, *H. gallinarum* is normally present in the upper respiratory tract and is associated with coryza, chronic respiratory disease and air-sac infections. Predisposing factors leading to the development of clinical disease with this organism include concurrent infection with the viruses of Newcastle disease, infectious laryngotracheitis or infectious bronchitis.

Diseases associated with *H. agni* include septicaemic infections in lambs, broncho-pneumonia in adult sheep and meningoencephalitis in cattle. Limited knowledge on the life history of these organisms indicates that they exist in many animals without causing disease, and that concurrent infections give rise to predisposing conditions leading to clinical disease.

Haemophilus-like organisms have also been isolated from goslings suffering from respiratory infection.

Symptoms and lesions

It is frequently the case that clinical signs of disease caused by most species of haemophilus organisms are related to both the bacterial infection and to concurrent disease produced by virus infections. Thus, in the majority of haemophilus infections the characteristic features of disease are not specific for the bacterial infection, alone.

In pigs, disease associated with *H. suis* frequently occurs concurrently with virus infections and causes a lobular pneumonia. *H. pleuropneumoniae*, on the other hand, produces a pneumonia characterised by a lymphocytic cellular reaction, particularly in the interlobular septa, and in the absence of a concurrent virus infection.

Glasser's disease in pigs arising from infection with *H. suis* may cause an arthritis of the carpal and tarsal joints, and the consequent lameness is not always accompanied by a rise in body temperature. More severe cases develop increased body temperatures as well as lameness, and post-mortem examination reveals excessive amounts of cloudy fluid in affected joints with thickened synovial membranes which may be hyperaemic. In addition, there may be a fibrinous pericarditis, pleuritis and peritonitis.

In poultry, infection with *H. gallinarum* develops characteristically in the upper respiratory tract and gives rise to catarrhal inflammation of the mucous membranes lining the infraorbital sinuses which become swollen and filled with purulent exudate. The organism has also been isolated from the trachea, bronchi and lungs of birds suffering from viral tracheitis, bronchitis and pneumonia.

Diagnosis

This is based on the isolation of haemophilus organisms from affected tissues. It should be emphasised that these organisms can exist in tissues without causing symptoms and that when isolated from disease conditions, they are frequently associated with viral infections. Their significance as primary aetiological agents of disease must be assessed in relation to predisposing factors and concurrent infections.

One method used for the primary isolation of these fastidious organisms is to inoculate suspected material on to sheep blood agar which has a staphylococcal culture already streaked across the diameter of the plate. This enables improved growth of haemophilus organisms to be readily observed as a result of satellitism.

Control and Prevention

A reduction in the incidence of *H. gallinarum* infections causing coryza and air-sac infections in poultry has been claimed from the use of vaccines prepared from cultures grown in egg yolk and inoculated intramuscularly.

Haemophilus infections have been successfully treated with sulphonamides, streptomycin, tetracycline and chloramphenicol.

MORAXELLA

Distribution in nature

This group of organisms is named after Morax who isolated and described in 1896, a bacterium associated with human conjunctivitis and corneal infections. This organism is now known as *Moraxella lacunata*. Other species in the group include *Moraxella bovis* (syn.: *Haemophilus bovis*) a cause of bovine keratitis and conjunctivitis; and *Moraxella liquefaciens* the cause of human conjunctivitis and corneal ulceration. These organisms used to be included in the *Haemophilus* group but as they do not require either the X or V factor for growth they have been classified separately as the *Moraxella* group.

Morphology and staining

The organisms are small bacilli measuring approximately $2\,\mu m$ in length and $1\cdot0\,\mu m$ in width, occurring in pairs, end-to-end as diplobacilli. Capsules are demonstrable in newly isolated strains. They are non-motile and do not develop spores.

The organisms stain Gram-negative.

Cultural characteristics

Moraxella bovis is an aerobe and can be isolated from infected material and propagated at 37°C on 5 per cent bovine blood agar. The colonies are smooth, circular, translucent and greyish in colour, reaching a diameter of 3-4 mm after 48 hours' incubation and surrounded by a zone of β-haemolysis. Haemoloytic strains produce both haemolytic and non-haemolytic progeny. Gelatin is liquefied. Growth in peptone broth develops as a granular deposit.

Moraxella lacunata grows aerobically at 37°C on nutrient agar containing blood or serum. The colonies on blood agar are pin-point size, transparent and produce β-haemolysis. The organism produces 'pitting' or 'lacunae' on the surface of Loeffler's coagulated serum. Failure to liquefy gelatin is a distinguishing feature between this organism and both *Moraxella bovis* and *Moraxella liquefaciens*.

Epidemiology and pathogenesis
Moraxella bovis is a cause of infectious bovine keratoconjunctivitis, a highly contagious disease of cattle which is transmitted by direct contact with infective material from one animal to another, or by indirect transmission of conjunctival or nasal exudates via flies or in the environment of cowbyres. The condition occurs in many countries, and in the United Kingdom has been referred to as New Forest disease. Although for many years the organism has been associated with the disease which tends to be more severe in younger animals, there is evidence to suggest that it may not be the sole cause of the condition. Experimentally, it produces only a very mild reaction, and it has recently been shown that the organism can exist in animals without causing any disease. The naturally occurring condition is more common in the summer when predisposing factors favouring an increased incidence of clinical infection may be flies, dust and ultraviolet light.

A comparatively rare condition of conjunctivitis in cats has been described, in which the causal organism closely resembled *Moraxella lacunata*.

Symptoms and lesions
The disease in cattle develops as a conjunctivitis followed by a keratitis, leading to ulceration of the cornea. One or both eyes may be affected.

Diagnosis
This is made from the characteristic lesions and by isolating *Moraxella bovis* from affected eyes. Swabs from the surface of the conjunctiva should be inoculated on to a blood agar plate.

Control and prevention
Satisfactory treatment has been reported from the use of chloramphenicol, tetracycline and the sulphonamides.

BORDETELLA

Distribution in nature
The name given to this group of organisms was in memory of Bordet who first described the causal organism of whooping cough (*Bordetella pertussis*) which requires blood in the medium for the establishment of primary cultures, but not the X and V growth factors required by haemophilus species.

The whooping cough organism and related bacteria used to be included in the haemophilus group but since *Bord. pertussis*, *Bord. parapertussis* and *Bord. bronchiseptica* are antigenically related to each other, they are now classified separately in the bordetella group. *Bord. parapertussis* is the cause of a mild form of whooping cough.

Bord. bronchiseptica is of veterinary importance because of its association with pneumonia in piglets and respiratory infections in dogs suffering from canine distemper. It has also been isolated from the respiratory tracts of guinea-pigs, ferrets, rabbits, cats and rarely from man.

Morphology and staining
Bord. bronchiseptica occurs in both tissues and primary cultures as a small, oval coccobacillus. The organism develops peritrichous flagella and is motile at 18–24°C but not at 37°C, as distinct from *Bord. pertussis* and *Bord. parapertussis* which are both non-motile organisms. Capsules are present in young cultures. Spores are not produced.

Bord. bronchiseptica stains Gram-negative.

Cultural characteristics
Bord. bronchiseptica is an aerobe and blood or serum is required in the medium for growth of primary cultures. On blood agar the colonies from most strains produce a zone of haemolysis. Subcultures will grow on media in the absence of blood or serum. The organism produces both catalase and urease, but does not ferment carbohydrates, does not hydrolyse aesculin but will utilise citrate as a sole source of carbon.

Resistance to physical and chemical agents.
The organisms are killed by a temperature of 55°C for 30 minutes.

Antigens and toxins
There are serological relationships between the surface antigens of the smooth form and the endotoxin of *Bord. bronchiseptica* with those of *Bord. pertussis* and *Bord. parapertussis*.

Epidemiology and pathogenesis
Bord. bronchiseptica often causes secondary infections in the lungs of dogs suffering from canine distemper. In young pigs it has been associated with pneumonia concurrently with virus diseases, and with rhinitis and atrophy of the turbinate bones concurrently with *Pasteurella multocida* infections. It can also

cause respiratory tract infections in a variety of other species, including rodents, cats, and occasionally man, and is particularly associated with pneumonia in guinea-pigs and snuffles in rabbits.

The organism is known to be a normal inhabitant of the respiratory tract and middle ear of domestic, laboratory and wild animals.

Symptoms and lesions

These are characteristic for penumonia and bronchopneumonia in various animal species, or atrophic rhinitis in pigs. The symptoms and lesions are not necessarily specific for infections with *Bord. bronchiseptica*.

Diagnosis

This depends upon the isolation of the organism from the respiratory tract where it is usually present with other bacterial species and sometimes viruses (e.g. distemper virus). A medium which has been used for this purpose consists of MacConkey's agar plus glucose, penicillin and mycostatin.

Control and prevention

Treatment with chloramphenicol or tetracycline may be beneficial.

Further reading

BRYAN, H.S., HELPER, L.C., KILLINGER, A.H., RHOADES, H.E. AND MANSFIELD, M.E. (1973) Some bacteriological and ophthalmologic observations on bovine infectious keratoconjunctivitis in an Illinois beef herd. *Journal of the American Veterinary Medical Association*, **163**, 739.

FARKAS-HIMSLEY H. (1963) Differentiation of *Pasteurella pseudotuberculosis* and *Bordetella bronchiseptica*. *American Journal of Veterinary Research*, **24**, 871.

FORMSTON C. (1954) New Forest Disease — Infective keratoconjunctivitis of cattle. *Veterinary Record*, **66**, 522.

HARRIS D.L. AND SWITZER W.P. (1968) Turbinate atrophy in young pigs exposed to *Bordetella bronchiseptica, Pasteurella multocida* and combined inoculum. *American Journal of Veterinary Research*, **29**, 777.

KEMENY, L.J. AND AMTOWER, W.C. (1973) Bordetella

agglutinating antibody in swine — a herd survey. *Canadian Journal of Comparative Medicine*, **37**, 409.

KENNEDY P.C., BIBERSTEIN E.L., HOWARTH J.A., FRAZIER L.M. AND DUNGWORTH D.L. (1960). Infectious meningo-encephalitis in cattle, caused by a haemophilus-like organism. *American Journal of Veterinary Research*, **21**, 403.

KENNEDY P.C., FRAZIER L.M., THEILEN G.H. AND BIBERSTEIN E.L. (1958). A septicaemic disease of lambs caused by *Haemophilus agni* (New species). *American Journal of Veterinary Research*, **19**, 645.

LITTLE T.W.A. (1970) Haemophilus infection in pigs. *Veterinary Record*, **87**, 399.

MATTHEWS P.R.J. AND PATTISON I.H. (1961). The identification of a haemophilus-like organism associated with pneumonia and pleurisy in the pig. *Journal of Comparative Pathology and Therapeutics*, **71**, 44.

NEIL D.H., MCKAY K.A., L'ECUYER C. AND CORNER A.H. (1969). Glasser's disease of swine produced by the intratracheal inoculation of *Haemophilus suis*. *Canadian Journal of Comparative Medicine and Veterinary Science*, **33**, 187.

PUGH, G.W., HUGHES, D.E. AND MCDONALD, T.J. (1971) Bovine infectious keratoconjunctivitis: serological aspects of *Moraxella bovis* infection. *Canadian Journal of Comparative Medicine*, **35**, 161.

WHITE D.C., LEIDY G., JAMIESON J.D. AND SHOPE R.E. (1964). Porcine contagious pleuropneumonia. III. Interrelationship of *Hemophilus pleuropheumoniae* to other species of Haemophilus: Nutritional, Metabolic, Transformation and Electron Microscopy Studies. *Journal of Experimental Medicine*, **120**, 1.

WILCOX G.E. (1968) Infectious bovine keratoconjunctivitis: A review. *Veterinary Bulletin*, **38**, 349.

WITHERS A.R. AND DAVIES M.E. (1961) An outbreak of conjunctivitis in a cattery (caused by *Moraxella lacunatus*). *Veterinary Record*, **73**, 856.

WRIGHT, N.G., THOMPSON, H. TAYLOR, D. AND CORNWELL, H.J.C. (1973) *Bordetella bronchiseptica*: a reassessment of its role in canine respiratory disease. *Veterinary Record*, **93**, 486.

CHAPTER 13

SPHAEROPHORUS

CHAPTER 13

Sphaerophorus

This genus contains eighteen species many of which exist as commensals in the intestinal tract, and *Sphaerophorus necrophorus* is the type species. They are characterised by staining Gram-negative, showing marked pleomorphism, and requiring strict anaerobic conditions for growth. The species of veterinary importance are *Sphaer. necrophorus* which is associated with the development of necrotic lesions in different sites in the body and in a variety of animal species; and *Sphaer. nodosus* which is the cause of foot-rot in sheep.

Sphaerophorus necrophorus

Synonyms
Fusiformis necrophorus; Bacteroides necrophorus; Bacillus necrophorus.

Distribution in nature
The organism was first described in 1884 by Loeffler who observed it in cases of calf diphtheria. It is now known to be widespread in nature, to have little or no host specificity, and has been identified in the intestinal tracts and faeces of a variety of animal species. The organism commonly exists as a commensal. Infections with *Sphaer. necrophorus* are responsible for severe economic losses to the agricultural industry in many countries.

Morphology and staining
The organism is very pleomorphic and a characteristic feature is the development of long, filamentous forms, sometimes measuring 80 μm or more in length. These filaments are produced by the organism when growing in tissues and in culture media, but there is a tendency for the filaments in old cultures to be shorter, about 5–10 μm in length, and sometimes the organism occurs as bacilli or coccobacilli, measuring 1–2 μm in length (Plate 13.1a, facing p. 164). The organism does not form spores, is non-motile and does not branch. L-forms have been described.

Sphaer. necrophorus stains Gram-negative and

unevenly, which gives the filaments a characteristic beaded appearance.

Cultural characteristics
Sphaer. necrophorus is a strict anaerobe and growth of a pure culture is sometimes difficult to obtain, particularly if the material to be examined is contaminated with other microbial species. Optimal growth occurs at a temperature of about 37°C. After 48–72 hours' incubation on blood agar or serum agar, the small colonies, about 1 mm in diameter, are convex and glistening. After prolonged incubation for 7–10 days the convex colonies will have become whitish in colour and surrounded by a flat filamentous edge. Production of haemolysis is not a constant feature but has sometimes been reported as occurring on sheep, ox, horse and human blood agar.

The organism is very susceptible to oxygen and is killed after exposure to the atmosphere for 4–5 days.

In fluid medium maximum growth is obtained in cooked meat broth, although there may be an initial lag phase of 2–3 days before the organisms begin to multiply. Growth will also occur in serum broth. Cultures growing in fluid media have an unpleasant smell of 'bad cheese' which is characteristic for these organisms, and the growth may develop as an even turbidity or as floccules.

Sphaer. necrophorus ferments some sugars, including glucose and maltose with production of acid and gas, but usually not lactose or sucrose. Indole is produced and the majority of strains also produce H_2S. Gelatin is not liquefied.

Resistance to physical and chemical agents
The organisms are killed by a temperature of 60°C for 15 minutes. A characteristic feature of *Sphaer. necrophorus* is its sensitivity to oxygen. Thus, exposure of a culture to the atmosphere will be lethal to the organisms in a period of 2–10 days, and for this reason cultures should not be stored in the

atmosphere at 37°C, room temperature or at 4°C. It is interesting to note, however, that under these conditions, *Sphaer. necrophorus* will survive longer when present in a mixed culture with *Staph. pyogenes*. In swampy pastures the organism can survive for at least 10 months.

Antigens and toxins

Serological studies of *Sphaer. necrophorus* have shown that these organisms are antigenically heterogenous. There is evidence to show that the organisms produce an endotoxin and an exotoxin. The endotoxin is closely associated with the bacterial cells which, when killed and inoculated intradermally into rabbits, cause necrosis. The exotoxin, after separation from the bacterial cells produces only a mild erythema when inoculated into the skin; but when injected intravenously it causes emaciation or sometimes death of rabbits in a few hours.

Epidemiology and pathogenesis

It has already been noted that *Sphaer. necrophorus* is widely distributed in nature and that normally it occurs as a commensal in a variety of animal species. Under certain conditions the organism becomes associated with the development of necrotic areas in various organs and tissues. These are sometimes referred to as lesions of necrobacillosis. The most common disorders in cattle are calf diphtheria, foot-rot ('foul-in-the-foot') and liver abscesses associated with lesions in the rumen. Secondary infections may also occur in cases of calf pneumonia and navel ill. In sheep the organism may be associated with the development of abscesses in the foot and liver and with ulcers on the lips. Similar necrotic lesions may develop on the skin of pigs, particularly around the snout, and in horses in the region of the lower limbs and hooves. In rabbits the organism causes a fatal contagious necrotic ulceration and abscess formation on the lips and skin. It will be noted from these typical examples that lesions commonly arise in areas of the skin which are especially subjected to trauma and superficial wounds through which the organism may be inoculated. Primary lesions usually contain other bacterial species in addition to *Sphaer. necrophorus*, but secondary metastatic abscesses containing only *Sphaer. necrophorus*, may arise in almost any site in the body. Experimental evidence indicates that *Sphaer. necrophorus* is widely distributed in nature and that its role as a pathogen depends upon the existence of favourable predisposing factors. The organism has been isolated from the intestinal contents of various animal species, and it has been postulated that liver abscesses arise from the passage of the organism from the intestines to the liver *via* the portal circulation.

Symptoms and lesions

Symptoms will vary according to the sites of the lesions. Animals which have developed lesions in the liver or some other organs may show no symptoms, and the lesions may not be observed until after death.

The characteristic features of lesions occurring in any tissues are central areas of pus and coagulation necrosis, surrounded by a well-marked inflammatory area in which *Sphaer. necrophorus* can be demonstrated.

Cattle

These animals are particularly susceptible to infections with *Sphaer. necrophorus* and lesions may develop at any site on the skin or in the digestive tract where the organisms may become inoculated. The most important conditions are calf diphtheria, foul-in-the-foot, and focal necrosis of the liver.

Calf diphtheria is a serious disease of cattle which affects both newly born calves and animals up to about 2 years of age. Symptoms include excessive salivation, a purulent discharge from the nose, coughing, increased body temperature and loss of appetite. The lesions may be situated in any part of the mouth or larynx, and consist of well defined areas of necrosis which are adherent to the surrounding and underlying inflamed tissue. In some cases the condition spreads to the lungs and liver where secondary necrotic lesions develop. In acute and severe cases death may occur within a week from the onset of symptoms.

Foul-in-the-foot develops as an acute, hot, painful swelling of a hoof with consequent lameness. Usually there is a superficial area of necrosis between the digits or in the heels which has a foetid odour. In severe cases the necrosis may spread to the adjacent tendons, ligaments and joints.

Liver necrosis develops in focal areas which may coalesce (Plate 13.1b, facing p. 164). Long standing lesions have a central core of pus. Usually the condition causes no clinical symptoms.

Sheep

Infection in this species causes lesions similar to those in cattle, including necrotic lesions of the feet. It should be noted, however, that the well-recognised condition of foot-rot in sheep is caused by *Sphaer. nodosus*.

Pigs

These animals may develop necrotic lesions on the skin associated with *Sphaer. necrophorus* especially around the snout or in the intestinal tract.

Other animal species

Necrotic lesions may develop in particular sites

where the predisposing factors are favourable for infection with *Sphaer. necrophorus* to become established. These include foot abscesses in reindeer, a condition in rabbits involving ulceration and necrosis in the region of the mouth, lips and skin; in horses an ulceration and necrosis of the skin on the lower part of the legs; in chickens, *Sphaer. necrophorus* has been reported as a secondary invader in lesions of fowl pox. Occasionally, infections in other species have been reported.

Dogs and cats show a marked degree of resistance to clinical disease associated with *Sphaer. necrophorus* infections.

Diagnosis
The nature of the lesion may be suggestive of infection with *Sphaer. necrophorus*. This can be confirmed by the preparation and examination of smears stained by Gram's method and by the isolation of the organism. Cultures should be made from the edge of lesions and incubated anaerobically for several days on blood agar or in cooked meat broth. Contaminated material containing a variety of bacterial species including *Sphaer. necrophorus* can be inoculated subcutaneously into rabbits or mice which are highly susceptible to infection. Lesions will develop in various sites throughout the body from which the organism can be obtained in pure culture before the rabbit dies from the infection.

Control and prevention
Attention to hygiene should be given to avoid or remove any conditions which may predispose towards clinical infection with *Sphaer. necrophorus*. The sulphonamides and penicillin have been used successfully for the early treatment of these infections, and a 5–10 per cent solution of $CuSO_4$ has been recommended for the treatment of foot lesions.

Public health aspects
Human cutaneous infections are most likely to occur among veterinary surgeons and others who handle infected animals and carcases, particularly through skin abrasions on the hands. Human infections may also arise following tonsillectomy, tooth extraction and other surgical operations. The organism has been associated with appendicitis, cystitis and infections of the female genital tract.

Sphaerophorus nodosus

Synonyms
Fusiformis nodosus; Bacteroides nodosus.

Distribution in nature
This organism was first described in 1941 by Beveridge who showed that it was the primary cause of foot-rot in sheep, and it has since been identified as the cause of a similar condition in cattle. A less severe form of foot-rot in sheep known as 'scald' or 'non-progressive foot-rot' has been described in Australia and the United Kingdom, and this condition is also caused by certain strains of *Sphaer. nodosus*. It is now known to be widely distributed in countries with extensive sheep industries. It is also known that the organism is unable to survive for long periods of time on pastures and that its natural habitat is on the feet of sheep and goats.

Morphology and staining
Sphaer. nodosus are rod-shaped organisms measuring 2–10 µm in length and about 0·5–1·0 µm in width. The organisms are straight or slightly curved and characteristically the ends of the bacilli become enlarged to give a dumb-bell appearance during growth in tissues; but this feature is often absent from organisms grown on laboratory media. Neither spores nor capsules are produced and the organisms are non-motile.

Sphaer. nodosus stains Gram-negative.

Cultural characteristics
Sphaer. nodosus is a strict anaerobe and requires an atmosphere of hydrogen containing 10 per cent CO_2 for cultivation. The optimum temperature for growth is 37°C. It is a difficult organism to cultivate in the laboratory, and one useful solid medium is Lemco agar containing pulverised hoof powder. Inoculated plates should be incubated for at least 3–4 days when the colonies will have developed to 0·5–1·0 mm in diameter, with convex translucent centres and flattened entire edges which later become fimbriate. A characteristic feature of the colonies is the indentation of the medium which can be observed after the removal of the colony.

Growth in fluid cultures is difficult to establish and large inocula are required. Usually the media employed consists of meat broth to which has been added hoof powder and horse serum.

The organism does not ferment carbohydrates.

Resistance to physical and chemical agents
Sphaer. nodosus is killed by a temperature of 50°C for 10 minutes. It is highly susceptible to atmospheric oxygen and will die within about 3 days when exposed to the air.

Antigens and toxins
Serological studies have shown that there are some antigenic differences between strains of *Sphaer. nodosus* isolated from foot-rot in sheep and from cases of 'scald' or 'non-progressive foot-rot'. Similarly, there are some common antigens which

occur on strains of the organism isolated from sheep and from cattle.

It is significant that *Sphaer. nodosus* produces keratinolytic enzymes which are produced in greater amounts by strains of organisms isolated from cases of ovine foot-rot than they are by strains isolated from cases of non-progressive foot-rot.

Epidemiology and pathogenesis

The epidemiology of foot-rot in sheep is affected by two features of the natural history of the causal organism; namely, that the natural habitat of *Sphaer. nodosus* is in the tissues of sheeps' feet, and that it can survive for only a few days in moist pastures and mud. Investigation into an outbreak often reveals that the disease originated on a farm subsequent to the introduction of fresh animals into the flock, some of which may have been carriers. In other cases the source of infection may have been from known infected animals which had been treated but had remained carriers.

There are a variety of conditions predisposing to the development of an outbreak of disease which may affect as many as 90 per cent of a flock in severe epidemics. The infection spreads rapidly when animals are grazing on damp pastures in warm weather and especially on lowland pastures. In contrast, the incidence of the disease may be markedly lower on these pastures during dry seasons. Similarly, the incidence of the disease among sheep grazing on mountain pastures in the United Kingdom is also comparatively low, and it has been postulated that this may be due not only to a reduced sheep population on these hill pastures, but also to the acid nature of the peaty soil which may inhibit the activity of the proteolytic enzymes produced by the organism.

The establishment of infection is facilitated by a number of factors including moist skin, minor abrasions and wounds which enable the organism to penetrate into the tissues adjacent to the horn. It has been suggested that one of these predisposing factors may be damage to the interdigital tissues caused by *Strongyloides* larvae; and it is known that the development of abscesses in the feet caused by *Sphaer. necrophorus* and *C. pyogenes* in particular, predispose to infection with *Sphaer. nodosus*, resulting in the separation of large sections of the hoof from the underlying soft tissue.

During the earlier studies of this disease it was noticed that *Sphaer. nodosus* in lesions was frequently accompanied by *Treponema penortha*, a motile, spiral-shaped organism, measuring about 5–10 μm in length and 0·3 μm in width. It was originally thought that this organism was one of the aetiological agents of foot-rot, but it is now known that this is not so, and that the disease can be established experimentally by *Sphaer. nodosus* in the absence of *Treponema penortha*.

The condition in sheep known as 'non-progressive foot-rot' is a mild form of the condition caused by strains of *Sphaer. nodosus* which produce smaller amounts of proteolytic enzymes and consequently less extensive inflammatory reactions of the feet. This milder condition often occurs in a flock either at the same time as an outbreak of foot-rot or soon afterwards.

Cattle have also been reported as suffering from foot-rot caused by *Sphaer. nodosus*. The disease is similar to that in sheep.

Symptoms

Foot-rot can occur in sheep of all ages and the most obvious symptom is an acute lameness on one or more feet. If both front feet are affected the animal will graze on its knees. Similar acute lameness occurs in cattle affected with foot-rot.

Lesions

The infection and consequent inflammatory reaction commences in the tissues adjacent to the margins of soft horn, and as a result of the spreading of the lesions and the action of the proteolytic enzymes, portions of horn become separated from the underlying tissues, and in severe cases this separation may involve the horn on the walls and the sole of the foot. Usually the germinal layer remains substantially intact, and this enables repair of horny structures to take place after the condition has been satisfactorily treated.

The lesions of 'non-progressive foot-rot' are comparatively mild and often consist of moist areas of skin in the interdigital spaces which may extend to the edges of the sole. The animal will be lame.

Diagnosis

A history of lameness in a flock of sheep is suggestive of foot-rot, and this can be confirmed from the clinical examination of typical lesions by someone familiar with the disease. Further confirmation of the diagnosis can be made by examining smears microscopically. These should be prepared from the edges of the lesion underneath the horn and stained by Gram's method or Loeffler's alkaline methylene blue. In many cases it may be difficult to observe *Sphaer. nodosus* and its characteristic morphology in one preparation, and it may be necessary to prepare and examine smears from other sites before the presence of the organism can be confirmed. In such smears it is usual to find a variety of other bacterial species, particularly *Treponema penortha*, *C. pyogenes*, *E. coli* and various fusiform bacilli.

Attempts to isolate the organism can be made,

but it should be recalled that growth is slow and often difficult to establish. Large inocula known to contain many *Sphaer. nodosus* organisms should be used and cultured anaerobically as already described. It is also an advantage if the cultures are sown with the material as soon after collection as possible because of the susceptibility of the organism to atmospheric oxygen.

Differential diagnosis

Foot-rot has to be differentiated from a number of other conditions, including:

(1) Foot abscesses caused by *Sphaer. necrophorus*. Usually only a few sheep in a flock are affected at any one time and only one digit on a foot. In severe cases the lesion may spread from the feet to the tendon sheaths and joints, and there is no separation of the hoof from the soft tissues.

(2) Strawberry foot-rot caused by *Dermatophilus spp.*, which develops as a severe dermatitis of the legs and feet of sheep, as well as on other parts of the body.

(3) Foot and mouth disease.

(4) A variety of pyogenic infections, particularly those associated with *C. pyogenes*.

Control and prevention

The affected hooves of diseased animals should be severely trimmed so that all infected tissue is exposed; and the area should then be treated with 10 per cent formalin or with chloramphenicol or tetracycline. Recent reports have suggested that parenteral treatment with a mixture of penicillin and streptomycin may be of value when used in conjunction with thorough paring of the hoof and local application of formalin. In all cases of treatment the sheep must be released on to dry ground. Vaccines are being developed for the immunization of young sheep,

and preliminary trials indicate that a substantial immunity may be developed after inoculation of two doses of alum precipitated vaccine at an interval of 4–6 weeks between each dose.

Further reading

ALBAEK, B. (1971) *Sphaerophorus necrophorus*. A study of 23 strains. *Acta Veterinaria Scandinavica*, **12**, 344.

ALBAEK, B. (1972) Gram-negative anaerobes in the intestinal flora of pigs. *Acta Veterinaria Scandinavica*, **13**, 228.

BEVERIDGE W.I.B. (1963). Foot-rot of sheep: its epidemiology and control. *Bulletin Office international des épizooties*, **59**, 1537.

EGERTON J.R. AND ROBERTS D.S. (1969). The aetiology and pathogenesis of ovine foot rot. I. A histological study of the bacterial invasion. *Journal of Comparative Pathology and Therapeutics*, **79**, 207.

FALES, W.H. AND TERESA, G.W. (1972) A selective medium for the isolation of *Sphaerophorus necrophorus*. *American Journal of Veterinary Research*, **33**, 2317.

FALES, W.H. AND TERESA, G.W. (1972) Fluorescent antibody technique for identifying isolates of *Sphaerophorus necrophorus* of bovine hepatic abscess origin. *American Journal of Veterinary Research*, **33**, 2323.

ROBERTS D.S. AND EGERTON J.R. (1969). The aetiology and pathogenesis of ovine foot rot. II. The pathogenic association of *Fusiformis nodosus* and *Fusiformis necrophorus*. *Journal of Comparative Pathology and Therapeutics*, **79**, 217.

SIMON P.C. AND STOVELL P.L. (1969). Diseases of animals associated with *Sphaerophorus necrophorus*. Characteristics of the organism – a review. *Veterinary Bulletin*, **39**, 311.

CHAPTER 14

STAPHYLOCOCCUS

Staphylococcus

This group of organisms develops characteristically as clusters of Gram-positive cocci which occur naturally in a great variety of sites related to animal and human environments. Some strains are pathogenic and characteristically produce coagulase, an enzyme causing the coagulation of blood plasma; other strains do not produce this enzyme and are non-pathogenic. Thus, the coagulase test which is used for detecting the enzyme, is a useful method for differentiating between pathogenic and non-pathogenic strains of the organism. Pathogenic strains are known as *Staphylococcus pyogenes* because they cause the production of pus in the tissues (i.e. pyogenic organisms); while others are for the most part non-pathogenic and sometimes referred to as *Staph. epidermidis* since they commonly occur as commensals on the skin of man and some species of animals. *Staph. hyicus* is, however, a pathogen occurring on the skin of piglets and causing an exudative dermatitis.

The production of pigment (carotenoids) is a variable but common feature of staphylococcal growth on solid media and has given rise to descriptive names for these organisms. For example, *Staph. aureus* refers to strains producing yellow-orange colonies, *Staph. albus* to white colonies and *Staph. citreus* to lemon coloured colonies. Since it has been shown that pigment production by some species is variable, and that many pathogenic strains of *Staph. aureus* do not produce yellow-orange pigment, *Staph. pyogenes* is now used as a more reliable and descriptive term for these pyogenic organisms. In addition, a few strains which develop characteristically as creamy white or lemon coloured colonies are coagulase producers, and they also, are classified as *Staph. pyogenes*.

Staphylococcus pyogenes

Synonyms
Staphylococcus aureus; Micrococcus pyogenes.

Distribution in nature
Staphylococci, including strains of *Staph. pyogenes*, constitute part of the bacterial environment of animals and man throughout the world; and these organisms occur commonly on the skin, anterior nares, saliva, intestines and faeces of man and many species of animals, as well as in water, soil and air. *Staph. pyogenes* is a pathogen which produces several toxins and is the cause of a number of pathological conditions including mastitis in several animal species, tick pyaemia in lambs, yolk-sac infection and arthritis in poultry, and a variety of skin lesions and other pyogenic infections in animals and man.

Morphology and staining
The organisms occur as spherical cocci, measuring approximately $1.0 \mu m$ in diameter. Characteristically, these cocci develop in groups or grape-like clusters, which tend to become partially disrupted during the preparation of films, so that it is not uncommon to see some organisms occurring singly, in pairs, or even in short chains as well as in clusters (Plate 14.1a, facing p. 164). The organisms are non-motile and do not form spores.

Staph. pyogenes stains Gram-positive and some organisms from old cultures readily decolourise and tend to stain Gram-negative.

Cultural characteristics
Staph. pyogenes are aerobes or facultative anaerobes and will grow satisfactorily on nutrient media at an optimum temperature of 37°C. Growth will occur more slowly over a wide temperature range of 10–42°C. Maximum growth rate occurs under aerobic conditions but growth will also take place in an atmosphere of reduced oxygen tension containing 10 per cent CO_2.

On nutrient agar growth is good and relatively large colonies measuring 2–4 mm in diameter, which develop after 24 hours' incubation at 37°C, are circular, convex, glistening, with an entire edge, sometimes pigmented and may resemble a drop of oil paint. The colour may vary from white to lemon yellow, and under aerobic conditions this pigmentation develops rapidly and intensely on milk agar, particularly when the cultures are incubated at 22–25°C. Some colonies may also be surrounded by a clear zone in the medium due to the digestion of casein by staphylococcal proteolytic enzymes. It is noteworthy that pigmentation is not always a constant feature of a particular strain of *Staph. pyogenes*. Strains which develop primarily as lemon-yellow colonies may also produce a proportion of white or cream coloured colonies, and a reverse form of this dissociation may also take place. In addition, some strains producing lemon-yellow pigment are coagulase-negative, and a small proportion of white strains are coagulase-positive. Thus, as already noted, pigment production is not a reliable indication of pathogenicity.

On blood agar prepared with cattle, sheep or rabbit erythrocytes in particular, the colonies of most pathogenic strains are surrounded by zones of haemolysis which become particularly well developed after the cultures have been incubated in an atmosphere containing CO_2 (Plate 14.1b, facing p. 164).

On MacConkey agar growth of *Staph. pyogenes* occurs as small pinkish-yellow colonies due to pigment production, while other strains develop as deep red or purple colonies. Gelatin medium is liquefied quickly by most pathogenic strains and coagulated serum more slowly.

Staph. pyogenes will grow in the presence of 5–10 per cent NaCl incorporated in solid or fluid media, and this characteristic feature is made use of for the selective growth of these organisms. Growth in nutrient broth develops as a uniform turbidity.

In 5 per cent egg yolk broth some strains of *Staph. pyogenes* cause a distinct opacity. This is due to a lipolytic enzyme produced by some coagulase-positive strains but not by coagulase-negative strains. The reaction is a common property of *Staph. pyogenes* strains derived from poultry and man, but occurs less frequently among strains isolated from other species.

Acid without gas is produced by most strains in glucose, lactose, maltose, sucrose and mannitol. Generally, nitrates are reduced to nitrites, and both urease and catalase are produced. Methyl red tests are usually positive but Voges-Proskauer reactions are variable. Indole and H_2S are not produced.

Resistance to physical and chemical agents.
Staphylococci are more resistant to heat and dehydration than most non-sporulating bacterial species, and the majority of strains are killed by a temperature of 60°C for 30 minutes, although some strains are more resistant and are not killed when subjected to a temperature of 70°C for 15 minutes. All strains are readily killed by disinfectants, including phenol, mercuric chloride and hypochlorite solutions, provided that they are not protected by an environment of pus, mucus or serum. Staphylococci will not grow in the presence of a 1:500 000 concentration of crystal violet which is incorporated in an inhibitory medium (Edwards' medium) for the isolation of streptococci from mixed cultures, since growth of the latter is not inhibited by this concentration of crystal violet. *Staph. pyogenes* can survive for many months in laboratory cultures, in dust and in a variety of environments in the absence of direct sunlight.

Antigens and toxins
Antigenic studies have been carried out mainly on human strains of staphylococci, and by using agglutination tests they have been divided into a number of different types and subtypes. Precipitation tests have shown that there are two distinct polysaccharides produced by these organisms. One is associated with virulence and pathogenic strains (type A) and the other with saprophytic strains (type B). A third polysaccharide (C) has also been described.

Pathogenic strains of *Staph. pyogenes* produce a variety of toxins and enzymes. The following is a brief summary of their characteristic properties.

Coagulase
A thermostable, filterable enzyme which interacts with a labile factor in plasma causing the production of fibrin from fibrinogen and the coagulation of plasma. Coagulase-positive strains of *Staph. pyogenes* can be identified by the coagulase test. A number of antigenically distinct coagulases have been identified.

Hyaluronidase
This substance is produced by most strains of *Staph. pyogenes* and is distinct from that produced by streptococci. This enzyme is known as a 'spreading factor' because it facilitates the distribution of *Staph. pyogenes* in the tissues and the diffusion of the various bacterial toxins produced.

Phosphatase
Produced by coagulase-positive cultures of *Staph. pyogenes* and capable of splitting phenolphthalein diphosphate, liberating free phenolphthalein which, in the presence of ammonia, results in the bacterial growth being coloured bright pink (Phenolphthalein test).

Fibrinolysin
An antigenically distinct, thermostable substance produced by the majority of coagulase-positive

strains isolated from horses, dogs and poultry, and by only a few strains derived from sheep and pigs.

Haemolysin

Most coagulase-positive strains of *Staph. pyogenes* from animals produce α, β and δ-haemolysins which are antigenically distinct and have different properties. An additional ε-haemolysin is often produced by coagulase-negative strains, only.

The α-haemolysin is commonly produced by strains derived from animals and man and causes lysis of rabbit, sheep and ox red cells at 37°C, and has little or no effect on horse, chicken or human erythrocytes.

The β-haemolysin produces a very large, clearly defined area of partial or incomplete haemolysis of sheep and ox red cells. This reaction develops progressively during storage at 4–20°C after preliminary incubation at 37°C, and gives rise to the formation of concentric peripheral rings of partially haemolysed cells which surround a central area of complete haemolysis. This phenomenon is known as hot-cold lysis. The β-haemolysin does not usually attack rabbit, chicken, horse or human red cells.

The δ-haemolysin causes lysis of many species of red cells and produces large, clearly defined zones on blood agar.

Coagulase-positive strains usually develop α- or δ-haemolysins together or in combination with β-haemolysins. Pathogenic strains from animals usually produce combinations of αβδ-, βδ- or αδ-haemolysins, in that order of decreasing frequency, and very few strains produce only β- or δ-haemolysin. Human strains, on the other hand, usually develop αδ- or αβδ-haemolysins, and a minority of strains produce either α or δ-haemolysin, singly. Coagulase-negative strains do not produce α or δ haemolysins. It is often difficult to distinguish on blood agar the different combinations of haemolysins produced by staphylococci and a method has been introduced to facilitate the identification of the different components. It consists of sowing the test organism in a streak across a blood agar plate at right angles to a strip of filter paper previously soaked in antibodies specific for α- or β-haemolysins and incorporated in the medium (Plate 14.2a, facing p. 164a). A second method which may also prove useful is based on the unusual property of growth products derived from either *Corynebacterium ovis* or *Corynebacterium haemolyticum* which inhibit the activity of the staphylococcal α- and β-haemolysins, have no effect on the δ-haemolysin, and enhance the activity of the ε-haemolysin (Plate 14.2b, facing p. 164a). Although the lytic effects of staphylococcal β toxin are inhibited by *C. ovis* and *C. haemolyticum* they are markedly enhanced by some other coryne-

bacteria including *C. renale*, *C. equi* and *C. pyogenes* (Plate 14.2c, facing p. 164a).

Necrotoxin

This toxin is the same as the α-haemolysin. After intradermal inoculation of the toxin into rabbits or guinea-pigs, an area of dermonecrosis surrounded by a zone of hyperaemia develops during the following 12–24 hours. The effect can be neutralised by specific antitoxin.

Lethal toxin

This toxin is the same as the α-haemolysin. It is lethal to mice after intravenous inoculation, and the greater the dosage the more rapid is the lethal effect, which can be neutralised by specific antitoxin.

Leucocidin

Produced by some strains of *Staph. pyogenes* and capable of destroying leucocytes. Three distinct leucocidins have been studied; one is identical with the α-haemolysin and another with the δ-haemolysin.

Enterotoxin

This is a thermostable toxin which can withstand heating to 100°C for 15 minutes, and is produced by strains of human origin belonging to phage groups III and IV. It causes acute gastroenteritis in man and is associated with cases of staphylococcal human food poisoning.

Bacteriophage typing

This technique has been developed extensively for studying the epidemiology of staphylococcal infections in man and subsequently in cattle and other animal species. There are 4 classified groups of phages used for this purpose and these are recognised internationally, so that comparisons can be made on the incidence and epidemiology of staphylococcal phage types in different countries.

Phage grouping is based on the lytic patterns produced by twenty-one different phages. Five of these phages are allocated to group I, five to group II, eight to group III, one to group IV and two are unclassified. The majority of staphylococcal strains isolated from human sources are susceptible to a lytic pattern produced by the phages belonging to one phage group, only. Human strains which are lysed by phages belonging to two or more groups are in a minority, provided that dilute solutions of phages are used for typing. The optimum amount is the Routine Test Dilution (RTD) which is the highest dilution of phage producing confluent lysis.

During recent years it has been shown that this phage typing scheme is inadequate when applied to strains of *Staph. pyogenes* from animal sources. For example, many bovine strains are sensitive to

TABLE 14.1. The system of phages used for typing human and bovine strains of *Staph. pyogenes* (Modified from Davidson, 1961).

Phage group	Individual phages for typing human strains	Phage group	Individual phages for typing bovine strains
I	29, 52, 52A, 79, 80	I–III	29, 52, 42E, 101, 110
II	3A, 3B, 3C, 55, 71	III	31B, 53, 77
III	6, 7, 42E, 47, 53, 54, 75, 77	IV	42D, 102, 107, 108, 111
IV	42 D	78 group	78, 115
Unclassified	81, 187		

phages belonging to both Groups I and III. A minority of human strains and a majority of bovine strains belong to Group IV, and many bovine strains can be so classified only when the individual phages allocated to this group for typing purposes are increased to include phages 102, 107, 108 and 111 (Table 14.1). Although this modified set of phages enables 90 per cent and more of bovine strains of *Staph. pyogenes* to be typed, it is of relatively little value for the typing of strains derived from sheep and other animal species. Further work on the phage typing of *Staph. pyogenes* from animal sources will be of value to epidemiological studies on the spread of infection from one host species to another. At the present time the evidence suggests that strains of *Staph. pyogenes* show a considerable degree of host species specificity.

Epidemiology and pathogenesis

From the foregoing section on antigens and toxins it will be realised that coagulase-positive strains of *Staph. pyogenes* are equipped with a formidable battery of enzymes and toxins to assist their penetration and establishment in animal host tissues, and attempts have been made to correlate the functions of these different substances with the initial colonisation of organisms in the body which leads to tissue damage.

Coagulase is a product of pathogenic staphylococcal strains and it may be that in the early stages of colonisation it is associated with the production of a layer of fibrin around the organisms which helps to protect them from phagocytosis. This anti-phagocytic activity may be enhanced by the presence on some staphylococcal strains of a recently identified antigen which appears to inhibit phagocytosis of these organisms. Other experimental evidence also indicates that coagulase protects bacteria from the bactericidal activity of normal serum. Leucocidin is an important additional factor which prevents phagocytosis of the organisms. It is well known that

pathogenic staphylococci which have become phagocytosed, will often survive intracellularly for long periods of time, and it is probable that this occurs as the result of the action of leucocidin on the metabolism of the leucocyte.

The part played by hyaluronidase (spreading factor) in the pathogenesis of staphylococcal infections is hard to assess. It may be that it assists the diffusion of toxins into the tissues surrounding the developing lesion, or it has been postulated that it helps to potentiate concurrent infections with other microorganisms by enhancing their distribution in the tissues.

After the initial colonisation of staphylococci in tissues, the subsequent development of lesions and damage to tissues may be attributed, in part at least, to the action of toxins. These have the collective effect of being haemolytic, necrotic and lethal, but at present their precise modes of action which vary in different host species, are not known. One characteristic feature, however, of tissue damage caused by staphylococcal toxins is the production of pus. It should be recalled that, in addition, an enterotoxin affecting man is produced by some strains of staphylococci. This toxin probably has a direct action on gastric mucosa.

It might be expected that because of the variety of toxic substances which can be produced by *Staph. pyogenes*, these organisms would not be found in animals except in association with pyogenic lesions. In fact, as in other host–parasite relationships, there is a variety of factors concerned with the establishment of a suitable environment which is ultimately favourable either to the host or to the parasite. Thus, toxin production by *Staph. pyogenes* can vary markedly from one strain to another. Some strains are active toxin producers and readily establish themselves in animal tissues. Other strains which are weak toxin producers cannot establish themselves in the host. Strains of *Staph. pyogenes* recently isolated from suppurative lesions, are usually highly toxigenic but after repeated subcultivation in laboratory media, toxin production may be greatly reduced.

The establishment of infection will depend upon not only the toxigenic capacity of the infecting strain of *Staph. pyogenes* but also on environmental conditions. These include the degree of specific immunity (antitoxin production) which the host may have developed against the toxic products of the bacteria, the incidence of *Staph. pyogenes* in the immediate environment of the host, especially on the skin surface, and the possibility of injuries to the skin from trauma or tick bites which will facilitate the inoculation of the organisms into the tissues.

The following are the major disease entities commonly associated with *Staph. pyogenes* infections.

Mastitis

This occurs particularly in cattle, sheep, goats and occasionally in other animal species. In cattle the disease may vary in intensity from an acute to a mild type of infection in which *Staph. pyogenes* are present in the milk secreted by a clinically normal udder. These organisms and also *Staph. epidermidis*, occur on the skin of cattle and in the environment of the cow byre and milking equipment where they can remain viable for many days or weeks. Infection of the udder with *Staph. pyogenes* occurs via the teat canal with organisms derived from the contaminated environment and particularly from the skin of the udder and teat where they commonly exist for weeks and months. It is also to be noted that some of the phage types of *Stah. pyogenes* associated with bovine mastitis are known to be pathogens for man and occur on human skin and the anterior nares. It is probable, therefore, that sometimes milkers may, themselves, be the sources of staphylococcal mastitis in cattle.

In sheep and goats, *Staph. pyogenes* is the cause of mastitis in lactating ewes and nanny-goats. The condition is typically acute and sometimes gangrenous but may also occur in a milder form. The phage types of *Staph. pyogenes* causing mastitis in these species are usually different from the types associated with bovine and human infections. Although the disease commonly occurs among sheep and goats in the Mediterranean area where they are often hand-milked, it is unlikely that the milkers act as sources of infection for these animals. *Staph. pyogenes* is a common inhabitant of the skin of sheep and goats, and infection probably arises mechanically from inoculation via the teat canal, since the phage types of the organisms occurring on the skin are similar to the types associated with mastitis.

Horses, pigs, dogs and sometimes other animal species suffer relatively infrequently from staphylococcal mastitis which can develop either as an acute suppurative or a chronic granulomatous form of the disease.

Lamb pyaemia (tick pyaemia)

This is the name given to staphylococcal infections of lambs which occur on farms infested with the sheep tick, *Ixodes ricinus*, especially during the spring and early summer when the ticks are active. Infection arises from the inoculation of *Staph. pyogenes* into lambs via tick bites. The consequent infection may give rise to an acute pyaemia followed by a fatal toxaemia, or to a more chronic form of pyaemia which causes the formation of abscesses in various sites of the body. The phage typing of strains of *Staph. pyogenes* involved in this disease has shown that the ticks do not act as vectors but mechanically inoculate into lambs the organisms already resident on the skin surface.

Staphylococcosis in poultry

This disease affects a variety of species, particularly chickens, turkeys, pheasants, ducks and geese. It occurs as a yolk-sac infection of embryos and young chicks and also as an acute septicaemia in older birds followed by the development of chronic arthritis, sometimes air-sac infections and, less frequently, spondylitis among survivors. The term 'bumble-foot' is sometimes used to describe localised lesions which occur on the feet of birds. During recent years the incidence of the disease, particularly the arthritic form, has increased. Many of the strains of *Staph. pyogenes* associated with staphylococcosis belong to phage group III and are similar to those which occur on the skin and upper respiratory tracts of birds. However, the phage patterns of these strains are dissimilar to the patterns of strains isolated from cattle, sheep and man; and present evidence suggests that the disease is caused by resident strains of *Staph. pyogenes* which actively invade the tissues of birds whose resistance is lowered by various predisposing factors, including concurrent diseases, skin wounds and modern methods of husbandry.

Botryomycosis

This term has been used to describe chronic granulomatous lesions associated with *Staph. pyogenes* infections in the udders of horses, cattle and pigs, and also infection of the spermatic cord in horses following castration.

Miscellaneous staphylococcal infections

It is important to remember that in addition to the major disease entities already referred to, pyogenic infections caused by *Staph. pyogenes* can develop in a variety of situations in the animal body consequent upon the presence of predisposing factors. These infections are occasionally associated with metritis, enteritis, infections of the ears and conjunctivae, but are most frequently recognised as the cause of infected skin wounds in animals consequent upon trauma and injury to the integument.

Symptoms

Disease may develop as an acute generalised pyaemia or a chronic localised infection, and the symptoms will vary accordingly.

Acute staphylococcal mastitis is characterised by a sudden rise in body temperature, loss of appetite, enlargement and hardening of the affected quarters with cessation of milk secretion. Small quantities of blood-stained fluid are secreted which later become thickened and contain pus and shreds of necrotic tissue. If the animal survives, the damaged quarters will remain functionless. Sometimes the affected quarters become dark in colour, cold, gangrenous and finally slough. Fatal cases die from a toxaemia in 3–4 days following the onset of symptoms, when the body temperature will have become subnormal and the animal more deeply comatose during the few hours preceding death.

The symptoms of chronic staphylococcal mastitis include induration of the udder, particularly near the base of the teat, and the milk will contain clots as well as an increased cell count. Otherwise the animal appears normal.

Lamb pyaemia may be acute and cause sudden deaths during the first few days of life. A more chronic form develops during the first four weeks after birth when affected lambs become lame as a result of infection of the joints which become hot, swollen and painful. Many lambs may survive but remain permanently crippled.

Deaths among poultry suffering from acute staphylococcosis usually occur within 3–4 days of the birds first showing symptoms of diarrhoea and acute infection of the joints which become hot, swollen and painful. Lame survivors remain chronically affected with arthritis and become emaciated. Birds affected with spondylitis remain crouched on their hocks and seldom move unless disturbed.

Botryomycotic and other superficial staphylococcal infections develop as chronic abscesses which sometimes involve the local lymph nodes.

Lesions

Cases of acute mastitis show necrotic and sometimes gangrenous areas in the affected quarters over which the skin has become discoloured. The interstitial tissue of the gland contains large quantities of blood-stained gelatinous exudate. Microscopically, the glandular cells are necrotic and the lesion is infiltrated with leucocytes and large numbers of Staph. pyogenes which occur in characteristic clumps.

Less acute cases develop areas of fibrosis in the glandular tissue and around the base of the teat.

Lamb pyaemia is characterised by the presence of abscesses, particularly in the liver, kidneys, joints and occasionally the central nervous system and other sites including the skin and muscle. Abscesses will not have had time to develop in the acute form of the disease when death occurs suddenly.

Staphylococcosis in poultry occurs as an arthritis of the hock joint and less frequently of other joints which show inflammation and sometimes necrosis of the articular surfaces and distention of the joint with fluid containing pus and fibrin. In addition, the carcases of chronic cases are emaciated. In cases of spondylitis, lesions have been reported as occurring in the region of the 6th/7th thoracic vertebrae and cause compression of the spinal cord.

Botryomycotic lesions are chronic inflammatory reactions consisting of granulation tissue surrounded by a layer of fibrous tissue. Within the granulation tissue are areas of pus which may penetrate to the surface via sinuses. The yellowish pus contains many staphylococci which are often situated in small granules contained in the pus.

Diagnosis

Staph. pyogenes can be readily observed in stained smears prepared from lesions, particularly in preparations of pus and exudate. Suitable media for isolation and identification of the organism are sheep or rabbit blood agar on which haemolysis is marked, particularly after growth in an atmosphere containing 10 per cent CO_2. Microscopical examination of stained smears prepared from these cultures will confirm identification of the organism. For the isolation of Staph. pyogenes from heavily contaminated material it may be necessary to use a differential medium. Phenolphthalein diphosphate agar allows the growth of pathogenic phosphatase-producing strains, and tellurite agar permits pathogenic strains to grow but inhibits non-pathogenic strains and many other bacterial species. All suspected strains of Staph. pyogenes should be tested for coagulase production by means of either the slide or tube test.

Coagulase slide test

Emulsify a staphylococcal colony with a drop of saline on a slide. Add one drop of undiluted human or preferably rabbit plasma and mix gently. If the organisms are coagulase-positive they will become clumped after a few seconds because fibrinogen becomes precipitated on the bacterial surfaces by the coagulase and renders them sticky. A control test consisting of saline and bacteria without plasma should be carried out to ensure that the organisms do not clump spontaneously.

Coagulase tube test
To each of two small tubes add 0·5 ml of a 1:10 saline dilution of human or rabbit plasma. To one tube add 5 drops of an overnight broth culture or saline suspension of bacteria to be tested, and incubate both tubes at 37°C. Examine frequently for the formation of a clot by coagulase-positive organisms. This usually occurs within 1–3 hours but occasionally takes longer. The control tube without bacteria should show no clot formation.

Control and prevention

Immunization
Many attempts have been made to develop vaccines and toxoids which would stimulate an immunity of sufficient level to be of practical value in the prophylaxis of staphylococcal infections. Although it has been shown that toxin inactivated by β-propiolactone is more immunogenic than toxin inactivated by formaldehyde, the results of these experiments have not been encouraging and at the present time there is no reliable method for immunizing animals against this disease. The most that has been achieved is a level of immunity which will inhibit the development of acute pyaemic infections but has little effect on the more chronic forms of the disease characterised by abscess formation.

Chemotherapy
Penicillin preparations, streptomycin, tetracycline, erythromycin, neomycin and novobiocin, are of value for treating *Staph. pyogenes* infections. At the present time, many strains show a marked resistance to penicillin, streptomycin or tetracycline. Resistance to benzyl penicillin is due to the ability of an increasing number of strains to produce penicillinase, whereas resistance to other drugs probably arises from mutations. It is important to remember that the chemotherapeutic effect may be greatly reduced when staphylococci are in an environment of pus and protein. The treatment of staphylococcal mastitis by intramammary inoculation of penicillin preparations is not always satisfactory and is often less reliable than the treatment of streptococcal mastitis. Similarly, the subcutaneous injection of penicillin preparations for the control of lamb pyaemia and infections in poultry is sometimes beneficial but not always satisfactory, particularly when the diseases are acute and toxaemic.

Public health aspects
Staph. pyogenes is a frequent cause of human pyogenic infections, including mastitis, superficial skin lesions and wound infections. In addition, man is susceptible to food poisoning caused by staphylococcal enterotoxin which may be produced in certain foodstuffs, especially meat and milk products, which have been re-heated or stored under conditions of temperature and humidity suitable for the elaboration of enterotoxin by staphylococci present in the foodstuff. This is one of the commonest forms of microbial food poisoning.

The most usual sources of infection and contamination of foodstuffs are human carriers. *Staph. pyogenes* is normally present on the skin surfaces and anterior nares of a high proportion of healthy persons, and the incidence of infection in the anterior nares of nurses, patients and especially babies in hospital is often considerably higher than 50 per cent.

Further reading
BLAIR, J.E. (1962) What is a Staphylococcus? *Biological Reviews of the Cambridge Philosophical Society*, **26**, 375.

DAVIDSON I. (1961) A set of bacteriophages for typing bovine staphylococci. *Research in Veterinary Science*, **2**, 396.

DAVIDSON, I. (CHAIRMAN) (1971) Working group on phage-typing of bovine staphylococci. *International Journal of Systematic Bacteriology*, **21**, 171.

DAVIDSON, I. (1972) A collaborative investigation of phages for typing bovine staphylococci. *Bulletin of the World Health Organisation*, **46**, 81.

DEVRIESE, L.A., DEVOS, A.H., BEUMER, J. AND MAES, R. (1972) Characterization of staphylococci isolated from poultry. *Poultry Science*, **51**, 389.

EASMON, C.S.F., HAMILTON, I. AND GLYNN, A.A. (1973) Mode of action of a staphylococcal anti-inflammatory factor. *British Journal of Experimental Pathology*, **54**, 638.

ELEK S.D. (1959) *Staphylococcus pyogenes and its Relation to Disease*, p. 239. Edinburgh: Livingstone.

FORBES D. (1969) The pathogenesis of bovine mastitis. *Veterinary Bulletin*, **39**, 529.

FRASER G. (1964) The effect on animal erythrocytes of combinations of diffusible substances produced by bacteria. *Journal of Pathology and Bacteriology*, **88**, 43.

HARRY E.G. (1967) The characteristics of *Staphylococcus aureus* isolated from cases of staphylococcosis in poultry. *Research in Veterinary Science*, **8**, 479.

HILL, M.J. (1968) A staphylococcal aggressin. *Journal of Medical Microbiology*, **1**, 33.

HOLMBERG, O. (1973) *Staphylococcus epidermidis* isolated from bovine milk. Biochemical properties, phage sensitivity and pathogenicity for the udder. *Acta Veterinaria Scandinavica*. Suppl. 45, 144pp.

LACEY, R.W. (1973) Genetic basis, epidemiology and future significance of antibiotic resistance in *Staphylococcus aureus*: a review. *Journal of Clinical Pathology*, **26**, 899.

LIVE, I. (1972) Differentiation of *Staphylococcus aureus* of human and of canine origins: coagulation of human and of canine plasma, fibrinolysin activity and serologic reaction. *American Journal of Veterinary Research*, **33**, 385.

MADOFF, M.A. (1965) The staphylococci: ecological perspectives. *Annals of the New York Academy of Sciences*, **128**, 122.

MARKHAM N.P. AND MARKHAM J.G. (1966). Staphylococci in man and animals. Distribution and characteristics of strains. *Journal of Comparative Pathology and Therapeutics*, **76**, 49.

Symposium on staphylococcal mastitis (1961). *Veterinary Record*, **73**, 1011.

OJO, M.O. (1972) Bacteriophage types and antibiotic sensitivity of *Staphylococcus aureus* isolated from swabs of the noses and skins of dogs. *Veterinary Record*, **91**, 152.

SATO, G, MIURA, S. AND TERAKADO, N. (1972) Classification of chicken coagulase-positive staphylococci into four biological types and relation of the types to additional characteristics including coagulase-antigenic type. *Japanese Journal of Veterinary Research*, **20**, 91.

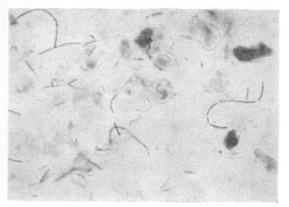

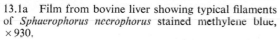

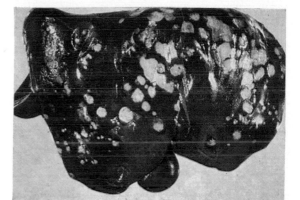

13.1a   Film from bovine liver showing typical filaments of *Sphaerophorus necrophorus* stained methylene blue, ×930.

13.1b   Focal areas of necrosis in bovine liver infected with *Sphaerophorus necrophorus*.

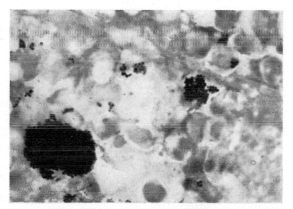

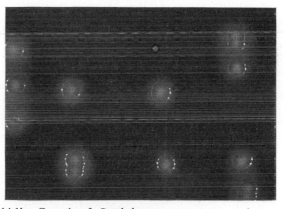

14.1a Gram-stained film of staphylococci showing characteristic groups of organisms, ×930.

14.1b Growth of *Staphylococcus pyogenes* on horse blood agar showing the characteristic colonies surrounded by zones of haemolysis.

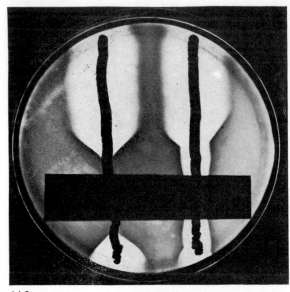

14.2a

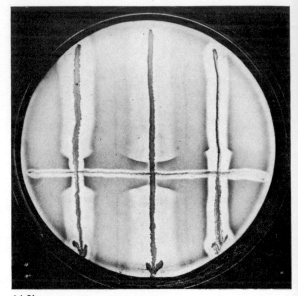

14.2b

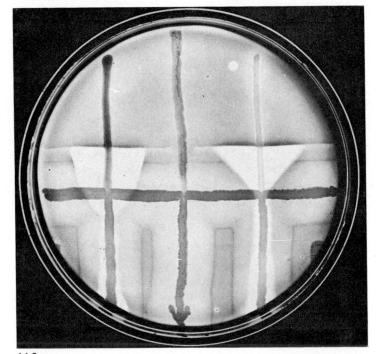

14.2c

14.2a Inhibition of the α-lysin of an α-strain (left) and an αδ strain (right) of staphylococcus, by means of a filter-paper strip soaked in α-antitoxin, The δ-lysin of the αδ strain is unaffected.

14.2b Effects produced on sheep blood agar by a horizontal streak culture of *C. ovis* on αδ, β and ε strains of staphylococci (left to right). The α and β haemolysins are inhibited, the ε-lysin is potentiated but the δ-lysin is unaffected.

14.2c Haemolytic effects obtained on sheep blood agar by drawing cultures of *C. equi, C. ovis* and *C. renale* (left to right) downwards across a horizontal streak culture of a β-toxin producing staphylococcus. The zone of incomplete β haemolysis is enhanced by *C. equi* and *C. renale* but is inhibited by *C. ovis*.

CHAPTER 15

STREPTOCOCCUS AND PNEUMOCOCCUS

Streptococcus and Pneumococcus

STREPTOCOCCUS

This group of organisms which includes saprophytic and parasitic species, develops characteristically as spheres or oval forms, approximately 1 μm in diameter, arranged in pairs or chains. The organisms stain Gram-positive. They have a world-wide distribution and are commonly associated with animal and human environments; their natural habitats being the skin, mouth, nose, throat, intestinal tract and genital tract. They are the causes of a variety of acute and chronic pyogenic infections and the most important of these disease entities in animals are bovine mastitis, strangles in horses and a variety of pyogenic infections in other animal species. In man, they are associated with scarlet fever, tonsillitis, otitis media, puerperal fever, erysipelas, arthritis and infected wounds.

The streptococcal group consists of a large number of organisms displaying considerable variation in their properties, and this has led to some confusion in establishing a concise method for differentiating between the species. For example, the majority of species are aerobes or facultative anaerobes and others are strict anaerobes. Some produce clear zones of haemolysis on blood agar; they are known as β-haemolytic streptococci and include many of the species associated with diseases in animals and man, and are differentiated into groups (Lancefield's groups A to T) serologically on the basis of the carbohydrate constituents in their cell walls. Other streptococcal species produce partial haemolysis with a greenish pigmentation of the medium and are classified as α-haemolytic (*Streptococcus viridans* group). A number of species fail to produce any haemolysis on blood agar media, and others are obligate anaerobes and are not important causes of animal disease.

Distribution in nature

As already noted, streptococci occur throughout the world and their natural habitats are the skin, the mouth, nose, throat, intestinal and genital tracts of animals and man. Pathogenic streptococci which are mainly the β-haemolytic species cause acute and chronic pyogenic infections. Economically, the most important disease entity in animals is bovine mastitis. Other animal diseases are strangles in horses and a variety of pyogenic infections including acute septicaemias, endocarditis, pneumonia, otitis media, polyarthritis and various wound infections.

Morphology and staining

Individual organisms are spherical or ovoid, measuring approximately 1·0 μm in diameter, and they develop characteristically in pairs or chains varying in length from two to twelve or more cocci (Plates 15.1a & 15.1b, facing p. 176b). Capsules are occasionally demonstrable with some species after growth in tissues or on primary isolation (e.g. *Str. bovis* belonging to group D and in young cultures of *Str. equi* group C), but cannot usually be observed after repeated sub-cultivation on laboratory media. These organisms do not produce spores. Motile strains occasionally occur, particularly among group D organisms and variant strains of *Str. lactis* (group N). It is noteworthy that motility is most apparent for only a limited period of time during growth, and can be observed most easily during the period from 4–18 hours' incubation at 37°C. An L phase of streptococci has also been described.

Streptococci stain Gram-positive and some organisms from old cultures decolourise easily and tend to stain Gram-negative.

Cultural characteristics

Streptococci are mostly aerobes or facultative anaerobes, capable of growing poorly on ordinary laboratory media at an optimum temperature of 37°C but developing more rapidly on media containing blood, serum or a fermentable carbohydrate. The maximum temperature for growth is 42°C but some organisms belonging to group D are thermophilic and will grow at a temperature of

TABLE 15.1 Some characteristic properties of group D streptococci (including enterococci).

Species	Growth at 10°C	45°C	50°C	pH 9·6	Growth in 40% bile	6·5% NaCl	Resistance to 0·05% tellurite	Reduction of tetrazolium	Fermentation of Mannitol	Sorbitol	Arabinose
Str. faecalis	+	+	−	+	+	+	+	+	+	+	−
Str. faecium	+	+	+	+	+	+	−	−	+	−	+
Str. durans		−	V	−	+	+	−	−	−	−	+
Str. equinus	−	+	−	−	+	−	−	−	−	−	−
Str. bovis	−	+	−	−	+	−	−	V	V	−	V

V = variable reaction.

45°C or higher (Table 15.1). After 24 hours' incubation on blood agar, colonies are about 1 mm in diameter, circular and greyish in colour. Some colonies have a distinctly mucoid or matt appearance and this is often but not always characteristic of a virulent strain.

Haemolytic reactions on horse blood agar cultures help towards the characterisation of streptococcal species isolated from animal sources, but it is important to remember that the quality and quantity of the haemolytic reaction can vary not only from one strain to another but also will be affected by the conditions of growth, including the species of blood and type of peptone used in the media, the thickness of the agar and the oxygen tension of the atmosphere in which the cultures are grown. To obtain uniformity of results, blood agar plates prepared from horse blood are used for determining haemolytic reactions. Growth under anaerobic conditions sometimes results in an increased colony size and a more intense haemolytic reaction on blood agar than when grown aerobically. The production of haemolysin reaches its maximum after approximately 8 hours of active growth and, conversely, the destruction of haemolysin can occur rapidly as a consequence of oxidation, particularly of those lysins which are oxygen-labile. Haemolysins which are relatively oxygen-stable can be demonstrated more readily than oxygen-labile haemolysins in centrifugates prepared from fluid cultures. Thus, the two varieties of β-haemolytic streptococcal strains are those producing haemolysins which are either demonstrable or not demonstrable in the presence of oxygen.

The types of haemolytic reactions which can develop on horse blood agar are as follows (Plates 15.1c & 15.2b, facing pp. 176a & 177):

(1) β-haemolysis refers to a narrow or wide zone of complete haemolysis around a colony growing on blood agar.

(2) α-prime haemolysis refers to a hazy zone of partial haemolysis, containing a proportion of unlysed cells and is less clearly demarcated from the surrounding medium than β-haemolysis. The zone extends during storage in a refrigerator.

(3) α-haemolysis refers to the development of a narrow or wide zone of partially lysed greenish coloured cells immediately adjacent to the colony and sometimes surrounded on the periphery by a clear zone of completely lysed cells. This latter zone often develops more intensely when the cultures are stored overnight at room temperature or in a refrigerator instead of at 37°C. It is important to remember that some pathogenic strains of streptococci do not produce haemolysins, others are haemolytic only when grown anaerobically, and that by common usage, the term 'haemolytic streptococci' usually refers to organisms which produce β-haemolysis.

The majority of streptococcal species do not grow on MacConkey's agar. Those which do include *Str. faecalis, Str. bovis, Str. uberis* and *Str. lactis* which produce very small colonies after 48 hours' incubation at 37°C.

Growth is slow in fluid medium and may produce either a faint, evenly dispersed opacity usually associated with short chains of cocci, or a fluffy deposit adherent to the side of the tube and a clear supernatant which is characteristic of long chains of cocci (e.g. *Str. agalactiae*).

Biochemical reactions are usually of secondary importance to Lancefield's serological method for grouping streptococci. The sugars commonly used are lactose, trehalose, sorbitol, raffinose, salicin, inulin and mannitol. Other tests sometimes employed are reduction of tetrazolium for differentiating between members of the enterococci (group D), growth at 45°C and 50°C, growth in the presence of 6·5 per cent NaCl or in 40 per cent bile, and growth at pH 6·9, all of which are characteristic properties of group D organisms (see Table 15.1).

Other tests include hydrolysis of sodium hippurate and hydrolysis of aesculin which is incorporated in Edwards' medium.

Resistance to physical and chemical agents

Usually these organisms are killed after exposure for 30 minutes to a temperature of 56°C, but some strains are thermophilic and will resist a higher temperature. They are relatively susceptible to the lethal action of disinfectants when this is not reduced by the presence of pus or protein. In the absence of direct sunlight the organisms can survive for weeks and months in dust and in the environment of animal houses.

Antigens and toxins

Following the original work of Lancefield in 1933, it has been shown that streptococci can be classified serologically into groups on the basis of group-specific polysaccharides which constitute part of the cell walls, with the exception of group C antigen whose location is not known. The usual method for preparing the polysaccharides is by hot acid extraction. Other methods of preparation involve the use of formamide or enzyme extraction.

Acid extraction of polysaccharides

The culture to be extracted is grown for at least 24 hours in broth and then centrifuged. The deposit from 10 or 30 ml of culture (depending on the density of growth) is resuspended in 0·4 ml of 0·2 N HCl, and placed in a boiling waterbath for 10 minutes. After cooling, 1 drop of 0·02 per cent phenol red is added, the fluid neutralised with 0·2N NaOH and then centrifuged. The clear supernatant contains the extract which is a hapten and, therefore, cannot be used for the preparation of antisera. Group specific antisera are prepared by inoculating rabbits with whole organisms, and the procedure for typing consists of carrying out precipitin ring tests in narrow tubes to reduce the volumes of antisera and polysaccharide extracts required.

On this basis, pathogenic streptococcal strains have been classified into groups labelled with letters of the alphabet but omitting I and J which were not included in these designations. This Lancefield grouping system has the advantage that it is closely related to the different host species concerned, but it should be remembered that several investigators have reported that a considerable proportion of streptococcal strains derived from animals cannot be classified by this grouping system. The great majority of strains pathogenic for man occur in group A; group B strains are commonly associated with chronic bovine mastitis; group C strains are particularly frequent in horses as well as occurring in other animal species; and strains belonging to

group G are often related to infections in dogs. Table 15.2 summarises the groups and names of streptococcal species and the diseases they cause in animals and man.

In addition to group-specific polysaccharide antigens, there are type-specific antigens enabling streptococci comprising a Lancefield group to be serologically distinguished one from another. These serotypes were investigated and described in detail by Griffith who showed by agglutination tests that group A organisms, in particular, can be divided into a large number of different serotypes. The difficulties which have often been experienced in developing satisfactory vaccines for the prevention of streptococcal diseases are due largely to the probability that strains used in the preparation of vaccines have had type specific antigens different to those of the infecting organisms. Group A streptococci possess additional protein antigens labelled M, T and R which occur on the surfaces of some group A strains. The M antigen which is an alcohol-soluble protein, is closely associated with virulence and is produced by matt or mucoid colonies but not by avirulent glossy colonies. It is type specific and used in agglutination and precipitation tests for identifying the many different serotypes which comprise group A. The T antigen which is alcohol-insoluble and the R antigen are neither type specific nor associated with virulence.

Phage typing of streptococci has been investigated, particularly in relation to the study of streptococcal antigens and their disposition on the cell surface. More recently, phage typing of group D strains has been examined but attempts to distinguish between the different species in this group have not proved satisfactory.

Pathogenic streptococci produce a variety of extracellular toxins and enzymes including the following which are of significance in the pathogenesis of animal infections.

O-streptolysin

This is an oxygen-labile haemolysin at room temperature which can be reactivated by reducing agents (e.g. sodium hydrosulphite). It has a toxic action on both erythrocytes and leucocytes, and is lethal for mice, guinea-pigs and rabbits. It is antigenic and combines with its specific antibody which is developed during infection with streptococcal strains producing O-streptolysin. The antibody prevents the haemolytic effect and this has been used as the basis of a serological test to detect whether an individual has recently sustained a streptococcal infection.

S-streptolysin

This is a serum-soluble, oxygen-stable haemolysin

TABLE 15.2. Summarising the occurrence of streptococci as pathogens or commensals in animals and man.

Serological group	Specific name	Haemolysis on blood agar	Host species	Streptococcal diseases — Disease entity	Natural habitats and sites where the organism may exist without causing disease
A	*Str. pyogenes*	β	Man	Scarlet fever, septic sore throat, puerperal fever, erysipelas, wound infections	Nose and throat
			Animals	Mastitis in cattle (rare) and other species (rare)	
B	*Str. agalactiae*	β-, α- or non-haemolytic	Cattle	Mastitis	Bovine skin, udder and milk
			Horses, dogs, rabbits, guinea-pigs, mice	Various infections (rare)	
			Man	Endocarditis (rare), puerperal fever (rare)	Throat and vagina (rare)
C	*Str. equi*	β	Horses	Strangles	Nose and throat
	Str. zooepidemicus	β	Dogs, cats and man	Various infections (rare)	
			Cattle	Mastitis	Milk
			Poultry	Avian streptococcosis (septicaemia)	
			Other animals	Infections of respiratory and urogenital tracts, wounds and polyarthritis	Nose, throat and vagina; horse faeces
	Str. equisimilis	β	Pigs	Septicaemia, joint infections (rare)	Lungs, liver, vagina, joints (rare)
			Cattle and horses	do.	do.
			Man	Septicaemia and local infections (rare)	Nose and throat
	Str. dysgalactiae	β or α	Cattle	Mastitis	Nose, throat, vagina and milk
			Lambs	Polyarthritis and endocarditis	
D	*Str. faecalis* var. *zymogenes* var. *liquefaciens*	α-, β- or non-haemolytic	Cattle	Mastitis, endocarditis, various infections	Liver, kidney, intestines, faeces and milk
	Str. faecium	α	Sheep and lambs	Pneumonia, arthritis, endocarditis	Intestines and faeces
			Pigs	Various infections	Various tissues, especially intestines and faeces
	Str. durans	α or β	Poultry		Lung, liver, joints, intestines and faeces
			Man	Cystitis, endocarditis (rare)	Throat, intestines, faeces, vagina (Enterococci also occur in water, soil, sewage and vegetation)

(*Str. faecalis*, *Str. faecium* and *Str. durans* are bracketed together as **enterococci**.)

	Species	Haemolysis	Host	Disease	Habitat
	Str. equinus	α	Horses and pigs		Intestines and faeces
	Str. bovis	α or non-haemolytic	Cattle and pigs		Intestines, faeces and milk
E	*Str. uberis*	α- or non-haemolytic	Cattle and sheep	Mastitis	Throat, rumen, faeces, milk, skin, vagina, soil
F	*Str. infrequens*	β	Cattle	Mastitis	Milk
			Pigs	Endocarditis, abscesses	Throat
G	*Str. minutus*		Man and dogs	Tonsillitis, glomerular nephritis	Nose, throat, faeces and vagina
	Str. canis	β	Dogs	Tonsillitis, otitis, metritis, mastitis, septicaemia	Throat, mammary gland, vagina
			Cattle	Mastitis	Milk
H			Cats	Puerperal fever	Nose, throat, faeces, vagina
			Man	Endocarditis (rare)	Nose, throat, faeces
K	*Str. salivarius*	α- or non-haemolytic	Man	Mastitis (rare)	
			Cattle		Liver and lung
L		β- or α-	Pigs	Tonsillitis, metritis, septicaemia	Nose and throat
			Man	Mastitis	Throat
			Dogs	Septicaemia and pneumonia	Kidney, muscle and milk
			Cattle		Lung, vagina
			Pigs		Anterior nares, boned poultry meat
			Poultry		Tonsils and urogenital tract
M	*Str. lactis*	β- or non-haemolytic	Dogs		Faeces, milk, dairy products
N	*Str. cremonis*	α- or non-haemolytic	Cattle		Liver and kidney
			Sheep		Heart and lung
			Pigs		Milk
O		β- or α-	Cattle	Mastitis	Nose and throat
			Man	Tonsillitis	
P		β or non-haemolytic	Pigs	Broncho-pneumonia, polyarthritis	
Q	*Str. avium*	α- or non-haemolytic	Cattle	Mastitis (rare)	Milk
			Poultry, other animals, Man		Faeces (especially poultry)
R		α-, β- or non-haemolytic	Cattle	Septicaemia and pneumonia	Milk
			Pigs		Various tissues
S		α-, β- or non-haemolytic	Pigs (especially piglets)	Septicaemia, arthritis, meningitis, encephalitis and enteritis	Various tissues
T		α-, β- or non-haemolytic	Pigs	Septicaemia	Various tissues

causing β-haemolysis on blood agar cultures in-cubated aerobically. It has an anti-inflammatory reaction.

Fibrinolysin (*streptokinase*)

This causes lysis of human fibrin clots and is only demonstrable in freshly isolated strains. It is produced particularly by groups A, C and G, and has an anti-inflammatory reaction.

Streptodornase

This causes liquefaction of purulent exudates by de-polymerisation of nucleo-protein and thus facilitates their removal. It has been employed therapeutically to liquefy viscous exudates.

Hyaluronidase

This is a 'spreading factor' causing increased perme-ability of tissues by hydrolysis of hyaluronic acid. This enzyme is distinct from that produced by staphylococci.

Erythrogenic toxin

This causes the rash (erythema) that is characteristic of scarlet fever which is produced only by group A strains elaborating this toxin. It is antigenic and has been used in the Dick test in man to measure the immunity of individuals to scarlet fever. Persons with antibodies to the toxin will not react to the antigen and are not susceptible to scarlet fever.

Epidemiology and pathogenesis

The biology of streptococci is closely associated with the way of life of their host species, and particularly with the conditions which facilitate the transfer of infection from one individual to another, the existence of the carrier state, and the predisposing factors which lead to the development of clinical disease from the carrier state. Although these conditions vary from one host species to another, there are certain features common to the development of streptococcal infections in all species of animals and man.

Pathogenic streptococci resemble pathogenic staphylococci in the variety of toxins and enzymes they can develop which facilitate their establishment in host tissues. As already noted, those substances include streptolysins which are both inhibitory to the cellular responses of the host to infection and also lethal. The dispersal of the disease process in the tissues is facilitated by hyaluronidase (spreading factor) which increases the permeability of the tissues. In addition, fibrinolysin (streptokinase) inhibits the inflammatory responses of the tissues, and the action of streptodornase assists the removal of purulent exudates. Furthermore, virulent organisms possess antigens which help to protect them from the defence mechanisms of the body. These have been characterised in relation to group A *Str. pyogenes* as the mucoid (M) antigen. It has also been postulated that additional unidentified toxins may be produced in the tissues consequent upon the interaction between host and parasite.

The natural habitats generally associated with streptococci are the skin, throat, nose, digestive tract and urogenital tract of animals and man. More specifically, some streptococcal species have become adapted to an existence in certain of these sites. For example, *Str. faecalis* is a common inhabitant of the intestinal tract and is characterised by its ability to grow on MacConkey's agar in the presence of bile salts. Similarly, group Q (*Str. avium*) organi-sms are frequently found in the faeces of poultry and sometimes from other species. *Str. agalactiae* and *Str. uberis* can exist in the normal bovine udder without causing disease and group A (*Str. pyogenes*) organisms frequently constitute part of the bacterial flora of the human nose and throat. It is also known that haemolytic streptococci are often present in the throats of healthy dogs. The likelihood of infection spreading from one individual to another will depend, therefore, upon a number of factors related to the host environment as well as to the adaptation which streptococcal species may have developed for particular sites in the body.

Bovine mastitis can be caused by a number of streptococcal species, the commonest being *Str. agalactiae*, *Str. dysgalactiae*, *Str. uberis* and *Str. zooepidemicus*. The normal habitat for *Str. agalactiae* and *Str. uberis*, in particular, is the skin of the belly and lips, and sometimes in the tonsils, rumen and faeces. Thus, when they are present in a herd it is practically impossible to eradicate infection. The bacteria may also be spread by suckling calves and possibly by flies, but the important vehicles which cause a rapid dissemination of infection are milk, milking utensils and the milkers' hands and clothing, because mastitis arises from infection which is introduced into the udder via the teat canal. By these various routes one animal which is a symptomless carrier can be the source of a severe and rapid build-up of infection in a herd. Less frequently, the origin of a streptococcal milk infection may be a human carrier harbouring the organisms in the throat, which is the natural habitat for group A *Str. pyogenes*. Mastitis caused by *Str. pyogenes* is often acute and the milk may contain large numbers of organisms.

The immunological response of the host to mastitis caused by bacteria has been studied in some detail, and it has been shown that immunoglobulins occur in colostrum and that these antibody globulin fractions are derived from serum and transferred to the mammary gland. The concentration of antibodies can reach a high level in colostrum and it is probable that a lower rate of transfer continues at a later stage, particularly towards the end of the lactation period. There is, in addition, some evidence to show that to a limited extent, local antibody production can take place in the mammary gland, itself. Nevertheless, it is a common experience to find that antibody concentrations in milk are low even in those animals which have high serum antibody titres.

Strangles in horses is primarily a disease of young animals caused by *Str. equi* and the initial colonisation of the bacteria takes place in the nasal and buccal mucous membranes. From these sites, infection spreads via the lymphatic system to local lymph nodes where abscesses develop and septicaemic infections in severe cases give rise to abscess formation in a variety of organs and tissues. The contents of abscesses contain large numbers of bacteria and when these discharge, infection can spread rapidly from one animal to another, particularly in stables where horses are in close contact with each other, where ventilation may be poor, and where droplet infection can occur directly from one animal to another or indirectly via drinking water, buckets, grooming tools and other equipment. Less frequently, infection is transmitted at coitus. Some infected animals remain carriers and potential sources of infection for other susceptible individuals.

Joint ill or navel ill is a streptococcal disease of young foals which may develop as an acute and fatal septicaemia or as a chronic infection giving rise to arthritis, pneumonia or enteritis. In addition to general wound infections in horses, endometritis in mares is another condition caused by streptococci.

Pigs are susceptible to infection with streptococci belonging to a number of different groups and particularly those belonging to group C which are frequently carried by symptomless animals. The infection may develop as a septicaemia followed by an endocarditis similar to that which is caused by *Erysipelothrix insidiosa*. Streptococcal infections may also cause meningitis, encephalitis or arthritis, particularly in association with group S organisms; and pigs may also suffer from streptococcal abscess formation in various organs and also from abortion.

Sheep are not particularly susceptible to streptococcal diseases but sometimes suffer from groups C and D infections which can give rise to pneumonia, polyarthritis and endocarditis.

Dogs may develop septicaemic infections, endocarditis, metritis and fatal neonatal infections in puppies. These diseases are commonly associated with groups G, C and L which are frequently carried by 50 per cent or more of dogs living in kennels. Strains belonging to group M are often present in the tonsils or urogenital tracts of dogs, but these organisms are non-pathogenic and do not cause disease. Cats are less frequently affected but may suffer from pneumonia and septicaemia associated with groups G and C.

Poultry are susceptible to streptococcal infections which cause pneumonia, endocarditis or abscess formation. Organisms belonging to a variety of groups may be responsible for these conditions; in addition, group D organisms are frequently present in the intestines of chickens and excreted in their faeces.

Many other animal species, including fur-bearers and laboratory animals are susceptible to pyogenic infections caused by organisms belonging to various groups. It is noteworthy that monkeys, like man, frequently carry streptococci in the throat and that it is not uncommon for these organisms to belong to group A.

Symptoms and lesions

Mastitis arises from the multiplication of streptococci in the teat sinus, extending into the ducts and secreting tissues of the mammary gland, and clinical signs of infection are detectable only after the lesions have become extensive. The condition may be chronic or acute depending upon the streptococcal species involved. *Str. agalactiae* causes a chronic, insidious form of the disease and during the early stages the milk will occasionally contain flakes. As the condition develops, milk secretion will become less and the normal consistency will change by stages into a thick purulent fluid containing fibrin and blood. During the infective process, polymorphs migrate to the interalveolar tissue which proliferates and may undergo fibrosis. The lumina of the alveoli become reduced in size and practically blocked with cellular material. There is thickening of the epithelial tissue of the ducts and some become occluded by the development of granulation tissue. These changes may not be permanent and from time to time the milk may revert to a more normal consistency for short periods before again becoming purulent. During the latter stages of disease, centres of fibrosis will have developed and these areas of induration can be palpated. Satisfactory treatment may result in the quarters returning to normal but the subsequent milk yield may be reduced. Mastitis caused by *Str. uberis* is clinically similar to *Str. agalactiae* infection but with a tendency to be less severe. In contrast, *Str. dysgalactiae* and *Str. zooepidemicus* usually cause a more acute and severe condition confined to one quarter and characterised by a hot swollen, painful udder and a purulent yellow secretion. The onset may be sudden, developing into severe symptoms within a few days and sometimes the disease spreads rapidly in a herd. Some animals also develop joint infections and become lame.

Recovery often results in atrophy of the affected quarter.

Equine strangles usually affects younger animals of 1–2 years of age and develops as a respiratory infection characterised by a mucopurulent nasal discharge accompanied by inflammation of the mucous membranes of the upper respiratory tract and the development of abscesses in the submaxillary glands and less frequently in the lymphatic vessels and glands of the forelegs. Joint ill in foals usually develops during the first week in life and acute septicaemic infections result in sudden death. More protracted infections may show various symptoms of enteritis, pneumonia and lameness associated with infection of the hock, stifle and knee joints.

The symptoms of streptococcal diseases in other species depend upon whether the infections are septicaemic or localised in various situations, including the heart, brain, visceral organs, urogenital tract and joints. A common form of the disease in dogs consists of severe septicaemic infections in puppies causing neonatal deaths.

Diagnosis

Mastitis

The methods to be employed will depend upon a variety of factors including the history of a particular outbreak and the acute or chronic nature of the infection. Diagnosis may involve clinical, microscopical and bacteriological examinations.

Palpation of the udder and supramammary lymph nodes will be helpful in distinguishing the chronic and insidious form of mastitis produced by *Str. agalactiae* and *Str. uberis* infections which cause the development of areas of palpable induration in the udder. In contrast, the more acute and often sporadic forms of streptococcal mastitis are caused by *Str. dysgalactiae* and *Str. zooepidemicus*, and these are usually characterised by a sudden onset of acute inflammation of one quarter only, sometimes associated with an acute systemic disturbance followed by joint infections and lameness. Clinical examination of the milk by a variety of methods for estimating the cell count and consistency, are of additional value for determining the presence and severity of mastitis.

Microscopical examination of milk samples may be useful for the diagnosis of streptococcal mastitis, but it is important to remember that in a large proportion of examinations from such cases, streptococci may not be observed. Conversely, when long chains of organisms are detected in milk samples derived from cases of chronic mastitis, it is almost certain that the causal organisms are *Str.agalactiae*.

Bacteriological examinations may require the use of a variety of media for the detection of various properties characteristic for different streptococcal species (Table 15.3). Blood agar inoculated with 0·1 ml of secretion is a useful method for estimating not only the type of haemolytic reaction but the approximate degree of infection in a milk sample. Edwards' medium containing blood agar, crystal violet and aesculin may be of value in some investigations since the crystal violet inhibits the growth of staphylococci and the incorporation of aesculin in the medium helps to differentiate between streptococcal species which do or do not hydrolyse aesculin. Thus, on Edwards' medium colonies of *Str. agalactiae* from cases of chronic mastitis are small, transparent, bluish-grey in colour and may be haemolytic or non-haemolytic. In comparison, colonies of *Str. uberis* from cases of chronic mastitis appear as dark-coloured colonies surrounded by black or brown zones of discolouration in the medium caused by the hydrolysis of aesculin by this organism (Plate 15.2c, facing p. 177). *Str. dysgalactiae* produces a non-haemolytic green discolouration of the medium (See Table 15.3).

The CAMP test, named after the initials of those who originated the method (Christie, Atkins and Munch-Petersen, 1944), is based on the observation that ruminant red blood cells partially lysed by the β-toxin of staphylococci at 37°C are completely lysed in the presence of *Str. agalactiae* (group B). There are various techniques for carrying out this test and one of these includes the use of an aesculin blood agar plate which has an inoculum of a β-toxin-producing staphylococcal strain across the full width of the plate. Suspected streptococcal strains under examination are then sown at right angles to the staphylococcus. A number of strains can be tested on each plate which is examined for areas of complete haemolysis after incubation (Plate 15.2d, facing p. 177). Although this test is useful for the diagnosis of *Str. agalactiae* (group B), a similar reaction may be produced occasionally by some strains of *Str. dysgalactiae* (group C) and *Str. uberis* (group E).

It is important to remember that milk samples may become contaminated with *Str. thermophilus*. This organism produces α-haemolysis and is a saprophyte occurring in dust and manure. It grows at a temperature as high as 60°C and will survive heating at 65°C for 30 minutes. Because of these thermophilic properties it is not destroyed by pasteurisation.

Other streptococcal infections

The general approach to diagnosing the great diversity of streptococcal infections in animals consists of the microscopical examination of suspected materials, the isolation of the organisms and their serological identification by using Lancefield's grouping methods. The choice of media used for

TABLE 15.3. Comparing some of the characteristic properties of streptococcal species which occur in bovine milk.

Group	Species	Appearance of growth on Edwards' medium	CAMP test	Hydrolysis of aesculin	Hydrolysis of hippurate	Growth in 40% bile salts	Growth at 45°C	Fermentation of Lactose	Trehalose	Sorbitol	Inulin
A	Str. pyogenes	β Moderate zone	−	−	−	∓	−	+	+	−	−
B	Str. agalactiae	β Narrow zone or non-haemolytic	+	−	+	±	−	+	+	−	−
C	Str. zooepide-micus	β Wide zone	−	−	−	−	−	+	−	+	−
C	Str. dysgalactiae	Green colour	∓	−	−	−	−	+	+	±	−
D	Str. faecalis (enterococcus)	Dark colonies	−	+	−	+	+	+	+	+	−
D	Str. bovis	Dark colonies	−	+	−	+	+	+	±	−	+
E	Str. uberis	Dark colonies; browning of medium	∓	+	+	+	−	+	+	+	+
E	Str. infrequens	β Wide zone	−	+	−	±	−	+	+	+	−
G		β Wide zone	−	±	−	∓	−	+	±	−	−
L		β Wide zone	−	∓	−	−	−		+	−	−
N	Str. lactis	Green colour	−	+	±	+	−	+	+	−	−
O			−		−		−	+	∓	−	−

± = usually positive and rarely negative. ∓ = usually negative and rarely positive.

isolations and the subsequent tests for observing the cultural characteristics of the isolates will be governed partly by the nature of material and whether it is heavily contaminated with other bacterial species, and partly by its source and animal species of origin which may give an indication of the streptococcal organisms involved (e.g. *Str. equi* (group C) and equine strangles; *Str. canis* (group G) and canine infections; *Str. pyogenes* (group A) and scarlet fever, septic sore throat or erysipelas, etc.).

Control and prevention

For the treatment of all forms of streptococcal infections in animals, including mastitis, the most satisfactory method is antibiotic therapy using penicillin preparations in preference to other substances because streptococci develop resistance to penicillin comparatively infrequently.

Vaccines are of very limited value for the im-munization of animals against streptococcal infections, with the possible exception of equine strangles (*Str. equi* infections). One probable reason for this situation is that there are often several different serological types of some of the important pathogenic streptococcal species, and unless a vaccine is prepared from the corresponding type of organism to that causing disease in an outbreak, the resultant immunity derived from its use will be inadequate to protect the animals at risk from infection. This may be the explanation for the unreliable results obtained from the use of vaccines for the prevention of mastitis caused by *Str. agalactiae*, which has several serological types, in comparison with the more satisfactory results recorded from the use of vaccines for the control of equine strangles caused by *Str. equi*, since only one serological type of this latter organism has been identified.

Additional general control and preventative measures include draining abscesses, giving strict attention to cleanliness, disinfection of animal environments and equipment, and careful nursing of affected animals.

Public health aspects

Str. pyogenes (group A) is the most usual cause of human infections which often give rise to suppurative lesions occurring in a wide variety of sites throughout the body. In general, however, the streptococcal species commonly responsible for disease in animals relatively seldom affect man, but occasionally, human disease may be derived from animal sources, the commonest being infected milk and other foodstuffs.

PNEUMOCOCCUS

Diplococcus pneumoniae

Synonyms
Streptococcus pneumoniae

Distribution in nature
These organisms are closely related to the strepto- cocci and share some common antigens with them. The pneumococcus is usually associated with infec- tions of the human respiratory tract, and they have also been isolated from the respiratory tracts of some species of healthy animals, and also from cases of pneumonia and of bovine mastitis.

Morphology and staining
The organisms are cocci, approximately $1 \cdot 0$ μm in diameter, usually oval or lanceolate in shape, occurring in pairs end-to-end and surrounded by capsular material. (Plate 15.2e, facing p. 177) After subcultivation the organisms tend to become more spherical in outline, sometimes developing in short chains in fluid culture, and capsular material may be absent. They do not produce spores and are non-motile.

The organisms stain Gram-positive. Old cultures easily decolourise and have a tendency to stain Gram-negative and to lyse spontaneously.

Cultural characteristics
The pneumococcus is aerobic and facultatively anaerobic; the optimum temperature for growth is 37°C but growth will take place over a temperature range of 25–40°C. Growth will occur on ordinary media but is enhanced in the presence of blood, serum or glucose, and in an atmosphere of 5–10 per cent CO_2.

On blood agar after 48 hours' incubation the small round dome-shaped translucent colonies of about 1 mm in diameter, which later become flattened with raised edges, are surrounded by a zone of α-

haemolysis similar to that produced by strains of *Str. viridans*. This haemolytic effect is more pro- nounced when cultures are grown on chocolate agar.

In enriched fluid cultures growth takes place diffusely for about 48 hours and then autolysis may occur and the broth culture becomes clear.

Differentiation between the pneumococcus and *Str. viridans* organisms is based on bile solubility and the optochin test.

Bile solubility test
Autolysis of pneumococcal cultures takes place within 15 minutes at 37°C in the presence of 10 per cent ox bile or 10 per cent sodium desoxycholate. These substances have no effect on *Str. viridans* organisms.

The Optochin test
The majority of pneumococcal strains are sensitive to optochin (ethyl hydrocuprein hydrochloride) whereas *Str. viridans* organisms are not. The test consists of placing a small circular piece of filter paper, impregnated with a 1:4000 aqueous solution of optochin, in the centre of a blood agar plate after sowing the test cultures in streaks across the full width of the medium. The growth of pneumo- coccal strains will be inhibited to a distance of some 5 mm from the circumference of the filter paper, whereas *Str. viridans* cultures will grow up to the margin of the paper.

Acid without gas is produced in a variety of carbohydrate media but it should be noted that the fermentation of inulin is not a reliable method for differentiating between the pneumococcus and *Str. viridans* organisms. Catalase is not produced and gelatin is not liquefied.

Resistance to physical and chemical agents
The organisms are killed when subjected to a temperature of 55°C for 15 minutes. Their suscep- tibility to disinfectants is similar to pathogenic species of streptococci.

Antigens and toxins
The capsular material of the pneumococcus contains immunologically distinct polysaccharides and on the basis of these substances, the organisms can be serologically classified into serotypes. There are now recognised to be some eighty different serotypes. The typing of these organisms is carried out either by means of an agglutination test, a precipitation test or more usually by the Quellung reaction which is a 'capsule-swelling' test.

Capsule swelling test (Quellung reaction)
For this test a loopful of bacterial suspension (i.e. broth culture or saline suspension prepared from growth on a blood agar plate) is mixed with a

loopful of diagnostic antiserum to capsular poly-saccharide and a coverslip superimposed. The diagnostic serum is mixed beforehand with methylene blue. The film is examined with reduced light and under an oil-immersion lens. When the antibody in the serum corresponds to the capsular polysaccharide of the bacterial strain under test, the enlarged unstained capsules can be observed easily after 2 minutes. When the antiserum does not correspond to the capsular substance, the capsules remain invisible. For routine testing, cultures are first mixed with a number of pooled antisera, each of which contains antibodies to a number of different capsular substances; and thereafter the cultures are tested against type-specific antisera.

It has been shown that isolated capsular material is non-toxic when injected into susceptible hosts, and that the organism does not produce a detectable soluble toxin.

Variation

Smooth cultures of the pneumococcus are those which produce variable amounts of capsular material. Most cultures contain a proportion of rough organisms which are those that are devoid of capsules. When a culture is grown in the presence of type-specific antiserum, the rough forms will predominate. Conversely, inoculation of rough cultures into mice will result in the development of predominantly smooth forms. This is because a small proportion of organisms in a rough culture will, in fact, be in the smooth encapsulated form, and will be able to resist the defence mechanisms of mice, especially the action of the phagocytes.

It has also been noted that transformation from one species to another can occur in mice. For example, if a mixture of living type 2 (rough form) and heat-killed type 3 (smooth capsulated form) is inoculated into mice, the animals die from infection with living type 3 organisms. Comparable results have also been obtained from other similar experiments in which the isolated capsular polysaccharide has been used in place of the heat-killed whole organisms. This transformation phenomenon is caused by the DNA from the killed encapsulated organisms being taken up by and stimulating the production in the living rough cells of capsular substance corresponding to that of the killed smooth culture.

Epidemiology and pathogenesis

Pneumococcal capsular substance plays an important role in the life history of these organisms by enabling them to survive, and multiply in host tissues. It has long been known from experiments in mice, which are particularly susceptible to pneumococcal infections, that smooth encapsulated organisms are able to resist phagocytosis, whereas rough non-capsulate bacteria are highly susceptible. It seems from more recent investigations that the reason for the resistance shown by capsulated organisms is that they can produce such large quantities of capsular material that antibodies concerned with the opsonic effect are largely neutralised, and this reduces the ability of phagocytes to remove and destroy these organisms.

Various investigations have failed to detect the production of a soluble toxin by the pneumococcus, and it has been postulated that the pathogenic effects produced by the organism are caused either by a hitherto unidentified soluble toxin or by toxic products resulting from the interaction between host tissues and the encapsulated bacteria. A study of the pathogenesis of pneumococcal infections shows that it is common for these to develop as secondary infections to respiratory virus diseases or other predisposing factors, and it is evident that the production of inflammatory reactions, especially excessive bronchial secretion and oedema, facilitates the development of the pneumococcus in the affected area.

The pneumococcus has been detected with varying frequency in the bacterial flora of the upper respiratory tracts of animal species which suffer from these infections, and it is significant that studies on the epidemiology of these animal diseases has shown the importance of the human carrier as the source of infection. A number of detailed studies on the pneumococcal types associated with pneumonic infections in calves and the types resident in the throats of people tending these animals, has illustrated this important epidemiological feature. It has also been found that a considerable proportion of these animal attendants have shown clinical evidence of influenza, mild pneumonia, acute colds and other signs of disease usually associated with pneumococcal infections at times when the disease was developing in the animals they were tending. It is also significant that where the source of an outbreak of pneumococcal mastitis occurs in a herd, the animal attendants are also found to be carriers of the organism in their throats, and that the cause of the mastitis is often the pneumococcal type 3 organism which is a frequent inhabitant of the human throat. The form of mastitis which develops is usually acute and the milk may contain large numbers of organisms. It has been postulated that this heavily infected milk, when fed to calves, may constitute another mode of calf infection leading to pneumococcal pneumonia.

Symptoms and lesions

Pneumococcal bovine mastitis is usually acute. The disease may affect one, two or all four quarters of the udder which becomes hot, swollen and painful. There is a sudden, severe drop in milk yield and the secretion becomes purulent, contains fibrin clots and is heavily infected with organisms. There is usually a general systemic disturbance reflected by increased body temperature and a loss of appetite. In severe cases, death from a septicaemic infection may take place on the sixth to seventh day following the onset of disease.

Pneumonia in young calves is often acute and the animal shows symptoms characteristic of this type of disease. Deaths of severe cases occur a few days after the onset of symptoms.

Diagnosis

This is based on microscopical examination of suitable material (e.g. milk) for the presence of characteristic Gram-positive diplococci, observations on cultural characteristics, especially haemolysin production on blood agar or chocolate agar, and differentiation from *Str. viridans* organisms by the use of bile solubility and optochin tests. Finally, the serological typing of the organism may be of value in tracing the origin of infection. It should be noted that when death follows a septicaemic infection, the organisms rapidly disappear from the circulation and may be difficult to identify in blood samples.

Control and prevention

The use of penicillin, chloramphenicol or sulphonamides is of value for treatment of acute disease provided that it is commenced as early as possible. Drug resistance to broad spectrum antibiotics has been reported.

Public health aspects

The pneumococcus is the cause of lobar pneumonia in man and is a secondary pathogen in cases of bronchopneumonia. Other infections associated with this organism are conjunctivitis, otitis media and less frequently peritonitis, meningitis and arthritis. In the United Kingdom more than 50 per cent of cases of lobar pneumonia are caused by types 1, 2 and 3, all of which are commonly carried in the human throat.

Further reading

BROWN, J., FARNSWORTH, R., WANNAMAKER, L.W. AND JOHNSON, D.W. (1974) CAMP factor of group B streptococci: production, assay and neutralization by sera from immunized rabbits and experimentally infected cows. *Infection and Immunity*, 9, 377.

CHRISTIE R., ATKINS N.E. AND MUNCH-PETERSEN E. (1944) A note on a lytic phenomenon by group B Streptococci. *Australian Journal of Experimental Biology and Medical Science*, 22, 197.

CULLEN G.A. (1969) Streptococcus uberis: A review. *Veterinary Bulletin*, 39, 155.

DEIBEL R.H. (1964) The group D Streptococci. *Bacteriological Reviews*, 28, 330.

FORBES D. (1969) The pathogenesis of bovine mastitis. *Veterinary Bulletin*, 39, 529.

GREER, D.O. AND PEARSON, J.K.L. (1973) *Streptococcus agalactiae* in dairy herds. Its incidence and relationship to cell count and inhibitory substance levels in bulk milk. *British Veterinary Journal*, 129, 544.

KRAUSE R.M. (1963) Symposium on relationship of structure of microorganisms to their immunological properties: IV. Antigenic and biochemical composition of haemolytic streptococcal walls. *Bacteriological Reviews*, 27, 369.

KUREK, C. AND RUTKOWIAK, B. (1971) Dog carriers of *Streptococcus pyogenes* on the mucus membrane of the tonsils. *Epidemiological Review*, 25, 234.

LANCEFIELD R.C. (1933) A serological differentiation of human and other groups of haemolytic streptococci. *Journal of Experimental Medicine*, 57, 571.

NATIONAL MASTITIS COUNCIL (1963) *Current Concepts of Bovine Mastitis*. Illinois: Kinsdale.

RØMER O. (1959) Bovine mastitis due to *Streptococcus pneumoniae*. *Nordisk Veterinärmedicin*, 11, 361.

RØMER O. (1960) A comparison between Pneumococcal infection in calves and man with special reference to the possibility of a causal relationship. *Nordisk Veterinärmedicin*, 12, 73.

SCHMITZ, J.A., OLSON, L.D., SCHUELER, R.L. AND GROSSER, H.S. (1972) Isolation of group E streptococcus from the blood of swine with streptococcic lymphadenitis. *American Journal of Veterinary Research*, 33, 449.

SHUMAN, R.D., NORD, N., BROWN, R.W. AND WESSMAN, G.E. (1972) Biochemical and serological characteristics of Lancefield groups E, P and U streptococci and *Streptococcus uberis*. *Cornell Veterinarian*, 62, 540.

STARK, D.M. (1971) Cross-reactive antigens of bovine streptococci. *Cornell Veterinarian*, 61, 617.

WANNAMAKER, L.W. AND MATSEN, J.M. [Editors] (1972) Streptococci and streptococcal diseases: recognition, understanding and management. New York and London: Academic Press.

WOOLCOCK, J.B. (1973) The immunology of streptococcal infections. *Australian Veterinary Journal*, 49, 85.

CHAPTER 16

CORYNEBACTERIUM

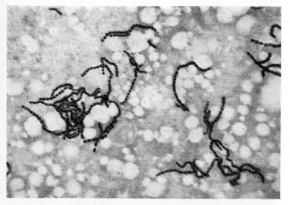

15.1a

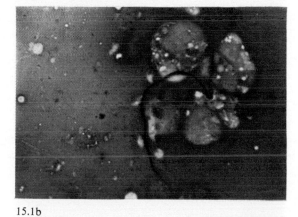

15.1b

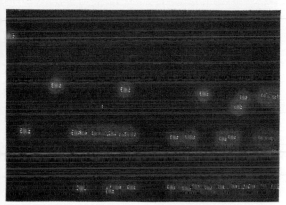

15.1c

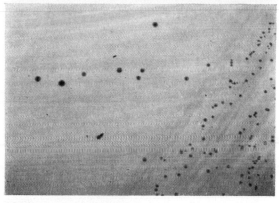

15.1d

15.1a   Gram-stained milk film of *Streptococcus agalactiae* showing chains of cocci, ×930.

15.1c   Colonies of *Streptococcus viridans* on blood agar showing haemolysis and greenish discolouration of the medium.

15.1b   Gram-stained tissue film of *Streptococcus equi* showing a characteristic long chain of cocci, ×930.

15.1d   Growth of *Streptococcus faecalis* on MacConkey's agar showing small pink-coloured colonies.

15.2a

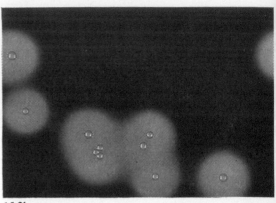

15.2b

15.2c

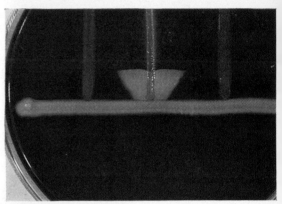

15.2d

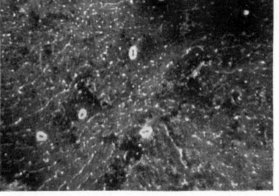

15.2e

15.2a Colonies of *Streptococcus faecalis* on horse blood agar showing no haemolysis.

15.2b Colonies of group G streptococci on horse blood agar showing wide zones of β haemolysis.

15.2c *Streptococcus uberis* growing on Edwards' medium showing dark-coloured colonies surrounded by brown zones of discolouration.

15.2d CAMP phenomenon on sheep blood agar. Note the increased haemolytic effect produced near the junction of *Streptococcus agalactiae* (central streak) with a β-toxin producing staphylococcus (horizontal streak). No effect is produced by other streptococcal strains (left and right).

15.2e India ink film of pneumococci, stained with methyl violet, to show capsules (colourless), × 930.

CHAPTER 16

Corynebacterium

These organisms are non-motile, non-sporing, non-capsulated Gram-positive rods arranged in pairs or pallisades. Some species produce potent exotoxins. The group includes *Corynebacterium diphtheriae* the cause of human diphtheria and a number of other organisms, sometimes referred to as diphtheroids, which are associated with disease in animals (see Table 16.1). In addition, *C. ulcerans* which occasionally causes tonsillitis in man has recently been isolated from some cases of bovine mastitis; *C. murium* may cause caseous lesions in mice; and *C. haemolyticum* has been identified in samples of bovine semen and isolated from pneumonic lungs in sheep. Two features common to all these corynebacterial infections in animals are that disease is characterised by the development of

TABLE 16.1. Comparing the characteristic properties of some corynebacteria

Characteristic properties	C. pyogenes	C. ovis	C. equi	C. renale	C. suis	C. bovis
Major disease processes	Mastitis (cattle & sheep); suppurative lesions in many animal species	Caseous lymphadenitis (sheep & goats); ulcerative lymphangitis (horses)	Purulent pneumonia (foals, calves, pigs & sheep)	Pyelonephritis and cystitis (cattle)	Pyelonephritis and cystitis (sows)	Mastitis (cattle)
Production of filterable toxin	+	+	—	—	—	—
Haemolysis on blood agar	+	V	—	—	—	—
Liquefaction of inspissated serum	+	—	—	—	—	—
Casein hydrolysis on milk agar	—	—	—	+	—	—
Pigment production on milk agar	—	—	pink	—	—	—
Volutin granules (Neisser's or Albert's stain)	—	+	—	+	—	—
Lactose	1	1	—	—	—	—
Glucose	1	1	—	1	V	1
Maltose	1	1	—	—	1	—
Mannitol	—	1	—	—	—	1

+ = Positive reaction   V = variable reaction   — = negative reaction   1 = acid production.

177

suppurative lesions, and that these clinical mani-festations do not develop in the absence of predis-posing factors.

Corynebacterium pyogenes

Distribution in nature

This organism is a cause of mastitis in cattle and sheep and of various suppurative lesions in these and other animal species. *C. pyogenes* has a world-wide distribution and is known to exist on the mucous surfaces of healthy animals.

Morphology and staining

C. pyogenes derived from young cultures or from infected tissues appears as short coccobacilli or rods with a maximum length of 2 μm and arranged in bundles or clusters. A variety of pleomorphic forms can occur, including club-shaped and globular forms (Plate 16.1a, facing p. 188b). The organisms are non-motile, and do not produce spores or capsules.

Young cultures stain Gram-positive but in older cultures a number of organisms will readily deco-lourise and appear Gram-negative.

Cultural characteristics

C. pyogenes will grow aerobically and anaerobically at an optimum temperature of 37°C. Blood or serum added to the medium enhances growth. On blood agar the colonies are greyish in colour, about 1 mm. in diameter, and surrounded by a zone of haemolysis (Plate 16.1b, facing p. 188b). Similar colonies develop on inspissated serum, but after 48–72 hours' incubation a slight depression develops around the colonies as a result of liquefaction of the medium. Liquefaction also occurs on inspissated egg and gelatin.

Glucose and lactose are fermented. Mannitol is not fermented. In litmus milk the organism produces acid and clot after about 3 days' growth, and thereafter the clot is digested.

Resistance to physical and chemical agents

C. pyogenes is killed rapidly at a temperature of 60°C and is very susceptible to disinfectants.

Antigens and toxins

C. pyogenes is antigenically homogenous and produces a filterable haemolytic toxin when grown in cooked meat media or in milk. This toxin is lethal for mice and rabbits when inoculated in-travenously.

Epidemiology and pathogenesis

There is evidence to show that *C. pyogenes* occurs in normal healthy cattle, pigs, sheep and goats, and it is in these species that the organism is a frequent cause of a variety of suppurative lesions.

Mastitis

Bovine mastitis caused by *C. pyogenes* occurs most frequently in heifers and dry cows during the summer months and is often referred to as 'summer mastitis'. It has been suggested that flies may be responsible for the transmission of infection. The evidence, however, is more in support of the view that the organism is latent within the host and that as the result of unidentified predisposing factors, rapid multiplication takes place in the udder, giving rise to an acute mastitis.

Other suppurative conditions

C. pyogenes causes suppurative conditions in a variety of animal species but more particularly in cattle, pigs, sheep and goats. The circumstances and sites at which these conditions occur vary widely, and there is little doubt that they develop as a result of predisposing factors which stimulate endogenous *C. pyogenes* to multiply rapidly and produce toxin in localised areas giving rise to suppurative lesions. Pyometra and endometritis in cattle associated with *C. pyogenes*, is an infection which develops as the result of predisposing factors related to calving, retention of the placenta and to different stages in the oestral cycle. *C. pyogenes* has been isolated from the normal bovine uterus and it has also been demonstrated that during oestrus the uterus is resistant to infection with this organism, whereas in the luteal phase it is susceptible and pyometra may develop.

Abscess formation from *C. pyogenes* infection in various sites in the body can result from trauma, including surface wounds, from penetration of the bovine reticulum by a foreign body, and following a primary infection with other species of bacteria (e.g. *Sphaerophorus necrophorus*).

Nephritis in cattle occasionally develops as an infection with *C. pyogenes* consequent upon an obstruction in the urinary tract.

Pneumonia in calves caused primarily by a virus may become secondarily infected with *C. pyogenes*. The latter may also occur in the seminal vesicles of bulls and cause a lowered fertility.

Symptoms

These vary according to the localised site of infection and the extent of the suppurative lesion. Mastitis caused by *C. pyogenes* is often acute and the affected quarter or quarters become enlarged and firm. In some cases the suppuration taking place within the tissue may break to the surface. The animal will also be fevered and show signs of a general toxaemia. In these acute cases the mortality rate may be high and among survivors the affected quarters may permanently cease to function.

Lesions

These are characteristically suppurative. Abscesses can develop in almost any site in the body and contain thick greenish-yellow foul smelling pus.

Diagnosis

The microscopical examination of thin films of pus stained by Gram's method will usually reveal large numbers of *C. pyogenes*, some of which may be intracellular. Inoculation of a blood agar plate with pus and subsequent incubation at 37°C for at least 48 hours will result in the characteristic growth of *C. pyogenes*, and further identification of its properties can then be made.

Control and prevention

Although *C. pyogenes* is sensitive to penicillin and other antibiotics, the effectiveness of treatment with these substances is greatly reduced by the presence of pus which inhibits their direct contact with the bacteria. The use of alum precipitated toxoid has not proved to be of practical value in the prevention of these infections because the antitoxin does not appear to protect the host against infection.

Corynebacterium ovis

Distribution in nature

This organism which is also known as the Preisz-Nocard bacillus or *Corynebacterium pseudotuberculosis ovis*, is the cause of caseous lymphadenitis in sheep and goats, and ulcerative lymphangitis in horses. The organism has occasionally been associated with orchitis and epididymitis in rams and also with suppurative lesions in monkeys. The disease in sheep is particularly common in the important sheep rearing areas of Australia, New Zealand and South America. The disease in horses occurs sporadically in the African and American continents.

Morphology and staining

The organism frequently occurs as filamentous rods measuring 1–3 μm in length, arranged in groups or clusters. Sometimes these rods show a beaded appearance and in ageing cultures may break up into small cocci. Club-shaped forms also occur. Capsules are not formed and the organism is non-motile.

C. ovis stains Gram-positive and when stained by Albert's or Neisser's method, volutin granules can be demonstrated. These granules contain phosphorus compounds and because of their peculiar staining properties are also referred to as metachromatic granules.

Cultural characteristics

C. ovis grows on nutrient media aerobically and anaerobically at an optimum temperature of 37°C. After 24 hours' incubation the colonies on nutrient agar are small, greyish in colour and have a dry granular appearance. On serum agar the colonies are pale yellow and there is no liquefaction of the medium. Haemolysis on blood agar is variable but large zones develop in the presence of *C. equi*. Growth in fluid medium develops as a granular deposit with a surface pellicle.

Acid is usually produced in lactose, glucose, mannitol, maltose and dextrin, but not in salicin. Urea is hydrolysed, catalase is produced, nitrates are reduced and litmus milk is unchanged.

Resistance to physical and chemical agents

C. ovis has properties similar to those of *C. pyogenes*.

Antigens and toxins

C. ovis produces a filterable toxin which partially resembles that produced by *C. diphtheriae*. The toxin has some properties in common with the cell-bound haemolysin, and guinea-pigs are particularly susceptible to its lethal effect.

Epidemiology and pathogenesis

It is probable that animals become infected with *C. ovis* through superficial wounds and tick bites. Although it is known that infection can develop in sheep following ingestion of contaminated food and water, there is at present no clear evidence to show that this is naturally a common route of infection. Some clinically normal animals may carry *C. ovis*, excrete it in the faeces and contaminate the ground. The mode of action of *C. ovis* in causing disease is not clearly understood but it is probable that the pathogenicity of the organism is associated with the toxin, the haemolysin and with an additional somatic factor closely associated with the bacterial bodies. This latter substance probably has pyogenic properties.

Symptoms

Caseous lymphadenitis in sheep can be a mild infection unrecognised until a post-mortem examination has been carried out. In some cases, however, the condition can be recognised in the living animal as suppurating skin wounds and enlarged lymphatic glands.

Ulcerative lymphangitis occurs as a chronic infection in horses and rarely in cattle. Initially, animals show signs of pain and swelling of the hind limbs. Lymphatic vessels become enlarged, ulcers may develop in the region of these vessels and discharge purulent material. In severe cases the condition spreads to the abdomen, forelegs and neck, causing death of the animal. The ulcers heal slowly in surviving animals.

Lesions
Caseous lymphadenitis in sheep is characterised by lesions in the superficial nodes which contain a mass of greenish-yellow caseation deposited in concentric layers. Calcification is not usual. In advanced cases similar lesions occur in the lungs, kidneys, liver and spleen.

Diagnosis
The nature of the lesions, their distribution and the animal species affected may be suggestive of infection with *C. ovis*. Confirmation may be obtained by isolating the organism from lesions and identifying its morphological and cultural characteristics.

Control and prevention
The difficulties experienced in preventing this infection are similar to those related to the prevention of *C. pyogenes* infections. An antibody response against the toxin does not provide protection but only gives evidence of infection. Antibiotics are prevented from being effective by the situation of organisms in caseous material.

Corynebacterium equi

Distribution in nature
This organism has been identified in a number of countries including Europe, Australia, India, America and rarely in the United Kingdom. It has been isolated from a variety of conditions in animals, particularly pneumonia in foals and less frequently from cases of pyometra in cattle, purulent pneumonia in sheep and calves and from tuberculous-like lesions in pigs and other animal species.

Morphology and staining
C. equi is a pleomorphic organism and may occur as large rods, oval coccobacilli or club-shaped forms arranged in groups or clusters. The organism is non-motile.

C. equi stains Gram-positive and some strains have been reported to be weakly acid-fast. No granules are observed when stained by Neisser's method.

Cultural characteristics
C. equi will grow aerobically on nutrient media at an optimum temperature of 37°C. Colonies on nutrient agar have a glistening, mucoid appearance and are pale pink in colour (Plate 16.1c, facing p. 188b).

Pigmentation is accentuated on potato or milk agar. No haemolysis occurs on blood agar. A characteristic feature of the organism is that primary cultures may take many days to produce growth but subcultures develop more rapidly and become visible after 24–48 hours' incubation.

Carbohydrates are not fermented by *C. equi*; indole is not produced and there is no liquefaction of inspissated serum or gelatin. The organism possesses the enzyme catalase and is urease positive.

Resistance to physical and chemical agents
C. equi is relatively insusceptible to heat and is not killed unless subjected to a temperature of 60°C for about 1 hour. The organism is usually resistant to oxalic acid and will survive in a concentration of 2·5 per cent for 1 hour.

Antigens and toxins
The antigenic composition of *C. equi* has not been clearly defined but there are known to be species and type specific antigens. No toxin has been identified.

Epidemiology and pathogenesis
C. equi is a pyogenic organism and subcutaneous inoculation results in the development of an abscess. It is, however, difficult to set up infection in laboratory animals. Little is known about the epidemiology of these diseases under natural conditions. For example, although infection is most frequently associated with pneumonia in foals and the organism is known to be present in certain studs or farms, there is no clear evidence that *C. equi* is carried from one premises to another by horses. The organism has been isolated from samples of soil and as it is relatively resistant it may survive in suitable climates for many months outside the animal body as a potential source of infection.

C. equi is known to exist in the United Kingdom although it has not been recorded in foals but has been identified only rarely in the lymph glands of pigs at slaughter. Similar isolations have been made from lesions in pigs in South Africa and Finland. Because of the difficulty of establishing primary isolations the incidence of *C. equi* may be greater than current information would suggest. Little is known about the predisposing factors which affect the pathogenicity of the organism.

Symptoms
Pneumonia in foals occurs most frequently in animals aged 2–4 months. They develop a cough, become dull and listless, the body temperature is raised and the respiration rate becomes increased. In severe cases there may be a purulent discharge from the nose shortly before death.

Lesions

In foals the most outstanding lesions are of a purulent broncho-pneumonia with abscesses in the lungs, associated lymph nodes and pus in the bronchi. In other animal species infection results in purulent lesions in various organs including the lungs, uterus and lymph nodes.

Diagnosis

This depends upon isolation of the causal organism from a suspected lesion and the identification of its characteristic properties. Material can be mixed with oxalic acid to give a final concentration of 2·5 per cent and after 15 minutes some of the mixture can be sown on media which should, if necessary, be subjected to prolonged incubation because of the characteristic delayed growth rate of C. equi on primary culture.

Control and prevention

There are no specific and reliable forms of treatment. Prevention of disease in foals can be attempted by ensuring that mares are moved away from known infected premises before foaling.

Corynebacterium renale

Distribution in nature

This organism is associated with pyelonephritis and cystitis in cattle, and has also been isolated from bull semen and occasionally from other animal species. C. renale is known to occur in a number of countries including the United Kingdom, Europe, Australia and America.

Morphology and staining

C. renale is a rod-shaped organism which occurs in groups or bundles. In older cultures some organisms may appear as coccoid forms. The organism does not produce a capsule and is non-motile.

C. renale stains Gram-positive and metachromatic (volutin) granules can be seen when stained by Albert's or Neisser's method.

Cultural characteristics

C. renale grows readily on nutrient media at an optimum temperature of 37°C. Growth on blood agar occurs as small, moist, greyish white colonies without any haemolysis (Plate 16.1d, facing p. 188b). Gelatin and serum agar are not liquefied. After 48 hours' incubation on agar containing 10 per cent sterilized milk, each colony is surrounded by a clear zone formed from the hydrolysis of casein (Plate 16.1e, facing p. 188b). Litmus milk is turned alkaline after 2–3 days' incubation.

Glucose is the only carbohydrate to be fermented regularly by all strains of C. renale. Indole is not formed. H_2S is not produced and nitrates are not reduced. The organism is catalase and urease positive.

Resistance to physical and chemical agents

C. renale has properties similar to those of C. pyogenes.

Antigens and toxins

The antigenic structure of C. renale has not been clearly defined but the precipitation test indicates that these organisms are serologically related.

Epidemiology and pathogenesis

C. renale is a specific cause of cystitis and pyelonephritis in cattle, and has been obtained in pure culture from these conditions. The organism can often be isolated from the urine, vagina and male genital tracts of healthy cattle, and it is usually considered that in this animal species the infection is not haematogenous but ascending from the urethra and ureters to the urinary bladder and kidneys. It is a characteristic feature of the disease that the necrosis and destruction of the medulla of the kidney is related to C. renale having a predilection for this site. Experimentally, it has been shown that after inoculation into mice the organisms are rapidly eliminated from the lungs and spleen but multiply in the kidneys. It is also known that C. renale has a particularly high urease activity and this may be the reason for the organism having a predilection site in the kidney. Moreover, urease is nephrotoxic and associated with the production of pyelonephritis.

From the limited knowledge available on the incidence of the organism it is evident that cattle may be symptomless carriers, and that it is only as the result of favourable conditions arising from undefined predisposing factors that infection becomes established in the upper parts of the urinary tract. The incidence is highest in females during or immediately after pregnancy, and it is probable that the unknown predisposing factors are closely associated with parturition.

Symptoms

The characteristic symptom of pyelonephritis in cattle is the frequent passage of turbid or blood stained urine by animals which are pregnant or have recently calved. The urine contains albumen, erythrocytes and pus cells.

Lesions

The kidneys are enlarged and contain areas of necrosis and suppuration in the medulla. Sometimes there are also wedge-shaped suppurative foci in the cortex. The kidney pelvis may contain pus and blood-stained urine. The location of bacteria varies with the severity of the lesions. In most cases they are present in the kidney calyces and in severe infections are found throughout the kidney tissue. Microscopically, there is cellular infiltration with lymphocytes, phagocytes and fibroblasts at the perimeters of necrotic lesions.

The bladder, containing urine mixed with pus and blood, has thickened walls showing petechial haemorrhages and sometimes ulceration. Similarly, the ureters may be filled with pus and the walls thickened.

Diagnosis
In cattle the symptoms and lesions are strongly suggestive of infection with *C. renale*. Confirmation is obtained by isolating the causal organism from either urine or lesions in the kidneys.

Control and prevention
C. renale is sensitive to penicillin but diagnosis of the infection is usually too late for subsequent treatment to ensure a complete recovery because a great deal of kidney tissue may already have been damaged.

Corynebacterium suis

Distribution in nature
This organism has been associated with cases of pyelonephritis and cystitis in sows in England.

Morphology and staining
C. suis is a pleomorphic organism usually appearing as slender rods measuring 2–3 μm in length and 0·3–0·5 μm in width, occurring characteristically in groups and clusters. It is non-motile.

The organism stains Gram-positive in infected tissues but has a tendency to decolourise readily after subcultivation. No granules are observed after staining by Albert's or Neisser's method.

Cultural characteristics
C. suis is an anaerobe and growth is slow on nutrient media but enhanced when 0·5–1·0 per cent maltose is added to the medium. After incubation for 3–5 days at 37°C on blood agar the colonies are small, round and translucent. There is no haemolysis. When grown on 10 per cent milk agar there is no zone of clearing around the colonies (cf. *C. renale*).

Maltose is the only carbohydrate which is regularly fermented by all strains with the production of acid. No fermentation occurs in lactose, salicin, mannitol, laevulose or galactose. The organism is urease positive, catalase negative, does not produce indole and does not liquefy gelatin or coagulate serum. Litmus milk becomes slightly alkaline after 7 days' incubation. Nitrates are not reduced.

Antigens and toxins
The use of the precipitin test has failed to show any antigenic relationships between *C. suis* and *C. renale*. No toxin has been identified.

Epidemiology and pathogenesis
C. suis has been isolated from the mucosa of the penile sheath and semen of healthy boars. It is probable that the organism has a wider distribution in the pig population than has hitherto been recognised. Although *C. suis* is associated with pyelonephritis in sows, the pathogenesis of the disease is closely related to predisposing factors which include pregnancy and parturition. Experimentally, it is difficult to produce infection in healthy animals unless the organisms are inoculated intrarenally with 5 per cent saponin to cause initial damage to the kidney. So far, these are the only experimental conditions under which the organism will establish itself in one kidney and give rise to a pyelonephritis which subsequently affects both kidneys.

Laboratory animals appear to be resistant to experimental infection with *C. suis*.

Symptoms
These occur most frequently in pregnant sows at about 4 weeks after service when a vaginal discharge develops and the urine becomes turbid and blood stained.

Lesions
The lesions are similar to those produced by *C. renale* infection in cattle.

Diagnosis
The lesions are suggestive of this infection and *C. suis* can be observed in stained smears prepared from lesions and sometimes from the urine. Confirmation is obtained by isolating and growing the organism anaerobically and observing its characteristic properties.

Control and prevention
Although *C. suis* is sensitive to penicillin, a diagnosis of the condition is usually made when the disease is so far advanced that treatment is of little value.

Corynebacterium bovis

Distribution in nature
This organism is known to occur in bovine milk from normal udders and also to be present in some cases of bovine mastitis. It has also been isolated occasionally from the reproductive tracts of healthy cows and from samples of bull semen.

Morphology and staining

A small rod-shaped organism having a morphology characteristic for corynebacteria and staining Gram-positive.

Cultural characteristics

After 48 hours' incubation on sheep blood agar the colonies appear small and smooth. Later they become crenated, and there is no haemolysis. Growth is very poor on nutrient agar but enhanced in the presence of 10 per cent serum, and particularly when yeast or liver extract is incorporated in the medium. On milk agar a clear zone is not formed around the colonies.

Acid is produced in glucose and mannitol after incubation for 5 days. There is no fermentation of lactose or salacin. Most strains are urease positive and all strains produce catalase.

Epidemiology and pathogenesis

For many years corynebacteria have been isolated in association with other pathogens from samples of bovine milk and it is only latterly that *C. bovis* has been identified in milk from clinical cases of bovine mastitis. However, the organism often occurs as a saprophyte and is not highly pathogenic. As stated above, it has been isolated frequently from normal bovine milk samples, occasionally from the reproductive tracts of healthy cows and from bulls' semen.

Public health aspects

C. diphtheriae is the cause of human diphtheria and does not produce disease in animals.

C. pyogenes has occasionally been reported as a pathogen for man but the other species discussed in this chapter are animal pathogens.

Further reading

BIBERSTEIN, E.L. AND KIRKHAM, C. (1972) The rate of urea hydrolysis as a diagnostic criterion for *Corynebacterium renale*. *Research in Veterinary Science*, **13**, 380.

CAMERON, C.M. AND ENGELBRECHT, M.M. (1971) Mechanism of immunity to *Corynebacterium pseudotuberculosis* (Buchanan 1911) in mice using inactivated vaccine. *Onderstepoort Journal of Veterinary Research*, **38**, 73.

CAMERON, C.M. AND PURDOM, M.R. (1971) Immunological and chemical characteristics of *Corynebacterium pseudotuberculosis* cell walls and protoplasm. *Onderstepoort Journal of Veterinary Research*, **38**, 83.

COBB R.W. (1963) Cultural characteristics of some corynebacteria of animal origin, with special reference to *C. bovis* and *C. pyogenes Journal of Laboratory Medicine Technology*, **20**, 199.

CRUTCHLEY M.J., SEAMAN A. AND WOODBINE M. (1961) Microbiological aspects of *Corynebacterium renale*. *Veterinary Reviews and Annotations*, **7**, 1.

DAWSON F.L.M. (1960) Bovine endometritis. A review. *British Veterinary Journal*, **116**, 448.

DUCKITT S.M., SEAMAN A. AND WOODBINE M. (1963) The bacteriology of *Corynebacterium bovis*. *Veterinary Bulletin*, **33**, 67.

GOEL, M.C. AND SINGH, I.P. (1972) Purification and characterisation of *Corynebacterium ovis* exotoxin. *Journal of Comparative Pathology*, **82**, 345.

HIRAMUNE, T., INUI, S. MIRASE, N. AND YANAGAWA, R. (1972) Antibody response in cows infected with *Corynebacterium renale* with special reference to the differentiation of pyelonephritis and cystitis. *Research in Veterinary Science*, **13**, 82.

PURDOM M.R., SEAMAN A. AND WOODBINE M. (1958) The bacteriology and antibiotic sensitivety of *Corynebocterium pyogenes*. *Veterinary Reviews and Annotations*, **4**, 55.

SORENSEN, G.H. (1974) Studies on the aetiology and transmission of summer mastitis. *Nordisk Veterinaermedicin*, **26**, 122.

CHAPTER 17

ERYSIPELOTHRIX

CHAPTER 17

Erysipelothrix

This group includes a number of closely related bacterial species which cause disease in animals and man. These organisms are collectively known as *Erysipelothrix insidiosa*.

Erysipelothrix insidiosa

Synonyms
Erysipelothrix rhusiopathiae; Erysipelothrix muriseptica; Erysipelothrix erysipeloides.

Distribution in nature
Erysipelothrix insidiosa, the causal organism of swine erysipelas, has a world-wide distribution and the disease is of particular economic importance in Europe, the United Kingdom and the United States of America. The organism also causes disease in sheep, poultry, mice, and other animal species and in man. The distinction between species of *Erysipelothrix* according to their hosts of origin (e.g. *E. muriseptica* derived from mice and *E. erysipeloides* the cause of erysipeloid in man) is not generally considered to be justifiable on the grounds that the differences between species are insignificant and man can become infected from animal sources.

Morphology and staining
In the tissues of animals acutely infected with *E. insidiosa* the organisms are seen as slender rods, sometimes slightly curved, measuring 1–2·5 μm in length and 0·2–0·4 μm in width, occurring singly, in groups or in chains. In chronic lesions the organisms develop as a mass of long filaments and after growth on laboratory media a mixture of filamentous and bacillary forms may develop (Plate 17.1a, facing p. 189). They are non-motile and do not form spores.

E. insidiosa stains Gram-positive.

Cultural characteristics
E. insidiosa is microaerophilic but will grow aerobically as well as in an atmosphere of reduced oxygen tension. The optimum temperature for growth has been variously reported as 35–37°C, although the organism will develop within a temperature range of 15–44°C.

Growth is slightly enhanced by the addition of serum or blood to the medium and a narrow zone of partial haemolysis is produced on blood agar. Optimum growth requires the presence of certain unidentified growth factors. Good growth can be obtained by incorporating meat or liver extract in a special medium which includes casein or gelatin hydrolysate, riboflavin, oleic acid and saponin. In gelatin stab cultures growth occurs along the line of inoculation with lateral growths developing at intervals, giving rise to the so-called 'bottle-brush' type of growth.

Growth can develop in either the smooth or rough phase. On solid media smooth colonies are small, glistening, translucent and about 0·5–1·0 mm in diameter. Rough colonies have serrated edges, a granular appearance and are about 1–2 mm in diameter after 48 hours' incubation, increasing in size to 3–4 mm after several days' incubation. In broth cultures the smooth form, composed of short rods, produces a uniform turbidity, whereas the rough form of filamentous organisms grows as a granular sediment.

The considerable variations which have been reported in the fermentation reactions of *E. insidiosa* are probably due to the difficulty in establishing adequate growth in some batches of peptone water in which the carbohydrates are incorporated, and to the probable variation in growth factors. Most strains ferment lactose, glucose, fructose and galactose with production of acid. The reactions in other carbohydrates are variable.

Resistance to physical and chemical agents
E. insidiosa are relatively resistant organisms capable of surviving for nearly a year in putrefying meat and for several months in smoked ham. They are comparatively resistant to alcohol, hydrogen

peroxide, formaldehyde, brine, phenol and cresol, but are susceptible to caustic soda and hypochlorites. They are killed in moist heat at a temperature of 55°C for 10 minutes.

Antigens and toxins

The antigenic structure of *E. insidiosa* is complex and composed of both heat-stable and heat-labile antigens. Detailed antigenic studies have shown that the various serotypes can be classified into groups labelled A, B, C, D, E, F, G and N. Although there are group specific antigens which form the basis for this classification, there are also other antigens common to the various groups. In addition, it has been observed that there is no clear antigenic distinction between serotypes isolated from different host species. For example, the heat-stable antigens of strains derived from man are similar to the heat-stable antigens of organisms isolated from animals.

Epidemiology and pathogenesis

Infection in pigs

Swine erysipelas is a widespread disease and causes serious economic loss. Although it occurs in pigs of all ages, those of 3 months to 1 year are most susceptible, and the acute form of the disease in unweaned pigs has become increasingly common.

The incidence of infection is variable and may be particularly high in some areas. There are a variety of clinical manifestations of the disease which are recognised as either acute and fatal infections or as more chronic forms of the condition. In all cases, however, the environment is likely to become infected from organisms present in the faeces, urine or vomit of clinically diseased animals, and in the faeces and urine of symptomless carriers. Thus, spread of infection among in-contact animals occurs either from ingestion or more rarely from contamination of skin wounds.

E. insidiosa can persist in the soil and may even multiply under suitable climatic conditions which might prevail during the summer months in temperate climates. For this reason some epidemiologists claim that soil infection may be an important feature in the spread of this disease. However, although the organism is known to survive in soil for periods of weeks or months under various conditions, there is little positive evidence that it leads a saprophytic existence in this situation. Concerning wound infections, it has been shown that biting flies (e.g. *Stomoxys calcitrans*), having previously fed on material contaminated with *E. insidiosa*, are capable of transmitting infection to pigs, and that this mode of transfer may account, in part, for the seasonal incidence of the disease.

Possible sources of infection in addition to soil are diverse. *E. insidiosa* is known to persist for months in putrefying materials, and it has been isolated from the intestines and tonsils of clinically normal pigs and from bone marrow of apparently healthy pigs at slaughter. Strains belonging to groups A, B and N have all been isolated from the tonsils of wild pigs but the majority of strains originating from domesticated pigs belong to groups A and B. The carrier rate in these latter animals may be as high as 50 per cent in some districts. A further indication of the widespread distribution of *E. insidiosa* in the pig population is that samples of gamma globulin derived from many healthy pigs can give passive protection to mice against the infection. This is a particularly interesting observation since mice, like pigeons, are highly susceptible to experimental infection with *E. insidiosa*.

All the evidence on the epidemiology of *E. insidiosa* infections, when considered collectively, suggests that the organisms are ubiquitous, that they can exist as saprophytes in a variety of conditions particularly in carrier pigs, and that only under certain undefined circumstances do they cause clinical disease. The importance of predisposing factors is emphasised by the fact that it is often difficult to reproduce swine erysipelas experimentally by either feeding or inoculating the causal organism into apparently normal animals.

Infection in other animal species

Sheep are particularly susceptible under natural conditions to infection with *E. insidiosa* which is manifest by a polyarthritis in young animals up to the age of about 3 months. Lambs can become infected via wounds when being docked or castrated, and older sheep may derive infection from sheep dip contaminated with *E. insidiosa*. Various species of poultry are also susceptible to an acute septicaemic form of the disease which affects chickens, turkeys, ducks, pigeons and wild birds kept in captivity. *E. insidiosa* has been associated occasionally with arthritis in other animal species, with generalised infections in rats, mice and voles, and has been isolated from the skin of fish. It is noteworthy, also, that the organism has been identified in samples of fishmeal and presumably may survive the processing of this material which may become a potential source of infection for poultry when incorporated in foodstuffs.

Symptoms

Pigs

Swine erysipelas manifests itself in three forms known as the acute, urticarial and chronic forms of the disease. The latter includes both the cardiac and arthritic types.

The acute form develops suddenly with a rise in body temperature, conjunctivitis and prostration. The animal may vomit and there will be initial constipation followed by diarrhoea. Areas of bright pink discolouration of the skin may develop at the base of the ears, over the surface of the abdomen and on the inside of the thighs. The knee and hock joints may become hot and painful. Death may occur 3–4 days after the onset of symptoms and the mortality rate may be as high as 50 per cent in a group of pigs suffering from an acute outbreak of disease.

The urticarial form is milder than the acute form and the symptoms are similar but less severe. In addition, red diamond-shaped areas develop on the skin. These areas vary in size, number and situation, but in severe cases they may coalesce; necrosis may develop with subsequent sloughing of the skin and slow healing of the wound. In the majority of cases this form of the disease is not fatal.

The chronic form develops in those animals which have survived the acute or urticarial forms, and is associated with endocarditis or arthritis. Pigs suffering from endocarditis are disinclined to move, they develop a cough and show marked signs of dyspnoea. Death is due to heart failure. Symptoms of severe lameness are characteristic for the arthritic form which may affect the joints of both the fore and hind limbs.

Other animal species
Infection of sheep usually takes the form of lameness or stiffness of the limbs in lambs during the first 3 months of life. Affected joints are swollen and painful.

In poultry, including pigeons, the disease is generally sporadic, acute and fatal. No symptoms develop other than lowered egg production in broiler chickens. Mice are also susceptible to acute and fatal infection.

Occasionally cattle, horses, dogs and other animal species suffer from an arthritic form of infection.

Lesions

Pigs
In the acute form of swine erysipelas there is a septicaemia and a monocytosis. On post-mortem examination the most striking lesions include petechial haemorrhages in the pericardium, endocardium, kidneys and sometimes in the subcutaneous tissues. The lungs are congested and oedematous, the spleen is also congested and the liver enlarged. In some cases there is a gastroenteritis and lymphatic glands will be enlarged.

In the chronic form of the disease one of the characteristic lesions is an endocarditis which develops as vegetations on the mitral valves (Plate

17.1b, facing p. 189). Consequent upon the development of heart lesions there may be hyperaemia and oedema of the lungs with a hydrothorax. Another characteristic feature of the chronic form is an arthritis which develops as a result of organisms colonising in the synovial membrane and then spreading into the synovial fluid. Proliferative changes take place in the infected area with infiltration of plasma cells and lymphocytes. At a later stage the organisms disappear and either the lesion resolves or the proliferative changes persist and fibrosis develops.

Other animal species
The lesions depend upon the type of infection in the particular animal species but in general the acute and chronic arthritic forms are similar to those seen in pigs.

Diagnosis
The diagnosis of swine erysipelas may be suspected from the history of disease on a farm, and from the symptoms and lesions of affected animals. Confirmation depends upon the identification of the causal organism. In acute cases, *E. insidiosa* can be observed in stained smears prepared from blood or visceral organs. The organism can also be isolated from heart blood, endocardium, liver and, less frequently, from the kidney, lymph nodes and muscle. Confirmation of the chronic form of the disease is based largely on characteristic lesions including endocarditis and arthritis. In cases of endocarditis, smears from the lesions on heart valves will usually reveal *E. insidiosa* in the filamentous form. Examination of smears and the isolation of the organism from cases of chronic arthritis may be negative. The bacterial agglutination test has been used for detecting chronically infected animals in a herd.

Control and prevention
Vaccination is widely practised for the prevention of swine erysipelas. The development of various methods for immunizing pigs against the disease have been hampered by the difficulty in reproducing swine erysipelas experimentally in order to assess the value of different procedures, and also in obtaining preparations of *E. insidiosa* which are both highly immunogenic and safe to use.

Serum – culture method
This procedure which consists of inoculating immune serum with virulent culture has been widely used and gives good protection. The disadvantages are that there is a risk to the operator in handling live virulent culture, that the inoculated animals may become symptomless carriers and contaminate the

premises, and that it is an expensive procedure relative to other methods of immunization.

Killed vaccines.
One of the most successful of these inactivated vaccines is prepared by adsorbing the soluble protective substance produced by relatively few strains of *E. insidiosa* on to aluminium hydroxide and mixing with formolised bacteria. This may be incorporated with an emulsifying agent and mineral oil. Protection lasts for approximately 4 months after one dose of vaccine and for at least 6 months after two doses.

Attenuated vaccines
A variety of living avirulent vaccines has been prepared and tested in a number of countries with encouraging results which include good protection and relative cheapness.

At the present time the most reliable methods for immunological control of swine erysipelas are the use of killed or attenuated vaccines. Breeding stock should be inoculated twice yearly and fattening pigs for slaughter should receive one dose soon after weaning at about 8–9 weeks of age. It is important that any vaccination programme be accompanied by high standards of hygiene, including the isolation for 14 days of all pigs brought on to disease-free premises and ensuring that these animals have been vaccinated before purchase.

Acute cases of swine erysipelas can be treated by administering hyperimmune serum together with penicillin. There is the risk, however, that animals which survive as the result of treatment may become chronically infected, excrete the organisms and contaminate the environment.

Public health aspects
A condition known as 'Erysipeloid' in man arises from cutaneous infections with *E. insidiosa*. The lesion is an acute and painful inflammatory response with localised swelling of the area and a greyish discolouration of the skin. Erysipeloid is an occupational disease which develops as the result of handling infected materials. It is a particular hazard to veterinary surgeons, laboratory workers, slaughter-men and those who handle infected animals and carcases, including fish and fish products.

Further reading
AJMAL M. (1970) Chronic proliferative arthritis in swine in relation to human rheumatoid arthritis. *Veterinary Bulletin*, **40**, 1.
DOYLE T.M. (1960) Can swine erysipelas be eradicated? Epidemiological and immunological aspects. *Veterinary Reviews and Annotations*, **6**, 95.
SNEATH P.H.A., ABBOTT J.D. AND CUNLIFFE A.C. (1951). The bacteriology of Erysipeloid. *British Medical Journal*, **2**, 1063.
WOOD, R.L. (1973) Survival of *Erysipelothrix rhusiopathiae* in soil under various environmental conditions. *Cornell Veterinarian*, **63**, 390.

CHAPTER 18

LISTERIA

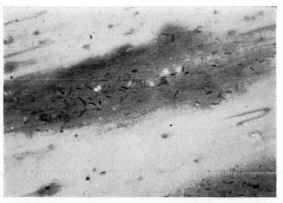

16.1a

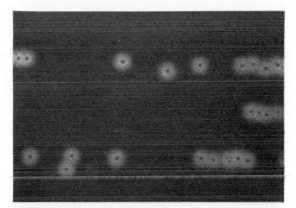

16.1b

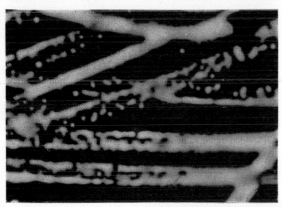

16.1c

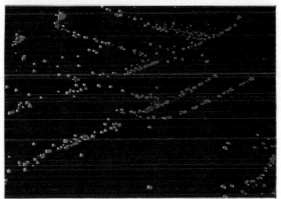

16.1d

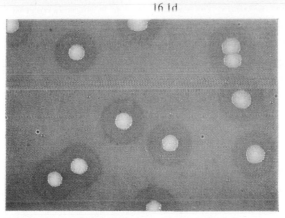

16.1e

16.1a Gram-stained film from abscess in a pig showing *Corynebacterium pyogenes*, × 930.

16.1b Colonies of *Corynebacterium pyogenes* on blood agar showing haemolysis.

16.1c *Corynebacterium equi* on blood agar, showing the typical pale pink, mucoid type of growth.

16.1d Growth of *Corynebacterium renale* on blood agar appearing as small colonies with no haemolysis.

16.1e Colonies of *Corynebacterium renale* after 48 hours' incubation on milk agar showing clear zones due to the hydrolysis of casein.

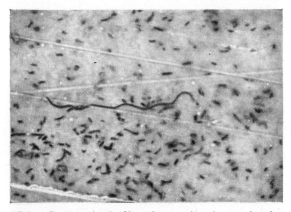

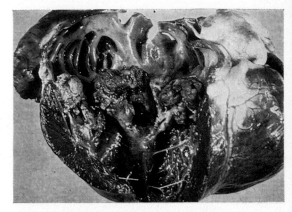

17.1a Gram-stained film from pig tissue showing *Erysipelothrix insidiosa* occurring as rods and filaments, ×930.

17.1b Pig heart valves showing vegetations due to chronic infection with *Erysipelothrix insidiosa*.

Listeria

Listeria monocytogenes

Synonyms
Bacterium monocytogenes; Listerella monocytogenes.

Distribution in nature
Listeria monocytogenes is the only species in this group of bacteria. The organisms are world-wide in their distribution and have a very extensive range of host species which includes mammals, poultry, fish, crustaceans and ticks as well as man. The name of the organism emphasises the relationship between infection and the development of a monocytosis in the host. This characteristic reaction was observed originally in rabbits more than 40 years ago, but it is now known to be an inconstant feature of listeriasis in all animal species. The manifestation of disease in animals may include a localised encephalitis or meningoencephalitis, a generalised septicaemic form of infection with hepatic necrosis, abortion in mammals and myocardial degeneration in fowls. Man is also susceptible to similar forms of *L. monocytogenes* infections.

Morphology and staining (Plate 18.1, facing p. 202)
The smooth form of *L. monocytogenes* is usually rod-shaped, sometimes slightly curved, measuring 1·0–2·0 μm in length and about 0·5 μm in width. The rough form occurs as longer rods measuring 5·0–7·0 μm in length or in chains. In smears from young cultures the organisms are often arranged in palisade formation and closely resemble *Corynebacterium*. Occasionally, coccoid forms are seen which must be distinguished from *Streptococcus*. The organisms are actively motile, showing a characteristic tumbling movement when grown in glucose broth at temperatures ranging from 6–25°C for a period of 6–18 hours, and are sluggishly motile at 37°C unless grown in an atmosphere of 20 per cent CO_2 at this warmer temperature. They do not produce spores and are not acid-alcohol-fast.

The organisms stain Gram-positive but old cultures have a tendency to stain Gram-negative.

Cultural characteristics
L. monocytogenes will grow moderately well on ordinary media under aerobic conditions and the growth of some strains may be increased in an atmosphere of CO_2. The growth of all strains is enhanced in the presence of serum, blood, glucose or liver extract. After overnight incubation at 37°C on solid media the colonies of the smooth form are about 1 mm in diameter, round, translucent with a smooth edge and bluish-grey in colour. After further incubation they increase in size to a diameter of about 3 mm. Rough colonies are larger, measuring 3–6 mm in diameter with uneven edges and roughened surfaces. On horse, cow, sheep, rabbit or human blood agar the majority of newly isolated strains develop a narrow zone of complete haemolysis. *L. monocytogenes* characteristically produces a diffusible substance which causes a haemolytic effect with *Corynebacterium equi*, and in this way can be readily distinguished from *Erysipelothrix insidiosa* which has no such effect (Plate 18.2, facing p. 202).

In fluid medium a slimy, tenacious precipitate forms after incubation for several days and growth is enhanced in the presence of glucose. The organism does not liquefy gelatin or serum. Nitrates are not reduced, indole is not formed and urea is not hydrolysed.

Most strains produce acid in glucose, laevulose, maltose, rhamnose, trehalose and salicin after 24 hours' incubation, and delayed acid production occurs after 7–10 days' incubation in lactose, sucrose and sorbitol. Mannitol is not usually fermented but a variant strain has been isolated from the faeces of chinchillas which ferments mannitol but not rhamnose.

Resistance to physical and chemical agents
L. monocytogenes is killed by moist heat at a temperature of 55°C for 40 minutes and is readily susceptible to the lethal effects of disinfectants. On old and dried laboratory media the organisms remain viable for periods of several months, and

under natural conditions they survive in fodder for approximately 1 month during the summer and for at least 3–4 months during the winter.

Antigens and toxins
L. monocytogenes possesses both O (somatic) and H (flagellar) antigens, represented by Roman numerals and letters of the alphabet, respectively. Studies of

deer, pigs, horses, dogs and cats; a variety of laboratory animals may be affected, particularly rabbits and occasionally guinea-pigs, rats, mice and ferrets. Other susceptible species are fur-bearing animals, especially chinchillas, zoo animals and poultry, including chickens, turkeys, ducks, geese, pigeons and pheasants. There are also reports of the organisms having been identified in fish. Improved

TABLE 18.1. The antigenic structure of *L. monocytogenes* serotypes.

Serotypes	O antigens	H antigens
1a	I, II, (III)	A, B.
1b	I, II, (III)	A, B, C.
1c	I, II, (III)	B, D.
3a	II, (III), IV	A, B.
3b	II, (III), IV	A, B, C.
3c	II, (III), IV	B, D.
4a	(III), (V), VII, IX	A, B, C.
4b	(III), V, VI	A, B, C.
4ab	(III), V, VI, VII, IX	A, B, C.
4c	(III), V, VII	A, B, C.
4d	(III), (V), VI, VIII	A, B, C.
4e	(III), V, VI, VIII, IX	A, B, C.
5	(III), (V), VI, VIII, X	A, B, C.
6	(III), VII, VIII, XI	A, B, C.
7	(III), XII	A, B, C.

( ) = antigen occurs irregularly.

these antigens in strains isolated from a variety of host species in different countries has enabled the organisms to be classified into serotypes (Table 18.1). These investigations have shown that contrary to earlier beliefs there is no relationship between particular serotypes derived from different host species.

Eight phage types of *L. monocytogenes* have been identified and these are closely related to the different serotypes. It is noteworthy that phages specific for *L. monocytogenes* cultures do not react with strains of *Erysipelothrix insidiosa*.

No toxin has been demonstrated although a number of attempts have been made to associate one as a cause of monocytosis. From recent studies it appears that the substance responsible for this characteristic cellular reaction in rabbits is a non-toxic, non-antigenic lipid material associated with the cell wall.

Epidemiology and pathogenesis
In recent years the study of *L. monocytogenes* infections has shown the world-wide distribution of the organisms in a variety of hosts, including man. Some of the more important animal host species are cattle, sheep, and less frequently, goats, buffaloes,

methods for isolating these bacteria and more intensive studies of their natural habitats have shown that they are widely distributed in nature, exist in symptomless carrier animals, and may be excreted in the faeces. *L. monocytogenes* has also been isolated from the milk of some cattle for as long as a year or more, and the organisms are sufficiently resistant to remain viable in animal faeces, human sewage, soil, silage and dust for periods of several weeks or months.

In the light of these more recent observations on natural habitats for *L. monocytogenes*, it is evident that precise knowledge on the epidemiology of listeriasis is still confused, since the organisms are known to be ubiquitous in both man and animals throughout the world, and there is evidence to show that they do not produce clinical infection in the absence of predisposing factors. Under experimental conditions these factors in mice may include an increased concentration of iron in the tissues which enhances the growth of the organism, and a haemolytic anaemia which increases the hosts' susceptibility to infection.

Under natural conditions clinical infection among farm animals is closely related to certain predisposing factors. The incidence of the disease is higher in winter months than it is during the spring and summer. This may be associated with the absence of green food, since the addition of grass to the diet of an affected group of animals may restrict the development of further cases. There have also been many reports that infection of cattle and sheep may result from the sudden change of diet to silage and that listeriasis may be avoided when the incorporation of silage into the diet is gradual. *L. monocytogenes* may be present in soil and herbage of certain districts, and has been isolated from poor quality silage, and very frequently from grass silage prepared on known infected premises. Although animals may become infected in this way, it is a characteristic feature of the disease that only a few individuals in a group of adults show signs of infection and that epidemics are not common but may occur particularly among young lambs. It is also probable that blood-sucking arthropods may spread infection among cattle since *L. monocytogenes* has been isolated from cattle ticks. The organism is also known to be able to multiply in Tabanid flies (horse flies) and is excreted in the faeces.

Preliminary studies on the serotypes of *L. monocytogenes* affecting animals have shown that cattle and sheep are commonly infected with serotypes belonging to group 1 and with 4b, and that on infected premises the same serotypes may be present in silage. Infections of chinchillas are also commonly associated with these serotypes. Further examination of the serotypes present in different animal species and their environments will give additional information on the epidemiology of listeriasis in both animals and man because many human infections are, also, associated with serotypes belonging to group 1 and with type 4b. In some countries sheep are considered to be a reservoir of infection and also a hazard to human health.

The organisms have a predilection for certain tissues, particularly the brain, gravid uterus, liver and spleen. In ruminants the disease usually develops as an encephalitis in adults or as a septicaemia in young animals. Infection of the fetus leads to death and abortion. In other species of mammals the disease may also occur either as an encephalitis or as a septicaemia, and younger animals are more susceptible than adults.

Among poultry, young birds are more susceptible than adults. and serious epidemics may occur in the former with a high mortality rate. The mode of spread of infection is not known but it is presumed that the organism is ingested from food and soil contaminated with faeces from infected poultry or other animal species. Studies of outbreaks suggest that *L. monocytogenes* infections may develop as a result of a variety of predisposing factors which lower the general resistance of birds. These may include parasitic infestations, Newcastle disease, salmonellosis, lymphomatosis and possibly other conditions. The probable importance of predisposing factors in the development of avian listeriasis is emphasised by the difficulty of producing the disease experimentally by infecting normal chickens with the organism.

Symptoms

In mammals the disease usually occurs towards the end of the winter and during early spring. The first signs of encephalitis are usually stiffness of the neck, the head is held on one side, movement of the limbs becomes incoordinated and the animal has a tendency to move in circles in the same direction or to lean against a fence or wall. In some cases there is conjunctivitis in one or both eyes and an apparent blindness. In addition, there may be paralysis of the muscles of the jaw and pharynx, partial paralysis of one ear, protrusion of the tongue, marked salivation, and an inability to swallow. Incoordination of the limbs becomes progressively more severe until the animal can no longer stand. When lying on the ground there may be spasmodic paddling movements of the hind limbs and respirations are deep and rapid. Some cattle which are not severely affected may survive but continue to show permanent signs of torticollis or other damage to nervous tissues. Abortions associated with *L. monocytogenes* infections have been reported in both cattle and sheep, and usually occur after 4–8 months' pregnancy in cattle and at a comparatively later stage in sheep. A few cases of bovine mastitis have been reported. In pigs and horses, clinical signs of infection are not common but may develop as an encephalitis, a general septicaemia or rarely in pigs as pox-like lesions on the skin. The symptoms of the encephalitic form are similar to those in cattle and sheep. The disease is usually fatal in sheep, pigs and horses.

In poultry the disease usually causes sudden death particularly among younger birds. Occasionally there are signs of torticollis, weakness and incoordination of the legs. In rodents the disease occurs as the septicaemic form, and mice, rabbits and chinchillas are particularly susceptible.

Lesions

There are seldom any macroscopic lesions in mammals which have died from the encephalitic form of the disease. Occasionally, the meninges may be congested and slightly oedematous. Microscopically, the most obvious lesion is perivascular cuffing with mononuclear cells in the cerebellum, medulla and anterior spinal cord. In addition, there may be pin-point haemorrhages, aggregations of neutrophils in small purulent areas and more general areas of hyperaemia and oedema. Lesions associated with the septicaemic form as reported in young lambs, for example, usually consist of focal areas of necrosis in the liver and spleen with infiltrations of mononuclear cells and neutrophils, petechial haemorrhages on serous surfaces and excess fluid in body cavities. Occasionally, the mesenteric lymph nodes are congested and there may be areas of necrosis in the myocardium. It is a characteristic feature of abortion in cattle and sheep associated with listeriasis that both the fetus and placenta become decomposed before abortion occurs.

In poultry there may be areas of necrosis in the myocardium which are often extensive and associated with hyperaemia of the heart muscle, pericarditis, excess fluid in the pericardium and abdominal cavity, and oedema of the skeletal muscles. Focal areas of necrosis may also be seen in the liver, spleen and lungs of some birds and inflammation of the air sacs. A few birds may show lesions of enteritis and ulceration of the ileum and caeca.

Infection in mice gives rise to a marked proliferation of lymphoid cells, the fixed macrophages in the liver undergo intense mitosis and it has been suggested that this latter reaction may be an important stage in the development of an immunological response.

Diagnosis

Histopathology
The encephalitic form of the disease may be diagnosed from the examination of sections of the cerebellum, medulla and anterior spinal cord. These will show characteristic perivascular cuffing with mononuclear cells together with areas of oedema and hyperaemia containing small haemorrhages.

Bacteriology
In farm animals the symptoms may be suggestive but a final diagnosis must depend upon the isolation of *L. monocytogenes* from infected tissues. Samples of brain tissue should be ground in a mortar with a small quantity of nutrient broth and sown on to tryptose agar or on blood agar prepared from horse or sheep cells containing meat extract and nalidixic acid. Polymyxin is sometimes added to inhibit the growth of contaminants. The remainder of the inoculum should be stored at 4°C. After the plates have been incubated at 37°C for 24 hours they should be viewed by oblique light using a hand lens to identify the characteristic growth of minute blue-green colonies. The colour of these colonies can be more readily observed on tryptose agar than on blood agar plates. If no growth has occurred on primary culture, additional cultures should be made

from the material stored at 4°C. Positive cultures may not be obtained from some material until it has been stored for several weeks at 4°C, and this is especially apparent with infected faecal and silage samples. The reason for this effect of cold storage is not established but it has been variously ascribed to the known ability of many strains of the organism to multiply more rapidly than contaminants at 4°C, or to the possible inactivation of unidentified inhibitory substances, possibly derived from other bacterial species, or to the presence of lactic acid and a low pH.

In cases of the septicaemic form of the disease the organism can be isolated from the liver, spleen, kidney, or lung. When tissues are contaminated with post-mortem invaders, isolation of *L. monocytogenes* may be facilitated by storing tissues in 50 per cent glycerol before making cultures, or by preparing primary cultures on media containing 0·05 per cent potassium tellurite. In addition, primary cultures may grow more readily in an atmosphere of 10 per cent CO_2. Recent trials have indicated that the isolation of *L. monocytogenes* from contaminated material may be more effective when the media for primary cultures consists of either nutrient broth or nutrient agar containing glucose (0·2 per cent w/v), thallous acetate (0·2 per cent w/v) and nalidixic acid (40 mg/ml or 60 mg/ml, respectively), adjusted to pH 7·0, and incubated at 30°C.

Fluorescent antibody techniques are being developed for the detection of *L. monocytogenes* in a variety of situations. They have the advantage of being rapid compared with cultural methods and further improvement of the techniques may result in the method becoming acceptable for routine diagnosis.

The developing chicken embryo is highly susceptible to infection which causes the development of focal necrotic lesions on the chorioallantoic membrane. Mice have also been used for isolating and identifying *L. monocytogenes*. Suspected material is inoculated intraperitoneally and the animals are observed for at least 7 days afterwards. Infection gives rise to focal necrosis of the liver and spleen and the organism can be isolated from the organs and from heart blood.

Serology
Antibody production is very variable except in rabbits and, therefore, the routine use of serological tests (bacterial agglutination and complement-fixation) in larger animals is unreliable. Preliminary trials using an indirect haemagglutination test suggest that this method is particularly sensitive for the detection of *L. monocytogenes* antibodies in infected animals.

Control and prevention

When outbreaks of disease occur, all affected animals should be slaughtered and either buried or burned. Litter and bedding should be burned and buildings thoroughly disinfected. Since antibody production by infected farm animals is so variable, serological tests are of little value for the detection of infected individuals.

Many attempts have been made to immunize animals using a variety of killed and living vaccines. In general, the results have been disappointing and have had little effect on the pathogenesis of infection under natural conditions. Tetracyclines are the most reliable antibiotics to employ for the treatment of listeriasis.

Public health aspects

Recent evidence suggests that *L. monocytogenes* may be present in apparently healthy individuals. It can also cause serious human infections, including meningoencephalitis and uterine infections associated with repeated miscarriages. In young infants the infection may be septicaemic.

Since it is now known that the different serological types of the organism can occur in both animals and man, it is probable that contact with infected rodents, farm animals and poultry constitute an important potential source of human disease. However, it seems that the ingestion of meat is not an important route of human infection, but probably under certain conditions raw milk may be a source of human listeriasis. It should also be emphasised that although milk which may be contaminated with *L. monocytogenes* is usually rendered safe for human consumption by pasteurisation, some organisms in heavily contaminated samples will survive this heat treatment. Pasteurisation cannot, therefore, be regarded as a procedure which will unfailingly render milk from being a potential source of human infection. There is also evidence to suggest that dogs may act as potential reservoirs of infection in cases of listeriasis in man, and especially when infected pets have close contact with members of households.

Further reading

BEAUREGARD M. AND MALKIN, K.L. (1971) Isolation of *Listeria monocytogenes* from brain specimens of domestic animals in Ontario. *Canadian Veterinary Journal*, **12**, 221.

BUSCH, R.H., BARNES, D.M. AND SAUTTER, J.H. (1971) Pathogenesis and pathologic changes of experimentally induced listeriosis in newborn pigs. *American Journal of Veterinary Research*, **32**, 1313.

GRAY M.L. AND KILLINGER A.H. (1966) *Listeria monocytogenes* and listeric infections. *Bacteriological Reviews*, **30**, 309.

JONES SUSAN M. AND WOODBINE M. (1961) Microbiological aspects of *Listeria monoctyogenes* with special reference to listeriosis in animals. *Veterinary Reviews and Annotations*, 7, 39.

KRAMER P.A. AND JONES D. (1969) Media selective for *Listeria monocytogenes*. *Journal of Applied Bacteriology*, **32**, 381.

LADDS, P.W., DENNIS, S.M. AND NJOKU, C.O. (1974) Pathology of listeric infection in domestic animals. *Veterinary Bulletin*, **44**, 67.

LANE, F.C. AND UNANUE, E.R. (1972) Requirement of thymus (T) lymphocytes for resistance to listeriosis. *Journal of Experimental Medicine*, **135**, 1104.

LARSEN H.E. (1969) *Listeria monocytogenes*: Studies on isolation techniques and epidemiology, p. 256. Copenhagen: Mortensen.

PEARSON, L.D. AND OSEBOLD, J.W. (1974) Effects of antilymphocyte sera and antimacrophage sera on cell-mediated immune reactions in Listeria-infected mice. *Infection and Immunity*, **9**, 127.

Proceedings 3rd International symposium (1966) *Listeriosis*, p. 461. Bilthoven.

SIDDIQUE, I.H., LIN, I-FONG AND CHUNG, R.A. (1974) Purification and characterization of hemolysin produced by *Listeria monocytogenes*. *American Journal of Veterinary Research*, **35**, 289.

CHAPTER 19

BACILLUS

Bacillus

This group consists of a large number of species which are saprophytes, with the exception of *B. anthracis* the cause of anthrax in animals and man. All the species are Gram-positive rods which produce spores. Some are motile and some develop capsules. All members of the group have a number of other common characteristic properties which necessitate the differentiation between the pathogenic species, *B. anthracis,* and some of the other members of the group being based on detailed comparative tests.

only be made when comparable numbers of each species are inoculated into laboratory animals. Differences in lecithinase production between *B. mycoides* or *B. cereus* and *B. anthracis* may be only a matter of degree. Similarly, the anthracoid organisms produce marked haemolysis on blood agar compared with only slight haemolysis produced by some strains of *B. anthracis*. Occasionally, some strains of anthracoid organisms are non-motile and in this respect resemble *B. anthracis*; and some

TABLE 19.1. Comparing the properties of *B. anthracis* and anthracoid organisms.

Differential Test	B. anthracis	Saprophytic species (anthracoid organisms)
Motility	Non-motile	Usually motile
Susceptibility to anthrax phage	Susceptible	Not susceptible
Haemolysis on blood agar	None or slight	Usually marked
Position of spores	Central. Do not bulge bacillus	Central, subterminal or terminal. May bulge bacillus.
Lecithinase production	Absent or slight	Marked
Gelatin liquefaction	Slow	Rapid
Pathogenicity for animals (similar dosages)	Pathogenic	Non-pathogenic

The type species of the non-pathogenic organisms is *B. subtilis* and these saprophytes are sometimes referred to as the subtilis group. They include *B. mycoides, B. megaterium, B. mesentericus, B. cereus* and many others. Their natural habitats are soil, water, decaying vegetable matter, dust and air.

The characteristic properties of some of these saprophytes (e.g. *B. cereus*) are so similar to those of *B. anthracis* that they have been termed the anthracoids. Table 19.1 which compares the properties of *B. anthracis* and the anthracoid organisms, emphasises the similarity between the two. In some instances the differences are only a matter of degree. For example, a comparison of pathogenicity can

capsulated forms of *B. megaterium* show a close resemblance to similar forms of *B. anthracis*. Although there are these similarities between *B. anthracis* and certain other members of the group, the differences which do exist and the unique nature of anthrax and its characteristic features have resulted in agreement on the recognition of the species *B. anthracis* as the cause of that disease.

Bacillus anthracis

History
The early studies on anthrax by Pasteur and others, form an important section of the history and develop-

ment of bacteriology. Descriptions of the disease, particularly in sheep and cattle, have been recorded in increasing detail since the middle of the nineteenth century. There is little doubt, however, that some earlier references to epidemics of animal diseases were, in fact, descriptions of anthrax, and that this was one of the diseases referred to by classical writers and described in the history of cattle diseases in the early and middle ages. Anthrax is also historically important because it was the first disease which was shown to be caused by a bacterial species, and it was with this species that the first demonstrations were made of the use of avirulent strains as immunizing agents.

Distribution in nature

Anthrax has a world-wide distribution and chiefly affects cattle, sheep, horses, pigs and, less frequently, other species of domesticated animals. The disease also occurs in a variety of wild animals. Man is susceptible but is not a primary host. Anthrax occurs in various degrees of severity from an acute and fatal septicaemia to a more chronic type of infection developing either as localised pustular lesions or as a transient febrile condition.

Morphology and staining

B. anthracis is a relatively large, straight, rod shaped, non-motile organism, measuring 4–8 μm in length by 1–1·5 μm in width. In laboratory cultures the bacilli develop into rectangular shaped cells with square-cut ends. Under *in vivo* conditions these vegetative organisms lose their rectangular shape and become more rounded. Sporulation occurs readily outside the body in the presence of oxygen and does not take place in the tissues. The spores do not bulge the bacilli. Bacilli in blood films which are kept in an atmosphere with a high humidity will sporulate in 8 hours at 37°C, 10 hours at 32°C, 18 hours at 26°C and in 24 hours at 21°C. Below this last temperature very little sporulation occurs. The organism can remain viable as a spore in an environment of reduced nutrients which is inadequate for growth of the vegetative form. Under favourable conditions the spores can develop into bacilli – each spore giving rise to one bacillus. When growing in tissues or blood the organism may produce a capsule which protects it from the action of opsonins and phagocytosis. The detection of a capsule is also of diagnostic importance.

B. anthracis stains strongly Gram-positive when it has been growing in tissue. After growth on laboratory media the reaction to the Gram stain becomes variable and older cells may stain frankly Gram-negative. Dormant spores will not stain by Gram's method and special spore staining techniques have to be used. Anthrax carcases decompose rapidly and simultaneously the morphological appearance of *B. anthracis* in the tissues no longer remains characteristic.

The presence of capsules revealed by special staining methods is of diagnostic importance. The most reliable methods are Wright's or Giemsa's stain. Methylene blue has been used widely for this purpose but the characteristic differentiation between the body of the bacillus and capsular material, known as the McFadyean reaction (Plate 19.1a, facing p. 203), may not be very obvious when some batches of stain are used. In this reaction, the capsular material is stained pale pink and the bacillary bodies are blue. The degree of heat used for the fixation of a blood film containing anthrax bacilli will affect the appearance of the stained film. Provided that a minimum amount of heat fixation has been employed, the capsular material will remain *in situ* surrounding the bacilli, but after more intense heat the capsular material will have become detached from the bacilli and appear as pale pink clumps interspersed between the blue stained organisms.

Cultural characteristics

B. anthracis grows readily on customary laboratory media under aerobic conditions and also in partial anaerobic atmospheres. The optimum temperature for growth of bacilli is 35–37°C although growth can occur within a range of 12–44°C. Sporulation will take place under aerobic conditions within a temperature range of about 15–40°C and optimally within temperatures of 25–30°C. Sporulation will also occur in an atmosphere containing a low partial pressure of oxygen but is greatly reduced in a high partial pressure of carbon dioxide. Spores will be activated to germinate and develop into bacilli in both aerobic and anaerobic atmospheres at a temperature of 65°C for as short a time as 15 minutes. Under defined conditions of growth in medium containing iron salts, *B. anthracis* produces a pink or purple coloured pigment which appears to be formed more readily by virulent than by avirulent strains.

On nutrient agar the 'wild', rough or virulent type produces a characteristic colony after 24 hours' incubation, which is flat with a frosted appearance about 3–5 mm diameter, with a roughened edge sometimes referred to as a 'medusa-head' type of growth (Plate 19.1b, facing p. 203). Microscopically, the edges of the colony consist of numerous chains or threads of bacilli protruding from the centre which is itself a mass of bacillary chains. When grown on 50 per cent serum agar in an atmosphere of 65 per cent CO_2 the growth develops as smooth, mucoid colonies which form roughened edges after prolonged incubation.

In gelatin stab cultures the growth pattern is often referred to as resembling an inverted fir tree. From the central perpendicular line of inoculum a number of fine filaments of growth develop laterally. Those nearer to the surface of the medium are the longest, and they become progressively shorter the further they are from the surface where there is less oxygen available. Liquefaction of the gelatin medium is slow.

In nutrient broth, cultures give rise to a flocculent deposit of long chains of bacilli. This is particularly well marked with newly isolated strains.

On blood agar B. anthracis produces only slight haemolysis compared with anthracoid organisms which usually are strongly haemolytic. There may be little capsule formation of B. anthracis when grown on blood agar, but capsules are produced more abundantly in fluid media containing blood or serum, and maximum capsule formation occurs more readily on both these solid and fluid media in an atmosphere with increased partial pressure of carbon dioxide.

Biochemical reactions
The following reactions are of importance for purposes of differential diagnosis. B. anthracis produces acid without gas in glucose, maltose, saccharose, laevulose, trehalose and dextrin. Nitrates are reduced to nitrites, indole is not produced, the Voges-Proskauer reaction is positive and methylene blue is reduced.

Variation
As early as 1881 Pasteur and his colleagues found that if a virulent rough culture of B. anthracis was incubated at 42°C for at least 2 weeks, most of the virulence was permanently and irreversibly lost. The colonies of these attenuated smooth strains differ in appearance from virulent strains, being smaller, more convex and smooth in outline, and consisting of bacteria in bundles instead of in chains. Thus, the anthrax organism is an exception to the general rule because rough strains of B. anthracis are virulent and smooth strains are avirulent. Many attenuated strains still maintain their capacity to produce capsules, and variants of virulent strains sometimes develop which are both rough and uncapsulated. It is evident that capsules alone are not responsible for virulence but that a strain which does not produce capsules cannot be virulent.

Resistance to physical and chemical agents
The bacilli or vegetative forms of the organism are killed by a temperature of 60°C for 30 minutes. By contrast, the spores of B. anthracis are highly resistant and will survive steaming or boiling at 100°C for 5 minutes; most strains are killed after 10 minutes under these conditions, and all strains

are killed after 10 minutes at 120°C. Spores will resist a dry heat temperature of 140°C for 2–3 hours, depending upon the variation in resistance shown by different strains. It is important to note that the common method for heat fixation of smears of anthrax organisms on to slides by passing the smears several times through a bunsen flame, may not be lethal to spores. Smears prepared in this way and stored for several years have been shown to contain viable spores capable of germination in media and of causing laboratory infections.

The spores of B. anthracis are relatively resistant to disinfectants, and it should also be remembered that the effectiveness of any particular disinfectant depends upon the temperature of the reaction, and on the presence and concentration of protein, mucus and other substances. For these reasons there is wide variation in the reported results of experiments which record and compare the efficacies of different bactericidal agents on the spores of B. anthracis. The following are some of the maximum figures for times of reaction and concentrations of disinfectants which are recorded as being lethal. Formaldehyde solution at 2–3 per cent concentration is claimed to be effective if the temperature of the reaction is kept at 40°C for 20 minutes. Similar results have been reported from treating material with 0·25 per cent formaldehyde solution for 6 hours at 60°C. These and similar methods are used for the disinfection of hair, wool and brushes. Spores may resist the lethal action of 5 per cent phenol for more than 5 weeks and of 5 per cent mercuric chloride for 3 weeks.

Antigens and toxins
The complex antigenic structure of B. anthracis includes a capsular polypeptide, a somatic protein and a somatic polysaccharide antigen. The capsular material consists mainly of polyglutamic acid which is only detectable in virulent strains. The capsule protects the organism from phagocytosis and blocks the natural anthracidal factor in normal serum. The somatic protein antigen is protective and found in the oedema fluid of lesions in infected animals. The somatic polysaccharide component is a hapten when in isolation and will react with antisera against the whole organism. In the cell wall the polysaccharide is combined with polypeptide.

B. anthracis produces an extracellular toxin which is composed of three components labelled Factors I, II and III by British workers and, respectively, oedema factor (EF) protective antigen (PA) and lethal factor (LF) by American workers. These three factors have now been isolated and examined individually. Factor I consists of a chelating compound containing phosphorus with protein and carbohydrate moieties; Factors II and III

TABLE 19.2. Showing the properties of the toxin components of *B. anthracis*

Toxin components	Oedema production	Lethality	Immunogenicity
I (oedema factor)	—	—	—
II (protective antigen)	—	—	++
III (lethal factor)	—	—	—
I & II	+++	+	+++
I & III	—	—	+
II & III	—	++	++
I & II & III	++	+++	++

+++, ++, + = Decreasing degrees of reaction
— = No reaction.

consist of proteins. It has been shown that the toxic properties of the toxin are not caused by any single factor alone, but by a combination of two or three factors. Thus, the individual Factors I, II or III when tested singly, are not lethal to mice or oedema-producing in either guinea-pigs or rabbits. However, mixtures of Factors I + II or I + II + III are synergistically oedema-producing after sub-cutaneous inoculation into guinea-pigs and rabbits. Similarly, lethality in mice is shown by the synergistic action of Factors II + III or I + II + III. A slight degree of immunogenicity in guinea-pigs is produced by Factor II and this is markedly increased by using Factor II with Factor I. Similarly, mixtures II + III and I + II + III are also immunogenic.

These experimental results indicate that both the toxic and immunogenic properties of the toxin are produced by combinations of the component factors, and that the most reliable anthrax vaccine should contain a mixture of all three of these components (Table 19.2).

Epidemiology and pathogenesis
The susceptibility of animals to anthrax shows considerable differences between the species. For example, under natural conditions cattle, sheep, horses, goats and pigs are attacked in that order of priority. Many other species of domesticated and wild animals, including deer, elephants, dogs and mink are less frequently affected. Birds are not susceptible except in captivity, but vultures and other carrion eaters may spread the infection. Although man is susceptible to anthrax, human infections are only derived secondarily from animal sources.

The epidemiology of anthrax and the perpetuation of the species *B. anthracis*, is closely related to the life cycle of these organisms. On exposure to an atmosphere containing oxygen and to an environment depleted of nutrients, the vegetative cells are stimulated to develop into spores. In this relatively resistant spore form the organisms can remain viable in soil for many decades. Only a very small proportion of all anthrax spores in an environment are deposited in sites where they are able to infect another host. It is also important for the completion of their life cycle that the strains of organisms are toxigenic. Thus, after entry into host tissues the spores are able to revert to the vegetative form, multiply in the tissues, produce toxin and kill the host. From the fatally infected animal large numbers of spores will be produced by organisms in tissues, blood and faeces which become exposed to the air, and these will maintain the species in the environment until some are able to infect and multiply in another host, and repeat the life cycle.

The likelihood of clinical infection developing in different animal species is affected by a variety of predisposing factors. These include the degrees of susceptibility of various animal species, the natural feeding habits of animals, the feeding of imported infected foodstuffs, climatic and seasonal conditions, and the relative populations of different animal species in a district.

Collectively, these factors are responsible for certain characteristic features of the epidemiology of anthrax in different countries and under particular local circumstances. For example, the incidence may be greater in sheep than in cattle or greater in goats than in sheep. In the United Kingdom the main source of animal disease is infected imported foodstuffs and artificial manures (bone meal, blood meal, etc.). In countries with warmer climates the disease is endemic and waterholes used by a variety of animal species often become centres for the dissemination of infection; and it is known from surveys that the incidence of *B. anthracis* in the total animal population, including wild animals, is greater than that recorded in national statistics. In these endemic environments, *B. anthracis* may also be disseminated by flies, rats and birds. Carrion eaters, especially vultures which feed on infected carcases, can carry *B. anthracis* and deposit the organisms in waterholes as a result of washing their feathers free from blood, regurgitation of excess food, and deposition of infected faeces. It has also been observed that in mountainous countries like Peru, the incidence of anthrax among susceptible animals on low lying ground is high, whereas the incidence of anthrax among similar animals living at altitudes of 2000 m or more above sea level is practically nil. It has been suggested that at these higher altitudes *B. anthracis* does not readily sporulate but the complete explanation of this epidemiological feature requires further investigation.

Among laboratory animals mice, guinea-pigs and rabbits are susceptible. Rats are generally more resistant except for a few highly susceptible strains.

Anthrax spores will germinate into bacilli in a localised area at the site of entry into the tissues. This may be in the intestinal tract after penetration of the mucosa or in the region of the throat. If the strain of organisms is highly virulent, capsules will be well formed and protect the organisms from phagocytosis and lysis. After the lesion has been developing for only 3–4 hours it will consist of a mass of well capsulated bacilli contained in an oedematous area of tissue. This zone of oedema will continue to spread outwards from the centre of the lesion. If the host shows sufficient resistance to infection, the borders of the lesion will be demarcated by large numbers of polymorphs and mononuclear cells which will inhibit the further encroachment of the lesion into the surrounding normal tissue. Following this stage, bacterial capsules will begin to disintegrate in the area of cellular infiltration, and then the bacterial bodies and some leucocytes will become destroyed. In the resistant animal these processes will continue until the cellular defences finally overcome the infection and the lesion heals with fibrosis.

Primary lesions which have developed in susceptible animals continue to overcome the local cellular defences. Bacilli become distributed, initially, via the lymphatics where secondary lesions develop in lymph nodes. The multiplication of bacteria continues at a rapid rate. Many pass into the blood stream, become distributed throughout the body and continue to multiply until the animal dies. Death may occur within 3 days in acute cases but may not take place until after 1–2 weeks following infection.

Earlier concepts on the cause of death from anthrax were associated with the large numbers of bacilli present in the tissues throughout the body. It was supposed that this high rate of multiplication resulted in the blockage of blood capillaries by bacteria, and that the oxygen requirements of so large a bacterial population in the tissues resulted in the animal suffering from a fatal anoxia. The results of more recent experiments have disproved these theories and revealed fresh information on the pathogenesis of this disease related to the development of the three components of the toxin. It is now known that plasma from animals fatally infected with *B. anthracis* contains the toxin which causes the development of oedema and shock, and that this reaction can be inhibited by specific antiserum. Furthermore, it has been shown that the typical symptoms of toxaemia and shock which are manifest in the terminal stages of anthrax can occur when the degree of bacteraemia is relatively slight or when the rapidly developing bacteraemia is halted by the administration of antibiotics.

Symptoms

Horses

The disease occurs in an acute form and death may take place about one day after oedematous swellings have developed in the region of the throat and neck. There may be also symptoms of colic. Some cases are less acute and the oedematous swellings become more extensive in the region of the throat, neck, shoulders and abdomen before death occurs in 2–3 days after the onset of symptoms.

Cattle

In acute cases death can occur within minutes of the animal collapsing to the ground and having convulsions. In less acute forms there is a sudden rise in body temperature, shivering, and signs of abdominal pain. Blood may escape from the rectum and nose immediately prior to death. Urine may also contain blood in the terminal stages of the disease. Occasionally, some infected animals develop oedematous swellings in the region of the throat and shoulders over a period of about one week before death occurs, while others suffer from only a raised body temperature before recovering.

Sheep

Usually the disease is acute and death occurs rapidly after convulsions.

Pigs

The symptoms are usually chronic since these animals have a greater natural resistance to anthrax than herbivores. The usual signs of infection are oedematous swellings in the region of the throat and neck which may interfere with normal respirations, or an enteritis giving rise to a mild or severe diarrhoea and sometimes dysentery. Other animals may suffer a rise in body temperature and loss of appetite for a few days. The disease is not always fatal.

Dogs

Infection in these animals commonly occurs as an acute gastroenteritis consequent upon the ingestion of heavily contaminated food. Sometimes the throat is also inflamed and swollen.

Lesions

The carcases of herbivores which have died from acute infection with *B. anthracis* rapidly decompose and become bloated. The blood is dark in colour, clots poorly and may have escaped from the natural orifices at the time of death. Droplets of blood-stained serum may have oozed through the skin, especially in the region of the ears, neck, forelegs and groin. Frequently, the spleen is enlarged, hyperaemic and dark red in colour. Haemorrhages may be seen on the serous and mucous membranes, and oedema is often visible in subcutaneous tissues and sometimes in the intestinal tract. In some cases there may be a severe haemorrhagic enteritis.

In pigs the most obvious lesions are oedema in the connective tissue of the throat and neck, together with enlarged haemorrhagic lymph glands. Sometimes there may be defined areas of enteritis consisting of thickened, haemorrhagic zones in the intestines, enlarged haemorrhagic mesenteric lymph nodes and a peritonitis.

The lesions in carnivores are associated with severe gastroenteritis or inflammation in the region of the throat, including the tongue and lips.

Diagnosis

There is a variety of techniques used for the diagnosis of anthrax in animals and the choice of which particular method to employ will depend upon a number of factors including the climate and rate of decomposition of the carcase, the species of animal involved, the sites of lesions situated superficially on the carcase, and the length of time between death and examination of the carcase. It should always be remembered that on post-mortem examination the exposure of anthrax bacilli to the atmosphere will result in the development of spores and an increased contamination of the environment around the carcase. The risk of infection becoming transferred to those who handle the carcase will also be increased. It is, therefore, required that a diagnosis should be attempted by methods which entail the least amount of manipulation and dissection of the carcase in countries like the United Kingdom where anthrax is a notifiable disease. To obtain a final diagnosis it may be necessary to use one or more of the following procedures.

Stained films of blood

In the majority of herbivores which have died from acute disease, many anthrax bacilli will be present in the peripheral blood at the time of death, and these organisms will usually possess well-formed capsules. Blood films prepared by puncturing a superficial vein of the ear or in the region of the foot, are fixed by heat and stained by Wright's or Giemsa's stain to reveal *B. anthracis* as large blue rods with capsules which stain characteristically dark pink or purple. Methylene blue gives a similar result except that the capsular material stains a paler shade of pink and may be more difficult to observe when the capsules are not well formed. After preparation of blood films a small pledget of cotton wool soaked in alcohol should be placed over the site of incision and ignited. This will help to seal the wound and prevent further exposure of bacilli to the atmosphere and subsequent sporulation.

Stained films of exudate and lymph glands

Deaths of horses and pigs from anthrax may take place when there are only small numbers of organisms in the peripheral blood. In these cases a diagnosis may be made by preparing films from oedematous fluid, particularly in the region of the throat and neck, and from local superficial lymph glands. These films should be stained and examined as described above for blood films.

Bacteriological examination of blood and exudate

Swabs of blood or exudate are prepared from superficial sites by making a small incision in the skin over a blood vessel or in the region of an oedematous lesion. These swabs are then placed in sterile tubes, plugged and transported to a laboratory. Defibrinated blood or serum is then added to each tube containing a swab, incubated for 6 hours at 37°C and examined for *B. anthracis* by preparing stained smears. Swabs can also be used for inoculating blood agar plates which are then incubated at 37°C for 24 hours before being examined for typical growths of *B. anthracis*.

Bacteriological examination of miscellaneous materials

It is usual for specimens of hair, wool, hide, bone, bone meal, blood meal and other materials to be heavily contaminated with a variety of bacteria in addition to possible infection with spores of *B. anthracis*.

Samples of these materials for examination should be added to saline and shaken intermittently for 3 hours in the cold. This will result in the suspension of anthrax spores and the cool temperature will ensure that they will not commence germination. The supernatant fluid should then be heated to 70°C for 10 minutes. This treatment will be lethal to vegetative organisms while the spores of *B. anthracis* and other spore forming organisms will remain viable. Some of this heated fluid can then be filtered through two layers of butter muslin, added to melted agar, poured into petri dishes, allowed to set and incubated at 37°C overnight. The cultures are then examined for the characteristic filamentous colonies of *B. anthracis*. It may be necessary to prepare a number of plates with different volumes of heated fluid in each, in order to obtain the optimum concentration for diagnostic purposes. It is also important not to incubate the plates for too long before examination. The maximum time for incubation is about 12 hours which enables the early characteristic colonial formation of *B. anthracis* to be observed without interference from the growths of other sporebearing bacterial species.

Precipitin test

This is often referred to as the Ascoli test and is used for the diagnosis of anthrax in a carcase which has begun to decompose and in which the anthrax organisms are beginning to disintegrate. The principle of the test is the identification of *B. anthracis* antigen in the tissues. There are a number of modifications to the method but the general procedure is as follows. A piece of tissue weighing 1–2 g is boiled for at least 5 minutes in about 5 ml saline containing 1/1000 acetic acid. The fluid which is then filtered, should contain anthrax antigen if these organisms had been present in the tissues. This is confirmed or otherwise by carefully running 0·5 ml of this filtrate on top of 0·5 ml anthrax antiserum in a narrow tube. A positive result indicating infection with anthrax is recorded when a distinct ring of precipitate develops at the interface of the two fluids within 15 minutes.

Fluorescent antibody test

This technique consists in applying a *B. anthracis* antiserum labelled with fluorescein isothiocyanate, to a film of the material suspected of being infected. This film is then inspected microscopically with u.v. light to observe the presence of *B. anthracis* which will fluoresce as a result of combination with the labelled antibody.

Bacteriophage typing

This is one of the more recent techniques developed for the differential diagnosis of *B. anthracis*. The test is based on the specificity of certain strains of bacteriophages for *B. anthracis* as distinct from other members of the genus *Bacillus*. The test is carried out by applying certain specific strains of bacteriophages to cultures of suspected *B. anthracis* and observing whether bacterial lysis occurs and growth is inhibited.

Animal inoculations

Guinea-pigs and mice are highly susceptible to anthrax and are used for the diagnosis of this disease. Material suspected of being infected with *B. anthracis* is inoculated by dermal scarification, subcutaneously or intramuscularly into these animals. If the amount of infection in the inoculum is heavy, the animals may die in less than 48 hours after inoculation, and all the tissues will be heavily infected with *B. anthracis*. In other instances infection may take longer to develop when the number of organisms contained in the inoculum is low.

Heat-treated material prepared for bacteriological examination (see above) can also be used for animal inoculation. The material (e.g. hair, bone meal, etc.) is prepared in the same way in saline, heated to 70°C for 10 minutes to kill vegetative bacteria, filtered through muslin and centrifuged. The deposit is used for animal inoculation either intramuscularly, subcutaneously or by scarification of the skin. Clear cut results may be difficult to obtain if the deposit is heavily contaminated with clostridia in addition to *B. anthracis* and other members of the genus *Bacillus*. In such cases clostridia may be responsible for the deaths of animals from toxaemia before the anthrax organisms have had time to produce disease. For this reason, it may be necessary to protect mice or guinea-pigs with clostridial antitoxins. For example, one day before the intramuscular inoculation of the prepared material, each guinea-pig should receive a polyvalent serum containing antitoxins to *Cl. septicum*, *Cl. oedematiens*, *Cl. welchii* and *Cl. tetani*. Provided that the inoculum contains approximately 50 or more viable spores of *B. anthracis*, death of the guinea-pig will occur in 2–3 days, and the organisms will be readily identifiable in the blood and tissues.

Control and prevention

Adequate measures for the control and prevention of anthrax which are both economic and practical when assessed in relation to the type of husbandry and the prevailing climatic conditions, will differ considerably from one continent to another. Countries situated in the northern hemisphere, including Europe and North America, which practise high standards of animal husbandry, experience a low and sporadic incidence of anthrax. Countries with warmer climates and poorer standards of animal husbandry, including Africa, the Middle East and Far East, where infected carcases of both domesticated and wild animals may be left to decompose and become a concentrated source of contamination of the environment, experience an increased incidence of the disease which may reach epidemic proportions. For these reasons, practical measures for controlling anthrax will be summarised separately for each of these differing circumstances.

Temperate climates

In the northern hemisphere anthrax occurs sporadically, affecting only small groups or individual animals in a district. The origin of infection may be from the environment or from infected foodstuffs and other materials imported from countries where the disease is endemic. These include bones and bone-meals, hair, wool and hides; and the effluents from factories in the importing countries which process these materials can also be an added source of infection. For these reasons the main features of control measures include the rapid identification of infected carcases and their adequate disposal by burning or burying to prevent contamination of the environment, particularly streams, ponds and other natural water supplies. It is important from the point of view of both animal health and public health, that consignments of imported foodstuffs, hides and other materials should be sterilised before being distributed. This can be done effectively by subjecting bone meal to high pressure steam. Anthrax spores exposed to the atmosphere on hides may be killed by exposure to liquid nitrous oxide gas. If a number of animals have died from anthrax in a particular area and it is suspected that the outbreak may continue, hyperimmune serum can be given to the in-contact animals. In areas where anthrax is known to be a risk, vaccination may be advantageous.

Tropical climates

In many tropical countries anthrax constitutes a serious and widespread disease problem. In these climates the conditions are particularly favourable for the sporulation of the organisms and many cases of anthrax are not diagnosed until an epidemic has become widespread. The only practical measure has been a programme of extensive immunization of animals with reliable vaccines. This procedure has proved to be of great value and has virtually eliminated the disease from some areas where previously it had reached epidemic proportions.

Vaccines

Since the original recognition of B. anthracis as the cause of anthrax in animals and man, many attempts have been made to produce an immunizing agent which is both safe to use and strongly protective. Some of the earlier attempts were the notable experiments of Pasteur and his colleagues during the last century who observed the attenuation of B. anthracis resulting from the incubation of cultures at 42°C. At the beginning of this century, Bail demonstrated that oedema fluid and tissues obtained from anthrax lesions which had been freed from viable organisms had protective properties. He termed the active substances 'aggresins' because they inhibited the natural defence processes of the body. At about the same time other workers were preparing experimental vaccines from spore suspensions derived from attenuated strains, using glycerin as the suspending fluid because it tended to prolong the protective effect and to inhibit the growth of contaminants. However, this type of vaccine occasionally produced severe reactions in some animals and the practice of using the vaccine in conjunction with hyperimmune serum was introduced to overcome this risk.

A more recent and useful development from these earlier experiments has been the production of living spore vaccines derived from avirulent uncapsulated strains of B. anthracis. This type of vaccine is safe to use in all species, irrespective of their differing degrees of susceptibility to the disease; it can be readily prepared in the laboratory, does not deteriorate rapidly, and has proved to be of great value in curtailing the incidence of anthrax in tropical countries. One dose of vaccine will give protection for one year and should be repeated annually. Vaccine prepared from non-living antigen gives a poorer immune response after two doses but it is probable that further research on this type of non-living vaccine will result in a more satisfactory product.

Chemotherapy

Antibiotics have no effect on the preformed toxins of B. anthracis, and for this reason treatment must be commenced as early as possible. Various penicillin preparations have been used successfully in the treatment of anthrax in pigs and in other animal species which show some natural resistance and in which the disease is not very acute. It is a less practical method of treatment for herbivores suffering from the acute form of the disease with a very short incubation period. However, under special circumstances infected cattle have been successfully treated in this way by giving large doses of penicillin intravenously.

Public health aspects

Human infections with B. anthracis are of animal origin and usually occur through abrasions of the skin or mucous membranes and less commonly from inhalation of spores. The incidence is relatively high among those who handle infected carcases and animal products, including bone-meal, feeding stuffs, hides, wool and hair. The risk is particularly great for veterinarians, farmers and personnel working in docks and factories, handling and processing these infected animal products. In underdeveloped

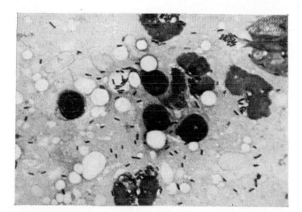

18.1   Brain impression film from mouse experimentally infected with *Listeria monocytogenes*, stained Leishman, × 930.

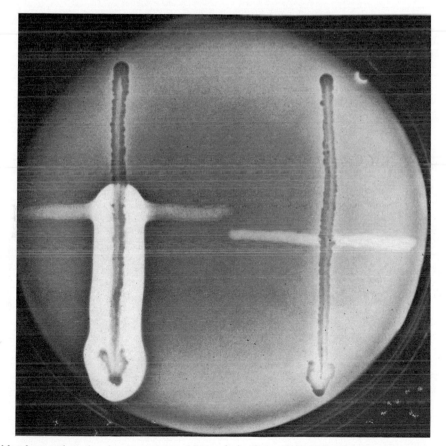

18.2   Sheep blood agar plate showing the increased haemolytic effect obtained by drawing a culture of *C. equi* across and at right-angles to a horizontal streak culture of *L. monocytogenes* (left) but not *E. insidiosa* (right).

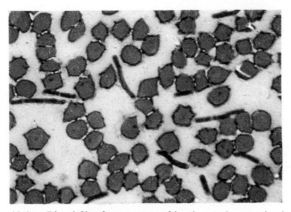 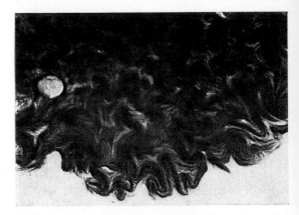

19.1a   Blood film from a case of bovine anthrax stained with methylene blue, showing blue bacilli surrounded by pink-coloured capsular material (McFadyean reaction), ×930.

19.1b   Impression smear of a rough colony of *Bacillus anthracis* stained with methylene blue, showing the roughened edge composed of numerous chains or threads of bacilli.

tropical countries infection may occur from the ingestion of meat from infected carcases.

The usual lesion is a malignant pustule which may take some 48 hours to develop subsequent to infection of a skin abrasion. Infection by inhalation of a spore-laden atmosphere can occur in certain commercial processes, for example, 'wool sorters' disease' among workers in wool factories, and similar infections have arisen from handling goat hair. Some individuals show a remarkable resistance to this route of infection since it has been assessed that they can inhale more than 1000 spores per day and not contract the disease. When clinical infection does become established it is acute and severe, with the development of haemorrhages and oedema involving both lungs and the local lymph glands. A septicaemia may develop.

Further reading

BUCHANAN, T.M., FEELEY, J.C., HAYES, P.S. AND BRACHMAN, P.S. (1971) Anthrax indirect micro-haemagglutination test. *Journal of Immunology*, **107**, 1631.

DAVIES, D.G. AND HARVEY, R.W.S. (1972) Anthrax infection in bone meal from various countries of origin. *Journal of Hygiene*, **70**, 455.

FISH D.C. AND LINCOLN R.E. (1967) Biochemical and biophysical characterisation of anthrax toxin. *Federation Proceedings*, **26**, 1534.

FOX, M.D., KAUFMANN, A.F., ZENDEL, S.A., KOLB, R.C., SONGY, C.G. CANGELOSI, D.A. AND FULLER. C.E. (1973) Anthrax in Louisiana, 1971: epizootiologic study. *Journal of the American Veterinary Medical Association*, **163**, 446.

GERHARDT P. (1967) Cytology of *Bacillus anthracis*. *Federation Proceedings*, **26**, 1504.

GLEISER C.A. (1967) Pathology of anthrax infection in animal hosts. *Federation Proceedings*, **26**, 1518.

GOLD H. (1967) Treatment of anthrax. *Federation Proceedings*, **26**, 1563.

HUGH-JONES, M.E. AND HUSSAINI, S.N. (1974) An anthrax outbreak in Berkshire. *Veterinary Record*, **94**, 228.

LINCOLN, R.E., WALKER, J.S., KLEIN, F. AND HAINES, B.W. (1964) Anthrax. *Advances in Veterinary Science*, **9**, 327.

NUNGESTER W.J. (1967) Symposium on progress in the understanding of anthrax. *Federation Proceedings*, **26**, 1483.

PIENAAR U. DE V. (1967) Epidemiology of anthrax in wild animals and the control of anthrax epizootics in the Kruger National Park, South Africa. *Federation Proceedings*, **26**, 1496.

SMITH H. AND STONER H.B. (1967) Anthrax toxic complex. *Federation Proceedings*, **26**, 1554.

WALKER J.S., LINCOLN R.E. AND KLEIN F. (1967) Pathophysiological and biochemical changes in anthrax. *Federation Proceedings*, **26**, 1539.

CHAPTER 20

CLOSTRIDIUM

CHAPTER 20

Clostridium

The clostridial group includes spore-forming bacilli which typically stain Gram-positive and grow in an atmosphere which is either anaerobic or microaerophilic. The natural habitat for most of these species is the soil, and they are frequently excreted in the faeces following ingestion from pastures, vegetables and fruit.

Spore formation constitutes an important part of the life cycle of clostridia. There is no doubt that the survival of spores under conditions which are adverse for the survival of vegetative forms of clostridial organisms is a significant feature in the dissemination of disease caused by pathogenic strains. Although one spore can give rise to only one bacterium, the latter can multiply rapidly and the resultant cell population can produce a vast number of spores. In this way, a heavy population of these bacteria can be developed and maintained in different environments under a wide range of conditions.

There are many species of clostridia and they can be divided into three groups according to their habitats and their natural history. Many of the species are saprophytes which live in the soil and are closely associated with the processes of putrefaction of plant and animal matter. Some species live as commensals in the intestinal tracts of animals and man. A few species produce substances toxic to host tissues and are pathogens.

The pathogenicity of these latter strains varies considerably according to the quantitative and qualitative activities of the toxins they produce. For example, *Clostridium tetani* multiplies in a localised area of the body at the site of inoculation, and produces a potent neurotoxin which is responsible for the characteristic symptoms of tetanus. *Cl. botulinum* also produces a very potent neurotoxin which is responsible for the disease known as botulism. Unlike *Cl. tetani*, *Cl. botulinum* cannot grow and produce its toxins in the tissues of living animals, but can do so in foodstuffs, carcases and other environments outside the living animal body. Botulism results from the ingestion of preformed toxin in contaminated foodstuffs. In contrast to

Cl. tetani and *Cl. botulinum*, other species of pathogenic clostridia exist in various organs of the body where certain predisposing conditions will stimulate rapid multiplication and toxin production by these organisms. Their toxins are comparatively milder than those of *Cl. tetani* and *Cl. botulinum*, and cause a lethal effect on tissues in the areas of bacterial multiplication. This type of reaction is characteristic for the group of organisms producing blackquarter lesions in cattle and sheep (e.g. *Cl. chauvoei*, *Cl. oedematiens*) similar to gas gangrene in man, and enteric infections in animals, including braxy (*Cl. septicum*), lamb dysentery and enterotoxaemia (*Cl. welchii*).

Clostridial organisms are able to actively decompose carbohydrates and proteins, and in most species one or other of these activities is predominant. On this basis it is possible to classify the organisms as being either saccharolytic (*Cl. welchii*, *Cl. septicum*, *Cl. chauvoei*) or proteolytic (*Cl. botulinum*, *Cl. tetani*, *Cl. histolyticum*, *Cl. sporogenes*). Clostridia ferment carbohydrates vigorously, producing large quantities of gas, and this is a characteristic feature of the fermentation of glucose by saccharolytic strains. The growth of these latter strains in cooked meat broth results in the rapid production of acid and gas, and the meat becomes pink but is not digested. In contrast, proteolytic strains are able to digest protein, causing decomposition and blackening of meat in cooked meat broth cultures.

Clostridium tetani

Distribution in nature

Cl. tetani is the cause of tetanus in animals and man, and the spores are distributed throughout the world in soil, faeces, dust, clothing and many other situations. The organisms have often been isolated from human and animal faeces, and they occur more frequently in richer soils which have been fertilised with human and animal faeces than they do in barren, uncultivated lands.

Morphology and staining

Cl. tetani is a long, slender rod-shaped organism measuring approximately 2–4μm in length and 0·5μm in width. Longer filamentous forms may also occur, particularly when the culture is growing on the surface of moist agar. The great majority of strains are motile, possessing peritrichous flagella, and all strains sporulate although some do so more readily than others. The fully developed spore of *Cl. tetani* is spherical, terminal and measures more than twice the diameter of the bacillus (Plate 20.1a, facing p. 216) giving it the characteristic 'drumstick' appearance. When attempting to differentiate *Cl. tetani* from *Cl. tertium* or any other species which produces fully mature terminal, oval spores, it is important to remember that the developing spores of *Cl. tetani* are also terminal and oval during development, and that they only become spherical when fully mature.

Cl. tetani stains Gram-positive in young cultures but in those which are more than 48 hours old, Gram-negative staining forms will often occur, particularly in nutrient broth cultures. Between these two extremes, a good deal of variation in staining quality can occur. Only the outer margins of mature spores will be stained by Gram's method and for thorough observation a special spore stain should be used. Immature developing spores often stain darkly by Gram's method. *Cl. tetani* does not form capsules.

Cultural characteristics

Satisfactory cultivation will only occur under strict anaerobic conditions. Maximum growth rate takes place at an optimum temperature of 37°C but will also occur within a temperature range of 14–44°C. Cooked meat broth will yield a good growth of *Cl. tetani* and there will be slight blackening of the meat after prolonged incubation. This medium is often used for storing cultures over a period of several months and for this purpose improved results have been reported from the addition of chalk and cooked minced egg-white to the medium. On blood agar the growth of young, actively motile cultures develops as partially translucent, greyish colonies, about 2–4 mm in diameter with filamentous edges which give them a fuzzy appearance. After further incubation the filamentous edges continue to extend from the colonies until the whole surface of the medium is covered by a film of growth which may be difficult to observe. A narrow zone of haemolysis caused by the production of tetanolysin toxin will develop beneath individual colonies but not under the spreading confluent growth. A similar type of spreading growth occurs on nutrient agar. Non-motile variants develop on these solid media as isolated colonies and do not produce a confluent type of growth.

Carbohydrates are not fermented by *Cl. tetani* and nitrates are not reduced to nitrites. Indole is formed but litmus milk remains unchanged except for delayed coagulation produced by some strains.

Resistance to physical and chemical agents

Spores are highly resistant to destruction by physical and chemical agents and those of some strains are particularly heat resistant. Boiling water may be lethal after 15 minutes but some more resistant strains may survive two or even three hours of this treatment. A moist heat temperature of 120°C for 20 minutes and a dry heat temperature of 150°C for more than one hour are usually lethal. In order to isolate *Cl. tetani* from cultures mixed with non-sporulating contaminants, the material should be heated to only 80°C for 10 minutes or 65°C for 30 minutes before inoculating the medium. Some strains resist the action of 5 per cent phenol for longer than 10 days and they are similarly resistant to a 1:1000 dilution of perchloride of mercury.

Antigens and toxins

Differences in the heat-labile flagellar antigens, detectable by agglutination tests, have enabled strains of *Cl. tetani* to be divide into 10 types. Some strains are non-flagellate and these comprise Type VI. The neurotoxins (tetanospasmin) produced by all types are antigenically similar and can be neutralized by one common antitoxin. There is one common heat-stable somatic antigen shared by all 10 types and a second somatic antigen shared by Types II, IV, V and IX.

Some strains of *Cl. tetani* are toxigenic and some are non-toxigenic. The former produce two toxic components known as tetanospasmin and tetanolysin. Tetanospasmin is an extremely potent neurotoxin which has been purified as a crystalline protein with a minimum molecular weight of 67 000. Maximum toxin production occurs in cultures which have been incubated for several days after growth has ceased, because the toxin is produced within the bacterial cell and is not released into the medium until the cell disintegrates. In this respect tetanospasmin may not be regarded strictly as an exotoxin since it is not secreted by the actively growing cell. An approximate dose of only $0·09 \times 10^{-3}$μg is lethal to a mouse, causing tetanic spasms which spread until the animal dies in a general tonic contraction. This highly purified form of toxin is unstable in solution and rapidly becomes converted into toxoid. The unpurified form of toxin in solution is destroyed by heating to 65°C for 5 minutes, but in the dried state will resist a temperature of 120°C for one hour. The horse is particularly susceptible to tetanospasmin and birds are relatively insusceptible.

Tetanolysin is the second toxic component

produced by *Cl. tetani* and causes lysis of red blood cells, particularly those of rabbits and horses. It is produced during the period of active growth of cultures and then becomes inactive. It is heat-labile, oxygen-labile and antigenically related to other oxygen-labile haemolysins, including *Cl. welchii* (theta toxin), *Cl. oedematiens* (delta toxin) and *Str. pyogenes* (streptolysin O).

Epidemiology and pathogenesis
Tetanus can affect many species of domesticated animals but occurs most frequently in horses and lambs, and less commonly in adult sheep, goats, cattle, pigs, dogs and cats. The disease occurs more rarely in poultry which are relatively resistant to the action of tetanospasmin. These differences in species susceptibilities may be accounted for partly by the development of a natural immunity and partly by the differences in diet between herbivores and carnivores. Young animals are more susceptible to infection than adults, and antitoxin can be detected in the sera of many adult healthy ruminants but rarely in samples from horses, pigs, dogs and cats. It has been suggested that *Cl. tetani* can produce small amounts of toxin in the rumen of cattle, sheep and goats, sufficient to stimulate the production of detectable levels of antitoxin in their sera, but that this does not occur in animal species having simple stomachs. In addition, the likelihood of ingesting *Cl. tetani* from pastures and soil is greater among herbivores than it is for carnivores.

Tetanus can be reproduced in laboratory animals, including rabbits, mice, rats, guinea-pigs and monkeys, all of which are susceptible to the action of tetanospasmin.

It is a characteristic feature of *Cl. tetani* that it has no powers of invasion in the tissues, and multiplication of the organism remains localised in a confined site. Moreover, the inoculation of washed spores into normal animals does not give rise to tetanus because they fail to germinate and are ingested by phagocytes. The development of tetanus in both animals and man depends entirely upon conditions suitable for the germination of spores into bacilli and for the subsequent production of the neurotoxin (tetanospasmin) in the confined site of the lesion and the subsequent action of this toxin on nervous tissue. Although satisfactory conditions for the multiplication of *Cl. tetani* can develop from the inoculation of spores into a deep wound contaminated with other bacterial species, there are additional conditions related to the establishment of a suitable environment which are necessary for the development of tetanus. For example, it is known from experiments that *Cl. tetani* can be present in the tissues of the body for several weeks without causing disease; and that the process of toxin formation will subsequently occur only when the organisms are in a suitable microenvironment. Such an environment must be sufficiently anaerobic and this can arise from traumatic conditions which involve reduced blood supply, necrosis and the multiplication of other species of bacteria which reduce the oxygen tension in the localised area. A suitable anaerobic environment can arise from a small zone of inflammation which may not be detectable, and for this reason no superficial wounds may be seen on some animals which develop tetanus. The disease may also arise from small areas of inflammation related to infected shallow wounds, superficial scratches, as well as from deep puncture wounds.

The method by which the toxin affects the hosts' tissues has been the subject of a great deal of research. In man the two most common manifestations of the disease are either the 'local' form or the 'general' form. The local form is characterised by spasticity of the muscles near to the site of infection, and although this is rare in animals under natural conditions it can be reproduced experimentally by inoculating toxin into the muscles of a limb. If a sufficient dose is inoculated, the condition will develop from the local form into the general form, which is characterised in animals and man by rigidity of the jaw, neck, limbs and trunk. Present evidence indicates that toxin generated by bacteria at the site of infection moves in the interneuronal tissue spaces of motor nerves and thence into the interstitial fluid of the central nervous system. The mode of action of the toxin is not precisely known but experiments indicate that the site of action is at the synaptic junction of the motor neurones with the interneurones of the inhibitory pathway resulting in uncontrolled activity of synaptic reflexes.

Symptoms
The incubation period is variable and can be as short as 5–6 days or of several months' duration before suitable conditions arise for the germination of spores. Sometimes there is a history of wounds or surgical interference related to castration, shearing, docking, or even injection. The symptoms are similar for all animal species and consist initially of mild stiffness and an unwillingness to move. This condition may last for 12–24 hours before being superimposed by more severe and characteristic signs of a general stiffness of the limbs and of the head, neck and tail which become rigid. Mild twitching of the muscles develops into obvious spasms of groups of muscles which can occur in response to sudden noises, often resulting in the animal falling over and being unable to rise. In the terminal stages the rigidity of the muscles may have extended from the limbs to the trunk, the nostrils become dilated, the ears erect, the nictitating membrane protruded, and mastication

becomes impossible because the mouth cannot be opened – hence the name lockjaw. Respiration becomes shallow and rapid before final respiratory failure occurs.

Lesions

There are no characteristic lesions of the disease but there may be superficial wounds which have developed from accidental injury or from surgery. In many cases, careful examination of the skin over the whole surface of the body will fail to show any injury.

Diagnosis

During life the disease is usually diagnosed from the characteristic symptoms. An attempt can be made to isolate *Cl. tetani* from an infected wound. For this purpose use is made of the properties of motility of most strains of *Cl. tetani* and of their ability to form spores. Material from the wound is cultured on blood agar and in meat broth for 2–3 days at 37°C. The broth is then heated to 65°C for 30 minutes to kill non-sporing organisms. The culture is inoculated either on to one half of a blood agar plate or into the water of condensation of an agar slope. The cultures are incubated anaerobically for 48 hours. If a motile strain of *Cl. tetani* is present it will be observed under a hand lens as a filamentous growth spreading over the surface of the medium. A subculture taken from the edge of this area of growth may give a pure culture of *Cl. tetani*. Confirmation may be obtained by inoculating mice subcutaneously or intramuscularly with some of the culture. Direct microscopical examination of the material from the wound for characteristic 'drum-stick' bacilli is not always reliable because the number of organisms may be relatively few in relation to contaminants.

Control and prevention

Active immunization of horses with tetanus toxoid has proved to be a valuable method for preventing the disease in that species. Horses are also used for the production of antitoxin on a commercial scale. The important steps in the preparation of toxoid are that a highly toxigenic strain is cultured under carefully controlled conditions to obtain the maximum amount of toxin production. The culture fluid containing the toxin is then filtered and incubated with formalin until all the toxin has become changed to toxoid. The concentration of toxoid can be increased by various methods (e.g. precipitation with ammonium sulphate) and reconstituted in a smaller volume. Adsorption of toxoid on to aluminium hydroxide gives a potent antigen which is absorbed over a longer period after injection. To stimulate the production of high concentrations of antitoxin in horses it is necessary to give at least two doses of toxoid at an interval of 3–4 weeks followed by repeated doses of toxin. Alternatively, the initial doses may be of toxin-antitoxin mixtures followed by repeated and increasing doses of toxin until a satisfactory antibody response has been stimulated.

Sheep are susceptible to disease caused by a variety of clostridia in addition to *Cl. tetani*, and for both economic and practical reasons a multi-component vaccine derived from several clostridial species is used for immunization (see Chapter 5). To obtain a satisfactory product of this sort, it is necessary to overcome a number of complications. In the first place the total volume of fluid containing a number of antigens has to be kept to a minimum and this entails preparing the component antigens sufficiently concentrated to keep the total volume of vaccine dose to a minimum. When using a multiple antigen it is also necessary to have each antigen as concentrated as possible in order to obtain maximum antibody response against each component, and to reduce the risk that the simultaneous production of antibodies against a number of distinct antigens will not result in the concentration of one or more being insufficient to give adequate protection. An additional difficulty is that the adsorption of antigen on to adjuvant enhances the duration of the immune response, but the use of very concentrated multiple antigens requires a relatively large quantity of adjuvant which may cause a severe reaction at the site of inoculation. To obtain a maximum degree of active immunity against each of the antigens of a multicomponent vaccine it is necessary to give more than one inoculation.

Animals which have received a wound that may be infected with *Cl. tetani* should be inoculated immediately with antitoxin as a precaution. The antitoxin will then combine with and neutralise toxin as soon as it is produced by the bacteria and before it has had time to become associated with nerve tissue. Treatment may also include dosing with penicillin parenterally and if possible, at the site of the lesion to overcome the localised infection. Dosing with central nervous system depressants, particularly acetylpromazine or chlorpromazine may also be employed when symptoms of the disease begin to appear.

Public health aspects

Man is susceptible to infection with *Cl. tetani* and the pathogenesis and pathology of the disease are similar to those in animals. Human infection can arise from wounds which become contaminated with spores from soil, animal faeces and dust. The incidence of *Cl. tetani* in human faeces varies from one part of the world to another, and may be particularly high in some countries where standards of personal hygiene are low. In these conditions, infection of wounds can occur from contaminated clothing or from spores present on the surface of the skin.

Clostridium botulinum

Distribution in nature

The usual habitat for *Clostridium botulinum* is the soil where it exists as a saprophyte. It is widely distributed throughout the world and is known to be present in both cultivated and barren lands. Consequently, the spores of the organism are also present in pastures, hay, vegetables, fruit and similar products which are in direct contact with the soil. When ingested by animals the organism passes through the intestinal canal without causing any pathological disturbance and is excreted in the faeces of healthy animals. The production of toxins by *Cl. botulinum* does not take place to any noticeable extent in living animals but can occur in carcases and in suitable environments outside the body. The disease of botulism which can affect many species of domesticated and wild animals and birds, arises from the ingestion of preformed toxin and not from the establishment of an infection with *Cl. botulinum* in the host. The organism produces a number of toxins which can be distinguished one from the other by immunological methods. On the basis of the antigenic differences of these toxins, strains of *Cl. botulinum* are identified as belonging to Type A, B, C, D, E or F.

Morphology and staining

The organisms grow as large rods measuring 4–6μm in length and 1μm in width, usually occurring singly, sometimes in pairs and occasionally in chains. Types C and D tend to be larger than other types and also more pleomorphic. *Cl. botulinum* produces spores which are oval, wider than the diameter of the bacillus, and usually situated subterminally but occasionally appear centrally or terminally (Plate 20.1b, facing p. 216). The bacilli have peritrichous flagella and are sluggishly motile. They do not produce capsules. The organisms stain Gram-positive but old cultures may contain some bacteria which have a tendency to stain Gram-negative.

Cultural characteristics

Cl. botulinum is a strict anaerobe. The optimum temperature for growth is 35°C but multiplication will take place at temperatures as low as 20°C. Growth occurs on ordinary laboratory media, and on solid media the colonies are large and semi-transparent with irregular edges. Most strains are haemolytic on horse blood agar but the zones of haemolysis are narrow. The organism grows well in cooked meat broth. The meat is digested and blackened by most strains of the toxigenic types A, B and F which are proteolytic. Types C, D and E are usually non-proteolytic and do not blacken the meat. Gelatin is liquefied rapidly by types A and B, and only slowly or not at all by types C, D and E. Lecithin is produced by all types and coagulated serum is liquefied slowly. All types ferment glucose and maltose with production of acid and gas except for types C and D which do not produce gas. Glycerol is fermented by types A and B but not by C. Salicin is fermented by type A but not by types B and C. Lactose is not fermented.

Resistance to physical and chemical agents

The spores of different strains of *Cl. botulinum* vary in their resistance to heat. Most strains are killed by moist heat at 100°C for 5–7 hours. The spores of type C are killed after 1 hour at 100°C and those of type E after a few minutes at this temperature. Autoclaving at 120°C for 20 minutes is lethal to all strains.

Antigens and toxins

Cl. botulinum possesses a number of H, O and spore antigens and it is possible on the basis of agglutination tests, to classify strains of the organism into a number of groups. However, this classification bears no relationship to the production of different toxins and it is in relation to the toxins that strains of the organism are typed.

Since the end of the last century it has been known that strains of *Cl. botulinum* produce highly potent neurotoxins which are more lethal than any other known substance. Like tetanospasmin produced by *Cl. tetani*, botulinum toxins are also produced intracellularly and liberated on rupture or autolysis of the cell wall. Continued immunological study of this dangerous material derived from animal and human sources has shown that there are important differences between toxins produced by various strains of the organism and that, unlike *Cl. tetani*, the antitoxin prepared against the toxin of one strain will not necessarily neutralise the toxin of another. On the basis of these observations at least six different toxins have been identified and labelled A, B, C, D, E and F. The preparations of purified toxin have shown that they consist of proteins. The molecular weight of type A toxin is in the order of about 1 000 000 and that of type B is about 60 000. The extremely toxic effect of type A toxin is illustrated by the fact that 1·0 mg of the purified product contains no less than approximately 40 million lethal doses of toxin for mice. Sometimes these toxins occur as prototoxins and develop into toxins from the action of trypsin or similar proteolytic enzymes. The toxins are absorbed by the small intestine but the amount absorbed is only a small proportion of the total concentration in the intestines. Botulinum toxin acts on the cholinergic nerve endings in the peripheral somatic and autonomic fibres, and does not appear to have any direct effect on the brain or spinal cord.

Epidemiology and pathogenesis

The epidemiology of botulinum intoxication emphasises the complex set of circumstances which are concerned with the likelihood of toxaemia occurring. In the first place the distribution of the organism is world-wide in soil, decaying vegetable matter, animal faeces and many other situations associated with the soil. The organism has little invasive power and when ingested, passes through the intestinal tract without producing a noticeable toxaemia or any pathological changes. It has already been noted that the toxins of *Cl. botulinum* are extremely lethal, particularly type A toxin, and it is remarkable that the incidence of botulism in animals should be as low as it is in relation to the wide distribution and the high incidence of toxigenic strains throughout the world. In this connection it is noteworthy that both toxigenic and non-toxigenic strains of *Cl. botulinum* occur, that under laboratory conditions toxigenic strains may also give rise to non-toxigenic strains but that non-toxigenic strains of type E, at least, do not produce toxigenic strains. It has also been observed that a bacteriocin (boticin E) produced by type E strains is lethal for the vegetative bacilli of toxigenic strains of that organism, and it may be that non-toxigenic bacteriocin-producing strains play an important part in the pathogenesis of botulinum infections.

Botulism can only occur within the following limited set of conditions which must be satisfied before the disease becomes apparent in animals.

(1) The disease arises from the ingestion of pre-formed toxin. *Cl. botulinum* does not usually invade the tissues and produces practically no toxin in the living body.

(2) A toxigenic strain of *Cl. botulinum* must contaminate material which is acceptable as animal foodstuff, including decomposing carcases of various animal species; and conditions must exist for the ingestion of the foodstuff containing toxin by susceptible animals.

(3) A suitable microenvironment must be present in the foodstuff to permit multiplication of *Cl. botulinum* and the production of toxin.

(4) There must be no loss or destruction of toxin from the foodstuff before being eaten.

Practically no cases of botulism in animals would occur unless these conditions were fulfilled, and it is probable that for these reasons the incidence of the disease is so low in contrast to the prevalence of the organism.

Lamsiekte is the South African name for botulism in cattle associated with type D toxin which occurs on the veldt where there is a phosphorus deficiency. Cattle which graze on these phosphorus-deficient pastures develop a depraved appetite and will eat pieces of decomposing carcases which they find lying on the veldt. If a decomposing carcase has become contaminated with a toxigenic strain of *Cl. botulinum* and has provided a suitable environment for the elaboration of toxin, cattle eating parts of that carcase containing the toxin will contract botulism. Similar forms of the disease also occur in sheep. The decomposing carcases of other animal species, including tortoises and rabbits in South Africa and Australia, respectively, have been incriminated as sources of botulinum toxin.

Forage poisoning in horses and cattle is the name given to suspected botulism arising from the ingestion of contaminated fodder or other foodstuffs.

Among poultry, the ingestion of fatal doses of botulinum toxin type C has given rise to diseases known as 'duck sickness' or 'western duck disease', limberneck in chickens and pheasants, and pseudo-limberneck or botulism among brooders. These toxaemic conditions are caused by type C toxin. With duck sickness it appears that under certain conditions infected decaying vegetation and marsh weed at the edges of lakes during periods of drought, provide a suitable environment for the production of toxin which is ingested by wild ducks. Limberneck in chickens and pheasants which derives its name from paralysis of the neck muscles, can arise from birds eating the larvae of the 'greenbottle' and other similar blowflies which have fed upon contaminated carcases. Botulism in broiler chickens can occur from pecking of litter and carcases in an environment where the earth and litter of broiler houses are contaminated with *Cl. botulinum* type C.

In mink, botulism can occur suddenly in a group of animals which has been given food contaminated with botulinum toxin. The disease is usually associated with type C but sometimes with types A and B. Foxes are usually affected by *Cl. botulinum* type E derived from fish meat but disease may also be caused by type A. They appear to be more resistant to type B.

Symptoms and lesions

In the larger domesticated animals the incubation period varies between 2–10 days but is usually not more than 6 days depending upon the dose of toxin ingested. The first symptoms are those of excitability followed by incoordination and latterly of paralysis, particularly of the hind limbs. In many cases there is paralysis of muscles in the region of the mouth, pharynx and neck, resulting in the animal being unable to swallow and the tongue protruding from the mouth. These symptoms increase in severity and are followed by coma and death.

Post-mortem examination may reveal pathological changes in the central nervous system, especially the brain stem and 3rd ventricle, catarrhal gastro-enteritis, hepatitis and nephrosis.

In poultry the main symptoms are paralysis of the wings, legs and neck, protrusion of the nictitating membrane, and in some cases birds become coma-tose and show signs of diarrhoea before recovering in 5–6 days' time.

Mink suffer from incoordination and paralysis, especially of the hind legs. The incubation period in these animals is about 1–4 days and varies according to the amount of toxin ingested.

Diagnosis

A diagnosis of botulism can only be established by detecting toxin in the suspected foodstuff, intestinal contents or serum of affected animals. It is important to remember that *Cl. botulinum* organisms are sometimes present in animal foodstuffs and unless conditions have been suitable for the production of toxin, the organisms by themselves remain harm-less. Similarly, the presence of *Cl. botulinum* in the intestinal canal, liver and other organs of animals immediately after death, is no proof that mortality was caused by these organisms because toxin production will not take place in the carcase until after the animal has been dead for some hours. Moreover, it may be difficult to differentiate between proteolytic strains of *Cl. botulinum* and *Cl. sporogenes* because of the similar cultural characteristics of the two organisms and also of the occurrence of non-toxigenic strains of *Cl. botulinum*. For these reasons, fluorescent antibody techniques have recently proved useful for differentiating between *Cl. botulinum* and other clostridial species, and especially between *Cl. botulinum* and *Cl. sporogenes* which have dissimilar somatic antigens.

The presence of toxin in a sample of material can be detected by macerating the material in saline and, if necessary, allowing to soak for several hours. The fluid should then be centrifuged and injected into a number of mice or guinea-pigs, some of which will have been protected with specific antitoxin beforehand. Similarly, the presence of toxin in serum can be detected by inoculating a sample of 0·5–1·0 ml intravenously into mice to test for lethality during the following 12–18 hours.

Control and prevention

The immunization of animals against *Cl. botulinum* toxins is not practised widely but only among particular groups which are exposed to special risks, particularly in South Africa and Australia. For example, the prevention of Lamsiekte in cattle

is attempted in South Africa by giving two injections of types C and D toxoid at an interval of several weeks, and sheep are similarly protected by one dose. Mink can be immunized against type C by giving one dose of an alum precipitated toxoid or a filtered preparation adsorbed on to calcium phosphate. Other methods for prevention concern husbandry and especially precautions to avoid the risk of foodstuffs containing preformed toxin being fed to animals.

Public health aspects

Botulism in man has been associated with a variety of foods containing toxin but which do not necessarily show any signs of spoilage. Sausage meats, hams and canned foods have sometimes been incriminated, and unsatisfactorily home-canned and preserved foodstuffs are a potential risk to human health. Type E botulism in man is almost always associated with fish or fish products.

Clostridium oedematiens

Synonyms

This organism is also known as *Clostridium novyi*.

Distribution in nature

This organism is a normal inhabitant of the soil and world-wide in its distribution. It is the cause of an infectious necrotic hepatitis in sheep and cattle known as black disease, and of gas gangrenous lesions arising from wounds. In Australia some of these infected wounds may occur around the heads and faces of rams as a result of fighting and the condition is referred to as 'big head'. *Cl. oedematiens* type D, also known as *Cl. haemolyticum*, is the cause of bacillary haemoglobinurea (red water disease) of cattle and sheep.

Morphology and staining

Cl. oedematiens is a large rod measuring approxi-mately 5–10μm in length and 1–1·5μm in width. Some strains of types B and C may be even larger, measuring 15–20μm in length. Spores are oval, situated either centrally or subterminally and distend the bacillary body. Capsules are not produced. The organism possesses peritrichous flagella and is motile under anaerobic conditions only, giving rise to a swarming type of growth.

Organisms from young cultures stain Gram-positive but after prolonged incubation many will stain Gram-negative. Sporulation occurs readily in culture, particularly if the medium contains serum. As with other clostridial species, developing spores stain darkly whereas only the outline of mature spores can be observed after staining by Gram's method.

Cultural characteristics

Cl. oedematiens is a strict anaerobe and may be difficult to grow on primary culture especially from a small inoculum. Growth on ordinary laboratory media can be enhanced by the addition of glucose or freshly prepared blood. The addition of fresh brain infusion to the medium has also been recommended for encouraging the growth of this fastidious organism. On the moist surface of solid media the organisms may develop colonial motility which becomes apparent after 3–4 days' incubation, is distinct from cellular swarming, and is characterised by the movement of daughter colonies away from larger parent colonies. This colonial movement takes place in spirals or arcs across the surface of the medium and often the daughter colonies return and fuse with the parent colony. On fresh horse blood agar the colonies are flat with irregular edges, often developing as a thin film of transparent growth. An area of haemolysis occurs initially beneath the colonies and develops into a wider zone after incubation for 48–72 hours. Only very slight haemolysis is produced on sheep blood agar. In cooked meat medium growth is slow and the meat is turned pink. Gelatin is liquefied and coagulated serum is not digested. When grown on egg-yolk medium the colonies of *Cl. oedematiens* types A, B and D produce an opalescent zone of precipitation (Nagler reaction) due to the presence of lecithinase in the gamma toxin of type A and the beta toxin of types B and D.

Fermentation of carbohydrates is variable. The great majority of strains produce acid and gas in glucose but do not ferment lactose. Many strains of types A and B ferment maltose which is not usually attacked by type D strains.

Resistance to physical and chemical agents

The spores of most strains survive heating to 95°C for 15 minutes but are killed in moist heat at a temperature of 120°C for 5 minutes. They are killed rapidly by exposure to hypochlorites but may remain viable for as long as 1 hour when exposed to 5 per cent phenol, 10 per cent formalin or 0·1 per cent merthiolate. Spores can remain viable for years in the soil or bones of dead animals.

Antigens and toxins

The somatic and flagellar antigens are not of importance for serologically identifying different strains of *Cl. oedematiens*. The species is divided into four types labelled A, B, C and D, according to the soluble antigens or toxins produced. The most important of these toxic components in relation to the aetiology of diseases are alpha, beta and gamma toxins, and their distribution among the four types of organisms is shown in Table 20.1. It will be noticed that type C is non-toxigenic and has been isolated from cases of osteomyelitis among buffaloes although not associated with the aetiology of the condition. The haemolytic activity of beta toxin is particularly active against horse and sheep cells, whereas the gamma toxin is active against horse cells but is markedly less haemolytic for sheep cells. Additional soluble antigens have been identified among different strains of *Cl. oedematiens*, including a tropomyosinase (eta toxin) from types B and D, and a lipase (epsilon toxin) produced by type A

TABLE 20.1. Showing the toxins and diseases produced by the different types of *Cl. oedematiens*.

| Type | Alternative name | Important soluble antigens | | | Animal species mainly affected | Disease |
| | | Alpha | Beta | Gamma | | |
		Lethal necrotizing	Lethal necrotizing haemolytic lecithinase	Necrotizing haemolytic lecithinase		
A	*Cl. oedematiens* (*Cl. novyi*)	+	—	+	Sheep; less frequently cattle	Gas gangrene and 'big head' in rams
B	*Cl. gigas*	+++	+	—	Sheep; less frequently cattle	Black disease (chronic hepatitis)
C	Kranefeld's bacillus *Cl. bubalorum*	—	—	—	Buffaloes	Associated with cases of osteomyelitis but not of aetiological significance
D	*Cl. haemolyticum*	—	+++	—	Cattle; less frequently sheep	Bacillary haemoglobinurea

strains which has the effect of producing an iridescent film (pearly layer) when the culture is grown on egg yolk medium. Delta and zeta toxins are haemolytic and produced by types A and G, respectively, and the theta toxin of type D is a lipase.

Epidemiology and pathogenesis

Cl. oedematiens can be the cause of gas gangrenous conditions in a variety of animal species, particularly horses, cattle, sheep, goats, pigs and laboratory animals. As a normal inhabitant of the soil and frequently present in the intestines of herbivores, the organism may become implanted in contaminated surface wounds on the skin and less frequently is associated with intestinal infections. Infected surface wounds develop as localised gas gangrenous lesions which may resemble infection with *Cl. septicum* and can only be differentiated by isolation and identification of the causal organism. This type of wound infection is more prevalent in areas or districts where there is a high incidence of the organism in soil and animal faeces in which it can remain viable for as long as one year; and such cases have been reported in cattle in the United Kingdom. Similar disease in pigs associated with intestinal infections occurs rarely.

A condition known as 'big head' in Australian sheep develops from wounds on the faces and heads of rams which have been fighting. These superficial wounds become infected with *Cl. oedematiens* type A, and the subsequent development of gas gangrenous lesions gives rise to severe localised swellings and death from toxaemia. The alpha toxin is responsible for the production of severe gelatinous oedema in the lesions and for the death of the animals.

Black disease is the name given to a condition of chronic hepatitis in sheep, occurring less frequently in cattle, which arises commonly in fluke infested areas in several countries, particularly Australia, New Zealand, the United Kingdom and some other European countries and the U.S.A. *Cl. oedematiens* is normally present in the soil, in the intestines of herbivores, and is often latently present as spores in the livers of healthy sheep and cattle in areas where black disease is endemic as well as in districts where the disease seldom arises. Black disease invariably develops in fluke infested areas, and the pathogenesis of the disease is related to the migration of immature flukes through the liver and the consequent inflammatory responses which provide a suitable environment for the growth of *Cl. oedematiens* already present in the tissues. The spores then develop into vegetative forms, the organisms multiply, produce large quantities of alpha toxin and the animal dies from a toxaemia. Occasionally, cases of infection with *Cl. oedematiens* type B occur in the absence of fluke infestations, and it seems probable that other causes of liver damage can also provide a suitable microenvironment for the stimulation of a latent infection and the consequent production of a toxaemia.

Bacillary haemoglubinurea, caused by *Cl. oedematiens* type D, occurs mainly in cattle and rarely in sheep. The epidemiology and pathogenesis of this disease are very similar to black disease, since the aetiology is related to the presence of bacterial spores in the liver which are provided with a suitable microenvironment to germinate and produce large quantities of beta toxin as the result of liver damage produced by infestation with liver flukes. These essential predisposing factors which exist in damp, fluke-infested grazing areas, give rise to disease most frequently in western areas of the U.S.A., in South America, and rarely in the United Kingdom.

Symptoms

The condition of 'big head' in sheep can be observed as a rapidly swelling gas gangrenous lesion around the face and head, followed by collapse and death of the animal. The mortality rate in susceptible animals is high and may be more than 90 per cent of cases.

Black disease is an acute toxaemia which results in the sudden death of animals after a brief period of symptoms. The first signs of disease are a rapidly decreasing ability to move, unsteady gait and collapse. The body temperature will be several degrees above normal and death may occur suddenly.

Bacillary haemoglobinurea usually occurs in the summer months and severely affected animals suffer from fever, abdominal pain, diarrhoea, sometimes dysentery and haemoglobinurea. The mortality rate may be as high as 90 per cent or more.

Lesions

In the carcases of animals which have died from black disease the most significant lesions are a number of clearly defined necrotic areas in the liver, several centimetres in diameter, usually superficial but occasionally situated within the substance of the organ. These lesions consist of a central core of necrosis surrounded by a zone of leucocytes in which are felt-like masses of *Cl. oedematiens*. If the animal has been dead for several hours many of the bacteria will have sporulated. In addition to these liver lesions there will be extensive subcutaneous and blood stained oedema which gives a dark colour to the carcase, and hence the name black disease. Straw coloured exudate will be present in both the pericardial and peritoneal cavities. Often there are areas of congestion in the duodenum and abomasum.

The most characteristic lesions occurring in bacillary haemoglobinurea are a number of anaemic infarcts in the liver arising from thrombosis of a branch of the portal vein. These infarcts are slightly raised, lighter in colour than the normal liver tissue, and may be several centimeters in diameter. Surrounding a central area of necrosis is a zone of leucocytes mixed with large numbers of rod-shaped *Cl. oedematiens*, many of them containing spores. Often there is a severe haemorrhagic enteritis with blood stained intestinal contents and dark coloured urine in the bladder. In addition, there will be marked icterus of the carcase, widespread oedema and haemorrhages in the myocardium.

Diagnosis

The history and lesions may be strongly suggestive of infection with *Cl. oedematiens*, and a final diagnosis will depend upon isolation of the organism which can also be identified in livers by immunofluorescence techniques. *Cl. oedematiens* can always be isolated from the liver but less frequently from other tissues of carcases affected with black disease. From cases of bacillary haemoglobinurea the causal organism can be isolated from the liver and often from other tissues.

It is advisable to carry out bacteriological examinations as soon after death as possible to reduce to a minimum the contamination of tissues with putrefactive bacteria. Direct smears from the periphery of liver lesions, stained by Gram's method, will show numbers of large Gram-positive bacilli with subterminal spores. Primary cultures can be made on blood agar, egg yolk agar to show the Nagler reaction, and in cooked meat medium. It is important to remember that the organism is a strict anaerobe and that it is often difficult to grow from a primary inoculum. For example, fluid medium may require an inoculum consisting of a piece of affected tissue emulsified in broth or 3–5 ml of exudate, in order to obtain satisfactory growth. After inoculation, the culture should be heated to 65°C for 15 minutes to kill vegetative contaminating bacteria, and following incubation anaerobically at 37°C for 24–48 hours, cultures are plated on solid media, incubated and examined for the growth characteristics of *Cl. oedematiens*. Inoculation into mice of the toxin produced in broth cultures after 48 hours' incubation causes very extensive subcutaneous oedema followed by death. Guinea-pigs are similarly susceptible to the toxin.

Control and prevention

Animals can be actively immunized against infection with *Cl. oedematiens* by using formalised whole cultures adsorbed on to aluminium hydroxide. At least two doses of vaccine may be required to stimulate a strong immunity which will last for at least one year. Vaccination is usually carried out in late summer in the United Kingdom. In addition, for the prevention of black disease and bacillary

haemoglobinurea every effort should be made to prevent animals from becoming infected with liver flukes.

Outbreaks of disease may be controlled by the prompt injection of hyperimmune sera.

Public health aspects

Cl. oedematiens type A is a cause of gas gangrene in man.

Clostridium septicum

Synonyms

Clostridium septicum was the first pathogenic clostridial species to be identified and was originally named *Vibrion septique* by Pasteur and Joubert in 1877. It was also named *Bacillus oedematis maligni* because of its association with a type of lesion originally described as malignant oedema but which is now usually termed gas gangrene. The characteristic properties of *Cl. septicum* are so similar to those of *Cl. chauvoei* that both species have been described recently as two types of a single species. Thus, *Cl. septicum* has been named as *Cl. chauvoei* type A and *Cl. chauvoei* as *Cl. chauvoei* type B.

Distribution in nature

Cl. septicum is a normal inhabitant of the soil and is frequently present in the faeces of herbivores and other animal species. It is associated with a condition known as braxy (or bradshot) in sheep and is the cause of a small proportion of blackquarter cases in cattle and sheep, as well as gas gangrenous infections arising from wounds in both animals and man.

Morphology and staining

Cl. septicum is a large rod-shaped organism measuring approximately 2–10 μm in length and 0·4–1·0 μm in width, with parallel sides and rounded ends. Sometimes it develops in the form of short or long filaments which are slightly curved, and this appearance is often seen in smears prepared from the livers of experimentally infected guinea-pigs (Plate 20.1c, facing p. 216). This characteristic shape may be of value in differentiating the organism from *Cl. chauvoei* which does not produce such marked filamentous forms. In naturally infected tissues it often develops into a variety of pleomorphic forms including cigar-shaped rods, swollen forms, citron forms with swollen centres and pointed extremities, sporulating bacilli and free spores. In these respects the organism is morphologically similar to *Cl. chauvoei*. *Cl. septicum* sporulates readily and the spores are oval, wider than the diameter of the bacillus and situated centrally or subterminally (Plate 20.1d, facing p. 216). The organism has peritrichous flagella and young cultures are actively motile. Capsules are not formed.

Cl. septicum stains Gram-positive when cultures are young and actively growing, but after 3–4 days' incubation many organisms will decolourise readily and a number will stain frankly Gram-negative. Developing spores stain darkly but only the outline of mature spores can be seen after staining by Gram's method. Pleomorphic forms stain irregularly and denser at one or both poles compared with the central area of the organism.

Cultural characteristics

Cl. septicum is a strict anaerobe. The optimum temperature is 37°C for growth on ordinary laboratory media which is enhanced in the presence of glucose. On the surface of solid media the colonies initially appear semi-transparent and rounded, but they soon become considerably larger, greyish-white in colour with irregular filamentous edges. On a moist surface this filamentous type of growth will spread over the entire surface of the medium and may be difficult to observe without careful examination. On horse blood agar the organism produces haemolysis. In cooked meat broth the meat is turned pink, there is no digestion and the culture has a rancid odour. Coagulated serum is not digested but gelatin is liquefied after 5–7 days' incubation. In litmus milk, acid and gas are produced but the so-called 'stormy fermentation' associated with some cultures of *Cl. welchii* is not so marked. The milk is clotted after 4–5 days' incubation.

Acid and gas are produced in glucose, lactose, maltose, and salicin. Mannitol and sucrose are not fermented. The reactions in salicin and sucrose are sometimes useful properties for differentiating between *Cl. septicum* and *Cl. chauvoei* but variants of both species do occur which give atypical fermentation reactions.

Resistance to physical and chemical agents

Probably similar to *Cl. chauvoei* but the details have not been recorded.

Antigens and toxins

Cl. septicum produces a variety of antigens enabling strains of the organism to be divided into six groups on the basis of two somatic and five flagellar antigens. The close antigenic relationship between *Cl. septicum* and *Cl. chauvoei* has been demonstrated by the presence of a common spore antigen produced by both species.

Cl. septicum produces four separate toxic components which have been labelled alpha, beta, gamma and delta toxins. The most important is alpha toxin which is lethal, necrotizing and also contains an oxygen-stable haemolysin; the beta toxin contains deoxyribonuclease and is toxic to leucocytes; the gamma toxin is a hyaluronidase, and the delta toxin is an oxygen-labile haemolysin antigenically related to streptolysin O and is also necrotizing. In addition, a thermolabile haemagglutinin for cattle, sheep and chicken red cells is produced and a fibrinolysin has been identified in culture filtrates.

Epidemiology and pathogenesis

Braxy in sheep is a characteristic infection of the abomasum and occurs particularly in the United Kingdom, Scandinavia and Iceland. The incidence of the disease is highest on farms in mountainous districts and among yearling sheep which are wintered on either hill pastures or old lowland grazings. The organism can remain viable in faeces for as long as 1 year. These conditions seem to provide the ideal factors which give rise to the rapid multiplication of *Cl. septicum* in the mucosa and submucosa of the abomasum. The precise conditions of the microenvironment which favour the growth of the organism in this area of the body are unknown and, moreover, it has never been established beyond doubt that *Cl. septicum* is the sole cause of the disease, since the condition has not been reproduced under experimental conditions. In view of the success in preventing the disease by specific immunization against *Cl. septicum* it would seem that the organism probably is the true cause of the disease, and that failure to reproduce it experimentally is due to a lack of knowledge about the predisposing factors, particularly those related to the microenvironment in the wall of the stomach which promotes the sudden multiplication of an organism which is a normal inhabitant of the intestines.

Some cases of blackquarter in cattle and sheep have been associated with *Cl. septicum* or with a mixed infection of both *Cl. septicum* and *Cl. chauvoei*. The epidemiology and pathogenesis of these infections are similar to those described for blackquarter caused by *Cl. chauvoei* and are not usually related to wound infections. However, wounds can become infected with *Cl. septicum*, causing the development of a gas gangrenous lesion often referred to as malignant oedema. Similar lesions of gas gangrene can occur in pigs.

Cl. septicum is pathogenic for laboratory animals, particularly guinea-pigs, mice, rabbits and pigeons. Following intramuscular inoculation of an actively growing culture into the thigh of a guinea-pig, the animal will die in 24–48 hours with an extensive oedematous lesion of the flank and abdomen with gas in the tissues. The organisms can be readily observed in smears from the lesion, heart blood and from the liver where they frequently occur in chains and filaments.

Symptoms

Braxy usually occurs in good conditioned yearling sheep. The affected animal becomes separated from the flock, loses its appetite and shows signs of abdominal pain for a period of a few hours before dying suddenly.

Infected wounds which become gas gangrenous are swollen and typically oedematous. When the skin over the centre of the lesion is rubbed with the fingers there is crepitation due to the gas produced subcutaneously by the organism.

The symptoms of blackquarter caused by *Cl. septicum* are similar to those associated with *Cl. chauvoei* infections.

Lesions

The characteristic lesion of braxy is an area of haemorrhagic inflammation in the wall of the abomasum. Histological examination of the fresh carcase reveals a mass of filamentous forms of *Cl. septicum* which have penetrated through the mucosa into the submucosa. In addition, there is usually an excessive quantity of blood-stained fluid in the peritoneal cavity.

Lesions of blackquarter are similar to those produced by *Cl. chauvoei*, and wound infections causing gas gangrene consist of a characteristic clostridial myonecrosis.

Diagnosis

Braxy may be suspected when sudden deaths occur among yearling sheep on hill or old pastures during the autumn and winter. An area of inflammation in the wall of the abomasum is also strongly indicative of the disease. Stained smears prepared from the surfaces of fresh lesions will reveal large numbers of *Cl. septicum* occurring as rods or filaments and staining Gram-positive. An additional and useful diagnostic method, particularly for differentiating the organism from *Cl. chauvoei*, is the fluorescent antibody technique using specific antisera conjugated with a fluorescent dye for microscopical examination under ultraviolet light of smears or frozen sections of tissue. It is important to remember that the carcase of an animal which has died from braxy will decompose rapidly and diagnosis becomes more difficult the longer a post-mortem examination is delayed after death. Similar methods are used for the diagnosis of blackquarter and gas gangrenous wound infections.

Control and prevention

Braxy can be controlled to a large extent by wintering sheep on new lowland pastures. Sheep can be effectively immunized against the disease and the vaccine is prepared in the same manner as a *Cl. chauvoei* vaccine and sometimes mixed with it in a multicomponent inoculum with other clostridial vaccines.

Penicillin alone or with hyperimmune antiserum can be used to treat infections with *Cl. septicum* if commenced promptly, but in practice the course of infection is so rapid that treatment is generally of no practical value.

Public health aspects

Cl. septicum is a cause of gas gangrene in man.

Clostridium chauvoei

Synonyms

Cl. chauvoei, sometimes referred to as *Cl. feseri*, has characteristic properties so similar to *Cl. septicum* that both organisms have been considered as two types of a single species. Thus, *Cl. chauvoei* has been named as *Cl. chauvoei* type B and *Cl. septicum* as *Cl. chauvoei* type A.

Distribution in nature

Cl. chauvoei is the common cause of a gas gangrenous condition known as blackquarter or blackleg which occurs in cattle and sheep and very occasionally in other animal species. Less frequently, other clostridial species have been incriminated as the aetiological agents of blackquarter, including *Cl. septicum, Cl. oedematiens* and *Cl. welchii*. The name blackquarter or blackleg is descriptive of the lesions in muscle which develop as dark and almost black coloured crepitant areas of infected tissue usually occurring in the area of the hind quarters.

The organism is world-wide in its distribution in soil and pastures where its incidence may be particularly high in certain districts or even in particular fields in which the annual occurrence of disease may be noticeably greater than in neighbouring areas.

Morphology and staining

The organism is rod-shaped with rounded ends, measuring about 3–8 μm in length and 0·5 μm in width and sometimes developing in a variety of pleomorphic forms, particularly as large cigar-shaped rods and as citron forms (Plate 20.1e, opposite). *Cl. chauvoei* stains Gram-positive in tissues and fresh cultures but has a tendency to stain Gram-negative when subcultured on laboratory media. Pleomorphic forms stain unevenly by Gram's method and sometimes only one pole of the organism will stain Gram-positive. Capsules are not formed but the bacilli have peritrichous flagella and are motile. Occasional non-motile variants occur. Spores are produced which are oval, wider than the bacillus and situated either centrally or subterminally. Mature spores do not stain by Gram's method.

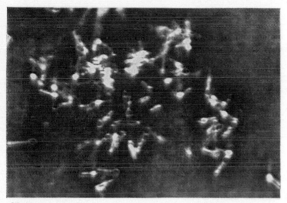

20.1a

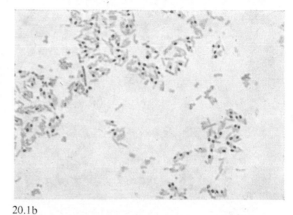

20.1b

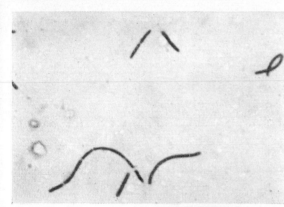

20.1c

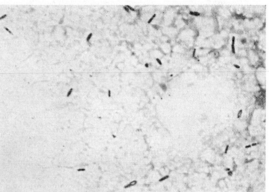

20.1d

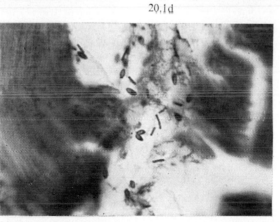

20.1e

20.1a Film of *Clostridium tetani* stained with strong carbol fuchsin and nigrosin showing spherical terminal spores, ×930.

20.1b Film of *Clostridium botulinum* stained by modified Ziehl-Neelsen method showing oval terminal and sub-terminal spores, ×930.

20.1c Gram-stained film from guinea-pig liver showing filamentous form of *Clostridium septicum*, ×930.

20.1d Gram-stained film of *Clostridium septicum* showing bacilli and unstained mature spores, ×930.

20.1e Gram-stained film from muscle showing *Clostridium chauvoei* occurring as rods, citron forms and developing spores, ×930.

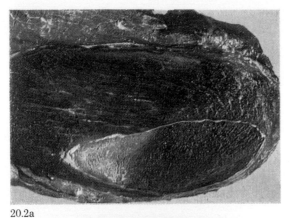

20.2a

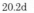

20.2b

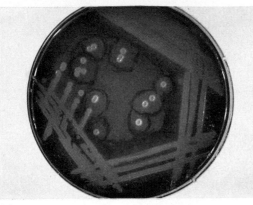

20.2c

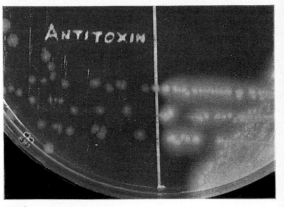

20.2d

20.2a Section of muscle showing blackquarter lesion caused by *Clostridium chauvoei*. The muscle is dark red in colour, dry and filled with small bubbles of gas.

20.2c Colonies of *Clostridium welchii* on blood agar showing narrow zones of complete haemolysis and wider zones of partial haemolysis.

20.2b Gram-stained film of *Clostridium welchii*. Note the absence of spores, × 930.

20.2d Nagler reaction showing opalescence on egg yolk medium produced by lecithinase of *Clostridium welchii* (right) and inhibition of the reaction by antitoxin (left).

Cultural characteristics

Cl. chauvoei is a strict anaerobe and growth is poor on ordinary laboratory media but enhanced by the addition of liver extract or glucose. The optimum temperature for growth is 37°C. On blood agar the whitish grey colonies have irregular edges, develop to about 2–4 mm in diameter and are surrounded by a zone of haemolysis. Growth in cooked meat broth is slow and the organism may show marked pleomorphism. The meat is turned pink and the culture has a sour odour. *Cl. chauvoei* ferments glucose, lactose, sucrose and maltose with production of acid and gas, but most strains do not ferment salicin (cf. *Cl. septicum*).

Resistance to physical and chemical agents

Spores of *Cl. chauvoei* are killed by steam in 40–50 minutes and in 20 minutes when autoclaved at 120°C. It has also been claimed that the spores are susceptible to 3 per cent formalin for 15 minutes.

Antigens and toxins

All strains of *Cl. chauvoei* have one common somatic antigen, but the organisms are divisible into two groups on the basis of their flagellar antigens. The organisms share a common spore antigen with *Cl. septicum*.

The supernatant from a broth culture of *Cl. chauvoei* contains toxin, particularly after growth in glucose broth to which has been added calcium carbonate to neutralise the acid produced. The properties of the toxic components include an oxygen-stable haemolysin (alpha toxin) for cattle, sheep and pig erythrocytes but not for those of horses or guinea-pigs. The alpha toxin is also a neurotoxin and causes dermonecrosis and fibrinolysis. The other toxic components are deoxyribonuclease (beta toxin), hyaluronidase (gamma toxin) and an oxygen-labile haemolysin (delta toxin).

The toxin is lethal for mice and guinea-pigs when given intravenously in sufficiently large doses. Rabbits show a marked resistance to the lethal effect of the toxin. These facts emphasise the low rate of lethality of this toxin compared with those of many other clostridial species, and underline the difficulty of carrying out neutralization tests and attempting to identify antigenic differences between the toxins of various strains.

Epidemiology and pathogenesis

The occurrence of blackquarter in cattle is associated with permanent pastures and it is a notable feature of the disease that the annual incidence among non-immunized animals in a particular district may be markedly higher than among similar cattle in a neighbouring district. The frequency of the disease is seasonal with the highest peak occurring during the summer months and it may be that animals at pasture during the spring and summer tend to increase the incidence of the organism in the soil. Although it has been suggested that infection of cattle arises from wounds contaminated with the organism, there are seldom any visible superficial wounds on the bodies of affected animals. It is probable that infection occurs from the ingestion of the organism and that these ingested bacteria remain as dormant spores in the tissues until predisposing factors arise which stimulate the development of vegetative forms and the rapid multiplication of the bacilli in a particular area of the tissues. This is commonly in the muscles of the hind- or fore-quarters. Evidence in support of this theory has been the demonstration that spores can be inoculated and left in the tissues for some 40 days without causing any noticeable effect. At the end of that time the injection of calcium chloride will activate the dormant spores and cause the development of a blackquarter lesion. The two interesting features are that an injection of washed spores alone, does not set up the disease, and the subsequent inoculation of any substance which damages tissue cells provides the trigger mechanism for stimulating the multiplication of the organisms and the development of a typical blackquarter lesion.

The incidence of blackquarter in sheep increases among animals grouped together in paddocks and fields which are heavily grazed, and may be the result of a higher frequency of oral infection among sheep kept under these conditions. However, it is more common for the disease in sheep to be related to a definite history of wounds and trauma associated with lambing, docking, castration, shearing or sometimes from inoculations.

Cl. chauvoei causes disease in guinea-pigs, mice and pigeons but is less virulent than *Cl. septicum*.

Symptoms

In cattle the disease usually occurs in younger animals of 6 months to about 2–3 years of age which are in good condition. These factors together with the occurrence of acute illness on pastures associated with a history of *Cl. chauvoei* infection may be suggestive of blackquarter. Sometimes animals are found dead without any premonitory symptoms having been observed. The most obvious sign is a crepitant swelling particularly in the hind- or fore-quarter, which crackles when rubbed with the fingers as a result of large quantities of gas produced subcutaneously by the organism. The fevered animal will be lame and the muscles in the affected region will show trembling and sometimes violent twitching. Death usually occurs suddenly and often within 24 hours of the symptoms first being observed.

In sheep an acute febrile condition develops within

1–2 days following an injury, and a typical black-quarter lesion can be observed near the site. In the case of ewes which have recently lambed, the lesion develops in the region of the perineum which becomes swollen and dark red in colour. Death occurs suddenly.

Lesions

In the central part of the lesion there is usually a well defined area of muscle which is dark red in colour, dry, necrotic and filled with small gas bubbles which give a swollen appearance to the muscle (Plate 20.2a, facing p. 217). The lesion has a characteristic rancid odour similar to that produced by cultures of *Cl. chauvoei* growing in cooked meat broth medium. Surrounding this central area the muscle becomes pinker and there is a variable amount of either yellow or blood stained oedematous fluid which is particularly obvious in the local connective tissue. Perineal lesions in ewes which have recently lambed include necrosis of the vaginal mucosa and skin, and extensive oedema often involving the hind limbs and thigh muscles which are swollen and dark in colour.

Diagnosis

The history of the disease and the symptoms may be strongly suggestive of blackquarter but the final diagnosis must depend upon the detection of the causal organism. *Cl. chauvoei* can be readily demonstrated in films prepared from the lesion and from the oedematous fluid. Most organisms will appear as Gram-positive rods when examined immediately following death of the animal, but after several hours the lesion will contain a greater preponderance of spores and pleomorphic forms.

In many cases the infection becomes septicaemic shortly before death and in a fresh carcase the organism can be cultured not only from the centre of the lesion and oedematous fluid but also from heart blood, liver and spleen. It is more difficult to obtain pure cultures from carcases which have been dead for several hours because of contamination with other anaerobic species, and in these cases the bone marrow may be a more satisfactory site from which to make a primary culture. Cultures of the organism can be examined for the characteristic properties of *Cl. chauvoei*. In addition, broth cultures or oedematous fluid from the lesion can be tested for toxicity and specific neutralization by antitoxin in mice or guinea-pigs.

When diagnosing blackquarter it may be important to be able to differentiate between *Cl. chauvoei* and *Cl. septicum* infections since the latter are occasionally associated with this type of condition. The morphology of *Cl. chauvoei* is usually more pleomorphic than *Cl. septicum* which appears as Gram-positive rods often occurring in chains of varying lengths. A more reliable differentiation between the two species can be made by using fluorescent antibody techniques. Antisera prepared against the bacilli of each species and labelled with fluorescein isothiocyanate or lissamine rhodamine are applied for 30 minutes to acetone-fixed smears or frozen sections of the lesion. The preparations are then examined by ultra violet light. Only *Cl. chauvoei* or *Cl. septicum* organisms in the preparation will fluoresce after applying the appropriate homologous antiserum. This is also a useful technique for diagnosing *Cl. chauvoei* infection in a carcase which has been dead for several hours when smears may contain a variety of other bacterial species. The technique has the additional advantage of providing a diagnosis more quickly than by other methods.

Control and prevention

Active immunization of animals to prevent blackquarter infection has proved to be of economic value, although there are difficulties in the standardization of vaccines on account of the low degree of lethality of the toxin produced by *Cl. chauvoei*. The most reliable results are obtained from using a formalised alum precipitated whole culture which confers an immunity against the bacteria as well as the toxin. Although the immunity derived from this vaccine may not be particularly strong it is adequate to protect animals exposed to infection under natural conditions and is preferable to an alum precipitated toxoid. It is now common practice to vaccinate animals before they are turned out to pasture in the spring and summer, and sheep are inoculated before lambing. For economic reasons it is usual to employ a multicomponent vaccine containing products from a variety of clostridial species in addition to *Cl. chauvoei*. These may include *Cl. septicum, Cl. welchii* type D and *Cl. tetani*. A stronger immunity is stimulated by two doses of vaccine instead of one, and a time interval of at least 2–3 weeks should occur between each dose of vaccine. On sheep farms the first dose of vaccine is often given in the autumn and the second dose a few weeks before lambing.

Hyperimmune serum can be prepared in horses but is not widely used for economic reasons. Moreover, the rapidity with which blackquarter develops often results in it being impossible to inoculate hyperimmune serum in time to save the life of the animal. Nevertheless, passive immunization has sometimes been used to advantage to control explosive outbreaks.

Cl. chauvoei is susceptible to penicillin which can be used for treatment when given promptly and inoculated into the site of the lesion or used in conjunction with hyperimmune serum. Oxytetracycline and chlortetracycline can also be employed effectively provided that they are given during the early stages of the disease.

Public health aspects
Cl. chauvoei does not cause disease in man.

Clostridium welchii

Synonyms
This organism is also known as *Clostridium perfringens*.

Distribution in nature
Cl. welchii was originally isolated by Welch and Nuttal in 1892 from a decomposing human cadaver. It is a common cause of gas gangrene in man and of a number of enterotoxaemic infections in sheep and less frequently in other animal species. Strains of *Cl. welchii* produce a variety of toxins which can be identified individually by neutralization tests. On the basis of toxin production these organisms are classified as types A, B, C, D or E and Table 20.2 summarises the toxins associated with the major diseases caused by each of these types. There are references in the literature to type F strains causing disease in man and rarely in animals. Since these strains differ from type C strains only in some of their minor toxins and not in their major lethal toxins, type F strains are referred to as type C.

Cl. welchii is present in the soil and in the intestines of healthy animals and man. Disease occurs when these intestinal organisms begin to multiply unusually rapidly and produce toxin, but little is known about the conditions which provide a suitable microenvironment for this to take place.

Morphology and staining
Cl. welchii is a rod-shaped organism varying in size from about 2–6 μm in length and 0·8–1·5 μm. in width (Plate 20.2b, facing p. 217). In carbohydrate media the bacilli may be shorter in length. The organisms usually occur either singly, in pairs and occasionally in short chains. In smears prepared from infected tissues, distinct capsules may often be observed surrounding the bacilli, and capsulated strains tend to produce colonies on solid media which are smoother and more mucoid than those of non-capsulated strains. *Cl. welchii* is non-motile. Spores, which are rarely produced in culture media or pathological material, are oval, central or subterminal and usually distend the sides of the bacillus.

Young cultures stain uniformly Gram-positive but in older cultures many organisms may appear granular and some will stain Gram-negative.

Cultural characteristics
Although *Cl. welchii* is an anaerobe it does not require such strict anaerobic conditions for growth as many other clostridial species. The organism will grow well on ordinary laboratory media within a temperature range between 37–47°C, the optimum being 43–47°C, and growth is enhanced in the presence of glucose or blood. On the surface of solid media the colonies of young cultures are round, 2–3 mm in diameter, smooth, evenly convex and opaque. Occasionally mucoid variants occur. Old laboratory strains sometimes develop as rough, relatively large, flat colonies with irregular edges. On blood agar the round colonies of smooth strains are surrounded by a narrow zone of complete haemolysis and a wider zone of partial haemolysis (Plate 20.2c, facing p. 217). Haemolysis is produced by the alpha, delta and theta toxins and the extent of the haemolytic reaction depends upon the amount of haemolytic toxin produced and the species of red cell incorporated in the medium. Sheep and ox cells are the most satisfactory. In addition, haemolytic zones may improve after incubation of the culture has been completed and during subsequent storage at lower temperatures. In cooked meat medium the meat becomes pink and is not digested. Gelatin is liquefied by the kappa and lambda toxins but coagulated serum is not liquefied. When grown on media containing human serum or filtered egg yolk, *Cl. welchii* produces a marked opalescence caused by alpha toxin (lecithinase) and referred to as the Nagler or lecithinase reaction (Plate 20.2d, facing p. 217).

Cl. welchii produces acid and gas in glucose, lactose, sucrose and maltose. In litmus milk there is acid and clot formation with a large amount of gas production which breaks up the clot to produce the 'stormy clot' reaction which is characteristic for many but not all strains of *Cl. welchii*.

Enterotoxaemic infections are characterised by the presence of very large numbers of *Cl. welchii* in the intestines of diseased animals and this feature can be of diagnostic value. Smears prepared immediately after death from intestinal contents or from lesions in the wall of the intestine and stained by Gram's method, will show abnormally large numbers of *Cl. welchii*.

For the isolation of *Cl. welchii* from a fresh sample of heavily infected material, a loopful of intestinal contents should be inoculated on to blood agar and incubated anaerobically for 24–48 hours. An almost pure culture of *Cl. welchii* will develop. Alternatively, a loopful of intestinal contents should be inoculated into cooked meat broth which has been heated previously in a water bath at 100°C to reduce free oxygen, and then cooled to 37°C. A characteristic feature of *Cl. welchii* is the high rate of growth and production of large quantities of gas. After a few hours' incubation, bubbles of gas will be seen rising

TABLE 20.2. Showing the various toxins of *Cl. welchii* associated with diseases.

Type	Occurrence	Toxic and enzymic substances produced by *Cl. welchii*											
		α Alpha — Lethal necrotizing Lecithinase Haemolytic	β Beta — Lethal necrotizing (destroyed by trypsin)	γ Gamma — Lethal	δ Delta — Lethal Haemolytic	ε Epsilon — Lethal necrotizing (activated by trypsin)	η Eta — Lethal (doubtful)	θ Theta — Lethal Haemolytic (O_2-labile)	ι Iota — Lethal necrotizing (activated by trypsin)	κ Kappa — Collagenase Gelatinase lethal necrotizing	λ Lamda — Proteinase	μ Mu — Hyaluronidase	ν Nu — Deoxyribonuclease
A	Gas gangrene (man). Intestinal commensal (man and animals). Soil	+++	−	−	−	−	±	+	−	+	−	±	+
B	Food poisoning (man)	+++	−	+	−	−	−	±	−	+	−	±	+++
	Lamb dysentery	+++	+++	++	±	++	−	++	−	−	+++	++	+++
	Haemorrhagic enteritis of sheep and goats (Iran)	+++	+++	−		++		++	−	++			++
C	'Struck' in sheep	+++	+++	+	++	−	−	++	−	+++	−	−	++
	Enteritis in lambs, calves and piglets	+++	+++	−		−	−	++	−	++	−	+	++
D	Enteritis necroticans (man). Enterotoxaemia of sheep and pulpy kidney disease	+++	+	++	−	−	−	−	−	−	+	+	+++
		+++	−	−	−	+++	−	++	−	++	++	±	++
E	Enterotoxaemia in lambs and calves	+++	−	−	−	−	−	+	+++	++	+	±	+

+++ = produced by all strains ++ = produced by most strains + = produced by some strains ± = produced by very few strains.
− = production of large amounts of toxin. Alpha, beta, epsilon and iota are the major lethal toxins.

▢ = production of large amounts of toxin.

from the base of the medium. A loopful of the culture should then be sown on to blood agar and incubated anaerobically. The rapid growth of *Cl. welchii* in the meat broth will have swamped other bacterial species and the subsequent culture on blood agar will yield practically a pure growth of *Cl. welchii*.

Resistance to physical and chemical agents

The spores of most strains of *Cl. welchii* are not highly resistant to heat and are killed by boiling for 5 minutes. In contrast, the spores of some strains of type A associated with human food poisoning and some strains of type C are highly resistant to heat and will survive a temperature of 100°C for more than 1 hour.

Antigens and toxins

Cl. welchii possess somatic antigens and a capsular polysaccharide antigen which are not of major importance for the identification of different strains. The recent introduction of fluorescent antibody techniques has been applied to the recognition of *Cl. welchii*, but owing to the serological heterogeneity of this group of organisms the method will probably not become reliable for the routine diagnosis of infection with these bacteria.

Cl. welchii produce a variety of toxic and enzymic substances which have been studied in detail because of their importance in relation to the identification of strains and the pathogenesis of disease. Table 20.2

isolated from cases of human enteritis necroticans, which used to be classified as type F on account of their lack of production of theta, kappa and mu toxins, are included in type C since their major lethal toxins (i.e. alpha, beta and gamma) correspond closely to this latter group. The important properties of the toxins and enzymes are described in Table 20.2.

Alpha toxin

This is a major lethal toxin which is an enzyme, lecithinase C, produced by all types of *Cl. welchii* and in large amounts by type A strains. It is relatively heat-stable and is a highly lethal toxin which causes the development of a yellowish-green area of necrosis surrounded by a zone of congestion after intradermal inoculation.

In the presence of free Ca and Mg ions it can split lipoprotein complexes in serum or egg yolk media causing opalescence (Nagler reaction). The lecithinase toxin produces haemolysis of many species of red blood cells except those from horses and goats, by its action on phospholipid constituents. However, it is the theta toxin of type A strains which causes the typical clear zones of haemolysis.

Beta toxin

A major lethal and necrotizing toxin produced by *Cl. welchii* types B and C which is absorbed from the intestinal tract. When inoculated intradermally, the toxin from type C produces a well defined

TABLE 20.3. Showing the neutralization reactions which occur between *Cl. welchii* toxins and antitoxins.

Type	Cl. welchii Major lethal toxins	A	B	C	D	E
A	Alpha	+	+	+	+	+
B	Alpha, beta, epsilon	—	+	—	+	+
C	Alpha, beta	—	+	+	—	—
D	Alpha, epsilon	—	+	—	+	—
E	Alpha, iota	—	—	—	—	+

+ = neutralization of toxin.
— = no neutralization of toxin.

shows the various toxins produced by each type of *Cl. welchii* and emphasises the variations which can occur both quantitatively and qualitatively between different types and also between different strains within a particular type. For example, strains of type B isolated from cases of haemorrhagic enteritis in sheep and goats from Iran differed from the classical lamb dysentery strains by producing collagenase (kappa toxin) but not proteinase (lambda toxin) or hyaluronidase (mu toxin). Strains of *Cl. welchii*

purplish, circular necrotic lesion and that from type B produces a more diffuse and irregular lesion due to the co-existence of hyaluronidase (mu toxin) with the beta toxin of these latter strains. The beta toxin is destroyed by trypsin compared with epsilon and iota toxins which are also dermonecrotic but are activated by trypsin.

Gamma toxin

A minor lethal toxin produced by types B and C.

Delta toxin

A lethal toxin and haemolytic for red blood cells of cattle, sheep, goats and pigs, produced characteristically by type C strains isolated from cases of 'struck' in sheep.

Epsilon toxin

A major lethal and necrotising inert heat-stable prototoxin produced by types B and D, which is activated by trypsin at an alkaline pH to become a heat-stable toxin, (cf. iota toxin). It is absorbed from the intestinal tract and under natural conditions may become auto-activated by kappa and lambda toxins produced by the organisms, themselves.

Eta toxin

A minor lethal toxin produced by some strains of type A.

Theta toxin

A lethal heat-labile haemolytic toxin produced by all types of Cl. welchii isolated from diseased animals. The haemolysin is oxygen-labile and acts on the red blood cells from horses, cattle, sheep and rabbits. The toxin adsorbs on to meat and when grown for toxin assay, the organisms should not be cultured in cooked meat broth. Theta toxin can be produced in the absence of alpha toxin in a peptone-salt-beef-extract medium at pH 7·5. Addition of glucose to the medium causes increased production of theta but also allows development of alpha toxin.

Iota toxin

A major lethal and necrotizing inert prototoxin produced by type E strains of Cl. welchii, which is activated by trypsin at an alkaline pH and becomes a heat-labile toxin (cf. epsilon toxin). It can become auto-activated by lambda toxin produced by the organisms, themselves. Iota toxin is absorbed from the intestinal tract and causes an increase in capillary permeability.

Kappa toxin

A collagenase which attacks collagen, hide powder and gelatin. It is a proteolytic enzyme which specifically attacks collagen fibres of muscle and leaves the myofibrils intact.

Lambda toxin

A proteinase and gelatinase which attacks hide powder, casein, haemoglobin and gelatin but not natural collagen.

Mu toxin

An enzyme with the properties of hyaluronidase which is produced in large amount by all strains of Cl. welchii type B isolated from cases of lamb dysentery. It breaks down the polysaccharide cementing substance present in most tissues. It is antigenically distinct from hyaluronidase produced by staphylococci, streptococci and Cl. septicum.

Nu toxin

A deoxyribonuclease which consequently can also be classified as a leucocidin.

Additional enzymic substances are produced by some strains of Cl. welchii which have a variety of effects on red blood cells. For example, one substance causes panagglutination of red blood cells. Another enzyme is responsible for destroying virus receptors on the surfaces of red blood cells, thus making them inagglutinable by myxoviruses. Cl. welchii also produces a diffusible haemagglutinin after repeated subculture, a fibrinolysin and a histidine decarboxylase which converts histidine to histamine.

Neutralization tests for the detection of toxins

The different types of Cl. welchii can be identified by carrying out neutralization tests for the lethal or necrotizing activities of the four major lethal toxins, alpha, beta, epsilon and iota.

It should be emphasised that epsilon and iota toxins occur as inactive prototoxins and must be activated by trypsin before their toxic activities can be assessed, and that beta toxin is destroyed by this treatment. The general principles of the tests which can be performed on intestinal contents and also on culture fluids are outlined as follows.

Lethal activity

Intestinal contents should be collected immediately after death of the animal, and chloroform added as a preservative prior to the sample being diluted with broth or saline and then centrifuged. Broth cultures for testing should be incubated for 6–8 hours until active growth and gas production have declined. The fluid should then be cooled and centrifuged or filtered. To activate epsilon and iota toxins the supernatant fluid from intestinal contents or the prepared broth culture filtrate may be treated with 0·05 per cent (w/v) crystalline trypsin for one hour at 37°C after adjusting the pH to a neutral or slightly alkaline reaction. Subsequently, not less than 0·2 ml is injected intravenously into the tail veins of two mice and the animals observed for lethal activity of toxin. In most cases deaths from toxaemia will occur within 4–6 hours but the animals should be observed for several days if necessary. When the material is known to be toxic, a volume of 0·5 ml is mixed with 0·2 ml of specific antitoxin, the mixture kept at room temperature for 1 hour to allow possible combination of toxin and antitoxin, and then 0·3 ml of the mixture is inoculated intravenously into two mice. The animals are observed for neutralization of the lethal activity of the toxins over a period of at least 24 hours.

Necrotizing activity

The test is carried out in a similar manner for the detection of lethal activity except that volumes of 0·2 ml of material are inoculated intradermally into the depilated skin of albino guinea-pigs. The sites of inoculation are observed over a period of 48 hours for the development of necrotic lesions by toxins and for the prevention of necrosis by appropriate antitoxins incorporated in the inocula. A more recently developed technique makes use of chick embryo and mouse embryo monolayers for detecting toxin-antitoxin reactions by observing cytopathic effects (CPE). Only about one quarter to one twentieth of an MLD of toxin for mice is required to produce a CPE.

Epidemiology and pathogenesis of diseases caused by Cl. welchii type A

These are mainly human infections associated with gas gangrene and human food poisoning. A few cases of gas gangrenous lesions in animals caused by type A have been reported. A variety of toxins are produced by this organism and the pathogenesis of the local lesion of gas gangrene and the systemic disturbances of shock and fatal toxaemia have been studied in some detail and apply fundamentally to blackquarter and enterotoxaemic infections in animals. For these reasons the following outline is given of the probable actions on tissues of the different toxins which collectively cause the development of these lesions.

Gas gangrene

Lesions of gas gangrene which are derived from wound infections with *Cl. welchii* type A usually have an incubation period of 12–24 hours, sometimes less and occasionally lasting several days. Pain soon develops in the region and this is associated with the development of oedema. Within an hour or two gas bubbles will form in the tissues together with an extensive haemorrhagic exudate. Initially, the area will appear superficially pale, soon becoming brown, and later dark green or blackish in colour. In addition, there are general systemic symptoms of shock and toxaemia.

These pathological processes are closely related to the activities of the various toxins produced by the causal organism, and it is possible to assess the probable contribution of these substances to the pathogenesis of the lesion. Most tissue cell walls contain lecithin in their lipoprotein complexes, and alpha toxin which is a lecithinase, will have a disruptive action on cell walls causing death of the tissues. This lethal action on capillary cell walls will increase the permeability of the vessels, giving rise to the formation of oedema, a consequent reduction in blood supply, and an increased anaerobic environment which will encourage the growth of *Cl. welchii* in the lesion. At the same time, kappa toxin which is a collagenase, attacks the collagen and reticulin in diseased muscle and around capillaries, which will have the effect of increasing the diffusion of toxic substances and infecting organisms, and promote the development of haemorrhages and thrombi. The destruction of cell structure and nuclei will also be enhanced by other toxins. Mu toxin is a hyaluronidase known as 'spreading factor', and attacks the intercellular cementing substance (hyaluronic acid) present in the tissues. In addition, there is a fibrinolysin which may also be associated with the development of the lesion. The absence of polymorphs from a lesion of gas gangrene is a notable feature and probably arises from the action of alpha toxin, possibly theta toxin, and also from nu toxin which is a deoxyribonuclease and consequently a leucocidin.

In addition to the local lesion there is always a general systemic disturbance which can develop rapidly to become a fatal toxaemia. The cause of the systemic disturbance is not understood since it has not been directly associated with the known toxins produced by the causal organism; neither has it been prevented under appropriate experimental conditions by inoculation of large doses of antitoxin. These observations have given rise to the theory that as a result of the action of known toxins on the tissues, an unidentified toxic factor is produced which is responsible for the symptoms of systemic shock and toxaemia.

Epidemiology and pathogenesis of diseases caused by Cl. welchii type B

Lamb dysentery

This is an acute disease affecting young lambs of about 2–5 days of age caused by the rapid multiplication of *Cl. welchii* type B in the intestines and a resultant fatal toxaemia. Although the causal organisms are present in the soil and ingested by lambs when suckling, this cycle of infection is not solely responsible for clinical disease since the organisms are normal inhabitants of the intestines of healthy animals. There are important predisposing factors providing an environment which encourages the rapid and unusually high rate of growth of *Cl. welchii* type B in the intestines with the consequent production and absorption of relatively large amounts of toxin. The microenvironment necessary for these events to occur has not been defined but a number of factors which predispose animals to disease are known. For example, lambs which ingest large quantities of milk are more susceptible than those which have a more restricted supply. This is confirmed by the higher incidence of the disease among lambs bred from heavy milking hill breeds compared with the lower incidence among lambs from lighter milking breeds with a higher lambing crop kept under similar conditions but with less milk available to each lamb. The incidence of the disease is highest in flocks which graze on the hills during summer and are moved to lowland pastures during the winter and spring. In the United Kingdom, therefore, the disease is particularly prevalent in the mountainous areas of Wales and in the border country between England and Scotland. When no prophylactic measures have been taken it is a characteristic feature of the disease that few lambs are affected during the early part of the lambing season, and that the incidence increases abruptly during the middle and latter part of the season. This disease pattern has been variously attributed to the incidence of the organism in the environment of lambing pens which increases during the lambing season, resulting in greater rates of infection for susceptible lambs during the latter half of the season. It has also been suggested that the increased incidence of the disease is possibly related to the time when milk yield in the flock is greatest.

Symptoms. The acute form of the disease commonly occurs in strong and healthy lambs at about 2–4 days of age. The animals show signs of abdominal pain, bleat repeatedly, cease to suck, collapse and die within a few hours. The faeces are blood stained. Some cases are less acute and the symptoms more protracted.

Lesions. In the peracute condition there may be no obvious lesions to be seen at autopsy. In the majority of cases, however, the lesions which are usually confined to the small intestine consist of intense haemorrhagic areas and sometimes ulcers. The stomach usually contains a large quantity of milk.

Diagnosis. The age of affected lambs, the symptoms, lesions and sometimes the history of the flock, together may provide strong supporting evidence that the disease is lamb dysentery. Confirmation is obtained by identifying the presence of toxins in the intestinal contents, observing dense masses of *Cl. welchii* in ulcers by direct smears or sections, and culturing the organism from intestinal lesions, bowel contents and sometimes from heart blood, bone marrow, liver or spleen. The type of *Cl. welchii* can be confirmed by identification of toxins.

Prevention and control. To prevent outbreaks of lamb dysentery, advantage is taken of the fact that lambs derive a passive immunity from their dams through the colostrum. Before the lambing season, ewes are vaccinated with formalised whole culture or alum precipitated vaccine. The resulting passive immunity which unweaned lambs derive from colostrum is adequate to protect them for approximately the first 3 weeks of life. Alternatively, lambs can be protected by injection with hyperimmune serum immediately after birth.

Enterotoxaemia in calves, sheep and goats
A few cases of enterotoxaemic infections caused by *Cl. welchii* type B have been reported in calves in the United Kingdom and in sheep and goats in the Middle East. It is interesting to note that the strain of organism isolated from affected animals in Iran and subsequently in Turkey differed from the classical lamb dysentery strains of *Cl. welchii* type B by producing kappa but not lambda or mu toxins.

Epidemiology and pathogenesis of diseases caused by Cl. welchii type C

Enterotoxaemia in sheep (Struck)
The disease known as struck which affects adult sheep, is an acute and fatal enterotoxaemia arising from the high rate of multiplication of *Cl. welchii* type C and the consequent absorption of increased amounts of toxin from the intestines. The disease has been known to be prevalent among sheep on the fertile farms of the Romney Marsh area of Kent for more than 30 years and probably existed even earlier. Sporadic outbreaks have been reported from other European countries, the U.S.A. and from New Zealand, but it remains of particular and perennial economic importance in the Romney Marsh area of the United Kingdom. Little is known about the predisposing factors of this disease. Although *Cl. welchii* type C is prevalent in the soil, the essential factors which promote the multiplication of these organisms and especially the permeability of the intestinal wall to the toxin are not understood. In many cases a fatal toxaemia develops before obvious lesions of ulceration have appeared in the intestines and at a time when the intestinal wall seems to be intact. The problem is one which concerns the mode of transfer of toxin through the intestinal wall, since healthy animals can be dosed orally with large concentrations of toxin and remain unaffected.

Symptoms. The disease occurs mainly during early spring and affects adult sheep only. Death often takes place suddenly and occurs soon after the animal has developed symptoms of rigidity and immobility. Sometimes there are signs of abdominal pain but seldom any diarrhoea.

Lesions. These include an acute enteritis and some-times ulceration in the small intestine with areas of necrosis. There may be acute inflammation of the abomasum. Other lesions include excessive fluid in the abdominal cavity and sometimes in the pericardial sac and thoracic cavity. There may be degenerative changes in the kidneys, particularly in carcases which are not examined very soon after death. *Cl. welchii* type C may be present in large numbers in the peripheries of some of the intestinal necrotic areas. The organism invades the carcase soon after death and when post-mortem examination is delayed, the muscles and subcutaneous tissues take on a typically gas gangrenous appearance.

Diagnosis. The disease history of the flock and the symptoms and lesions of a typically enterotoxaemic condition in adult sheep in spring are strongly suggestive of infection with *Cl. welchii* type C. Confirmation can be obtained by identifying the toxin present in the intestinal and abomasal contents. The causal organism can be isolated from the intes-tinal contents, from the edges of necrotic lesions, and sometimes from visceral organs.

Prevention and control. Vaccination with formalised whole culture during the autumn and early spring is of value. A lamb dysentery vaccine can be used as an alternative to a type C vaccine because of the similarity of several of the toxic components.

Enterotoxaemia in lambs, calves and piglets
A few cases have been recorded of enterotoxaemia associated with *Cl. welchii* type C occurring in lambs and calves in the U.S.A. The disease in lambs is clinically indistinguishable from classical lamb dysentery associated with *Cl. welchii* type B. In calves the disease occurs rarely and animals less than 1 week of age are the most susceptible. The symptoms and lesions are similar to lamb dysentery.

Outbreaks of enterotoxaemia in young pigs have been described in the United Kingdom. The acute form of the disease occurs in piglets aged 1–3 days. Some animals may show weakness and dysentery before death. Post-mortem examination reveals acute inflammation of the intestines, especially the jejunum, with necrotic areas in the intestinal mucosa. The wall of the intestine usually contains large numbers of *Cl. welchii* type C. It is probable that the piglets become infected orally at the time of suckling from organisms present in the faeces of the sow and on the skin at the time of farrowing. It is known that *Cl. welchii* type C occurs in the intestines of some 5–10 per cent of normal pigs and there is evidence to suggest that this organism may be associated with swine dysentery when the incidence

of infection increases to 65–70 per cent of animals in an affected herd.

Enterotoxaemia in fowls
This is not a common disease of fowls. It has been described in birds aged from 6 weeks to 3 months which show symptoms of sudden weakness and dysentery. The mortality rate is usually low. In acute cases there are lesions of haemorrhagic necrosis of the intestine and congestion of the liver. Beta toxin has been identified in the intestinal contents. Predisposing factors are stress associated with overcrowding and the mixing together of birds of different ages.

Epidemiology and pathogenesis of diseases caused by Cl. welchii type D

Enterotoxaemia in sheep (pulpy kidney disease, overeating disease)
This is a toxaemia which develops as the result of the rapid multiplication of *Cl. welchii*, type D in the abomasum and small intestine. It occurs in sheep of different ages, particularly in lambs aged 3–8 weeks, in fattening lambs aged 6 months to 1 year, and in adult animals. The disease is common in those countries where sheep farming forms a substantial or major part of the agricultural industry, particularly the United Kingdom, the U.S.A., Scandinavia, Australasia, the Middle East and South America.

Cl. welchii type D is a normal inhabitant of the soil and also of the intestines of healthy sheep where it produces small amounts of toxin without affecting the well-being of the host. It is only under particular circumstances that the organism multiplies at an unusually high rate and produces sufficient con-centrations of toxin to cause a fatal toxaemia. These predisposing conditions are associated with con-centrated feeding or overeating, and the incidence of the disease is closely related to any method of sheep farming concerned with intensive rearing of lambs and high level feeding. A sudden change to a more concentrated diet may result in the rapid develop-ment of enterotoxaemia in a group of fattening lambs. High production sheep farming which involves these predisposing methods of husbandry are practised in parts of Wales, the border country between England and Scotland and in the U.S.A. on farms rearing feedlot lambs. It is in these areas that the incidence of enterotoxaemia is particularly high.

The explanation of the relationship between these predisposing factors and the development of a fatal toxaemia is not precisely known. It has been variously conjectured that the feeding of concentrated protein diets reduces the acidity of the stomach and thus favours rapid bacterial multiplication and production of toxin. Alternatively, it has been suggested that as a result of overfeeding, some undigested starch passes from the stomach to the small intestine, thus providing ideal conditions for the rapid multiplication of *Cl. welchii* type D which is already present in the intestines.

There still remain the unknown factors which affect the permeability to toxin of the intestinal wall. It is known that the low concentrations of alpha toxin, insufficient to cause necrosis of the tissues, will produce an increased permeability of blood vessels. Similarly, epsilon toxin increases the permeability of blood vessels in the brains of sheep, and this may be related to cerebral oedema which is sometimes observed in affected animals. Epsilon toxin also increases the permeability of the intestinal wall of mice but there are other unknown factors which are also involved in the process of absorption of toxin through the bowel wall.

Symptoms. Deaths may occur suddenly and un-expectedly. When symptoms are observed the animals become dull, weak, and soon collapse. The head is often retracted, and there is spasmodic struggling before the animal becomes comatose and dies.

Lesions. In lambs there is often a characteristic degeneration of the kidney cortex which will be more advanced in carcases which are not examined until several hours after death. The kidney becomes extremely soft and pulpy and immediately after death the only microscopic change seen in sections is a marked hyperaemia of the kidney cortex. This is soon followed by toxic degenerative changes which develop in the organs of a carcase a few hours after death. Lesions in the kidney are uncommon and frequently absent from older sheep affected with this disease. Additional lesions include excessive quantities of straw coloured fluid in the pericardium, endocardial haemorrhages and areas of congestion in the abomasum and small intestine.

Diagnosis. The association of disease with a sudden change in diet to a concentrated ration is strongly suggestive of enterotoxaemia. Confirmation depends upon the identification of high concentrations of epsilon toxin detectable in the intestinal contents. It may be necessary to activate the toxin with trypsin so that the maximum activity of the toxin can be demonstrated. Unusually large numbers of *Cl. welchii* type D can be seen in smears prepared from intestinal contents soon after death, and practically pure cultures will be obtained in cooked meat broth or blood agar plates incubated anaerobically. Urine should be tested for the presence of glucose which is a constant feature of the disease.

Prevention and control. Alum precipitated formalin-killed culture is a good antigen for stimulating an active immunity. Similarly, an alum-precipitated trypsin-treated toxoid is also satisfactory. Vaccination of pregnant ewes will result in a strong passive immunity being transferred to lambs during the first 3–5 weeks of life. Lambs can also be vaccinated and they will develop their own active immunity to a satisfactory level when the first dose is given within 72 hours of birth and repeated at 4 weeks of age.

Enterotoxaemia in cattle
Cl. welchii type D has occasionally been reported as the cause of enterotoxaemia in calves, and young cattle. The disease is similar in all respects to enterotoxaemic infections in sheep. However, it is important to emphasise that the nervous symptoms shown by some infected animals are very similar to those associated with lead poisoning.

Diseases caused by Cl. welchii type E
These infections are not of major economic importance. Enterotoxaemia in calves and lambs give rise to symptoms and lesions characteristic for this type of disease.

Public health aspects
The two most common human diseases caused by *Cl. welchii* are gas gangrenous lesions and food poisoning. Some strains of *Cl. welchii* type A are characterised by their inability to produce haemolysis on horse blood agar and by the unusual heat resistance of their spores which may survive boiling for 1–5 hours. This degree of heat resistance means that the spores in meat and meat products may survive the temperatures used for cooking, and the subsequent ingestion of large numbers of organisms may result in symptoms of food poisoning.

Some additional clostridial species
The clostridial group includes a large number of species in addition to the pathogens already described. The following is a brief summary of the important characteristic features of four of these additional species which are occasionally associated with disease or commonly occur as contaminants in anaerobic cultures.

Clostridium bifermentans and Cl. sordellii
The properties of these organisms are so similar that they will be considered as two types of a single species. The name *Cl. bifermentans* originates from the ability of these organisms to decompose both carbohydrates and proteins. The two organisms can be differentiated one from another by the production of urease by *Cl. sordellii* only, and also by the

fermentation of mannose, sorbitol and salicin by *Cl. bifermentans* but not by *Cl. sordellii*, although these latter reactions are not always constant for all strains.

The organisms are large Gram-positive rods, 2–5 μm in length and 0·5–1·0 μm in width. Spores are oval, subterminal or central, do not usually swell the bacilli and are developed readily in cultures. Both organisms are slightly proteolytic and digest meat. They liquefy gelatin, produce a lecithinase serologically related to the alpha toxin of *Cl. welchii*, and an oxygen-labile haemolysin related to the theta toxin of *Cl. welchii*, but unlike the latter species they fail to ferment lactose. Some strains of *Cl. sordellii* produce a necrotizing lethal toxin and both organisms produce a proteinase. *Cl. sordellii* has been isolated from a few cases of gas gangrene in man and from cattle and sheep in which it has been associated with lesions resembling blackquarter and 'big head' disease in rams.

Clostridium histolyticum

This organism is morphologically similar to *Cl. sporogenes* and readily sporulates on media producing oval, subterminal spores. Most strains are motile by means of peritrichous flagella, and all strains are actively proteolytic but not saccharolytic. They are not strict anaerobes and most strains will grow aerobically. A number of toxins are produced. The alpha toxin is lethal and necrotizing, the beta toxin is a collagenase, the epsilon toxin is haemolytic, and both the gamma and delta substances are proteinases. *Cl. histolyticum* has occasionally been associated with gas gangrene in man.

Clostridium sporogenes

This organism is widely distributed in soil and is frequently present as a normal inhabitant in the intestines of animals and man. It is one of the primary causes of decomposition of proteins under natural conditions. It is a Gram-positive, motile bacillus measuring 3–6 μm in length and 0·5 μm in width, and is not pathogenic but may occur as a contaminant in anaerobic cultures. The organisms sporulate readily, producing oval, subterminal spores which can survive boiling for several hours.

Cl. sporogenes produces a pseudo-haemolysis but not true haemolysis on horse blood agar and liquefies coagulated serum and gelatin. In cooked meat medium the meat is blackened, digested and the culture has an unpleasant odour of sulphuretted hydrogen. Acid and gas are produced in glucose and maltose but no fermentation occurs in lactose and saccharose. *Cl. sporogenes* produces proteinases and this property results in the organism being able to enhance the pathogenicity of *Cl. chauvoei*, *Cl. welchii* and other clostridial species.

Further reading

ANON. (1960) *Clostridium welchii* food poisoning. *British Medical Journal*, **1**, 711.

BAGADI, H.O. AND SEWELL, M.M.H. (1973) An epidemiological survey of infectious necrotic hepatitis [black disease] of sheep in southern Scotland. *Research in Veterinary Science*, **15**, 49.

BAGADI, H.O. AND SEWELL, M.M.H. (1973) Experimental studies on infectious necrotic hepatitis [black disease] of sheep. *Research in Veterinary Science*, **15**, 53.

BAGADI, H.O. AND SEWELL, M.M.H. (1974) A study of the route of dissemination of orally administered spores of *Clostridium novyi* Type B in guinea-pigs and sheep. *Research in Veterinary Science*, **17**, 179.

BATTY I., BUNTAIN D. AND WALKER P.D. (1964) *Clostridium oedematiens*. A cause of sudden death in sheep, cattle and pigs. *Veterinary Record*, **76**, 1115.

BATTY I. AND WALKER P.D. (1963) Differentiation of *Clostridium septicum* and *Clostridium chauvoei* by the use of fluorescent labelled antibodies. *Journal of Pathology and Bacteriology*, **85**, 517.

BULLEN J.J. (1952) Enterotoxaemia of sheep. *Clostridium welchii* type D in the alimentary tract of normal animals. *Journal of Pathology and Bacteriology*, **64**, 201.

BULLEN, J.J. (1970) Role of toxins in host-parasite relationships. In "*Microbial Toxins*", vol. 1. *Bacterial Protein Toxins*. Edit. Ajl, S.J., Kadis, S. and Montie, T.C. p. 233. Academic Press.

CHANDLER, H.M. AND GULASEKHARAM, J. (1974) The protective antigen of a highly immunogenic strain of *Clostridum chauvoei* including an evaluation of its flagella as a protective antigen. *Journal of General Microbiology*, **84**, 128.

CLAUS K.D. AND MACHEAK M.E. (1972) Characteristics and immunizing properties of culture filtrates of *Clostridium chauvoei*. *American Journal of Veterinary Research*, **33**, 1031.

COLLEE, J.G. (1961) The nature and properties of the haemagglutinin of *Clostridium welchii*. *Journal of Pathology and Bacteriology*, **81**, 297.

COLLEE, J.G. (1965) The relationship of the haemagglutinin of *Clostridium welchii* to the neuraminidase and other soluble products of the organism. *Journal of Pathology and Bacteriology*, **90**, 13.

DEMELLO, F.J., ANDERSON, W.R., HITCHCOCK, C.R. AND HAGLIN, J.J. (1974) Ultrastructural study of clostridial myositis. *Archives of Pathology*, **97**, 118.

FJØLSTAD, M. (1973) The effects of *Clostridium botulinum* toxin type Cβ given orally to goats. *Acta Veterinaria Scandinavica*, **14**, 69.

FREDETTE V., ed. (1968) *The Anaerobic Bacteria*. Proceedings of an International Workshop, p.

261. Montreal: Institute of Microbiology and Hygiene.

GARCIA M.M. AND McKAY K.A. (1969) On the growth and survival of *Clostridium septicum* in soil. *Journal of Applied Bacteriology*, **32**, 362.

GARDNER, D.E. (1972) The stability of *Clostridium perfringens* type D epsilon toxin in intestinal contents in vitro. *New Zealand Veterinary Journal*, **20**, 167.

GARDNER D.E. (1973) Pathology of *Clostridium welchii* type D enterotoxaemia. I Biochemical and haematological alterations in lambs. II Structural and ultrastructural alterations in the tissues of lambs and mice. III Basis of the hyperglycaemic response. *Journal of Comparative Pathology*, **83**, 499, 509 and 525.

GRINER, L.A. (1961) Enterotoxemia of sheep. I. Effects of *Clostridium perfringens* type D toxin on the brains of sheep and mice. *American Journal of Veterinary Research*, **22**, 429.

HARTLEY, W.J. (1956) A focal symmetrical encephalomalacia of lambs. *New Zealand Veterinary Journal*, **4**, 129.

JAMIESON S., THOMPSON J.J. AND BROTHERSTON J.G. (1948) Studies in black disease. I The occurrence of the disease in sheep in the north of Scotland. *Veterinary Record*, **60**, 11.

JANSEN, B.C. (1971) The toxic antigenic factors produced by Clostridium botulinum types C and D. *Onderstepoort Journal of Veterinary Research*, **38**, 93.

KEYMER I.F., SMITH G.R., ROBERTS T.A., HEANEY S.I. AND HIBBERD D.J. (1972) Botulism as a factor in waterfowl mortality at St. James Park, London. *Veterinary Record*, **90**, 111.

KERRIN J.C. (1929) The distribution of *B. tetani* in the intestines of animals. *British Journal of Experimental Pathology*, **10**, 370.

LAMANNA C. AND SAKAGUCHI G. (1971) Botulinal toxins and the problem of nomenclature of simple toxins. *Bacteriological Reviews*, **35**, 242.

MACLENNAN J.D. (1962) The histotoxic clostridial infections of man. *Bacteriological Reviews*, **26**, 177.

McCLUNG L.S. (1956) The anaerobic bacteria with special reference to the genus *Clostridum*. *Annual Review of Microbiology*, **10**, 173.

MORGAN, K.T. AND KELLY, B.G. (1974) Ultrastructural study of brain lesions produced in mice by the administration of *Clostridium welchii* type D toxin. *Journal of Comparative Pathology*, **84**, 181.

ROBERTS, T.A. AND COLLINGS, D.F. (1973) An outbreak of type C botulism in broiler chicken. *Avian Diseases*, **17**, 650.

ROBERTS T.A., KEYMER I.F., BORLAND E.D. AND SMITH G.R. (1972) Botulism in birds and mammals in Great Britain. *Veterinary Record*, **91**, 11.

ROBERTS, T.A., THOMAS, A.I. AND GILBERT, R.J. (1973) A third outbreak of type C botulism in broiler chicken. *Veterinary Record*, **92**, 107.

Second World Symposium of the International Office of Epizootics on Diseases caused by Anaerobes, Paris (1967) *Bulletin de l'Office international des Epizooties*, **67**, 1161.

SMITH L.D. AND HOLDEMAN L.V. (1969) *The Pathogenic Anaerobic Bacteria*. Springfield, Illinois: Charles C. Thomas.

SMYTH, C.J. AND ARBUTHNOTT, J.P. (1974) Properties of *Clostridium perfingens* [*welchii*] type-A alpha-toxin [phospholipase C] purified by electrofocusing. *Journal of Medical Microbiology*, **7**, 41.

UEMURA, T., SAKAGUCHI, G. AND RIEMANN, H.P. (1973) In vitro production of *Clostridium perfringens* enterotoxin and its detection by reversed passive haemagglutination. *Applied Microbiology*, **26**, 381.

WILLIAMS B.M. (1964) *Clostridium oedematiens* infections (Black disease and bacillary haemoglobinurea) of cattle in mid-Wales. *Veterinary Record*, **76**, 591.

WILLIS A.T. (1969) *Clostridia of Wound Infection*. London: Butterworth.

CHAPTER 21

MYCOBACTERIUM

Mycobacterium

This group of organisms includes a number of different species occurring characteristically as thin rods which, although difficult to stain because of waxy components in the walls of the bacilli, will withstand decolourisation with acid or acid-alcohol. For this reason they are sometimes referred to as acid-fast or acid-alcohol-fast organisms. Some species, particularly those which are pathogenic to man and animals, grow slowly on artificial media. Infection with these pathogenic mycobacteria results in the development of typically chronic granulomatous lesions which sometimes become necrotic, caseous and calcified.

Major diseases produced by mycobacteria include, tuberculosis in man and animals caused by the human, bovine, avian, murine and cold-blooded types of *Mycobacterium tuberculosis*; Johne's disease in cattle and sheep caused by *Myco. paratuberculosis*; and leprosy in man caused by *Myco. leprae*.

There are many other species of these organisms which are referred to as 'anonymous' or 'atypical' mycobacteria. On the basis of pigment and catalase production, morphology, resistance to drugs and other properties, these anonymous bacteria have been classified into groups. Some species grow rapidly on laboratory media, are non-pathogenic, and include *Myco. phlei* which occurs in soil and water, and *Myco. smegmatis* found in smegma and on the skin. Other species (e.g. *Myco. kansasii, Myco. fortuitum, Myco. ulcerans*) produce yellow-orange or red pigments when grown in the light but not in the dark and are referred to as photochromogens. These organisms can be distinguished from other species which produce yellow pigment in the dark and are known as scotochromogens. The apparent incidence of some of these anonymous bacteria in relation to diseases in animals and man is low but is being recognised more frequently than in the past in those areas where the incidence of tuberculosis has been reduced. During recent years *Myco. kansasii* has been isolated from bovine lungs, and occasionally, *Myco fortuitum* and *Myco. smegmatis*

have been associated with bovine mastitis and the former with skin lesions in pigs and calves. *Myco. ulcerans* grows within a temperature range of 25–35°C, and can cause lesions in rats, mice and guinea-pigs in sites where the body temperature is low (e.g. tip of the nose, tail or scrotum).

Mycobacterium tuberculosis

Distribution in nature
Tuberculosis in man and animals has a world-wide distribution. The human type of the organism (*Myco. tuberculosis*) is primarily a pathogen for man but can cause disease in cattle, pigs, dogs, monkeys, parrots, canaries and other species. Under experimental conditions guinea-pigs are highly susceptible. The bovine type (*Myco. bovis*) is a common cause of disease in domestic animals particularly cattle, pigs, cats, dogs and horses. It also causes human tuberculosis. Rabbits are more susceptible to infection with the bovine type than they are to the human type. The avian type (*Myco. avium*) is especially pathogenic for birds and sometimes causes disease in mammals. This organism can also cause tuberculosis in man. *Myco. intracellulare*, formerly known as the Battey bacillus, is closely related to *Myco. avium* and is sometimes regarded as the same species. The murine type (*Myco. murium*) also known as the Vole Bacillus, causes tuberculosis in voles and similar species; and the cold-blooded types (*Myco. piscium; Myco. marinum; Myco. platypoecilis*) produce a similar condition in fish and other cold-blooded animals.

Morphology and staining
The different types of *Myco. tuberculosis* cannot be distinguished one from another on morphological features alone (Plates 21.1a–c, facing p. 230). They appear in the tissues as slender rods which may be straight, curved or in the form of clubs, measuring 1·0–4·0 μm in length and 0·2–0·3 μm in width, occurring singly, in pairs or as small bundles.

Under experimental conditions it has been noted that in the early stages of infection the organisms may develop initially as cocci. After growth on laboratory media, they can appear in a number of forms varying from cocci to long rods measuring 6–8 μm in length. The organisms do not produce capsules or flagella.

Mycobacteria are not readily stained by the aniline dyes and it is difficult to demonstrate that they are Gram-positive. The organisms are stained pink with hot carbol fuchsin and they will then resist decolourisation with 3 per cent HCl in 95 per cent alcohol (i.e. acid-alcohol-fast) because of the presence in the intact organisms of a waxy substance known as mycolic acid. After washing, the films can be counterstained with methylene blue or another contrasting stain. This is known as the Ziehl-Neelsen method of staining and is widely used as a diagnostic procedure. Sometimes these organisms show beaded staining.

Cultural characteristics

Human and bovine types (Myco. tuberculosis and Myco. bovis)
These organisms are aerobes and the optimum temperature for growth is 37–38°C. Growth does not take place on simple laboratory media but occurs slowly (10–14 days) on media containing serum, potato or egg (Dorset egg medium). It has been estimated that the generation time is approximately 18 hours and primary cultures are particularly slow in developing. The addition of glycerine (e.g. Lowenstein-Jensen medium) enhances the growth of human strains but has no effect on, and may even inhibit, the growth of bovine strains (Plate 21.1d, opposite). On these media the difference in growth rate between human and bovine strains is striking. The relatively luxuriant growth of human strains is termed 'eugonic', and the less luxuriant growth of bovine strains is known as 'dysgonic'. Human strains are also characterised by producing a yellowish pigment on culture. Stonebrink's medium is useful for the isolation of *Myco. bovis* because it contains inspissated egg with malachite green to prevent growth of contaminants, and sodium pyruvate to enhance the growth of bovine strains.

A characteristic feature of both human and bovine strains is that the organisms are strongly adherent to each other, giving rise to tenacious and friable bacterial masses which do not easily produce a homogenous suspension. This feature is particularly apparent with human strains. A useful fluid medium is one containing casein hydrolysate, bovine serum albumen, asparagin and various salts. The difficulty of suspending the friable growth which normally develops on the surface, can be overcome by incorporating a detergent, Tween 80, which reduces surface tension and results in submerged growth.

Avian type (Myco. avium)
The optimal temperature for growth of these aerobes is 40°C and unlike the mammalian types, growth will also take place at 42–43°C. Avian strains develop poorly or not at all on ordinary media but growth is satisfactory on Dorset egg medium and enhanced in the presence of glycerine. Their rate of development is more rapid than that of the mammalian types and visible growth which occurs in 4–5 days, is less friable and more easily emulsified. Avian strains commonly produce a yellow or slightly pink coloured pigment. Some slow-growing avian strains which can be cultured on media containing an extract of *Myco. phlei* have been isolated from wood-pigeons.

Murine type (Myco. murium)
These organisms grow very poorly at their optimum temperature of 37–38°C. Growth does not occur on ordinary media and takes 3–4 weeks to develop on potato or Dorset egg. Growth is inhibited in the presence of glycerine.

Cold-blooded type (Myco. piscium)
This organism will develop at an optimal temperature of 25°C. Good growth will take place in 2–3 days on ordinary media and is enhanced in the presence of glycerine.

Resistance to physical and chemical agents

The various types of *Myco. tuberculosis* are killed at a temperature of 60°C for 15 minutes and are slightly more resistant to the lethal effects of disinfectants than many other species of bacteria. The organisms are particularly susceptible to ionic detergents and to sunlight. They can remain viable for long periods in the dark, in putrefying material, faeces and sputum, where the lethal effects of disinfectants may be delayed for several hours.

Antigens and toxins

The application of various serological techniques to the study of the antigens of *Myco. tuberculosis* has shown the close relationship which exists between the various types. The human, bovine and murine types are indistinguishable and they also have some antigens in common with saprophytic mycobacteria. The avian type has an antigen in common with the mammalian types and additional specific antigens which enable the avian strains to be subtyped. Because of the complicated antigenic structures of mycobacteria, it is easier to distinguish between the various types of *Myco. tuberculosis* by cultural instead of by serological methods.

No soluble exotoxins have been demonstrated.

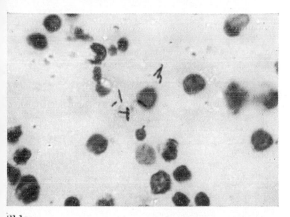

21.1a

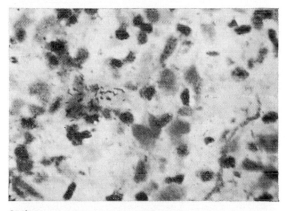

21.1b

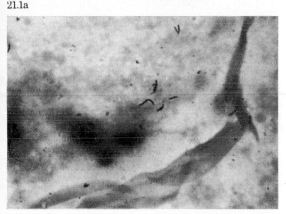

21.1c

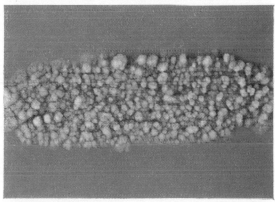

21.1d

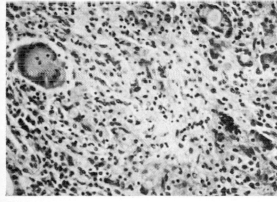

21.1e

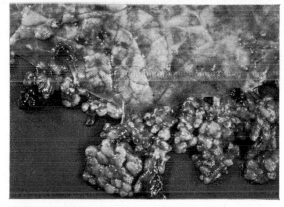

21.1f

21.1a   Film of centrifuged milk deposit stained Ziehl-Neelsen, from a case of bovine tuberculous mastitis. Note the acid-alcohol-fast pink coloured rods of *Mycobacterium tuberculosis* (bovine type) surrounded by blue-stained cells, ×930.

21.1c   Ziehl-Neelsen stained film of human sputum showing acid-alcohol-fast *Mycobacterium tuberculosis* (human type), ×930.

21.1e   Histological section from bovine udder infected with *Mycobacterium tuberculosis* (bovine type) showing giant cell formation. Haematoxylin and eosin stain.

21.1b   Ziehl-Neelsen stained film from spleen of tuberculous chicken, showing acid-alcohol-fast *Mycobacterium tuberculosis* (avian type), ×930.

21.1d   Macroscopic appearance of *Mycobacterium tuberculosis* (bovine type) growing on Löwenstein-Jensen medium. Note the roughened surface of the growth.

21.1f   Macroscopic appearance of tuberculosis in bovine lung and pleura showing characteristic granulomatous grape-like nodules.

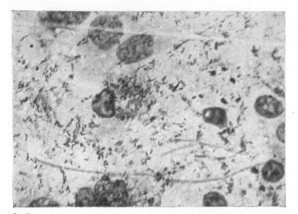

21.2a

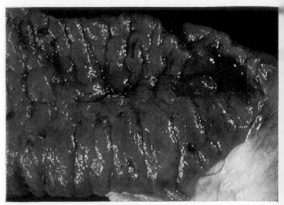

21.2b

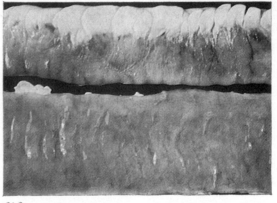

21.2c

21.2a Ziehl-Neelsen stained film prepared from bovine intestine in the region of the ileo-caecal valve from a case of Johne's disease. Note the large numbers of acid-alcohol-fast *Mycobacterium paratuberculosis* organisms appearing as small pink-staining rods, ×930.

21.2b Macroscopic appearance of bovine intestinal mucosa in the region of the ileo-caecal valve from a case of Johne's disease. Note the characteristically wrinkled, congested appearance of the mucosa.

21.2c Macroscopic appearance of ovine intestinal mucosa from a case of Johne's disease. Note the wrinkled surface and yellow-orange discolouration of the mucosa which shows areas of haemorrhage.

Epidemiology and pathogenesis

Reference has already been made to the different host species which are susceptible under natural conditions to infection with the various types of *Myco. tuberculosis*. A great deal of information has been accumulated on the pathogenicity of these organisms which clearly reveals that under particular conditions various animal species are susceptible to infection with one or other of the different types of organisms. The common routes of infection are by inhalation or ingestion. Less frequently, the bacilli may gain entrance into the tissues via the skin, and congenital infection of the bovine fetus via the placenta has occasionally been reported. It is a feature of infection with pathogenic mycobacteria that entrance of the organisms into the tissue does not necessarily result in the development of clinical disease. The defence mechanisms of the host may successfully contain these organisms and although they remain viable the bacilli will not proliferate until some undetermined predisposing factors prevail in the tissues.

The ability of mycobacteria to proliferate in the tissues is also related to the virulence of the organisms which is known to vary, although the mechanism involved in the development of virulence is not clearly understood. A characteristic feature of virulent strains is that the organisms develop in parallel formation as cords, whereas avirulent strains develop in clumps. The virulent corded bacilli are surrounded by a lipid material which inhibits leucocytic migration and also has a toxic effect on leucocytes.

The incidence of tuberculosis in different host species depends upon a variety of factors related to husbandry, hygiene and environment, which allow survival of the organisms outside the body and suitable conditions for transference of infection from one individual to another of the same or different species.

Among cattle the common sources of infection with the bovine type (*Myco. bovis*) are contaminated environments and contact with other infected cattle. During recent years attempts to eradicate this disease in the United Kingdom, some European countries and in the U.S.A. have been particularly successful, and the incidence of infection is now becoming very low. Occasionally, infection of cattle with the bovine type has been derived from human cases of pulmonary infection with this organism, and only rarely do cattle become clinically infected with the human type. Infection of cattle with the avian type (*Myco. avium*) can result from contact with infected poultry, but the few lesions which develop remain small and do not give rise to widespread infection of the organs as occurs with the bovine type.

Sheep and goats are not commonly infected with tuberculosis. It would appear that this is because of the conditions of husbandry which seldom give rise to a highly infected environment. The pathogenesis of infection is similar to that in cattle. Cases of natural infection with the bovine and avian types have been recorded in both sheep and goats.

Horses have a high natural resistance to tuberculosis and the incidence of the disease is low. They are infected more commonly with the bovine type than with either the avian or human type. Disease arises from contact with infected individuals or from ingestion of contaminated foodstuffs, and results in primary lesions which develop in lymph nodes associated with the pharynx or intestines. Generalised infections may develop subsequently through the blood stream.

Pigs become infected with tuberculosis mainly from ingestion of foodstuffs contaminated with infected bovine or avian faeces or from infected milk. Pigs are susceptible to infection with bovine, avian and human types of *Myco. tuberculosis*, in that order of frequency, but under natural conditions disease caused by the human type is rare. The frequency of infection with the different types varies according to the incidence of these organisms in their primary host species in any particular district, and also to the degree of contact between pigs and their potential sources of infection. There is epidemiological evidence to indicate that the incidence of tuberculosis in pigs becomes reduced in areas where the disease in cattle is satisfactorily controlled. In pigs, the bovine and avian types can each give rise to generalised haematogenous spread of infection to many tissues. On the other hand, infection with the human type causes the development of a primary lesion, only.

Dogs and cats are naturally susceptible to human and bovine types of the organism. Although precise information on the incidence of tuberculosis in these animals is not known, it is related to the occurrence of open cases of human disease and of infected bovine milk. On some occasions the diagnosis of infection in dogs may be the first indication of tuberculosis being present in the owner's household. Primary lesions in these animals can occur in the respiratory or digestive tracts, and the disease soon becomes progressive and affects various organs.

Poultry are susceptible only to *Myco. avium* and infection arises from the ingestion of contaminated food and water. The faeces of diseased birds often contain large numbers of bacilli and the spread of disease in a flock arises from faecal contamination of the environment.

A variety of other animal species are susceptible to infection with *Myco. tuberculosis*, particularly wild animals living in zoological gardens. The human type of the organism has been isolated from canaries, parrots and other exotic birds. Voles and similar animal species are susceptible to the murine type (*Myco. murium*) which produces typical tubercular lesions in these animals. Murine strains have been used for the preparation of trial vaccines because they have a low virulence for different host species and possess antigens in common with other mammalian types of *Myco. tuberculosis*. *Myco. piscium* causes disease in cold-blooded animals.

Symptoms

The symptoms will depend upon the organs involved and the extent of the lesions. In cattle, pulmonary infection gives rise to a dry cough which increases in frequency as the disease develops and is accompanied by loss of weight. Infection of the udder sometimes causes no definite symptoms although the tubercular mastitis may be extensive. Similarly, tuberculosis of other organs may not give rise to diagnostically reliable symptoms.

In other mammals the symptoms of disease are similar to those in cattle. In dogs and cats the infection may be associated with the digestive tract, and cause symptoms which are not suggestive of tuberculosis. Tuberculosis in poultry is primarily a disease of the digestive tract and the symptoms consist of severe emaciation, pale mucous membranes and intermittent diarrhoea.

Lesions

Cattle

Lesions develop most commonly in the lungs, pleura and local lymphatic nodes. A progressive cellular, granulomatous type of lesion develops initially as a concentration of polymorphs. This is soon replaced by an intense mononuclear reaction in which a number of giant multinucleated cells (cells of Langhans) can be seen (Plate 21.1e, facing p. 230). The lesion becomes delineated from the surrounding normal tissue by a concentration of macrophages, lymphocytes, plasma cells and finally a layer of fibrous tissue. As the lesion increases in size, necrosis and caseation develop centrally, and later the caseous material containing bacilli may be discharged, spreading infection to other sites, and the lesion becomes a cavity. There is a tendency for calcification to occur in these lesions. Alternatively, a more acute exudative type of lesion may develop which is characterised by an inflammatory exudate containing neutrophils, eosinophils, macrophages and fibrin. Both the cellular and exudative types of lesion may develop in the lungs and pleura (Plate 21.1f, facing p. 230).

When there is an extensive distribution of tubercle bacilli via the blood stream, miliary lesions (i.e. resembling millet seeds) may develop in almost any site of the body, including the spleen, kidneys, joints, uterus, central nervous system and udder.

Sheep and goats

The lesions are similar to those in cattle.

Horses

Lesions usually develop as tumour-like masses in which it is difficult to demonstrate the causal organisms. Common sites for these lesions are liver, spleen, and lungs.

Pigs

Infection with the bovine type of *Myco. tuberculosis* gives rise to caseous lesions which may also undergo calcification, whereas disease associated with the avian type causes the development of tumour-like areas in affected tissues. The skeleton, especially the vertebrae and long bones, are common sites for tuberculosis. Lesions may also develop in the liver, spleen and lungs; and areas of caseation in the submaxillary lymph nodes are sometimes associated with acid-alcohol-fast bacilli which may be difficult to isolate on laboratory media. It should also be recalled that similar caseous lesions in the lymph nodes may be caused by *Corynebacterium equi* as well as by the avian type of *Myco. tuberculosis*.

Dogs and cats

Primary infection in both species develop in the lungs or digestive tract. In dogs infection usually arises in the lungs in the form of nodules which develop into bronchopneumonia with areas of intense congestion and cavitation. There is commonly an accompanying pleurisy. Primary infection of the intestines, which is more usual in cats, gives rise to excessive quantities of fluid in the abdominal cavity and to enlarged mesenteric lymphatic nodes. There may be intestinal ulceration.

Poultry

Infection usually occurs from ingestion and lesions develop most commonly in the spleen, liver, intestines and, less frequently, in the lungs as greyish-white granulomatous areas. The liver and spleen become enlarged and contain either many lesions or a few relatively large nodules. Smears prepared from these organs contain many tubercle bacilli. Lesions in the intestines are relatively large and there may be ulceration of the mucous surface.

Diagnosis

Microscopical examination

Diagnosis by this method depends upon the identification of *Myco. tuberculosis* in suspected materials including lesions, sputa, milk, uterine discharges, pleural and peritoneal fluids, urine or faeces. The usual method is to prepare smears, stain by the Ziehl-Neelsen method and examine microscopically for tubercle bacilli. Films prepared from sputa may need to be examined extensively before observing a single tubercle bacillus, and a negative result does not necessarily preclude the possibility of infection. Conversely, it should also be remembered that saprophytic acid-fast bacilli may be present in sputa and milk. Samples of milk, urine, uterine discharges, pleural and peritoneal fluids should be centrifuged and films prepared from the deposits, stained and examined. Volumes of at least 25–50 ml should be used for obtaining these deposits. Films of milk should be treated with alcohol-ether for 30 seconds and washed to remove fat before staining. Tubercle bacilli often occur in clumps and several microscopic fields may have to be searched before one or more organisms are identified. In the centrifuged deposits of milk samples the bacilli are frequently found in fields containing clumps of epithelioid cells, and when examining these samples, cell groups should be searched particularly thoroughly for tubercle bacilli.

Bacteriological examination
Material infected with *Myco. tuberculosis* usually contains a variety of other microorganisms which can be destroyed by treating the material with an equal volume of 5 per cent oxalic acid, although this may not always kill contaminating moulds. Alternatively, 10 per cent trisodium phosphate, 4 per cent caustic soda or 20 per cent antiformin (sodium hypochlorite) can be used with subsequent cultivation on Dubos' solid medium containing penicillin. It should be remembered, however, that these methods of treatment will also kill some of the tubercle bacilli, and the concentrations and times of application may have to be varied for different samples. Stonebrink's medium is preferable to Lowenstein-Jensen medium for the isolation of *Myco. bovis*.

Animal inoculation
Suspected materials, especially milk samples which are not heavily infected with *Myco. bovis*, can be inoculated into the thighs of guinea-pigs to diagnose the presence of infection. It is preferable to inoculate two animals with each sample. Animals are killed 4–6 weeks after inoculation and examined for typical lesions of tuberculosis in the liver, spleen and lymphatic nodes draining the site of inoculation. These lesions should not be confused with those of pseudotuberculosis (see page 128).

Typing of bovine, human and avian strains can be carried out by animal inoculation methods.

Rabbits usually die from generalised infection with the bovine type 4–5 weeks after intravenous injection but survive similar inoculations with the human type. Guinea-pigs are highly susceptible to both the bovine and human types. The reliability of this test depends upon the use of weighed doses of culture. The avian type is less virulent for rabbits and guinea-pigs and produces a more chronic form of disease unless inoculated in unusually large doses by the intravenous route. It does not cause the production of macroscopically visible tubercles, although the spleen and liver become enlarged and contain many tubercle bacilli which can be readily seen in stained smears. This is sometimes referred to as the Yersin type of infection. Chickens are not affected by the human or bovine types but will die after inoculation of most strains of the avian type. Recently, it has been observed that some atypical strains of the avian type are not pathogenic for chickens but possess other characteristic properties in common with the species.

Control and prevention

Tuberculin test
This test is widely used throughout the world for the control of tuberculosis in cattle and to a lesser extent in other animal species. The basis of the test is that animals infected with tuberculosis develop a hypersensitivity to *Myco. tuberculosis* so that when an extract of the organism (i.e. tuberculin) is subsequently injected into the skin, a localised hypersensitive reaction occurs at the site of inoculation. No reaction occurs in healthy animals.

The history of the preparation and use of tuberculin goes back to the days of Robert Koch who was the first to observe the potential value of tuberculin as a diagnostic aid. Since that time many different methods for preparing tuberculin have been studied. One of the earlier preparations known as old tuberculin (OT) was prepared by evaporating a glycerinated broth culture to one-tenth of its volume. This yielded a tuberculin which had only a small proportion of active principle mixed with non-specific material, and the proportions varied from one batch to another. These disadvantages were overcome by using synthetic media which are free from meat protein and by developing variations on methods for producing purified protein derivative tuberculin (PPD). In these techniques the protein, which is the active principle, is separated by precipitation with trichloracetic acid or some other precipitant. The yield from consecutive batches can be readily standardised and impurities are removed. PPD tuberculins can be prepared from different organisms and especially from the human, bovine and avian types of *Myco. tuberculosis*.

Various methods for carrying out the test in cattle have been used, including the subcutaneous test with subsequent observations on increases in body temperature, the double intradermal comparative test using both mammalian and avian tuberculins, or the single intradermal test recording the amount of skin swelling 72 hours after injection of 0·1 ml of mammalian or avian PPD. The last of these methods is the one now in general use. When the test is carried out in the skin of the neck a swelling of 3 mm is a doubtful reaction and one of 4 mm or more is positive. The presence of an oedematous swelling at the site of inoculation is also regarded as a positive reaction.

Cattle are liable to become sensitised to tuberculin as a result of infection with the human, bovine or avian type of *Myco. tuberculosis*, with *Myco. paratuberculosis*, or with some other mycobacterial species. To overcome this difficulty of cross-reactions, animals may be tested simultaneously or consecutively with mammalian and avian tuberculins. Infections with the avian type or with *Myco paratuberculosis* will result in a more marked reaction against the avian than against the mammalian tuberculin. Conversely, bovine infections will give rise to a greater reaction to mammalian than to avian tuberculin.

The tuberculin test in other animal species is not so widely employed but the general principles and methods are similar. When testing poultry, the wattle is often used as the preferred site for inoculation. Recently, a whole-blood rapid agglutination test has been developed experimentally for the detection of tuberculosis in poultry and preliminary trials indicate that it is a useful supplementary test to the wattle tuberculin test.

Vaccination

Many attempts have been made to control tuberculosis in animals by using killed vaccines but none of them have been as successful as eradication programmes employing the tuberculin test and the slaughter of reactors. An alternative method has been the preparation of a living vaccine from an attenuated strain of the bovine type (Bacille Calmette Guérin) known as BCG. The inoculation of this vaccine may give rise to positive reactions to the tuberculin test in cattle, and although harmless the degree of immunity which develops subsequent to vaccination is uncertain. For these reasons it has not been generally accepted as a method for controlling tuberculosis in cattle.

Public health aspects

Tuberculosis is a major disease problem in the human population of the world, and man is susceptible to infection with the human, bovine and avian types of *Myco. tuberculosis*. For these reasons the control of tuberculosis in animals forms an integral and essential part of the control of the disease in man, because there are many environmental conditions in which man may derive infection from contact with his animals. One important route is by ingestion of milk infected with mycobacteria. The risk of this type of infection occurring can be removed by pasteurisation of milk supplies. There is also evidence to show that animals, particularly domestic pets, may contract infection from human sources. The risks of infection are considerable for those who handle and examine infected animals, and they are particularly serious for laboratory workers. It is always wise to manipulate cultures and infective materials in the laboratory with great caution and under protective hoods of proven efficiency.

Other mycobacteria causing disease in man are *Myco. kansasii*, which has also been isolated from cattle, *Myco. ulcerans* and *Myco. balnei* both of which produce ulcerative skin lesions in man; and *Myco. fortuitum* which occurs in man and occasionally in cattle. *Myco. leprae* is the cause of leprosy in man. It is specific for the human species and cannot be transmitted to animals under natural conditions. A comparable condition which occurs in rats is caused by *Myco. lepraemurium*, an organism which is distinct from the leprosy bacillus.

Mycobacterium paratuberculosis

This organism was originally named *Mycobacterium johnei* after Johne who, with Frothingham, was the first to study this infection in cattle known as Johne's disease.

Myco. paratuberculosis is the cause of a chronic, contagious enteritis in cattle, sheep, goats, camels, reindeer and occasionally in pigs and other animal species. It is world-wide in its distribution and is a disease of considerable economic importance.

Morphology and staining

Myco. paratuberculosis is a short rod measuring approximately 1–2 μm in length and 0·5 μm in width with rounded ends. On artificial media there is a tendency for the organism to be shorter and for occasional club-forms to develop. It is non-motile and does not form spores. The organisms stain Gram-positive and as they are also strongly acid-alcohol-fast, they stain well with the Ziehl-Neelsen method (Plate 21.2a, facing p. 231).

Cultural characteristics

It is a feature of *Myco. paratuberculosis* that it is an obligatory parasite and particularly difficult to cultivate on laboratory media. The organism will grow slowly on media containing killed acid-alcohol-fast organisms or extracts prepared from them. The optimum temperature for growth is 38–39°C and primary cultures will require some 4–8 weeks' incubation before minute greyish-white, friable, irregular colonies on solid media become visible to the naked eye. Further incubation results in the colonies becoming larger and pale yellow in colour. Subcultures produce slightly improved growths.

The first isolations of this organism were made on glycerine egg medium containing killed *Myco. tuberculosis*. Later, it was shown that extracts from saprophytic mycobacteria were as satisfactory as those from *Myco. tuberculosis*, and it is now the usual practice to incorporate extracts prepared from *Myco phlei* (known as mycobactin) in the media. Because of these difficulties it is not surprising, therefore, that many attempts have been made to find more satisfactory media for the cultivation of these fastidious organisms. It is possible to train laboratory strains to grow on synthetic media in the absence of mycobacterial extracts; but as a practical routine, satisfactory results are obtained with a basic medium of whole egg to which is added either killed *Myco. phlei* or mycobactin. A semi-synthetic medium incorporating bovine serum and penicillin as well as mycobactin has also been developed.

Three strains of *Myco. paratuberculosis* have been isolated from sheep. They include the bovine strain described above, an Icelandic strain which also occurs in the United Kingdom, and the yellow or orange pigmented strain. Both the Icelandic and pigmented strains can infect cattle as well as sheep.

Epidemiology and pathogenesis

Under natural conditions the disease in cattle spreads by the ingestion of *Myco. paratuberculosis* from a contaminated environment. It also seems that infection occurs more commonly during the earlier months of life than during adulthood. However, when assessing age susceptibility it must be remembered that one potential source of infection for calves, in particular, is contamination of milk with infected faeces from diseased cows. Primary infection of milk with *Myco. paratuberculosis* is uncommon. Also, adult animals which have not come in contact with the organism during early life are susceptible to infection, and the long incubation period, extending from at least 12 months to several years, makes it difficult to be precise as to the most susceptible age at which infection occurs under natural conditions. Any attempt to try to assess the susceptibility of different age groups must also take account of the fact that, like tuberculosis in animals, infection does not necessarily lead to recognisable symptoms but may result in either eventual recovery or symptomless carriers in which clinical manifestations of the disease may develop some time later.

The epidemiology of the disease in sheep is similar to that in cattle and the clinical disease frequently develops when animals are 3–5 years old and especially soon after lambing.

Pigs can become infected when in contact with diseased cattle and experimentally they can be infected wih organisms or with diseased bovine intestines.

Under experimental conditions, infection can be reproduced in mice and hamsters.

Symptoms

Characteristic symptoms in cattle are chronic diarrhoea and emaciation. Infected sheep show a loss of condition with or without diarrhoea which may be suggestive of parasitic infection as well as Johne's disease.

Lesions

The carcases of chronically infected cattle are emaciated and show varying degrees of anaemia. Localised lesions occur most frequently in the vicinity of the terminal portion of the small intestine and the ileocaecal valve. In the earlier stages of the disease this area may be oedematous and show haemorrhagic streaks. In more chronic cases the intestinal mucosa may be wrinkled or corrugated (Plates 21.2b & c facing p. 231), but this is not a constant feature of these cases. The lymphatic nodes draining the area may be enlarged and oedematous.

The lesions in sheep are similar to those in cattle. Infection with the pigmented variety of *Myco. paratuberculosis* gives rise to an orange discolouration of the mucous surface. Necrosis and caseation may develop in mesenteric lymphatic nodes of infected sheep and goats.

Microscopically, the lesions consist of an infiltration of the mucosa with plasma cells and especially endothelioid cells. Giant cell formation is not common (cf. tuberculosis). *Myco. paratuberculosis* may be present in other parts of the small intestine as well as at the site of the lesions, and the concentration of bacilli bears no relationship to the severity of the lesions.

Diagnosis

Microscopical examination of faeces

When Johne's disease is suspected a faecal smear should be prepared, stained by the Ziehl-Neelsen method and searched carefully for *Myco. paratuberculosis*. It is important to remember that the examination of only one sample from each suspected case may result in little more than 30 per cent of infected animals being diagnosed. It may be necessary to examine a number of samples from an individual before being able to make a positive diagnosis.

Bacteriological examination of faeces
Under certain conditions it may be considered of value to carry out bacteriological examinations of faecal samples. The methods are similar to those used for the isolation of *Myco. tuberculosis* from contaminated material. Faecal material can be treated with 20 per cent antiformin for 20 minutes at room temperature, or with malachite green and oxalic acid. In addition, penicillin may be incorporated in the media.

Johnin test
Johnin is prepared from *Myco. paratuberculosis* in a manner similar to that used for the preparation of tuberculin from *Myco. tuberculosis*. Many attempts have been made to control Johne's disease by using the Johnin test but in general the results have been disappointing, because it seems that the degree of hypersensitivity occurring in infected animals takes a comparatively long time to develop and is of low degree. Avian tuberculin can be used in place of Johnin and gives comparable results.

Complement-fixation test
This test has been applied to the control of Johne's disease, and various modifications of the basic method have been introduced. One method is to use heat-killed *Myco. paratuberculosis* as antigen and allow antibody to be adsorbed on to the antigen before the latter is washed, resuspended in saline and complement added.

The complement-fixation test is of value for the confirmation of infection in clinically diseased animals provided that bovine tuberculosis is not present. The test is also of some value for detecting infection in diseased animals which show no symptoms but it cannot be relied upon to keep a herd free from disease.

Control and prevention
A live vaccine has been developed which consists of non-pathogenic strains of *Myco. paratuberculosis* mixed with an adjuvant which includes liquid paraffin, olive oil and a small quantity of ground pumice. The vaccine is inoculated subcutaneously into calves soon after birth and before they are 4 weeks of age. There is evidence to show that vaccination reduces the incidence of clinical Johne's disease. The vaccine has also been used in sheep.

Further reading

AHO, K., BRANDER, E. AND ESTOLA, T. (1973) Agglutinins against Group III atypical mycobacteria. *Acta Pathologica et Microbiologica Scandinavica*, **81B**, 589.

BOUGHTON E. (1969) Tuberculosis caused by *Mycobacterium avium. Veterinary Bulletin*, **39**, 457.

COLLINS C.H. (1966) Revised classification of anonymous mycobacteria. *Journal of Clinical Pathology*, **19**, 433.

CROWLE A.J. (1958) Immunizing constituents of the tubercle bacillus. *Bacteriological Reviews*, **22**, 183.

DANNENBERG A.M. (1968) Cellular hypersensitivity and cellular immunity in the pathogenesis of tuberculosis: specificity, systemic and local nature, and associated macrophage enzymes. *Bacteriological Reviews*, **32**, 85.

DUBINA, J., SULA, L., KUBIN, M. AND VAREKOVA, J. (1974) Incidence of *M. avium* and *M. intracellulare* in cattle and pigs. *Journal of Hygiene, Epidemiology, Microbiology and Immunology*, **18**, 15.

HOLE N.H. (1958) Johne's Disease. *Advances in Veterinary Science*, **4**, 341.

JORGENSEN J.B. (1969) Paratuberculosis in pigs. *Acta Veterinaria Scandinavica*, **10**, 275.

LUKE D. (1958) Tuberculosis in the horse, pig, sheep and goat. *Veterinary Record*, **70**, 529.

MERKAL, R.S. (1973) Laboratory diagnosis of bovine paratuberculosis. *Journal of the American Veterinary Medical Association*, **163**, 1100.

MIDDLEBROOK G., Ed. (1969) Biology of mycobacterioses. *Annals of New York Academy of Science*, **154**, 243.

PARISOT T.J. (1958) Tuberculosis of fish. A review of the literature with a description of the disease in Salmonid fish. *Bacteriological Reviews*, **22**, 240.

ROSWURM, J.D. AND RANNEY, A.F. (1973) Sharpening the attack on bovine tuberculosis. *American Journal of Public Health*, **63**, 884.

SCHAEFER, W.B., BEER, J.V., WOOD, N.A., BOUGHTON, E., JENKINS, P.A. AND MARKS, J. (1973) A bacteriological study of endemic tuberculosis in birds. *Journal of Hygiene*, **71**, 549.

SUTHER, D.E., FRANTI, C.E. AND PAGE, H.H. (1974) Evaluation of a comparative intradermal tuberculin test in California dairy cattle. *American Journal of Veterinary Research*, **35**, 379.

TUFFLEY, R.E., LEGGO, J.H., SIMMONS, G.C. AND TAMMEMAGI, L. (1973) Studies on the virulence of *Mycobacterium intracellulare* serotype VI for pigs. *Journal of Comparative Pathology*, **83**, 467.

VOGEL H. (1958) Mycobacteria from cold-blooded animals. *American Review of Tuberculosis and Pulmonary Diseases*, **77**, 823.

WINBLAD, B. AND DUCHEK, M. (1973) Comparison between microscopical methods and cultivation for demonstration of tubercle bacilli in experimental tuberculous infection. *Acta Pathologica et Microbiologica Scandinavica*, **81A**, 824.

YACHIDA, S., SHIMIZU, K., HOROSE, T. AND SATO, M. (1973) Studies on mycobacteria isolated from skin lesion tuberculosis of the bovine udder. *Japanese Journal of Veterinary Science*, **35**, 357.

CHAPTER 22

ACTINOMYCES AND NOCARDIA

ACTINOMYCES

NOCARDIA

Actinomyces and Nocardia

ACTINOMYCES

There has been some confusion about the taxonomy of the group *Actinomyces* which consists of filamentous anaerobic or micro-aerophilic organisms. The pathogenic species are *Actinomyces bovis* and *Actinomyces israeli* which cause granulomatous conditions in animals and man known as actinomycosis. These organisms commonly occur as commensals and both species have very similar properties and can be distinguished from each other only with difficulty. Neither of them occurs outside the animal or human body.

Actinomyces bovis

Synonyms
This organism is also known as ray-fungus because of the characteristic arrangement of the organism in lesions. The species *Actinomyces israeli* is almost indistinguishable from *Actinomyces bovis*.

Distribution in nature
In 1877 the causal organism of a condition known as 'lumpy jaw' or actinomycosis was described and named *Actinomyces bovis*. A year later, Israel gave an account of a similar condition in man caused by an organism known as *Actinomyces israeli*.

In the past there has been some confusion as to the natural habitats and distribution of *Actinomyces bovis* but it is now generally agreed that it is an obligatory parasite occurring in the region of the mouth, pharynx and tonsils in animals and man, and that it does not exist outside the body. The infection has been reported from a variety of countries including the United Kingdom, Russia, Scandinavia and less frequently in other European countries. It has also been reported from some parts of the United States of America.

Morphology and staining
The organism shows considerable pleomorphism according to the conditions of growth. In lesions of actinomycosis the pus contains small pale yellow granules, sometimes referred to as 'sulphur granules', each about the size of a pin-head. Although these granules are sometimes hard and calcified, they contain colonies of bacteria. When crushed between two glass slides or observed in sections, the organisms can be seen as a central mass of filaments, about 1 μm. in width, which show true dichotomous branching, together with some shorter rods or coccoid forms (Plates 22.1a & b facing p. 242). These organisms stain Gram-positive.

Around the periphery of this filamentous mass is a circle of club-shaped bodies, arranged radially with their narrow ends pointing in towards the centre of the lesion (hence the name 'ray fungus') (Plate 22.1c, facing p. 242). These clubs form the main characteristic feature of older lesions, and probably arise from interaction between the filaments and host tissues at the periphery of each colony. These clubs stain Gram-negative.

After growth on laboratory media the organism occurs mostly as short bacilli or diphtheroid forms. A few filaments and branching forms may also be seen particularly in old cultures.

Cultural characteristics
Growth occurs anaerobically in an atmosphere containing 5 per cent CO_2 on agar enriched with glucose, serum or blood, on Dorset egg medium, Loeffler's serum, or in heart broth or glucose broth. The organism is non-haemolytic and non-proteolytic. The optimum temperature for growth is 37°C. After 4–6 days' incubation, colonies of *Actinomyces bovis* are round, flat, pale yellow in colour, about 1 mm in diameter, and they do not adhere to the medium. It should be noted that under similar conditions colonies of *Actinomyces israeli* have a rougher surface, a harder consistency, and are markedly adherent to the media.

In fluid media growth occurs in the form of small granules about 1 mm in diameter at the bottom and sides of tubes.

Acid without gas is produced in glucose and a variety of other carbohydrates.

Resistance to physical and chemical agents
The organism is killed by moist heat at a temperature of 60°C for 20 minutes.

Antigens and toxins
Strains of *Actinomyces bovis* isolated from cattle are antigenically homogenous and distinguishable serologically from the antigenically homogenous strains of *Actinomyces israeli* derived from human sources.

Epidemiology and pathogenesis
Present evidence indicates that *Actinomyces bovis* inhabits the digestive tract, particularly the mouth and pharynx as an obligatory parasite in the crypts of the tonsils, and in carious teeth. Lesions will develop only as the result of damage to the buccal epithelium and subsequent inoculation of the organism into the site. Thus, the common areas for infection are the cheek muscles, the lower jaw, the submaxillary region, and less frequently other areas in the region of the throat and head.

In pigs a frequent site for infection is the mammary gland and it may be that this arises from the organism being in the mouths of piglets and becoming inoculated through abrasions of the skin during suckling. The lungs and other organs are occasionally affected.

In dogs and cats the condition may arise in a variety of tissues including the liver, lungs, skin and subcutaneous tissues.

In the horse there is definite evidence that *Actinomyces bovis* occurs in lesions of fistulous withers and poll-evil in association with *Br. abortus* infections.

Symptoms
These vary according to the site and extent of the lesion. In cases of 'lumpy jaw' in cattle there are marked swellings associated with a suppurating osteitis in the region of the cheek and mandibular region, and extensive lesions may interfere with mastication. Another chronic form of infection occurs in the mammary glands of pigs which become enlarged, indurated and finally soften with the escape of pus containing the characteristic granules. In horses the infection is usually associated with fistulous withers or poll-evil, which develop as swellings containing pus at these sites.

Lesions
The typically chronic lesions arising from infection with *Actinomyces bovis* consist of areas of suppuration accompanied by the formation of granulation tissue, erosion of old bone and formation of new bone. The pockets of pus increase in size, develop sinuses or fistulae and discharge to the surface. The pus characteristically contains small granules (sulphur granules) which contain colonies of the organism.

Secondary sites of infection in the liver, bone and lungs may develop as the result of metastases which become distributed via the blood stream. In dogs and cats there is a tendency for the tissue reaction to be more rapid and exudative in type.

Microscopically, the typically chronic type of lesion consists of a central area of necrosis surrounded by granulation tissue which is enclosed in a compact layer of fibrous tissue.

Diagnosis
This depends upon the demonstration of *Actinomyces bovis* as the causal organism. A diagnosis can be made by squashing and examining microscopically the granules in the pus which contain the organisms. Alternatively, the isolation and growth of the organism on laboratory media under anaerobic conditions enables it to be differentiated from organisms belonging to the genus *Nocardia* which grow aerobically. Cultures can be made on blood agar, glucose agar or Dorset egg medium.

Control and prevention
Actinomyces bovis is sensitive to penicillin and the most satisfactory form of treatment consists of repeated daily injections with penicillin until the symptoms of infection have disappeared. Other methods of treatment have included administration of sulphonamides or streptomycin.

NOCARDIA

Distribution in nature
Nocardia differ from *Actinomyces* in being aerobic organisms. Many are acid-fast and chromogenic. The majority of species are saprophytes but a few are pathogenic and produce chronic suppurative conditions in animals and man. *Nocardia farcinica* (*Actinomyces farcinicus*) is the cause of bovine 'Farcy' and was first described in 1888 by Nocard, after whom the group of organisms is named.

Morphology and staining
These are long filamentous, branching organisms which produce mycelia with terminal spores (Plate 22.1d, facing p. 242). After subcultivation on laboratory media there is a tendency for the filaments to fragment into oval, coccoid or bacillary forms.

The organisms stain Gram-positive and some strains are acid-fast.

Cultural characteristics
The organisms grow aerobically but not anaerobically on a variety of media at 37°C or at room

temperature. After 4–7 days incubation on solid media the colonies of *Nocardia farcinica* are opaque, wrinkled, yellowish-white and of a dry consistency. Some other members of the group produce colonies which become yellow or pink in colour. In broth cultures the organisms develop as irregular, whitish clumps dispersed throughout the medium.

Resistance to physical and chemical agents
The organisms are killed by heating to a temperature of 70°C for 10–15 minutes.

Epidemiology and pathogenesis
Little is known about the pathogenesis of these infections but it is probable that *Nocardia farcinica*, the cause of Farcy in cattle, gains entry into the body through superficial wounds. As a result of infection the lymphatic vessels and glands in the legs become enlarged, corded and nodular, due to the slow formation of caseous material which sometimes breaks to the surface. Bovine mastitis associated with *Nocardia asteroides* has been des-cribed and this organism may also cause a severe pneumonia in debilitated dogs. (Plate 22.1e, facing p. 242).

Nocardia madurae is a cause of an infective granulomatous condition in man known as 'madura foot'.

Further reading

AINSWORTH G.C. (1962) Classification of actinomycetes. *Veterinary Annual*, **4**, 70.

AINSWORTH G.C. AND AUSTWICK P.K.C. (1958) *Fungal Diseases of Animals*. Farnham, England: Commonwealth Agricultural Bureau.

COPE Z. (1962) Actinomycosis. *Veterinary Annual*, **4**, 5.

MOSTAFA I.E. (1966) Bovine nocardiosis (cattle farcy): A review. *Veterinary Bulletin*. **36**, 189.

PINE L., HOWELL A. AND WATSON S.J. (1960) Studies of the morphological, physiological and biochemical characters of *Actinomyces bovis*. *Journal of General Microbiology*, **23**, 403.

CHAPTER 23

PSEUDOMONAS

CHAPTER 23

Pseudomonas

This group of organisms includes a large number of different species of non-sporulating aerobic bacilli which stain Gram-negative. With the exception of *Pseudomonas mallei*, all species are motile by means of one or more polar flagella. The only pathogenic species for animals are *P. aeruginosa*, associated mainly with pyogenic infections and enteritis, *P. mallei* the cause of glanders, and *P. pseudomallei* the cause of melioidosis.

Pseudomonas aeruginosa

Synonyms
Pseudomonas pyocyanea, Bacillus pyocyaneus.

Distribution in nature
This organism has a wide distribution, occurring as part of the normal bacterial flora of the intestines of animals and man. It is known to be associated with a wide variety of infections in many animal species and man, and is frequently the cause of suppurative lesions.

Morphology and staining
P. aeruginosa is rod-shaped, usually measuring about 1·5 μm in length by 0·5 μm in width, but sometimes longer forms develop. The organisms are actively motile and possess polar flagella. Capsules and spores are not produced.

   P. aeruginosa stains Gram-negative and is non-acid-alcohol-fast.

Cultural characteristics
The organism grows well on ordinary nutrient media at 37°C but growth will also occur over a wide temperature range of 5–43°C.

   On agar the colonies are convex, glistening, with a tendency for the edges to be translucent and spreading. The majority of strains appear fluorescent due to the production of the pigments pyocyanin and fluorescin which diffuse through the media

(Plate 23.1a, facing p. 243). These pigments possess limited antibacterial activities; both of them are soluble in water and pyocyanin is also soluble in chloroform.

   In nutrient broth there is abundant growth with discolouration of the medium resulting from pigment formation. All cultures develop a characteristic sickly odour.

   Acid without gas is produced in glucose. Gelatin is liquefied and urea is hydrolysed slowly. The organism gives negative Voges-Proskauer and methyl red reactions, does not produce H_2S or indole, and fails to reduce nitrates to nitrites. The alkaline phosphatase of this organism and of *P. pseudomallei* resist a temperature of 70°C for 20 minutes, whereas the phosphatases of non-pathogenic species of *Pseudomonas* are thermolabile.

   Unlike *P. pseudomallei*, *P. aeruginosa* does not ferment sucrose but grows on desoxycholate citrate agar.

Resistance to physical and chemical agents
P. aeruginosa is relatively susceptible to the lethal effects of heat and disinfectants. The organisms are killed by a temperature of 55°C for 1 hour.

Antigens and toxins
Attempts have been made to use the somatic and flagella antigens for serotyping strains of *P. aeruginosa* isolated from animals. Several 'O' groups have been described and phage typing has also been studied.

Epidemiology and pathogenesis
P. aeruginosa is widely distributed in nature and is a common inhabitant of the soil. Although not a highly pathogenic organism, its virulence is increased by the production of extracellular slime which is known to contain proteases. *P. aeruginosa* is associated with the development of abscesses and wound infections characterised by the formation of

greenish-yellow pus in a variety of animal species. It has been isolated from cases of bovine mastitis, from infections of the uro-genital tract of adult animals, and from cases of enteritis in calves and pigs. It has also been associated with liver abscesses, peritonitis and arthritis in calves, with pneumonia in pigs and calves, and with similar infections in rabbits, mink and chinchilla. The organism is frequently present as part of the intestinal bacterial flora of normal calves during the first four weeks of life and, thereafter, its incidence decreases.

Laboratory animals, including rabbits, guinea-pigs, rats, mice and pigeons are susceptible to subcutaneous, intraperitoneal or intravenous inoculation of the organism. Small doses tend to produce localised abscess formation and larger doses cause a generalised and fatal infection.

Symptoms and lesions

The symptoms depend upon the degree and site of infection. In severe cases there is a rise in body temperature and additional symptoms are related to the organs affected. Characteristically, localised lesions contain greenish-yellow pus and are sometimes associated with other bacterial infections, particularly pyogenic organisms. Non-specific symptoms are those associated with bovine mastitis which may be either chronic or acute and fatal in 3–4 days, and with enteric infections in young animals, particularly calves and pigs.

Diagnosis

A final diagnosis depends upon the bacteriological examination of material from suspected cases, and the isolation and identification of the causal organism.

Control and prevention

Various chemotherapeutic agents have been employed with mixed results. The organism is particularly susceptible to polymyxin B.

Public health aspects

P. aeruginosa may occur normally on the skin and in the intestine and faeces of healthy individuals. It is the cause of localised infections in adults arising as secondary infections to surgical trauma or as concurrent infections with other microbial species. Common sites of infection are skin wounds, the urinary tract following catheterisation, otitis media, enteritis and pneumonia.

Pseudomonas mallei

Synonyms

Actinobacillus mallei, Loefflerella mallei, Pfeifferella mallei, Malleomyces mallei, Bacillus mallei.

Distribution in nature

This organism is the cause of glanders in equine species and in man. The disease which was originally described by Loeffler and Schutz as long ago as 1882 has been eradicated from the United Kingdom, some other European countries, the U.S.A. and Canada, but occurs in a number of countries in Eastern Europe and Asia.

Morphology and staining

In infected lesions and on primary culture the organism occurs in the smooth form as rods measuring 2–4 μm in length and 0·5 μm in width. After repeated subculture, rough pleomorphic forms may develop as filaments, sometimes showing branching. The organism is non-motile and does not produce capsules or spores.

P. mallei stains Gram-negative and sometimes shows uneven or beaded staining.

Cultural characteristics

P. mallei is aerobic but under strict anaerobic conditions growth will also occur in the absence of glucose and in the presence of nitrate. Growth occurs slowly on ordinary laboratory media at an optimum temperature of 37°C, and is improved on media containing glycerol. After 48 hours' incubation on glycerol agar the colonies are small, yellowish in colour and slimy. Prolonged incubation results in the development of larger brownish colonies. Inspissated serum or serum agar can also be used for growing these organisms. On glycerol potato medium most strains appear characteristically after 3 days' incubation as pale yellow colonies which, after prolonged incubation, become brown or chocolate coloured. There is no growth on MacConkey's agar.

Broth cultures yield moderate growth with uniform turbidity, and after several days' incubation areas of slimy growth develop on the surface pellicle.

Glucose is fermented slowly by some strains. Other carbohydrates are not fermented.

Resistance to physical and chemical agents

P. mallei is highly susceptible to moist heat and exposure to a temperature of 55°C for 10 minutes is lethal. The organisms are also killed by mercuric chloride, phenol and other disinfectants after contact with these substances for 15–30 minutes, depending upon the prevailing conditions. Organisms in pus will be protected to some extent from the rapid lethal effects of disinfectants.

Antigens and toxins

Strains of *P. mallei* can be divided into three antigenic groups on the basis of antigens which are specific for these organisms. In addition, there is a common

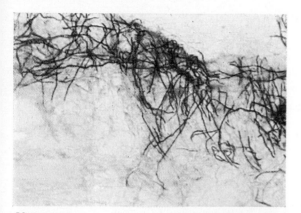

22.1a

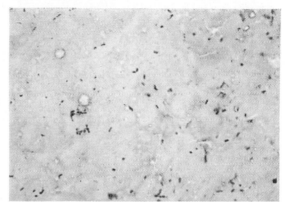

22.1b

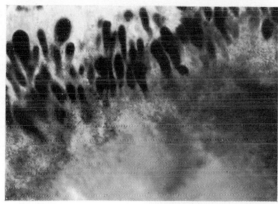

22.1c

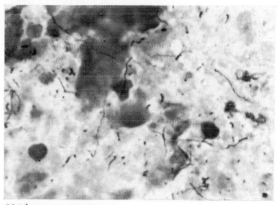

22.1d

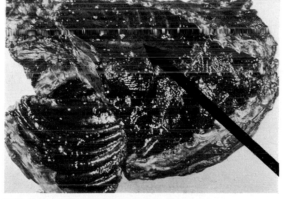

22.1e

22.1a Gram-stained film of *Actinomyces bovis* showing the organisms as branching filaments, × 930.

22.1b Gram-stained film of *Actinomyces bovis* showing the organisms as short bacilli or coccoid forms, × 930.

22.1c Crushed granule from pus stained Ziehl-Neelsen, showing radially arranged club-shaped bodies surrounding a filamentous mass of *Actinomyces bovis* organisms, × 930.

22.1d Gram-stained film from peritoneum of dog showing the branching filaments of *Nocardia asteroides*, × 930.

22.1e Macroscopic appearance of a dog's thorax infected with *Nocardia asteroides*, showing miliary lesions (arrowed) associated with severe pneumonia and haemorrhages.

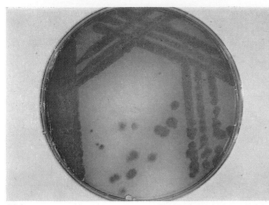

23.1a

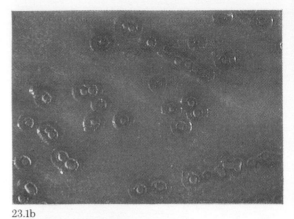

23.1b

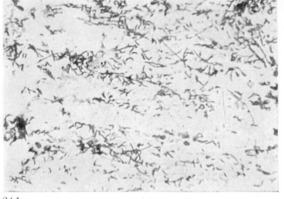

24.1

23.1a Growth of *Pseudomonas aeruginosa* on agar showing green colouration due to the pigment pyocyanin.

23.1b Colonies of *Pseudomonas pseudomallei* after 24 hours' incubation on an agar medium.

24.1 Gram-stained film of *Campylobacter fetus* in stomach contents of aborted bovine fetus. Note the comma- and filamentous-shapes of the organisms, ×930.

protein antigen produced by strains of *P. mallei*, *P. pseudomallei* and *Actinobacillus lignièresi*. *P. mallei* is described as showing S (smooth) $\longrightarrow$ R (rough) variation. The S form grows on solid media as moist, circular colonies, whereas the R form develops as smaller, yellow, crenated colonies with a drier consistency. There is a tendency for the S colonies to be composed of short rods and R colonies to consist of bacillary chains or filaments. It should also be noted that the virulence of a particular strain of *P. mallei* may become markedly reduced as a result of repeated subcultivation on laboratory media. Conversely, an avirulent strain may develop increased virulence as a result of animal passage.

Epidemiology and pathogenesis

Under natural conditions glanders affects horses, mules and donkeys. The disease is also known to have occurred occasionally in lions, tigers and leopards as a result of eating meat from horse carcases infected with *P. mallei*. Cattle, pigs and poultry are resistant. In those areas of the world where glanders is still a problem the sources of infection are carrier animals. The clinical signs of infection may include the development of lesions containing large numbers of the causal organism in the nasal cavity and on the skin. These sites of concentrated infection are the sources for contamination of water, food, grooming utensils and harness. In this way, infection is spread to other animals by ingestion, inhalation or wound infection.

Although infection by ingestion of *P. mallei* can take place through the intact surface of the digestive tract, the process is greatly facilitated by wounds to the mucosa. It is unusual for primary infection of the lung to occur by inhalation of the causal organisms. It can only arise from the inhalation of fresh infected material since infectivity decreases rapidly as a result of dessication. In addition, the general susceptibility of individual animals to glanders is increased by overwork, poor nutrition, other debilitating diseases and possibly by the size of the infective dose.

Initially, the distribution of organisms in the body occurs via the lymphatic system and as the burden of infection increases in an individual, organisms are disseminated via the blood stream and settle in the lungs, the nasal mucosa, and less frequently in the skin and other organs.

Under laboratory conditions hamsters, guinea-pigs and ferrets are susceptible to infection; and mice, rats and rabbits are relatively insusceptible.

Symptoms and lesions

The incubation period depends upon the route of infection, the virulence of the organism, and the size of the infective dose. Under experimental conditions a rise in temperature takes place 2–3 days after inoculation of organisms into the skin or on to the nasal mucosa, and a day or two later after ingestion of infective material. Following infection under natural conditions, several weeks may elapse before definite symptoms develop, but during the incubation period there may be intermittent rises in temperature to about 40°C.

For convenience of description, the clinical forms of the disease in horses have often been classified as the pulmonary form, the nasal form and the cutaneous (farcy) form. However, it should be remembered that one form alone seldom occurs in an individual and that two or more forms may be present in one animal at the same time.

The pulmonary form first becomes manifest by a rise in temperature and coughing which may produce blood stained mucus. The nasal form develops initially as a reddening of the nasal mucosa and a mucoid discharge from one or both nostrils which later may become purulent, blood stained and adherent to the nasal margins as brown crusts. Ulcers may form on the nasal mucosa. The submaxillary lymph glands become enlarged.

The cutaneous form of glanders, also known as farcy, is characterised in the early stages by the development of small cutaneous or subcutaneous nodules, commonly occurring on the limbs or flanks. Later, these nodules develop into hollow ulcers exuding a yellow, oily pus. The local lymphatic vessels become corded.

Asses and mules infected with glanders usually suffer from an acute form of the disease which often terminates fatally after a few weeks.

Histologically, the development of a glanders lesion in the lung commences with an infiltration of neutrophils, and fragmentation of cellular nuclei (karyorrhexis). Endothelial cells develop around the central, necrotic area of older lesions which become walled-off by a fibrous capsule. Giant cells sometimes develop but calcification is rare. These lesions may appear as yellowish-grey nodules about 1 mm in diameter, frequently surrounded by small haemorrhagic areas. At a later stage they become larger, reddish-brown in colour and with a suppurative centre surrounded by an area of haemorrhage.

Diagnosis

Clinical cases of glanders may be diagnosed on the history of the disease in the particular environment together with symptoms of chronic coughing, nasal discharge, ulceration and lymphadenitis. Confirmation is obtained from bacteriological examinations. The mallein test and serological methods must be used for the diagnosis of the occult form of the disease.

Mallein test

This consists of an allergic test, basically similar to the tuberculin test. Mallein is the active principle prepared from cultures of *P. mallei*. Various sites can be used for inoculation, particularly the intradermopalpebral test in which mallein is injected into the skin of the lower eyelid. A positive reaction develops as an oedematous swelling of the eyelid and congestion of the conjunctiva after 36–48 hours following inoculation. A similar cutaneous test can be carried out in the skin of the neck in which a positive reaction develops as a delayed oedematous swelling. Mallein can also be inoculated subcutaneously in which case a positive reaction occurs as an extensive diffuse swelling with well-defined borders at the site of injection together with a rise in the body temperature.

Serological tests

The agglutination, precipitation, complement-fixation and conglutination tests have all been used for the detection of infected animals. Normal serum agglutinins are often present in titres of about 1/640 and infection cannot be reliably diagnosed unless the titre is about 1/1000. The precipitation test is used more frequently for the study of antigens than for the routine identification of infected animals. The complement-fixation test gives more specific results than the foregoing method and has been widely used for the diagnosis of infection in horses. The conglutination test is a sensitive method for diagnosing the disease and has the advantage that it can be used with samples from mules, asses and a proportion of horses whose sera may be anticomplementary. None of these serological tests should be applied to sera from animals which have received subcutaneous injections of mallein, since these cause rises in serum titres to diagnostic levels for periods of several months after injection.

Bacteriological tests

Pus from a cutaneous lesion can be examined microscopically for *P. mallei* and a differential diagnosis made between glanders and streptococcal or cryptococcal infections. It should be remembered, however, that it is sometimes difficult to demonstrate the glanders bacillus in pus. Cultures of *P. mallei* can be made from pus using glycerol agar or potato, inspissated serum or selective media incorporating malachite green and fuchsin or thionine.

Control and prevention

This disease is controlled by the identification and slaughter of infected animals and the thorough disinfection of contaminated premises.

Public health aspects

The disease occurs in man usually as a result of direct contact with infected animals and is often fatal. It commonly develops as a skin infection arising from a cutaneous wound. The infection spreads from the local primary lesion to produce a lymphangitis and finally a pyaemia.

Pseudomonas pseudomallei

Synonyms

Loefflerella pseudomallei; Pfeifferella whitmori; Bacillus whitmori; Malleomyces pseudomallei.

Distribution in nature

This organism is the cause of a human disease known as melioidosis. The infection has also been reported in the horse, cow, sheep, goat, pig, dog and cat. Melioidosis occurs mainly in Malaysia, Indo-China, India and Sri Lanka. A few cases have been reported among sheep and goats in Australia and in the Caribbean.

Morphology and staining

Morphologically, the organism resembles *P. mallei* except that it possesses one polar flagellum and is motile. It stains Gram-negative with a marked tendency to bipolar staining.

Cultural characteristics.

P. pseudomallei grows well on ordinary laboratory media at 37°C and growth is enhanced in the presence of glycerol. Cultures have a characteristic earthy odour. Colonies on solid media may be corrugated or mucoid, cream coloured and sometimes become pale brown after 7–10 days' incubation. Gelatin is liquefied slowly at 20°C and rapidly (3–4 days) at 37°C. The organism grows on MacConkey's agar, producing red colonies clearly visible after 48 hours' incubation (Plate 23.1b, facing p. 243). Growth is slower on all media incubated at 21°C.

Carbohydrate fermentation is variable. Some strains ferment glucose and sucrose only, with production of acid, especially after they have been subcultured several times on laboratory media. Catalase and ammonia are produced but indole and H_2S are not formed.

The alkaline phosphatases of this organism and of *P. aeruginosa* resist a temperature of 70°C for 20 minutes, whereas the phosphatases of non-pathogenic species of *Pseudomonas* are thermolabile.

Unlike *P. aeruginosa*, *P. pseudomallei* ferments sucrose and fails to grow on desoxycholate citrate agar.

Resistance to physical and chemical agents

Similar to *P. mallei.*

Antigens and toxins

All strains of *P. pseudomallei* have antigens in common with each other, and in addition there is an antigenic relationship between strains of *P. pseudomallei* and some strains of *P. mallei*. A complex exotoxin is produced which is both lethal and necrotizing.

Epidemiology and pathogenesis

Over 50 years ago it was suggested that wild rats were a reservoir for these organisms, but this has since been disproved following the failure to isolate *P. pseudomallei* from many thousands of rats examined in the area of Saigon where melioidosis is endemic. Present evidence indicates that *P. pseudomallei* is a normal inhabitant of water and soil, that it is not a highly pathogenic organism and has practically no invasive ability. Disease associated with this organism seldom develops in the absence of predisposing factors which lead to a lowered host resistance and to the inoculation of the organism into wounds via contaminated mud and water. Another characteristic epidemiological feature is that all cases of melioidosis have occurred within the parallels 20°N and 20°S of the equator and the disease has not been reported from temperate climates. It is becoming clear that domesticated animals are, themselves, reservoirs of infection because the majority of infected animals are symptomless carriers.

Symptoms and lesions

Infected sheep may show lameness, an unsteady gait, coughing and lesions resembling those of caseous lymphadenitis. Post-mortem examination shows numerous abscesses situated particularly in the lungs and less frequently in the spleen and kidney. Similar lesions occur in pigs. Infected goats may develop a mastitis, and in horses the symptoms may resemble those of glanders. The few reports of cases in dogs and cats refer to symptoms of acute gastroenteritis.

Diagnosis

This can be made from the symptoms and lesions of the condition as it occurs in tropical regions, together with bacteriological examination and isolation of the causal organism on 10 per cent blood agar or on MacConkey's agar. Special note should be taken of the organisms' motility, the frequently corrugated type of growth on solid media and liquefaction of gelatin. Slide agglutination tests can be used for screening suspected colonies.

Guinea-pigs often die after intraperitoneal inoculation with infected pus or tissue, and multiple abscess formation will have developed in the liver, spleen, omentum and sometimes in the lungs and kidneys.

Control and prevention

The complement-fixation test is of value for the detection of both acute and chronic infection in sheep. A titre of 1/20 indicates active or recent infection; and this level of antibody titre is known to develop within 7 days of infection. There is no cross-reaction with *P. aeruginosa*. A haemagglutination test can be used but is less sensitive.

The melioidin test has been applied to goats. The preferable site is intradermal inoculation into the caudal fold and examination of the lesion after 3–4 days.

P. pseudomallei is very sensitive to tetracycline and less sensitive to chloramphenicol and aureomycin.

Public health aspects

The disease often develops in man as a pulmonary infection resembling tuberculosis, followed by a septicaemia which gives rise to the formation of multiple small abscesses in the lungs, liver, spleen and other organs. This generalised type of infection is often fatal. The organism is not highly invasive and clinical melioidosis only develops in people whose general health and resistance have been reduced by concurrent disease. Among natives living in endemic areas the disease can be relatively benign.

Further reading

BERGAN, T. (1972) Bacteriophage typing and serogrouping of *Pseudomonas aeruginosa* from animals. *Acta Pathologica et Microbiologica Scandinavica*, **80B** 351.

CRAVITZ L. AND MILLER W.R. (1950) Immunologic studies with *Malleomyces mallei* and *Malleomyces pseudomallei*. I. Serological relationships between *M. mallei* and *M. pseudomallei*. *Journal of Infectious Diseases*, **86**, 46.

FARKAS-HIMSLEY H. (1968) Selection and rapid identification of *Pseudomonas pseudomallei* from other Gram-negative bacteria. *American Journal of Clinical Pathology*, **49**, 850.

GOULD J.C. AND McLEOD J.W. (1960) A study of the use of agglutinating sera and phage lysis in the classification of strains of *Pseudomonas aeruginosa*. *Journal of Pathology and Bacteriology*, **79**, 295.

LIU P.V., ABE Y. AND BATES J.L. (1961) The roles of various fractions of *Pseudomonas aeruginosa* in its pathogenesis. *Journal of Infectious Diseases*, **108**, 218.

REDFEARN M.S., PALLERONI N.J. AND STANIER R.Y. (1966) A comparative study of *Pseudomonas pseudomallei* and *Bacillus mallei*. *Journal of General Microbiology*, **43**, 293.

SANDVIK O. (1960) The serology of *Pseudomonas aeruginosa* from bovine udder infections. *Acta veterinaria Scandinavica.* **1**, 221.

SENSAKOVIC J.W. AND BARTELL P.F. (1974) The slime of *Pseudomonas aeruginosa*: biological characterization and possible role in experimental infection. *Journal of Infectious Diseases*, **129**, 101.

CHAPTER 24

CAMPYLOBACTER

CHAPTER 24

Campylobacter

The microaerophilic vibrios have been recently removed from the genus *Vibrio,* which still contains the aerobic species *Vibrio cholerae,* and reclassified in the genus *Campylobacter* (Gr. adj. *Campylo,* curved; Gr. n. *bacter,* rod).

There are a number of species of campylobacters associated with disease in animals and economically the most important of these is *Campylobacter fetus* (formerly *Vibrio fetus*) which causes infertility and abortion among bovine animals and abortion in sheep. *C. jejuni* has been isolated from cases of diarrhoea in cattle, *C. coli* has been identified with a form of severe dysentery in young pigs, and a distinct catalase negative species allied to *C.bubulus,* has more recently been associated with the lesions of porcine intestinal adenomatosis. A campylobacteral hepatitis has been described in chickens and turkeys. In addition, there are non-pathogenic species associated with animals and man.

The classification of campylobacters is still incomplete and knowledge on the incidence of pathogenic strains and on the disease processes they cause has been hampered by the technical difficulties of isolating and propagating some species in the laboratory. There is little doubt that further research into these organisms will reveal additional important knowledge concerning their natural history and more particularly their antigenic structures and the pathogenesis of the diseases they cause.

Campylobacter fetus

Distribution in nature
Campylobacter fetus is world-wide in its distribution and has been known as a cause of abortions in sheep for more than 50 years and of infertility in cattle for some 20 years. The natural habitats for these organisms are the genital and intestinal tracts of cattle and sheep, and there is evidence to show that some species of wild birds may harbour and disseminate infection.

Morphology and staining
C. fetus is characteristically comma- or S-shaped and is often described as having the appearance of a 'flying seagull' (Plate 24.1, facing p. 243). Sometimes longer forms of the organism consist of four or five coils. The length varies from 1·5 to 4·0 μm or more and the width is about 0·5 μm. In tissues and young cultures the shorter forms are more usual but in older cultures chains of organisms appearing as long spirals may be seen together with coccoid forms. It has been suggested that the latter which have some similarities to bacterial L-forms, could be a stage in the life cycle of *C. fetus*. The organisms have polar flagella and are motile. They do not form spores.

C. fetus stains Gram-negative.

Cultural characteristics
C. fetus is micro-aerophilic and requires a reduced oxygen tension for growth. This can be provided by an atmosphere of 10 per cent CO_2 with or without nitrogen to reduce the oxygen tension to 30 per cent. The optimum temperature for growth is 37°C.

For primary isolations blood agar is widely used with or without the addition of 0·1 per cent sodium thioglycollate, or with antibiotics, including bacitracin, novobiocin and cyclohexamide. Another medium sometimes employed is serum-dextrose-antibiotic broth containing horse serum, actidione, polymixin and bacitracin. Thiol medium has also been used for both isolation and maintenance of cultures. Chocolate agar is sometimes employed for the production of antigens. Growth on laboratory media is slow and inoculated plates may have to be incubated for 2-5 days before smooth strains are observed as small, delicate, circular and opaque colonies. Frequently, cultures consist of a mixture of small and large colonies and a number of these may have coalesced to produce a large mucoid mass which may be elongated along the line of inoculation. Other cultures may be difficult to observe as they produce only a frosted appearance over the surface of the medium. Rough strains develop as larger colonies with a drier consistency and slightly irregular margins.

A comparative study of the biochemical reactions of different strains of *C. fetus* (Table 24.1) has shown that *C. fetus* (*venerealis*) causing infertility and sometimes abortion in cattle is catalase positive and H_2S negative. *C. fetus* (*intestinalis*), causing enzootic abortion in sheep and sporadic abortion in cattle, is catalase positive and H_2S positive. Although further study is required on the criteria employed for subdividing strains of *C. fetus*, these two varieties are now generally accepted. These and other properties, including tolerance to 3·5 per cent NaCl and to 1·0 per cent glycine, enable strains of *C. fetus* (*venerealis*) and *C. fetus* (*intestinalis*) to be differentiated from saprophytic species including *C. bubulus* which is catalase negative.

Resistance to physical and chemical agents
C. fetus is relatively susceptible to heat and is killed by exposure to a temperature of 60°C for 5 minutes. It will survive for 10–20 days in soil, hay and manure, depending upon the conditions of humidity and temperature. The organisms are readily killed by disinfectants.

Antigens and toxins
C. fetus possesses O (somatic), H (flagellar) and K. (capsular) antigens. Strains are antigenically heterogenous and attempts to classify them serologically have led to some confusion. Several groups have been identified and some contain both bovine and ovine strains of the organism. The antigenic structures of *C. fetus* organisms are distinct from those of saprophytic catalase negative strains of other campylobacteral species. The H antigens of *C. fetus*

consist of some components which are related either to a group of strains or to only an individual strain. The K antigen which has been observed on some organisms inhibits O agglutination and this inhibition can be removed by heating to 120°C for 2 hours.

Comparisons between the antigens of bovine and ovine strains of *C. fetus* have shown that some derived from one animal species may be antigenically related to those isolated from the other species. Although there may be this common antigenic relationship between some bovine and ovine strains, there is little evidence to indicate that under natural conditions infection will spread from one animal species to the other. It has been shown that some strains of *C. fetus* have an antigenic relationship with *Brucella abortus*.

Epidemiology and pathogenesis

Cattle
C. fetus (*venerealis*) infection is a venereal disease. Healthy bulls may become infected during coitus with diseased cows, or from contaminated bedding. The site of infection is the epithelium of the prepuce and such animals show no clinical signs of disease and their conception rates may be normal. During coitus the transference of organisms will result in the development of either an acute or chronic infection of the uterus depending upon the immune status of the cow. It is generally believed that acute infection causes inflammatory changes in the uterus and subsequent death of the fertilized ovum, followed by either expulsion or absorption of the embryo in the early stages of development, and probably within three to four weeks of fertilization. In cows which have some immunity to *C. fetus*, the development of the embryo may proceed to a later

TABLE 24.1. Comparison of the properties of *C. fetus* (*venerealis*), *C. fetus* (*intestinalis*) and *C. bubulus*.

Characteristic properties	*C. fetus* (*venerealis*)	*C. fetus* (*intestinalis*)	*C. bubulus*
Production of catalase	+	+	−
Production of H_2S	−	+	+
Growth in presence of 3·5 per cent NaCl	−	−	+
Growth in presence of 1·0 per cent glycine	−	+	+
Predilection sites	Genital tract of cow. Preputial epithelium of bull	Intestinal tract and vagina of sheep	Vagina and preputial epithelium of cattle and sheep
Diseases	Infertility and abortion in cattle	Enzootic abortion in sheep Sporadic cases of abortion in cattle	Not pathogenic

stage in pregnancy before the inflammatory reactions of the uterus and placenta cause death and abortion of the fetus, which usually takes place at about the fifth month of pregnancy.

Sheep

C. fetus (*intestinalis*) infection in sheep is not a venereal disease. The common route of infection is by ingestion of the organism from contaminated pastures or water; and there is evidence suggesting that infection may be disseminated by chickens, turkeys, ravens, magpies, sparrows, starlings and other species of birds. The disease is characterised by abortion which usually occurs during the third to fifth months of pregnancy. Infection does not cause infertility. Sheep show a remarkable resistance to infection and it has been demonstrated on several occasions that abortions do not occur when healthy pregnant animals become infected with *C. fetus* before the second or third month of pregnancy. It is only during the later stages of pregnancy that infection will persist and cause abortion. There is also evidence to show that following an 'abortion storm' in a flock, sheep will subsequently develop an immunity and many animals will become symptomless carriers and a source of infection to other susceptible sheep. Unlike bulls, rams play little or no part in the dissemination of infection in a flock, and this is confirmed by the resistance of ewes to infection until after the third month of pregnancy.

The fact that *C. fetus* has been detected in the faeces of clinically normal sheep, in the vaginas of pregnant ewes which have not aborted, and also in the vaginas of virgin yearlings, illustrates clearly the resistance which sheep can develop against this type of infection.

The pathogenesis of infection leading to abortion is not known. From various investigations it has been shown that after oral infection a transient bacteraemia may develop and the organisms localise and multiply in the gravid uterus causing a placentitis. The actual cause of fetal death has been variously ascribed to the inflammatory responses of the uterus, to bacterial multiplication in that organ, to a toxaemia, or to a hypersensitive reaction related to the immune status of the host and the high concentration of bacterial lipopolysaccharide.

Symptoms

Cattle

Infertility caused by infection with *C. fetus* may become apparent only when the percentage of pregnancies in a herd is low after one mating and after several subsequent matings when a proportion of the herd remains barren. It is a feature of this disease that the infertility rate tends to be higher in heifers than in cows. Some infected cattle may show signs of long and irregular oestral cycles particularly if they have become recently infected, and there may be a transient inflammation of the vaginal mucosa and excess vaginal mucus.

Abortions resulting from infection with *C. fetus* occur usually between the fifth and sixth months of pregnancy but can also take place as early as two months or almost at full term.

Infected bulls show no symptoms and their semen is normal.

Sheep

The disease is characterised by abortion occurring towards the end of the gestation period and is usually preceded by a vaginal discharge for several days before abortion takes place, and for a few days afterwards. It is not unusual for an 'abortion storm' to develop in a flock at about one or two months before the normal lambing season is due to commence. The number of abortions may vary from about 5–60 per cent or more and often averages around 20 per cent. A small number of ewes may die subsequently as a result of septic infections of the uterus.

Lesions

Cattle

The carcase of an aborted fetus is oedematous and there is a serofibrinous peritonitis and pericarditis with petechial haemorrhages. In some cases there are miliary necrotic lesions in the liver. The fetal membranes are oedematous and there are haemorrhagic and necrotic areas on the cotyledons. The cow will be suffering from acute catarrhal inflammation of the vagina and cervix.

Sheep

The main features in the fetus are subcutaneous oedema with petechial haemorrhages on the serous surfaces and necrotic foci in the liver. Putrefaction may be advanced in some cases. The fetal membranes show severe hyperaemia of the cotyledons and general oedema with areas of haemorrhage between the cotyledons. The placenta often shows signs of decomposition and some cotyledons may be yellowish in colour. In many cases the ewe will appear normal but in some the uterus will be oedematous with areas of marked hyperaemia.

Diagnosis

Bacteriological tests

A history of sterility or abortion in cattle or of abortion in sheep may provide evidence suggestive of *C. fetus* infection, but a final diagnosis must depend upon a more detailed examination of the herd or flock and of aborted fetuses. The latter should be examined bacteriologically as soon as possible. Smears prepared from the stomach contents of fetuses and stained by Gram's method will show the characteristic morphology of *C. fetus*. Cultures should be made from the stomach contents or visceral organs, and when the fetus shows signs of decomposition the bone marrow or brain may be preferable sites for primary cultures. The organism can be readily seen in stained impression smears prepared from the fetal cotyledons of sheep provided the material is fresh.

Suspected infection in cows may be confirmed by bacteriological examination of vaginal mucus. Material should be collected in glass or plastic pipettes to avoid contamination. The most suitable time to obtain infected samples from heifers is soon after infection, namely, within 3 weeks of service or artificial insemination. *C. fetus* can be isolated from cervical mucus at all stages of the oestral cycle and especially during oestrus, and samples should be stored at −65°C until examined. Infection in bulls can be diagnosed by examining bacteriologically the semen and preputial washings. However, contamination of samples may cause difficulty in isolating *C. fetus* and one negative result should not be interpreted as indicating absence of infection. The identification of *C. fetus* can be facilitated by using fluorescent antibody techniques, particularly for the examination of preputial washings from bulls.

Vaginal mucus agglutination tests
Antibodies may be detectable in the vaginal mucus of diseased cattle for approximately 2–12 months after infection and occasionally longer. Tests should be carried out on a herd basis because of the lag period between the time of infection and the appearance of agglutinins in the mucus, and also because agglutinin titres in the mucus become reduced and sometimes negative during oestrus. Mucus is collected either in a glass pipette or with a gauze tampon and mixed with saline. Agar is used to extract the antibodies from the mucus in the following manner. A volume of 2·0 ml of mucus-saline (1:4) mixture which has been homogenised, is placed in a waterbath at 57°C, and 2·0 ml molten agar is added. The contents of the tube are thoroughly mixed and dispensed into a 30 ml screw-capped glass bottle and allowed to stand at room temperature. After the agar has set, 2·0 ml of 0·5 per cent phenol-saline is added to the bottle and the contents incubated at 37°C for 18 hours. The clear supernatant fluid will then contain the extracted antibodies, and is tested for agglutinins in doubling dilutions commencing at 1 in 2. The test is incubated at 37°C for 18 hours before being read. A positive reaction is recorded when at least 75 per cent agglutination has occurred in the first two tubes. Any lesser degree of agglutination is considered as suspicious of infection. This mixture is used in place of serum in a routine agglutination test. A similar test has been used for the examination of mucus derived from sheep.

Indirect haemagglutination test
This recently developed technique promises to become a widely acceptable method for the diagnosis of infection, and more reliable than the vaginal mucus agglutination test.

Serum agglutination test
The application of this test for the diagnosis of infection has shown that serum titres are so variable that the method is not reliable for the identification of infected cattle or sheep.

Mating test
The detection of an infected bull can be made by artificially inseminating virgin heifers with semen mixed with preputial washings from the suspected animal and examining the heifers' vaginal mucus during the following 3–4 weeks.

Control and prevention

Cattle
Most strains of *C. fetus* are sensitive to a variety of antibiotics, particularly aureomycin, streptomycin and penicillin, which have all produced cures in a proportion of treated animals, and will in any case reduce the level of infection and shorten the course of the disease concurrently with the development of specific immunity. Since the disease in cattle is venereal it is essential to ensure that bulls are free from infection. Many reports on the local and parenteral treatment of infected bulls with antibiotics have shown that this can be an effective method for controlling disease, whereas the antibiotic treatment of semen is not always reliable. Similarly, no completely reliable method for treating cows has been established. Clean herds should be maintained by the purchase of known non-infected virgin animals or by the use of artificial insemination using semen from known healthy bulls. Preliminary studies on the use of killed vaccines indicate that they may reduce the incidence of infertility in a herd but do not result in the eradication of infection.

Sheep
Ewes which have aborted should be isolated for 3–4 weeks until uterine discharges have ceased. Thereafter, they can be returned to the flock as they will lamb normally in the following year. It is advisable to keep infected flocks closed and not to introduce

healthy susceptible adult sheep. Preliminary studies on vaccination trials suggest that this may prove to be a useful method for controlling the disease. Various investigations have shown that the abortion rate can be reduced by antibiotic therapy and particularly by the use of chlortetracycline.

Other diseases of animals caused by Campylobacter

Cattle
C. jejuni has been described as the cause of infectious diarrhoea in cattle. The organism is morphologically and culturally similar to C. fetus but there are two antigenic types both of which are distinct from C. fetus. Affected animals become listless, show signs of abdominal pain and the faeces are fluid, dark brown in colour and often contain mucus and blood.

Pigs
C. coli has been described as a cause of dysentery in pigs in the U.S.A., Australia, Europe and the United Kingdom. The organism has morphological and some cultural properties similar to C. fetus venerealis and is catalase positive and reduces nitrates to nitrites.

The disease occurs as a severe dysentery in young weaners and causes a necrotizing colitis. Large numbers of vibrios can be seen in smears prepared from intestinal mucus. The death rate may be 50 per cent or more in young pigs. Older animals suffer from diarrhoea, rapid loss of weight and a mortality rate of about 2–10 per cent. Initially, when the disease develops on a farm as a result of the introduction of infected animals, pigs of all ages may be affected. Later, the disease becomes endemic particularly among weaners.

Attempts to transmit the disease experimentally have often proved difficult, suggesting that C. coli may not be highly pathogenic and that some predisposing factors are necessary for acute outbreaks to develop.

Chickens
An entero-hepatitis of chickens and turkey poults has also been described. The causal organism is morphologically similar to C. fetus and will grow on blood agar in an atmosphere of 10 per cent CO_2 and a reduced oxygen tension. The incubation period of the disease is approximately two weeks following ingestion of the organism and birds of all ages may be affected. The characteristic lesions include a catarrhal enteritis and enlargement of the liver with focal necrosis. Other macroscopic lesions may include hydropericardium, a pale myocardium and an enlarged spleen. The organism can be isolated most frequently from the caecum and small intestine.

Public health aspects
There have been a number of reports of human infections caused by organisms resembling C. fetus. The symptoms have included abortions and premature births, nausea, headaches, diarrhoea, vomiting and undulating temperatures similar to those produced by brucellosis and malarial infections. The epidemiology of the disease is not clearly understood and although some patients may have had direct contact with animals there has been no positive evidence concerning the sources of infection.

Vibrio cholerae, an aerobic species morphologically similar to the campylobacters, is the cause of Asiatic cholera and naturally affects man only. Under experimental conditions the organism can cause disease in young rabbits and guinea-pigs. Asiatic cholera is an acute disease in man causing vomiting, watery diarrhoea and collapse as a result of multiplication of the organisms in the small intestine. Infection results from the ingestion of contaminated water supplies in particular, and also from infected foods.

Further reading
ALLSUP T.N. AND HUNTER, D. (1973) The isolation of vibrios from diseased and healthy calves: Part I: laboratory. Veterinary Record, 93, 389.
BERG R.L., JUTILA J.W. AND FIREHAMMER B.D. (1971) A revised classification of Vibrio fetus. American Journal of Veterinary Research, 32, 11.
BRYNER J.H., DERRY P.A.O., ESTES P.C. AND FOLEY J.W. (1974) Studies on vibrios from gallbladders of market sheep and cattle. American Journal of Veterinary Research, 33, 1439.
BRYNER, J.H., RITCHIE A.E., BOOTH, G.D. AND FOLEY, J.W. (1973) Lytic activity of vibrio phages on strains of Vibrio fetus isolated from man and animals. Applied Microbiology, 26, 404.
CLARK, B.L. AND MONSBOURGH M.J. (1974) Serological types of Vibrio fetus var. intestinalis causing ovine vibriosis in Southern Australia. Australian Veterinary Journal, 50, 16.
DENNIS S.M. (1961) Vibrio fetus infection of sheep. Veterinary Reviews and Annotations, 7, 69.
FRANK F.W., WALDHALM D.G., MEINERSHAGEN W.A. AND SCRIVNER L.H. (1965) Newer knowledge of ovine vibriosis. Journal of the American Veterinary Medical Association, 147, 1313.
HOFSTAD M.S., McGEHEE E.H. AND BENNETT P.C. (1958) Avian infectious hepatitis. Avian Diseases, 2, 358.
LAING J.A. (1960) Vibrio fetus infection in cattle, Ed. J.A. Laing, p. 62. Rome: F.A.O.
MORRIS J.A. (1973) Haemagglutinating properties of Campylobacter species [microaerophilic vibrios] British Veterinary Journal, 129, lxxxvi.
MORRIS J.A. AND PARK R.W.A. (1973) A comparison

using gel electrophoresis of cell proteins of campylobacters (vibrios) associated with infertility, abortion and swine dysentery. *Journal of General Microbiology*, **78**, 165.

PARK R.W.A., MUNRO I.B., MELROSE D.S. AND STEWART D.L. (1962) Observations on the ability of two biochemical types of *Vibrio fetus* to proliferate in the genital tract of cattle and their importance with respect to infertility. *British Veterinary Journal*, **118**, 411.

PECKHAM M.C. (1958) Avian vibrionic hepatitis. *Avian Diseases*, **2**, 348.

ROWLAND A.C., LAWSON G.H.K. AND MAXWELL A. (1973) Intestinal adenomatosis in the pig: occurrence of a bacterium in affected cells. Nature, **243**, 417.

SCHURIG, G.D., HALL, C.E., BURDA, K., CORBEIL, L.B., DUNCAN, J.R. AND WINTER, A.J. (1973) Persistent genital tract infection with *Vibrio fetus intestinalis* associated with serotypic alteration of the infecting strain. *American Journal of Veterinary Research*, **34**, 1399.

SEBALD M. AND VERON M. (1963) Teneur en bases de l'ADN et classification des vibrions. *Annales de l'Institut Pasteur*, **105**, 897.

SHIRES, G.M.H. AND KRAMER, T.T. (1974) Filtration of bovine cervicovaginal mucus for diagnosis of vibriosis, using the fluorescent antibody test. *Journal of the American Veterinary Medical Association*, **164**, 398.

VERON M. AND CHATELAIN R. (1973) Taxonomic study of the genus Campylobacter Sebald and Veron and designation of the neotype strain for the type species, *Campylobacter fetus* (Smith and Taylor) Sebald and Veron. *International Journal of Systematic Bacteriology*, **23**, 122.

WILKIE, B.N., DUNCAN, J.R. AND WINTER, A.J. (1972) The origin, class and specificity of immunoglobulins in bovine cervico-vaginal mucus: variation with parenteral immunization and local infection with *Vibrio fetus*. *Journal of Reproduction and Fertility*, **31**, 359.

CHAPTER 25

LEPTOSPIRA

Leptospira

Distribution in nature

The clinical condition of Weil's disease in man was first described in 1886, and it was not until 1915 that *L. icterohaemorrhagiae* was identified as the causal organism in both Japan and Germany. In 1918 another leptospire (*L. hebdomadis*) was identified as the cause of a human condition known as seven-day fever, and in 1925 a third organism (*L. autumnalis*) was shown to be the cause of Japanese autumnal fever. In 1916 *L. icterohaemorrhagiae* was isolated for the first time from rats, but it was several decades before surveys in various animal species were carried out which revealed the wide distribution of these organsims in nature. This delay was due, partly, to the earlier concept that animals were a potential source of infection for man only, and partly to the fact that it was not realised for many years

accordingly, are classified into a number of different serogroups (Table 25.1). Leptospirosis is now known to be one of the most important and widespread zoonoses occurring in temperate and subtropical countries at the present time. For many years it has been recognised that rodents are a common host species for these organisms, but more recent evidence indicates that many other species of wild animals may act as carriers. Pigs, also, are frequent carriers of leptospires; they are susceptible to infection with various serotypes and may play a major role in the dissemination of infection among animals and man.

Morphology and staining

Leptospires are characteristically long, coiled or spiral-shaped filaments with hooked ends (Plate 25.1a, facing p. 266b). Their size varies in length from

TABLE 25.1. List of the serogroups of parasitic leptospires isolated from man and animals.

Icterhaemorrhagiae	Pomona
Javanica	Grippotyphosa
Celledoni	Hebdomadis
Canicola	Bataviae
Ballum	Tarassovi
Pyrogenes	Panama
Cynopteri	Shermani
Autumnalis	Semaranga
Australis	Andamana

that subclinical or inapparent forms of infection are common in several species of animals but unusual in man. It is now established that the leptospiral group has a world-wide distribution and can be divided into saprophytic and parasitic subgroups, represented by *L. biflexa* and *L. interrogans*, respectively.

The large number of different serotypes which are pathogenic for man as well as for animals, are identified on the basis of their antigenic structures by agglutination and agglutinin-absorption tests and

about 6–14 μm and their breadth is 0·1–0·2 μm. Electron microscopy has shown that leptospires consist of a cell wall, a cylindrical, granular protoplast, about 0·1 μm wide which is twisted into a spiral, and they also possess a very thin axial filament. The organisms are actively motile due to their flexibility and show rotary or gliding movements. Both their general morphology and motility are readily observed in fresh preparations using dark-ground illumination. The organisms can be seen in films stained by Giemsa's method and in tissue sections by silver impregnation using Levaditi's or Fontana's method. Fluorescent antibody techniques are particularly useful for demonstrating these organisms.

Cultural characteristics

Leptospires grow very poorly on solid media and better growth occurs slowly in fluid or semi-solid media. It is a characteristic feature that multiplication takes place just below the surface of solid and semi-solid media. Although leptospires need oxygen for growth it has recently been found that some strains also require small quantities of carbon dioxide. This may be the reason for growth developing below the surface of solid and semi-solid media. Pathogenic strains require the addition of serum to the medium. Rabbit serum is commonly used for this purpose but sera derived from other species, including sheep, cattle and guinea-pigs can also be used but are not so satisfactory. It is advisable to test all serum samples before use to ensure that they do not contain leptospiral antibodies.

The optimum temperature for growth is about 29–32°C but primary cultures from animal tissues may grow better at 37°C. It is important to remember that substances which inhibit the growth of leptospires occur in tissues and fluids of infected animals, and more satisfactory results from primary cultures may be obtained when only small volumes of inocula are used or when the material is diluted 1/10 before being added to the media. As soon as growth has been established, subcultures should be incubated at the lower temperatures.

Some of the media commonly used for growing leptospires are Korthof's medium which contains haemoglobin as well as serum, Fletcher's agar medium containing rabbit serum, Schuffner's medium and Dinger's semi-solid agar medium for maintenance of cultures. Medium containing albumen-Tween 80 has been used for the growth of leptospires in the preparation of antigens.

Resistance to physical and chemical agents

Leptospires are relatively susceptible to heat and are killed by a temperature of 50°C for 10 minutes or 60°C for less than 1 minute. Conversely, the organisms in tissues may survive at low temperatures of about —20°C for some 3 months or at 3–5°C for 7–14 days.

Present evidence indicates that multiplication of leptospires outside the animal body is rare and their survival under these conditions is markedly affected by slight changes in the environment. Moisture is essential for survival but the moist environment should not be more acid than approximately pH 6·6. Some serotypes can survive for several weeks in water and mud with a pH of about 7·0–7·4, and L. canicola can survive for about 1 week in undiluted pig urine at a pH of 6·0–7·4. The survival time of leptospires is shorter in sea water and in sewage, and they die rapidly when in an environment of dry soil.

Antigens and toxins

On the basis of their antigenic structures, members of the group have been divided into more than 120 different serotypes or subtypes belonging to 18 serogroups. Various attempts have been made to isolate different fractions from these organisms and to study in more detail their antigenic structures. Polysaccharide fractions have been isolated, some of which are common to all members of the group and others are restricted to certain serotypes. Erythrocytes modified with some of these fractions have been used for indirect haemagglutination tests in attempts to develop a more sensitive and reliable serological test for diagnostic purposes. Recent experiments have shown that pathogenic leptospires produce toxic substances which have haemolytic and lipolytic properties and that they possess endotoxin-like material. The relationship of these toxins to the pathogenesis of disease is not known.

Epidemiology and pathogenesis

Although serum antibodies to many leptospiral serotypes have been detected in a great variety of animal species in different countries, the majority of spontaneous disease cases is associated with the six serogroups represented by L. icterohaemorrhagiae, L. canicola, L. pomona, L. grippotyphosa, L. hebdomadis and L. tarassovi (formerly L. hyos). Table 25.2 summarises the most common reservoir hosts for these serogroups and the host species in which

TABLE 25.2. The leptospiral serogroups most commonly associated with infection in animals and the different host species usually involved.

Serogroup	Reservoir carrier hosts	Spontaneously diseased hosts
L. icterohaemorrhagiae	Rats, pigs	Rats, pigs, cattle, dogs, foxes, chimpanzees, man
L. canicola	Pigs, dogs, jackals, rats	Pigs, dogs, cattle, sheep, goats, man
L. grippotyphosa	Cattle, voles, field mice	Cattle, pigs, goats, dogs, man
L. tarassovi	Pigs, cattle	Pigs, cattle, man
L. hebdomadis	Mice	Cattle, pigs, dogs, man

these organisms usually produce spontaneous infection. All these organisms can cause disease in man.

In the carrier animal the organism usually localises itself in the kidneys, particularly the convoluted tubules, and is excreted intermittently in the urine. Thus, infected urine is responsible for the contamination of an environment and is the common source of infection for other hosts. Pigs and various species of rodents are frequent carriers of leptospires, and it follows that the risk of infection among domestic animals is greater in environments where the rodent population is high. This applies especially to infections with *L. icterohaemorrhagiae* which are carried primarily by the brown rat (*Rattus norvegicus*) and to a less extent by other species of rodents. *L. icterohaemorrhagiae* is a particularly virulent organism affecting animals and man, occurring in many countries throughout the world including the United Kingdom.

L. canicola also occurs throughout the world, including the United Kingdom, and the common species of carrier animals for this organism are the pig and the dog. The most common carriers of *L. pomona* are pigs and to a less extent cattle; and *L. grippotyphosa* is disseminated most frequently by field mice (*Microtus* spp.). More recently, hedgehogs in a number of countries have been shown to be carriers of various leptospiral serotypes, and infection in this species has also been associated with the blood-sucking nematode *Physaloptera clausa*, which parasitises the hedgehog stomach. On a more limited scale, other carrier species include bats, skunks, marsupials, poultry and aquatic birds, and probably some species of reptiles, especially frogs and snakes. Moreover, serological evidence suggests that hares, foxes and deer may also be carriers. There is little doubt that the extension of surveys in different parts of the world will result in the recognition of an even greater variety of host species known to be carriers and potential sources of infection for domesticated animals.

The primary mode of spread of infection from one host to another is known to involve contact with infected urine, which may contain many millions of organisms per ml. In some outbreaks the exact route of infection is not always apparent. The risk of disease occurring is increased under conditions of husbandry and hygiene which allow contamination of food and water with urine; and the habit, particularly among dogs, of sniffing and licking objects on which urine has been deposited, including the external genitalia of other individuals, may constitute an important mode of infection in this species. The killing and eating of infected rats by dogs and pigs may also give rise to infection in these latter species. Under particular circumstances, materials other than urine may be responsible for conveying infection from one individual to another. These may include aborted fetuses, placentae and sometimes milk from pigs and cattle infected with *L. pomona*. There is also evidence that in cattle, at least, there is a seasonal incidence of the disease related to climatic conditions. It is probable that the organisms can survive and be transmitted more readily from one host to another in a damp climate, and that the spread of infection is more restricted during dry spells of weather. There is at present some inconclusive evidence to indicate that under particular circumstances ticks may transmit leptospires from one host to another.

Leptospiral infection can take place not only through the intestinal tract after ingestion of the organisms but also through areas of the skin which have become damaged or softened by repeated contact with water and mud as may happen with pigs. The entry of leptospires into the body of a susceptible host results in a leptospiraemia which is followed in some infections by the establishment of localised colonies of leptospires in the kidney tubules. These local sites of infection may become chronic and result in the intermittent release of organisms into the urine of an individual for periods of several years and probably for the lifetime of rats infected with *L. icterohaemorrhagiae*.

The study of leptospiral infections in different species and in various countries has shown some unusual features relating to the virulence of these organisms which is subject to considerable variation. Differences in virulence and pathogenicity of a particular serotype may vary for a single host species depending upon the country of origin of that species. For example, *L. grippotyphosa* has been reported to be more pathogenic for ruminants in Russia than in some other countries. In the Middle East, serological evidence has shown that simultaneous infection with this organism of goats and cattle grazing on common pasture resulted in a serious disease among goats, only. A leptospiral serotype which becomes highly pathogenic for a species of laboratory animal as a result of repeated passage, may simultaneously lose its original virulence for a farm animal host. These and other similar observations emphasise that the virulence of a particular leptospiral strain for a host species is related less closely to the recognised antigens of the organism than it is to various and sometimes unidentified factors related to its environment. It is interesting to note that after prolonged cultivation in laboratory media containing leptospiral immune sera, there have been indications that the antigenic structure of the organisms may become modified. Further work on this problem is required to confirm these findings and to establish their relevance to naturally occurring infections.

Symptoms

Pigs

These animals are common carriers of leptospires and may show no clinical signs of disease. In some herds leptospirosis is the cause of infertility. Infection with *L. pomona* often causes only a transient rise in temperature, a slight conjunctivitis and some unthriftiness. Occasionally, more severe cases may show signs of jaundice and convulsions. Infection of pregnant sows may result in abortions.

Infection with *L. canicola* can give rise to a variety of symptoms. Some animals excreting these leptospires in their urine will show such mild symptoms that the infection may pass unnoticed. More acute cases are associated with a rise in temperature, weakness, loss of appetite and conjunctivitis. Abortions may occur. Infection with *L. icterohaemorrhagiae* may show similar symptoms together with jaundice, paralysis and a mortality rate which may be high.

Cattle

Infection may be manifest by a variety of symptoms depending upon whether the disease has developed as the chronic or acute form. The chronic form may produce few obvious symptoms other than some abortions in groups of infected animals. More severe cases are characterised by a loss of appetite and cessation of rumination. The milk may develop a pink discolouration, contain blood clots, and at the same time the yield becomes greatly reduced and may cease altogether. The animals become jaundiced but deaths do not occur frequently. Very acute forms of the disease are characterised by a rapid rise in temperature, depression, diarrhoea, severe jaundice and dark coloured urine containing haemoglobin and albumen. Abortions are common and may occur as epidemics. The mortality rate among acutely infected animals is high and deaths occur within about 1 week of the commencement of symptoms.

Sheep and goats

The symptoms are similar to those recorded for cattle.

Horses

Acute forms of the disease are characterised by a rapid rise in temperature, jaundice, haemoglobinurea and a high mortality rate. Present evidence indicates that lesions in the eye develop more frequently in horses than in other animal species, and that periodic ophthalmia may be associated with leptospiral infections.

Dogs

The consecutive stages in the pathogenesis of the disease consist of first, the invasive stage when there is a leptospiraemia; second, the primary renal stage which refers to the concentration of the organisms in the kidneys; and third, the secondary renal stage which is one of chronic nephritis. Symptomatically, the different manifestations of the disease have been described as the peracute, icteric and subacute types.

The peracute form is characterised by a sudden onset with a rise in temperature, severe depression, shivering, and sometimes vomiting. The temperature then begins to fall and haemorrhages develop in and around the mouth and lips, conjunctiva and skin. The animal becomes thirsty but only small quantities of urine are passed. Initially, there is constipation followed by the passing of loose, blood-stained faeces. Collapse and death may occur within a few hours or days after the onset of symptoms in severe cases.

The icteric form is characterised by similar initial symptoms, followed by a severe jaundice which develops after 3–4 days and is readily noticeable on the conjunctivae, mouth, tongue and gums. Intussusception of the small intestine is not uncommon. Haemorrhages are not so extensive as they are in the peracute form. Severe cases terminate in death after a few days. Less severe cases may not die until 7–10 days after the onset of symptoms and a few may survive.

The subacute form of the disease is also a severe illness in which there are signs of slight jaundice and symptoms of nephritis. The mortality rate is variable but in those animals which recover, convalescence is protracted.

It is important to emphasise that a very mild form of the disease can develop in which no symptoms are observed.

Cats

It is known that in some countries cats may become infected with leptospires but this does not usually result in the development of characteristic symptoms.

Lesions

Pigs

The entire carcase is usually jaundiced, particularly as a result of infection with *L. icterohaemorrhagiae*, and there may be petechial haemorrhages in the lungs, kidneys and intestines. Macroscopically, lesions in the kidneys usually appear as greyish-white areas, about 2–3 mm diameter, and these may be surrounded by zones of acute congestion. In some cases no macroscopic lesions are evident although the kidneys contain many leptospires. Microscopically, the most obvious lesions are focal infiltrations of mononuclear cells between the tubules. There is also damage to the epithelial cells of the tubules themselves, associated with the infiltration of large numbers of leptospires into the lumen of the tubules. In the liver there may be areas of cellular necrosis.

Cattle

The lesions which vary according to the severity of the infection, include a jaundiced appearance of the whole carcase, haemoglobinurea, an enlarged spleen, and congestion of the kidneys with petechial haemorrhages. Microscopically, the kidneys show a tubular nephritis with distension of the tubules which may contain cellular casts, and focal areas of infiltration with mononuclear cells occurring around the tubules. The liver may appear macroscopically normal, but microscopically there may be areas of necrosis and localised cellular infiltrations around the bile ducts.

Sheep and goats

Similar to those which occur in cattle.

Horses

Lesions are similar to those already described for other species, and in acute cases include jaundice of the whole carcase, petechial haemorrhages and ophthalmia in some cases.

Dogs

The lesions are similar to those already described for other species of animals. In addition to haemorrhages and jaundice, the more acute cases show petechial haemorrhages of the kidneys, with degeneration of the tubules which contain large numbers of leptospires. More chronic cases of nephritis are characterised by areas of fibrosis, thickening of Bowman's capsule in the glomeruli, and only a few leptospires within the badly damaged walls of the tubules (plate 25.1b, facing p. 266b).

Diagnosis

Microscopical examination

Blood examination can be made during the early septicaemic stage which occurs during the first week of clinical infection. To facilitate the detection of leptospires in the blood which vary in number according to the stage of infection, the serotype involved and the host species affected, the organisms can be concentrated in the plasma by differential centrifugation at 500 rev/min for 15 minutes after the addition of buffered (pH 8) sodium oxalate solution. Urine examinations are best carried out sometime after the first two weeks of clinical infection when the septicaemic phase has passed and infection has become localised in the kidney tubules.

Direct microscopical examination may reveal the presence of leptospires in plasma before or after concentration, or in the deposits of urine after centrifugation at 10 000 rev/min for 15 minutes. Immunofluorescence microscopy is becoming a more sensitive method of diagnosis than other micros- copical techniques, and is also more rapid than cultural methods provided that appropriate antisera are available. The technique is particularly useful for examination of urine samples. Dark ground microscopy is also widely used.

Cultural examination

Blood, urine or tissues can be cultured by using, for example, Korthof's, Schuffner's or Fletcher's medium containing 20 per cent rabbit serum and incubating the primary cultures aerobically at 37°C until growth becomes visible. This may take as long as 3–4 weeks to develop in some primary cultures. Subsequent cultures are incubated at a temperature of 29–32°C. It is often advantageous to dilute infected material 1/10 before inoculating culture media (See page 254.), and the addition of 5-fluorou- racil, a pyrimidine analogue, to the medium will inhibit the growth of other bacterial species.

Animal inoculation

Mice, guinea-pigs or hamsters can be used for the inoculation of suspected samples. More recently, it has been found that chinchillas are highly suscep- tible to infection with leptospires. The inoculum may consist of a saline emulsion of kidney, a mixture of tissues derived from kidney, liver and spleen, or the centrifugate from an infected urine sample. Animals are inoculated with 0·5 ml of suspension intraperi- toneally. An alternative route is to inoculate material on to an area of scarified skin. Young guinea-pigs or hamsters, aged one to two months, are more susceptible than adults, particularly to infection with *L. icterohaemorrhagiae*. Similarly, hamsters are more susceptible to infection with *L. canicola* than are guinea-pigs and will die about one week after infection. Although guinea-pigs may survive in- fection with *L. canicola* and *L. pomona*, they develop a transient septicaemia and the organisms can be isolated from the blood.

Serological examination

The most commonly used techniques are the following.

The agglutination test is carried out in the usual manner, using killed formalized antigens prepared from known serotypes, and standing the tubes at room temperature overnight or in a refrigerator at 5°C after preliminary incubation at 37°C for 2 hours.

The agglutination-lysis test consists of adding pure cultures or mixed strains of living leptospires to serial dilutions of serum, incubating the mixtures and then examining one drop from each tube by dark ground microscopy for agglutination or lysis of the organisms. With positive tests it will be noted that in the lower serum dilutions there will be agglutination of the leptospires, and in the higher dilutions this will be replaced by lysis.

Serum agglutinins usually become demonstrable towards the end of the second week of clinical illness and continue to be present in chronically diseased survivors for years. Titres of between 1/100 and 1/300 are considered to be indicative of chronic infection, and lower titres suggest a past infection. A rising titre in consecutive serum samples from an animal suffering from sudden illness is indicative of acute leptospirosis.

Other methods which are not used so widely but on a more experimental basis are the complement-fixation and erythrocyte-sensitization tests. With the former test there are difficulties in standardising the techniques in relation to the preparation and use of the different complement-fixing antigens which are prepared in various laboratories. An erythrocyte-sensitization test has been developed in which the antigen consists of erythrocytes modified with alcohol-extracted leptospiral antigen. The method is to carry out either a haemagglutination test or a haemolytic test in the presence of complement. The results are diagnostically less valuable than those obtained from the agglutination test.

Control and prevention

The widespread incidence of carriers among both wild and domesticated animals, and the various routes by which infection may be transmitted from one individual to another, makes it difficult in many circumstances to prevent individual animals or groups of animals from contracting infection under various conditions. The more generally accepted methods for preventing the spread of infection to groups of animals include:

(1) Efficient control of wild rodents.

(2) Maintenance of high standards of hygiene to prevent contamination of food and water.

(3) Detection by serological and bacteriological tests of infected domesticated animals, and their separation from apparently healthy individuals.

(4) Immunization and the use of antibiotics.

A variety of methods for the passive and active immunization of animals against leptospirosis have been attempted in different countries. The results are variable and there is no generally accepted procedure to be recommended at the present time. There is evidence to show that the degree of protection afforded by a hyperimmune serum is not necessarily related to the agglutinin titre of that serum. It is, therefore, not always possible to accurately assess and compare the protective values of particular batches of hyperimmune sera. Furthermore, the passive protection afforded by their use is short and probably of greatest value only when given in the very early stages of infection.

Killed vaccines prepared against different serotypes have been used with varying degrees of success in different species of animals, but to obtain the most beneficial results it is essential to combine vaccination procedures with strict attention to hygiene and elimination of wild rodents. Recent studies on the efficacy of vaccination in cattle, pigs and dogs indicate that immunization prevents the development of clinical infection and reduces the incidence of leptospiral abortions in cattle but may have little effect on symptomless carriers.

Leptospira are highly sensitive to penicillin, dihydrostreptomycin and the tetracyclines under *in vitro* conditions. However, the efficacy of these antibiotics under *in vivo* conditions is limited, and it is important that treatment be commenced during the very early stages of infection if diseased animals are to survive, and especially if the stage of chronic renal infection is to be avoided. Dihydrostreptomycin is a more reliable antibiotic to use for preventing the development of the chronic form of infection.

Public health aspects

Leptospirosis is a serious disease of man and its incidence in human populations varies in different countries according to climate, living standards and occupation of communities. The classical form of infection is Weil's disease, caused by *L. icterohaemorrhagiae*, which may occur as an acute haemorrhagic jaundice. Less acute and subclinical forms of this infection are also common. The many other serotypes which occur in various animal species are also pathogenic for man and may cause febrile conditions, meningitis, nephritis, lymphadenitis or mild forms of jaundice.

Some of the predisposing factors leading to human infections are conditions of poor living standards in areas with a high rodent population, and the contamination of food and water with infected urine. Contact between infected water and abrasions of the skin facilitates the penetration and invasion of the body by leptospires which can also penetrate mucous membranes. This latter mode of infection through skin abrasions constitutes a special risk for persons, particularly veterinary surgeons, who are in close contact with dogs infected with *L. canicola*. During the stage of acute leptospiral infection in cattle, the organisms may be present in the milk in which they can survive long enough to set up infection in people who are accustomed to drinking fresh, unheated milk; and in addition, these acutely infected animals are a health risk to veterinary surgeons and herdsmen attending them.

The incidence of human infections derived from wild rodents is particularly high among those who are sewage workers, miners or agricultural workers in rice fields or sugar cane plantations. There is a particular risk of infection for animal attendants and veterinary surgeons who handle infected animals and carry out post-mortem examinations on carcases of animals which have died from leptospirosis.

Further reading

ALSTON J.M. (1961) Recent developments in leptospirosis. *Proceedings of the Royal Society of Medicine*, **54**, 61.

ALSTON J.M. (1967) Leptospirosis in wild and domestic animals. *Veterinary Annual*, **8**, 19.

BABUDIERI, B., CASTELLI, M. AND PISONI, F. (1973) Comparative tests with formalized and irradiated vaccines against leptospirosis. *Bulletin of the World Health Organization*, **48**, 587.

BIRCH-ANDERSEN, A., HOUGEN, K.H. AND BORG-PETERSEN, C. (1973) Electron microscopy of Leptospira. I. Leptospira strain pomona. *Acta Pathologica et Microbiologica Scandinavica*, **81**, 665.

ELLINGHAUSEN, H.C. JR. (1973) Growth temperatures, virulence, survival and nutrition of leptospires. *Journal of Medical Microbiology*, **6**, 487.

HANSON, L.E., TRIPATHY, D.N. AND KILLINGER, A.H. (1972) Current status of leptospirosis immunization in swine and cattle. *Journal of the American Veterinary Medical Association*, **161**, 1235.

HODGES, R.T. (1974) The use of a polyvalent antigen in complement fixation tests for bovine leptospirosis. *New Zealand Veterinary Journal*, **22**, 21.

HODGES, R.T. AND EKDAHL, M.O. (1973) Use of fluorescent antibody technique for the serological differentiation of leptospiral serotypes in cultures and in bovine urine. *New Zealand Veterinary Journal*, **21**, 109.

HODGES, R.T. AND RIS, D.R. (1974) Complement fixing and agglutinating antibody responses and leptospiruria in calves inoculated with Leptospira serotypes pomona, hardjo, copenhageni and ballum. *New Zealand Veterinary Journal*, **22**, 25.

HOEDEN J. VAN DER (1958) Epizootiology of leptospirosis. *Advances in Veterinary Science*, **4**, 277.

International Colloquium on Leptospirosis (1965) *Annales des Sociétés Belges de Médicine Tropicale de Parasitologie et de Mycologie*, **46**, 1 and 135.

KNIGHT, L.L., MILLER, N.G. AND WHITE, R.J. (1973) Cytotoxic factor in the blood and plasma of animals during leptospirosis. *Infection and Immunity*, **8**, 401.

MCERLEAN, B.A. (1973) Leptospirosis in pigs: a serological survey. *Irish Veterinary Journal*, **27**, 157.

MICHNA, S.W. (1967) Animal leptospirosis in the British Isles. A serological survey. *Veterinary Record*, **80**, 394.

MICHNA, S.W. (1971) Leptospirosis in British cattle. *Veterinary Record*, **88**, 384.

MICHNA, S.W. AND CAMPBELL, R.S.F. (1970) Leptospirosis in wild animals. *Journal of Comparative Pathology*, **80**, 101.

NEGI, S.K., MYERS, W.L. AND SEGRE, D. (1971) Antibody response of cattle to *Leptospira pomona*: response as measured by haemagglutination, microscopic agglutination, and hamster protection tests. *American Journal of Veterinary Research*, **32**, 1915.

STANECK, J.L., HENNEBERRY, B.C. AND COX, C.D. (1973) Growth requirements of pathogenic Leptospira. *Infection and Immunity*, **7**, 886.

SZATALOWICZ F.T., GRIFFIN T.P. AND STUNKARD J.A. (1969). The international dimensions of leptospirosis. *Journal of the American Veterinary Medical Association*, **155**, 2122.

United Nations World Health Organisation (1967). *Current Problems in Leptospirosis Research*. Report of a W.H.O. Expert Group. Tech. Rep. Ser. No. 380. Geneva: W.H.O.

WIESMANN, E. (1967) Epizootiology, diagnosis and control of the leptospiroses of cattle, sheep and pigs. *Bulletin, de l' Office International des Epizooties*, **68**, 15.

CHAPTER 26

BORRELIA, TREPONEMA AND
SPIRILLUM

Borrelia, Treponema and Spirillum

BORRELIA

Distribution in nature

This group of spirochaetes consists of comparatively large, irregularly coiled organisms which are easily stained Gram-negative. The group comprises a number of species, some being commensals and others pathogens for man and animals.

The most widely recognised animal pathogen occurring in many countries is *Borrelia anserina* (syn: *Borrelia gallinarum, Spirochaeta gallinarum, Spirochaeta anserina*), the cause of spirochaetosis in poultry. The name is derived from the original observation of the organism in diseased geese in the Caucasus by Sakharoff in 1891. Since that time, it has been recognised in many countries throughout the world.

Borrelia-like organisms have also been observed in the intestinal tracts of a variety of animal species, including dogs and pigs in which the organisms constitute part of the normal bacterial flora of the intestines, and may increase in numbers during the development of dysentery and intestinal ulceration in these animals. *Borr. theileri* which is transmitted by ticks, occurs in cattle and solipeds in Kenya, South Africa, Australia and South America, causing a relatively benign disease producing only a transitory rise in body temperature.

In man, *Borr. vincenti* is associated with a fusiform bacillus in the development of ulcers and necrotic lesions on the gums, pharynx and tonsils. Human relapsing fever which has almost a world-wide distribution, is caused by *Borr. recurrentis, Borr. duttoni* and many other species and subspecies which have lice or ticks as their vectors. Additional species, including *Borr. buccalis* and *Borr. refringens* are human commensals occurring in the mouth and perineal regions.

Morphology and staining

Borr. anserina is a spiral-shaped organism varying considerably in length from 5–30 μm, but commonly they are approximately 14–15 μm long, 0·3 μm wide and composed of some five or six loose spirals (Plate 26.1, facing p. 266b). They are actively motile showing flexuous or serpentine movements. Borrelia-like organisms derived from other animal species are morphologically similar to *Borr. anserina* and *Borr. theileri* is approximately 10–20 μm in length. Borrelia-like organisms observed in pigs measure approximately 7–12 μm in length.

These organisms stain Gram-negative, and also stain readily with crystal violet, dilute carbol fuchsin and also by Leishman's or Giemsa's method.

Cultural characteristics

Considerable difficulties are still experienced in attempting to cultivate pathogenic species of borreliae in the laboratory and no successful method which ensures their multiplication has yet been devised. Although oxygen is not utilised by these organisms for growth it does not appear to be toxic to them. Cultures remain viable for only a few days in complex media in which tissue, ascitic fluid, blood and serum have been incorporated. Strains of the human pathogen *Borr. recurrentis*, remain viable for as long as 8 months when stored at 0–12°C in a complex medium consisting of coagulated egg albumen, human ascitic fluid, dextrose, buffer solution (pH 7·8), saline, and when the medium is covered by liquid paraffin to give anaerobic conditions for growth.

Some attempts at cultivation have indicated that the metabolic products of other bacterial species may help to maintain the viability of borreliae in culture. In this connection, it is interesting to note that non-pathogenic strains of borreliae which normally inhabit the rumen of cattle and sheep can be cultured in the laboratory, provided that the media contain ruminal contents and a fermentable sugar. Growth occurs under anaerobic conditions at pH 6·5–7 and at a temperature of 39°C. One technique recently developed, consists of suspending material containing borreliae in thioglycollate or other nutrient broth and transferring one drop to the surface of a membrane filter of 0·22 μm A.P.D. which is lying on a complex nutrient agar medium. After anaerobic incubation at 37°C for 5 days, the organisms develop as a zone of hazy growth around the filter membrane.

The organisms have been grown in the developing chicken embryo and this method has been used for producing formalised vaccines employed in the control of avian spirochaetosis. Material is inoculated on to the chorioallantoic membrane on the 10th day of incubation and harvested 5 days later. This route gives a higher yield than inoculation into the yolk sac. However, it has been reported that some strains derived from adult chickens develop less satisfactorily than strains derived from other host species when inoculated on to the chorioallantoic membrane of the developing chicken embryo; and that strains which are successfully adapted to growth in the developing chicken embryo have a lowered virulence after several passages.

Antigens and toxins
There is evidence for the existence of different antigenic groups of *Borr. anserina* but further studies are handicapped by the difficulty of growing the organism satisfactorily in the laboratory.

A significant feature of the growth of these organisms *in vivo* is antigenic variation which can develop during the course of infection. For example, in relapsing fever specific antibodies appear in the blood serum of patients recovering from an outbreak. During the recovery phase some organisms will survive in the tissues, and a mutant with a different antigenic structure may also develop which is unaffected by antibodies already produced by the host against the original strain. This variant will produce a septicaemia and cause a relapse of the disease.

Resistance to physical and chemical agents
Borreliae are highly susceptible to changes in their environment, although the degree of susceptibility is hard to assess because of the difficulty of cultivating the organisms in the laboratory. For example, it is common for *Borr. anserina* to be recovered from only about 60–70 per cent of birds that have recently died from spirochaetosis. Organisms may not be recoverable from infected avian carcases after 24 hours' storage at 37°C, after approximately 1 week at 22°C or after 1 month at 4°C. It has been claimed, however, that the organism will remain alive and virulent in infected citrated blood for some 3 months when stored at 4°C.

Epidemiology and pathogenesis
It should be remembered that any assessment of the relative importance of borrelia species as primary causes of disease in animals, must take into account the fact that compared to other pathogenic microbes the borrelia group has attracted less attention. Investigations into the epidemiology and pathogenesis of borrelia infections have been greatly handicapped by the lack of success which microbiologists have had in being able readily to isolate, propagate and study the characteristic features of the organisms under defined conditions. With the exception of *Borr. anserina*, the study of this group of organisms in animals has been directed largely towards finding other host species for those organisms which cause human relapsing fever. So far, natural animal hosts for *Borr. recurrentis* or *Borr. duttoni* have not been found, but other similarly pathogenic members of the group (e.g. *Borr. hispanica, Borr. crocidurae* and *Borr. persica*) have been identified in a variety of animal species, including wild rodents, dogs, horses, goats and sheep in various countries.

Since the beginning of the century it has been known that *Borr. anserina*, the causal organism of avian spirochaetosis, is transmitted from one bird to another by the fowl tick, *Argas persicus*. Soon after the ticks have ingested infected blood, *Borr. anserina* can be detected in the intestinal tract, whence the organisms migrate to the salivary glands. Thereafter, the ticks may remain infected for as long as 2 or 3 days, during which time the organisms may be transmitted via the eggs to the next generation of ticks. After *Borr. anserina* has been inoculated into a susceptible bird from the bite of an infected tick, the bacteria multiply by transverse fission in the liver, spleen, bone marrow, and can be detected in the blood stream 4–6 days later.

Investigations into the variety of vectors which may be associated with the transmission of this disease in different countries has produced some conflicting evidence, but it is probable that in addition to *Argas persicus* and the pigeon tick, *Argas reflexus*, the disease may be transmitted occasionally by the red mite, *Dermanyssus gallinarum* and only rarely by mosquitoes (e.g. *Culex pipiens*). It should be noted that spirochaetes ingested by mites and mosquitoes begin to lose their pathogenicity for poultry in 1–2 days, and it is probable that these vectors are of minor importance as disseminators of avian spirochaetosis. In addition to transmission of infection from the bite of infected vectors, the disease may also be spread by ingestion of infected ticks or of infected faeces from diseased or carrier birds.

Avian spirochaetosis is known to occur in various species of birds in many countries throughout the world. Those most commonly affected are chickens, geese, ducks and turkeys. The disease occurs less commonly among pheasants, guinea fowl, pigeons and other domesticated avian species. When studying the epidemiology of this disease it should be remembered that disease in a flock may be derived from infected poultry brought on to the farm or possibly from wild birds, since it is known that in some countries *Borr. anserina* occurs in sparrows, rooks and other avian species. Conversely, healthy susceptible poultry introduced on to an infected premises will suffer from an acute and fatal form of the disease. During the initial stages of infection a septicaemia develops when large numbers of organisms are present in the peripheral blood and can be ingested by vectors. In those birds which survive the acute stage of infection, the numbers of organisms in the peripheral blood will become reduced. This reduction is associated with the development of antibodies, and these include both agglutinins and lysins which also have the effect of immobilising the organisms. Recovered birds develop a solid immunity.

Borreliae occur in other animal species although its significance in relation to disease production is not known. In pigs, for example, borrelia-like organisms have been observed in intestinal ulcers of animals suffering from hog cholera and also in the intestines of pigs affected with dysentery. At the present time there is no substantial evidence to indicate that borreliae are associated with the aetiology of swine dysentery.

Spirochaetes, including organisms which are believed to belong to the borrelia group are known to constitute part of the intestinal bacterial flora of many other animal species, including dogs, cats, cattle, sheep, goats, rodents and monkeys. Although it has been noted in some instances that there may be a marked increase in the population of these organisms in the intestines, their role as pathogens is not known and cannot be effectively studied until more appropriate methods are available for isolating and cultivating these organisms under controlled conditions in the laboratory.

Symptoms

Avian spirochaetosis affects birds of any age and can cause a very high mortality rate. Following the inoculation of *Borr. anserina* from a tick bite, the incubation period varies from 4 to 10 days. The body temperature then rises to 43–44°C, and is accompanied by depression, weakness of the legs and wings, marked cyanosis and pallor of the comb and wattles, followed by jaundice. Emaciation develops rapidly in birds which do not die within 5–6 days following infection. The faeces are of watery consistency, usually greenish in colour and contain large quantities of urates. The mortality rate may be almost 100 per cent in a susceptible flock.

Lesions

The spleen is usually very enlarged and pale, having a mottled appearance and necrotic areas throughout its substance. The liver, also, may have areas of focal necrosis, particularly in birds which had reduced numbers of spirochaetes in the peripheral blood at the time of death. The livers from birds suffering from a severe septicaemic infection at death are usually enlarged, congested and haemorrhagic. Other lesions are variable but include jaundice, petechial haemorrhages throughout the carcase, enteritis but not dysentery, and congestion of the kidneys with lymphocytic infiltration of the interstitial tissue.

Diagnosis

Avian spirochaetosis can be diagnosed by observing the organism, *Borr. anserina*, in blood smears or sections of spleen, liver or kidney. Blood films can be stained by Giemsa's or Leishman's method, or simply by carbol fuchsin. In smears prepared shortly before death the organisms frequently occur as tangled masses but it is important to remember that in films made at the time of death they tend to have disappeared and care is required in making a diagnosis. Tissue sections can be stained by Giemsa's method. Dark ground or phase contrast microscopy may be used for observing the living organisms in fresh preparations of tissue.

Specific agglutinins may be detectable when *Borr. anserina* has disappeared from the blood of infected birds but antibodies are usually not demonstrable during the septicaemic phase of the disease.

Control and prevention

Arsenical preparations have been used successfully for treatment when administered promptly and, more recently, penicillin has proved effective under similar conditions. Attempts to limit the spread of disease must include the eradication of ectoparasites from the flock, particularly ticks, as well as attention to hygiene to reduce the possibility of the disease spreading by ingestion of infected faeces.

Vaccines have been prepared either from haemolysed blood or tissue derived from infected geese and preserved with phenol or formol saline, or from formalised chicken embryo cultures. These vaccines remain effective for at least 6 months and stimulate an immunity which prevents the development of clinical infection under natural conditions for approximately one year.

TREPONEMA

Distribution in nature

This group of spirochaetes includes many saprophytic species and a few which are pathogens for animals and man. They have a world-wide distribution. The most important animal pathogens are *Treponema cuniculi*, the cause of rabbit syphilis, and the recently described species of *T. suis*, associated with preputial infections in pigs, and *T. hyodysenteriae* isolated from cases of swine dysentery. Treponemes have also been observed in the digestive tracts of normal dogs and other animal species.

In man, the organisms cause the venereal disease, syphilis (*T. pallidum*), a tropical disease known as yaws (*T. pertenue*), and a skin disease occurring in the West Indies, Central and South America known as pinta (*T. carateum*).

Morphology and staining

T. cuniculi is a very slender spiral-shaped filament varying in length from 6–14 μm and about 0·15 μm in width, with pointed ends and having 6–10 small coils regularly spaced throughout its length. The organism is motile and shows corkscrew-like, flexuous movements, sometimes bending through an angle of 90°. *T. suis* shows similar morphology, measuring about 16 μm in length and 0·19 μm in width, consisting of 6–11 spirals, and *T. hyodysenteriae* varies from 6–10 μm in length and about 0·4 μm wide.

Treponemes do not stain readily with simple stains but are coloured pale pink by Giemsa's method which may require prolonged application to obtain optimum results. India ink may be used for the examination of fluid suspensions or Levaditi's method for tissue sections.

Cultural characteristics

No satisfactory method for cultivating *T. cuniculi* has been developed. *T. hyodysenteriae* is a strict anaerobe and can be grown in an atmosphere of carbon dioxide and hydrogen on blood agar. Small colonies, 1 mm in diameter, develop as hazy zones in the centres of haemolytic areas after 72 hours' incubation. The organism has also been grown in the yolk sacs of embryonated hens' eggs. Isolation of the organism from saline suspensions of intestinal contents has been achieved by filtration through membrane filters of 0·65 μm APD and inoculation of the filtrate on to blood agar followed by incubation for at least 72 hours. Alternatively, the inoculum is placed in the centre of membrane filters (0·65 μm APD) situated on the surface of blood agar. After 48–72 hours' incubation the filter is removed and the organisms subcultured from the exposed haemolytic area.

Resistance to physical and chemical agents

These organisms will not readily survive away from host tissues. They are killed rapidly at a temperature of 55°C but will survive for a few days in tissue at 5°C and for longer periods when stored at −65°C.

Epidemiology and pathogenesis

T. cuniculi, the cause of rabbit syphilis, is a venereal disease and is spread during coitus. The condition can also be transmitted experimentally by inoculating fluid from lesions into healthy rabbits. *T. hyodysenteriae* is ingested by pigs and the organisms develop in the mucosa of the large intestine and are subsequently excreted in the faeces.

Symptoms and lesions

The incubation period varies between 2–9 weeks. The first lesions develop on the prepuce or vagina, and often spread to the perineal area. Less frequently, lesions may also occur later on the lips, nostrils and eyelids. Typical lesions take the form of superficial, localised areas of erosion covered by thin scaly crusts, which tend to persist in the female for several months but resolve more quickly in the male.

T. suis is reported to cause ulceration on the surface of the prepuce of pigs.

Diagnosis

T. cuniculi and *T. suis* can be stained and observed in exudates or in sections prepared from the lesions. *T. hyodysenteriae* can sometimes be observed in faeces and sera of pigs using indirect fluorescent antibody techniques and can sometimes be isolated in pure culture.

Control and prevention

Penicillin and arsenical preparations have been successfully used for the treatment of rabbit syphilis.

SPIRILLUM

This group of organisms includes a number of relatively large saprophytic species occurring in putrefying material and stagnant water. The one pathogenic species is *Spirillum minus* which is a cause of rat-bite fever in man.

Morphology and staining

Spirillum minus organisms vary in length from 3–5 μm, are rigid and spiral-shaped, possessing regular coils at intervals of approximately 1 μm, and are actively motile by means of polar flagella. The organisms do not produce spores or capsules.

Spirillum minus stains Gram-negative and is also readily stained by Leishman's method.

Cultural characteristics

Spirillum minus has not been successfully cultivated on artificial media and has only been propagated by inoculating infected material into guinea-pigs, white rats and mice.

Epidemiology and pathogenesis

Spirillum minus is carried by rats, mice and possibly other animal species in Far Eastern countries and infection is transmitted to man as a result of being bitten by infected rats. A similar disease has been reported in cats. The organisms can be demonstrated microscopically in the local lesion or lymphatic glands draining the site and sometimes in the blood; and they may also be detected by inoculation of infected material into guinea-pigs or white rats which develop a generalised fatal infection. Inoculation of organisms into mice usually results in the transient appearance of a few organisms in the blood 7–10 days later.

Further reading

BEER R.J. AND RUTTER J.M. (1972) Spirochaetal invasion of the colonic mucosa in the syndrome resembling Swine Dysentery following experimental *Trichuris suis* infection in weaned pigs. *Research in Veterinary Science*, **13**, 593.

FELSENFELD O. (1965) Borreliae, human relapsing fever, and parasite-vector-host relationships. *Bacteriological Reviews*, **29**, 46.

DICKIE C.W. AND BARRERA J. (1964) A study of the carrier state of avian spirochaetosis in the chicken. *Avian Diseases*, **8**, 191.

GLOCK, R.D., HARRIS, D.L. AND KLUGE, J.P. (1974) Localization of spirochetes with the structural characteristics of *Treponema hyodysenteriae* in the lesions of swine dysentery. *Infection and Immunity*, **9**, 167.

HOUGEN, K.H., BIRCH-ANDERSEN, A. AND JENSEN, H-J.S. (1973) Electron microscopy of *Treponema cuniculi. Acta Pathologica et Microbiologica Scandinavica*, **81B**, 15.

KUJUMGIEV I. AND SPASSOVA N. (1968) Identification and taxonomy of a new species of the genus Treponema: *Treponema suis. Zentralblatt fur Bakteriologie, Parasietnkunde, Infektionskrankheiten und Hygiene*. I. (Orig.) **206**, 404.

LEACH, W.D., LEE, A. AND STUBBS, R.P. (1973) Localization of bacteria in the gastrointestinal tract: a possible explanation of intestinal spirochaetosis. *Infection and Immunity*, **7**, 961.

MEHTA, M.L. AND MULEY, A.R. (1972) *Borrelia anserina*: a survey of its antigenic types. *Indian Journal of Animal Sciences*, **42**, 139.

PINDAK F.F., CLAPPER W.E. AND SHERROD J.H. (1965). Incidence and distribution of Spirochaetes in the digestive tract of dogs. *American Journal of Veterinary Research*, **26**, 1391.

TAYLOR, D.J. AND ALEXANDER, T.J.L. (1971) The production of dysentery in swine by feeding cultures containing a spirochaete. *British Veterinary Journal*, **127**, lviii.

TODD, J.N., HUNTER, D. AND CLARK, A. (1970) An agent possibly associated with Swine dysentery *Veterinary Record*, **86**, 228.

CHAPTER 27

MYCOPLASMA, ACHOLEPLASMA AND L-PHASE OF BACTERIA

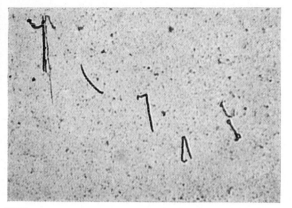

25.1a

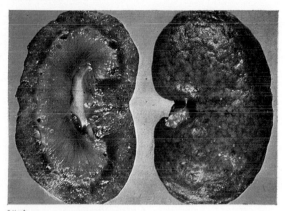

25.1b

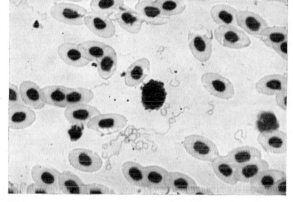

26.1

25.1a   Film of *Leptospira icterohaemorrhagiae* stained by Fontana's method, showing the characteristic spiral-shaped filaments with hooked ends, ×930.

25.1b   Macroscopic appearance of chronic nephritis from a case of canine leptospirosis.

26.1   Blood film stained Giemsa from a chicken infected with *Borrelia anserina*. Note the characteristic long, thin filamentous shapes of the organisms, ×930.

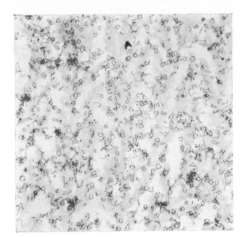

27.1a

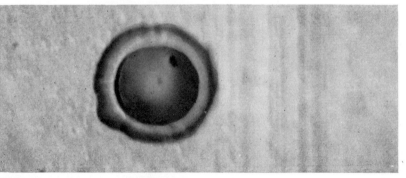

27.1b

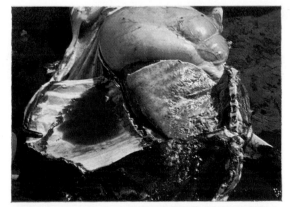

27.1c

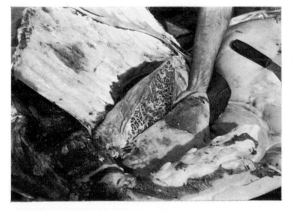

27.1d

27.1a   Impression smear from a colony of *Mycoplasma gallisepticum* stained Giemsa showing filaments, rings and stellate forms, × 645.

27.1b   Mycoplasmal colony growing on solid medium showing the characteristic 'poached egg' appearance.

27.1c Macroscopic appearance of the opened thorax from a case of bovine contagious pleuropneumonia, showing a quantity of pleural blood-stained fluid and fibrinous adhesions.

27.1d Macroscopic appearance of cut surface of lung from a case of bovine contagious pleuropneumonia, showing thickened interlobular septa giving the so-called 'marbling' appearance.

Mycoplasma, Acholeplasma and L-Phase of Bacteria

Mycoplasma and Acholeplasma

Synonyms

The first species of the Order *Mycoplasmatales* to be studied was *Mycoplasma mycoides* var. *mycoides*, the cause of contagious bovine pleuropneumonia. Earlier names given to this organism were *Asterococcus mycoides*, *Coccobacillus mycoides peripneumoniae*, *Micromyces peripneumoniae bovis contagiosae*, *Mycoplasma peripneumoniae*, *Asteromyces peripneumoniae bovis* and *Borrelomyces peripneumoniae*.

Classification

Recent research on these organisms indicates that the Order consists of over 43 species belonging to the *Mycoplasma* (sterol-requiring) and *Acholeplasma* (not sterol-requiring) groups. The characteristic properties of these groups include features which are not associated with either bacteria or viruses. For example, they differ from bacteria in not possessing a cell wall and most species, with the exception of *Acholeplasma laidlawii* and *A. granularum*, require sterols for growth. They differ from L-phase of bacteria in not being derived from bacterial parents and unlike L-phase bacteria they require sterol for growth. The majority of characterised species of *Mycoplasma* differ from viruses in that they grow both on artificial media in the absence of living cells, as well as in tissue cultures.

For these and other reasons the Subcommittee on Taxonomy of Mycoplasmatales proposed in 1966 that *Mycoplasma* should not be included with bacteria in the class *Schizomycetes* but allocated to a new class to be known as *Mollicutes* (Latin: *mollis* — soft, pliable; *cutis* — skin).

Distribution in nature

Mycoplasma are the aetiological agents of some important diseases of animals, including contagious bovine pleuropneumonia in cattle caused by *M. mycoides* var. *mycoides* (or *M. mycoides*), pleuro-pneumonia in goats caused by *M. mycoides* var. *capri* (or *M. capri*), and contagious agalactia of sheep and goats caused by *M. agalactiae*, an organism which is antigenically distinct from both *M. mycoides* and *M. capri*.

In addition to these well documented diseases, further species of *Mycoplasma* have been isolated from both ruminants and other animals suffering from disease, but the irrefutable classification of some of these further species as aetiological agents remains doubtful. Thus, mycoplasmas have been isolated from the genital tracts of cattle in association with inflammatory changes predisposing to infertility, from cases of bovine bronchopneumonia, from goats and pigs suffering from pneumonia, peritonitis and arthritis.

Pigs are frequently infected with *Mycoplasma*, including *M. hyorhinis* in association with atrophic rhinitis and *M. hyopneumoniae* related to chronic pneumonia. Other mycoplasmal species have been identified in dogs and cats.

Chronic respiratory disease (CRD) in chickens and turkeys is related to infection with the pathogenic organism *M. gallisepticum*, often in association with *Haemophilus gallinarum* or *Escherichia coli*; and this mycoplasmal infection should not be confused with *M. gallinarum* or *M. iners* which also occur in the respiratory tracts of these birds as commensals. *M. meleagridis* is the cause of airsacculitis in turkeys and *M. synoviae* produces synovitis in chickens and turkeys.

Mycoplasmas have been isolated from rats and mice suffering from bronchiectasis, bronchopneumonia and arthritis (*M. pulmonis*; *M. arthritidis*) and from mice affected with 'rolling disease' (*M. neurolyticum*). Many additional species have also been isolated from animals; some appear to be pathogenic and may not grow on artificial media, but the majority are non-pathogenic, probably lead a commensal existence and can be grown on laboratory media.

It has been suggested that because of the exacting

growth requirements of these organisms they exhibit a marked degree of host species specificity. However, recent work has provided some limited evidence to the contrary. For example, strains of *A. laidlawii* were originally isolated from soil and sewage and classified as saprophytes, but similar strains have now been isolated from various animal hosts, and one of the causes of arthritis in pigs is *A. granularum* which is closely related to *A. laidlawii*. *M. pulmonis*, a parasite of rats and mice, has also been isolated from man and rabbits. Similarly, pigs may harbour strains of *Mycoplasma* hitherto associated only with infections in goats and poultry.

Morphology

The absence of a cell wall means that these organisms are not rigid and show a great deal of plasticity. Consequently, a variety of bizarre shapes develop during their life cycles, including granules or cocci which are often referred to as elementary bodies, tear-drop shaped cells, clubs, filaments, rings and stellate forms. Variations in morphology are related to the composition of the media, and marked changes also occur when the organisms are filtered through membrane filters consequent upon the negative and positive pressures involved. During preparation for examination by electron microscopy some organisms may fragment and similarly, the preparation of colonies growing on solid media for microscopic examination may result in considerable morphological distortion unless handled with extreme delicacy. Although these features may account, in part, for the variety of pleomorphic appearances of these organisms, there are striking differences between the development of various strains even when observed under comparable conditions. Some workers believe that the production of filaments and their fragmentation into elementary bodies capable of further development of filaments, constitutes the normal life cycle; whereas others hold the view that filaments are artifacts produced during the preparation of specimens for examination or develop in exceptional environmental conditions and do not constitute part of the normal developmental cycle. When considering these two divergent views, it is relevant to emphasise that recent experimental results, obtained after taking considerable precautions to avoid the production of artifacts, suggest that the mode of reproduction may show marked differences between strains of *Mycoplasma*. For example, *M. mycoides* produces long slender filaments about 0·075 μm in diameter in which numbers of elementary bodies develop, and when subsequently released these bodies measure about 0·1 μm in diameter. *M. pulmonis* shows budding of the mature cell followed either by the release of elementary bodies or the development of filaments which then produce elementary bodies. This organism tends to include the filamentous stage less frequently in its life cycle than *M. mycoides* unless grown under special conditions. *A. laidlawii* also produces filaments which are very slender and smaller than those of *M. mycoides*. *M. gallisepticum* is unusual in that no filamentous stage in the growth cycle has been observed. Some strains of this organism replicate by a process of budding and others produce characteristic blebs about 0·1 μm diameter on the ends of cells which divide and form colonies (Fig. 27.1.

Composition

Mycoplasmas are procaryotic cells and differ from bacteria in not possessing a typical bacterial cell wall which is the reason for their plasticity. The plasma membrane forms the outer coat and is rich in lipids as well as protein, constituting some 30–40 per cent dry weight of the total cell and about half of this consisting of protein. Carbohydrate content varies and is particularly high in strains of *M. mycoides* which is encapsulated by galactan, and it has been suggested that this latter property may have an important relationship to the pathogenicity of these organisms. Carbohydrate content is considerably less in strains of *M. capri*, *M. gallisepticum* and *A. laidlawii*. Nucleic acids form about 15–20 per cent dry weight of *Mycoplasma* and consist of both RNA and DNA in the approximate proportion of 2:1. The organisms do not possess a nuclear membrane, and their cytoplasm contains ribosomes which, in the case of *M. gallisepticum*, are arranged in groups of about fifty in cylindrical formation.

Staining

Mycoplasmas are Gram-negative organisms but stain poorly with ordinary aniline dyes. More satisfactory results are obtained by staining with Giemsa after fixation with methyl alcohol or by staining negatively with nigrosin (Plate 27.1a facing page 267). Giemsa is also satisfactory for staining sections, particulary if they are first treated with a freshly prepared 1·0 per cent solution of potassium permanganate for 2 minutes which increases the intensity of subsequent staining. The sections are then washed in distilled water, stained for 18 hours with 1 in 25 Giemsa stain in phosphate buffer (pH 6·4) and finally differentiated in 0·5 per cent acetic acid. The preparations need to be examined promptly when the minute organisms are stained pink or purple.

Dienes' staining method is appropriate for the examination of colonies on agar. This stain consists of azure II (0·25 g), methylene blue (0·5 g), maltose (2·0 g), $Na_2 CO_3$ (0·05 g), benzoic acid (0·04 g) and distilled water (20·0 ml). A drop of the freshly

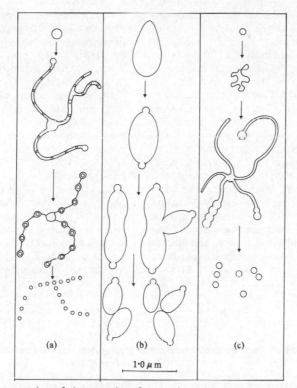

Fig. 27.1 Diagrammatic representation of three modes of mycoplasmal reproduction. (a) *M. mycoides* elementary body develops into a filamentous form and new elementary bodies develop within these filaments and are released when mature. (b) *M. gallisepticum* may develop from tear-drop shaped cells which form characteristic polar blebs, and these cells divide by fission. Other strains of this organism may develop by budding from large round cells measuring about 0.5 um. in diameter. (c) *M. pulmonis* develops from an elementary body by a process of budding, development of filamentous forms and the release of new elementary bodies.

filtered stain is placed on a coverslip and allowed to dry. A small, thin piece of agar containing the colony is cut out and delicately placed on the coverslip with the surface growth in contact with the stain. The colony of organisms stains moderately intensely and the surrounding agar remains unstained.

Cultural characteristics

General properties
Mycoplasmas are fastidious organisms and unlike bacteria, require cholesterol or a related sterol incorporated in the medium for growth. Exceptions are *A. laidlawii* and *A. granularum* which do not require a sterol. Some strains also require desoxyribonucleic acid and most cultures will grow aerobically but a minority need an atmosphere of 10 per cent CO_2.

Solid medium
A generally suitable solid medium for the primary isolation of mycoplasmal organisms includes agar containing 20 per cent unheated horse serum, 10 per cent fresh yeast extract which has not been heated above 75°C, 20 μg/ml of desoxyribonucleic acid, together with 50 units/ml of penicillin and 0·25 mg/ml thallous acetate to control the growth of bacterial contaminants. The medium should be adjusted to pH 7·0–8·0 by the addition of K_2HPO_4.

A variety of modifications to this solid medium have been devised, including an alternative basal medium of beef heart infusion in 1·5 per cent agar adjusted to pH 7·8. A 100 ml volume of this basal medium is heated, cooled to 50°C and packed, unwashed, horse blood cells added. The mixture is slowly brought to the boil and then heated in a waterbath at 56°C for 30 minutes. The clear supernatant is decanted from the precipitate and horse serum or ascitic fluid added to the former to give a concentration of either 10 per cent or 20 per cent, respectively, in a final concentration of 1·1–1·2 per cent agar. The medium is then dispensed in Petri dishes to a depth of 3 mm and allowed to set. If the primary inoculum is likely to be heavily contaminated with bacteria a solution of penicillin may be streaked over the surface of the agar to give a final concentration of a few hundred units of penicillin per ml of medium.

Solid medium used specifically for the isolation and cultivation of *M. mycoides* contains a digest of ox heart and liver plus serum and agar, including 500 units/ml of penicillin and a 1:4000 concentration of thallous acetate, or alternatively a basal medium composed of a papain digest of liver (Panmede) with added nutrients. The growth of *M. bovigenitalium* is enhanced by including vaginal mucus, probably because of its content of deoxyribonucleic acid.

The optimum temperature for growth is 36–38°C for pathogenic strains of *Mycoplasma*, and after 3–4 days' incubation some colonies will measure 0·5–1·0 mm diameter, with a yellowish, opaque centre which penetrates into the substance of the medium and is surrounded by a thin, translucent periphery giving a poached egg appearance (Plate 27.1b, facing p. 267). Smaller colonies can only be seen under a low-power microscope. When high magnification of a colony is required, a small piece of agar containing the colony may be cut out and placed carefully on a coverslip with the colony adjacent to the glass. This preparation can then be placed on a slide and sealed with paraffin wax for examination by either light or phase contrast microscopy.

A variety of characteristic features have been observed when different strains of *Mycoplasma* are cultivated on solid medium. For example, *M. mycoides* is haemolytic in the presence of bovine red blood cells, *M. agalactiae* will grow in medium containing milk instead of serum, *M. capri* has been grown on medium containing allantoic fluid from hens' eggs in place of serum, and *A. granularum* will grow more abundantly in media to which pig gastric mucin has been added. An important feature of laboratory media is that they may not support the growths of all pathogenic strains of *Mycoplasma*, and this has become particularly apparent in relation to the isolation of some strains causing chronic respiratory diseases in poultry.

T-strains (T = tiny) of *Mycoplasma* which have been identified in the urogenital and respiratory tracts of cattle, the urogenital tracts of dogs and man and in the throats of squirrel monkeys, possess certain characteristic properties. Growth will not take place in the absence of serum, and on solid media the colonies measure only about 5–10 μm in diameter with either a rough granular texture or a smooth appearance with a clearly defined central nipple. These strains metabolise urea but not glucose or arginine. Growth is not inhibited by penicillin but the organisms are slightly sensitive to thallous acetate.

Fluid medium

This consists of serum broth similar to the solid medium referred to above with the omission of agar. Growth may be difficult to observe unless examined by lateral illumination against a dark background. When a young, actively growing culture is gently shaken it produces characteristic swirls. However, if the original inoculum was small, visible growth may not develop for 6–7 days. *A. granularum* develops a particularly granular type of growth in fluid cultures, and this feature has been recognised in the name given to this species.

Embryonated eggs

Cultivation of *Mycoplasma* in embryonated hens' eggs is of particular value for the growth of fastidious strains which fail to develop in culture media, and also for the serial passage of *M. mycoides* as a method for preparing attenuated vaccines. Inoculation into the yolk sac of 7-day embryos is generally recognised to be a more satisfactory route than into either the allantoic or amniotic cavities, particularly for pathogenic avian strains which cause death of embryos in 2–4 days after inoculation, characterised by extensive cutaneous haemorrhages and generalised oedema. There is a risk that a small proportion of eggs used for cultivation may be contaminated with *Mycoplasma*. The incidence of avian strains of the organism may be as high as 1–6 per cent in eggs derived from flocks infected with chronic respiratory disease. Occasionally, strains of *Mycoplasma* serologically unrelated to the avian pathogens have also been isolated from chick embryos.

Cell culture

A variety of cell systems have been employed including monolayers of HeLa cells, chicken heart fibroblasts, explanted chick embryonic membranes and human conjunctival cells. Recently isolated strains of *M. bovigenitalium* often grow more satisfactorily in bovine cell cultures than in ordinary cell-free media. The nature of the growths vary with different strains of *Mycoplasma* and may occur intracellularly or extracellularly, and pathogenic strains may produce definite cytopathic effects. An important problem related to the use of cell culture techniques for the isolation and maintenance of these organisms, is the possibility of infection of cell lines with contaminant strains of *Mycoplasma* or *Acholeplasma* occurring in the laboratory (e.g. *A. laidlawii*). Contamination has been reported when using HeLa, human conjunctival and other cell lines, including some derived from monkey, mouse and chicken tissues. Occasionally, contamination may be derived from the use of originally infected cells or may arise during the preparation of monolayers.

Biochemical reactions

Carbohydrate fermentation tests using glucose enable *Mycoplasma* to be divided into two groups — the fermenting and the non-fermenting species. It is often necessary to carry out repeated subcultivation in carbohydrate media before fermentation takes place. Most species of *Mycoplasma* associated with animal infections and also *A. laidlawii*, ferment glucose, fructose, mannose and maltose with production of acid. Those which do not ferment carbohydrates include *M. arthritidis*, *M. hominis*, *M. salivarium* and *M. orale*. The non-fermenting strains break down arginine with the liberation of ammonia.

Two growth inhibition tests have been developed and are used for diagnostic purposes.

Growth inhibition test

This is based on the fact that mycoplasmal growth is specifically inhibited by strong concentrations of antibody incorporated in solid or fluid media, and the method is used as a technique for the identification of strains.

Metabolic inhibition test

This is similar to the above but based on the reduction in metabolic activities of *Mycoplasma* by specific antisera, in relation to fermentation of glucose, degradation of arginine or reduction of tetrazolium. This test can be used for detecting serum antibody levels as well as for the identification of strains.

Resistance to physical and chemical agents

Mycoplasmas are relatively susceptible to moist heat and are killed by a temperature of 55°C for 15 minutes and 60°C for 5 minutes or less. In contrast, the organisms may remain viable for several months in frozen lung, and freeze dried cultures can be satisfactorily stored for several years. Disinfectants are highly lethal to these organisms which are killed after exposure for a few minutes to 1 per cent phenol, 0·5 per cent formalin or 0·01 per cent mercuric chloride.

Antigens and toxins

The application of agar diffusion techniques has demonstrated the presence of multiple antigenic components occurring in *Mycoplasma*. Some of these components are shared between different strains and others are specific for each serological type. Strains derived from different host species can usually be distinguished by agglutination tests and grouped into several types according to their antigenic structures. Strains of *M. mycoides* possess at least three antigenic components constituting only one antigenic type, and the serological activity

of the organism is known to be associated with galactan.

A neurotoxin is produced by strains of *M. neurolyticum* and consists of a thermolabile protein which becomes attached to astrocytes in brain tissue, causing them to be distended with fluid. This lesion is associated with the characteristic symptoms of 'rolling disease' in mice.

Although it has not been demonstrated that *M. gallisepticum* produces a soluble exotoxin, there are similarities between the pathogenesis of this organism and *M. neurolyticum*. Washed suspensions of viable *M. gallisepticum* organisms have a neurotoxic effect on turkey poults. About 1 hour after intravenous inoculation the birds show symptoms of incoordination, torticollis, weakness, paralysis of the legs and finally death. The lesions developing in birds which survive for at least 24 hours consist of polyarteritis in brain tissue and fibrinoid necrosis followed by cellular infiltration of the walls of these arteries. It is not yet known whether the same toxic substance is responsible for both the nervous symptoms and the development of polyarteritis.

Some experiments have suggested that *M. mycoides* may produce a diffusible toxin but this property has not been established. Galactan produced by *M. mycoides* can be detected in the blood of acutely infected cattle, and experimentally it has been shown that high titres of galactan in the blood can affect the pathogenesis of subsequent infection with the organism, particularly in relation to the likely development of joint infections.

Acholeplasmal viruses

Two viruses infecting *A. laidlawii* have recently been identified and they are both capable of producing lysis similar to the reactions between bacteriophages and bacteria. This raises the probability that other viruses may exist which infect mycoplasmal species and could be of value in distinguishing, for example, between different strains of *M. mycoides* which at present can only be compared by animal inoculation.

Epidemiology and pathogenesis

Growing interest in *Mycoplasma* and the development of newer techniques for the isolation and study of these fastidious organisms, is revealing their widespread occurrence in many species of animals and their association with a variety of pathological processes. A general picture of the epidemiology and pathogenesis of these diseases is now emerging and shows that a common route of infection is via the respiratory tract which may constitute both the primary and main site of infection. The urogenital tract is another frequent site for some infections. Organisms may be disseminated in the body via

TABLE 27.1.   Summary of mycoplasmal and acholeplasmal infections occurring in various host species.

Host	Species of mycoplasma and acholeplasma	Nature of disease	Natural habitat of mycoplasma and acholeplasma
Cattle	*M. mycoides*	Contagious bovine pleuropneumonia	Respiratory tract
	M. bovigenitalium	Mastitis; vulvovaginitis	Genital tract
	M. bovirhinis	(Experimental mastitis)	Respiratory tract
	M. agalactiae var. *bovis* (*M. bovimastitidis*)	Mastitis; arthritis	Udder
	A. laidlawii	(Infertility?)	Sewage (saprophyte)
	T-strains		Urogenital tract; respiratory tract.
	Additional species	Pneumoenteritis; mastitis; arthritis in calves	Respiratory tract; udder; joints
Goats	*M. capri*	Contagious caprine pleuropneumonia; arthritis	Respiratory tract
	Oedema disease organism	Oedema; cellulitis; arthritis; mastitis	Throat; joints; udder
	Additional species	Arthritis; conjunctivitis; peritonitis; lymphadenitis in adults; septicaemia in kids	
Goats and Sheep	*M. agalactiae*	Contagious agalactia; mastitis; conjunctivitis; polyarthritis	Udder; conjunctiva; joints
	M. arginini	Arthritis in goats; brain of sheep	
Pigs	*M. hyorhinis*	Associated with atrophic rhinitis and chronic pneumonia; arthritis and polyserositis in young pigs	Respiratory tract
	A. granularum	Associated with arthritis in older pigs	Nasal cavity
	M. hyopneumoniae (*M. suipneumoniae*)	Enzootic pneumonia	Respiratory tract
	Additional species	Associated with mastitis and metritis	Udder; uterus
Dogs	*M. spumans*	(Infertility?)	Throat; vagina
	M. canis		Throat; urogenital tract; (commensal)
	M. maculosum		Throat; urogenital tract; (commensal)
Cats	*M. felis*	Conjunctivitis; catarrh	Saliva; conjunctiva
	M. gateae		Saliva
	M. feliminutum		Saliva
Lion	*M. leonis*	Pneumonia	Lung and brain (1 isolation)
Mice	*M. neurolyticum*	Rolling disease	Respiratory tract
Mice and rats	*M. pulmonis*	Infectious catarrh; pneumonia; otitis	Respiratory tract; also upper respiratory tract of rabbits
	M. arthritidis	Polyarthritis	Respiratory tract; joints
Chickens, turkeys, partridges, pheasants, pigeons	*M. gallisepticum*	Coryza; chronic respiratory disease; sinusitis; arthritis	Respiratory tract; eggs
Chickens & turkeys	*M. gallinarum*		Respiratory tract (commensal)
	M. iners		Respiratory tract (commensal)
	M. synoviae	Infectious synovitis; myocarditis; pericarditis airsacculitis	Respiratory tract
Turkeys	*M. meleagridis*		Respiratory tract; genital tract; eggs
Ducks	*M. anatis*		Respiratory tract (saprophyte)
Chickens, turkeys, ducks, pigeons	Additional species		
Man	*M. pneumoniae* (Eaton's agent)	Pneumonia	Respiratory tract
	M. pharyngitis		Throat; respiratory tract (commensal)
	M. salivarium		Respiratory tract; mouth (commensal)
	M. fermentans		Urogenital tract (commensal)
	M. hominis	(Urethritis?)	Urogenital tract
	T-strains	Urethritis	Urogenital tract

the blood stream and lymphatic vessels to the joints and mammary glands, causing arthritis and mastitis which are typical features of some mycoplasmal diseases. In addition, concurrent bacterial and viral infections may constitute significant predisposing factors to the development of mycoplasmosis.

Cattle

M. mycoides was first identified as the cause of contagious bovine pleuropneumonia in 1898. Before that date it is probable that the disease existed in Central Europe and spread to other parts of the Continent during the early part of the nineteenth century. In 1841 it reached the United Kingdom and in the following 20 years it spread to the U.S.A., Scandinavia, South Africa, Australia, and in the beginning of the twentieth century it appeared in India and the Far East. Effective control measures eradicated the disease from the U.S.A. in 1892, the United Kingdom in 1898, South Africa in 1916, Japan in 1932 and the U.S.S.R. in 1935. No cases have been reported from Australia since 1967 where vaccination was prohibited in 1972. However, the disease continues to exist in Spain, Portugal and several countries on the African continent.

The disease is almost entirely specific for cattle, and has only rarely been reported in buffaloes, bison and reindeer. Water buffaloes (*Bubalus bubalus*) are slightly less susceptible than cattle but they develop lung lesions earlier and these lesions resolve more quickly with the result that infected buffaloes are less likely to spread disease to cattle by contact. Similarly, the African or Cape buffalo (*Syncerus caffer*) is less susceptible to the disease than cattle and the importance of this species in the spread of infection is unknown. Under natural conditions it is a contagious disease spread by organisms derived from infected droplets expelled either from the respiratory tracts or from splashing of infected urine derived from diseased animals. In an infected animal the organism can also pass through the placental barrier. It is an important characteristic feature of the disease that many animals which recover from clinical infection continue to harbour the organisms in their lungs and remain sources of infection for other healthy animals. As many as 10 per cent of a group of infected animals may become symptomless carriers detectable only by serological methods, and they remain in this state for periods of up to 18 months and possibly longer.

The natural pulmonary form of the disease in cattle cannot be experimentally reproduced by any route of inoculation other than inhalation. Intramuscular, intradermal or subcutaneous inoculation causes extensive local oedematous reactions followed by a septicaemia and sometimes a polyarthritis, but the typical pulmonary manifestation of the natural disease does not develop. Sheep and goats are susceptible to subcutaneous inoculation with *M. mycoides* which causes the development of localised oedematous swellings, abortion and sometimes death of pregnant animals but no pulmonary lesions develop. Inoculation of *M. mycoides* on to the chorioallantoic membrane of embryonated chicken eggs causes oedema and death of the embryos. Rabbits, guinea-pigs, mice and hamsters are also susceptible.

M. bovigenitalium is a cause of bovine mastitis and has also been associated with vulvovaginitis and infertility. The organism was first isolated from cattle in the United Kingdom and has since been reported from other European countries, the U.S.A., Africa, India and Australia. The sites from which it has been isolated include the semen of apparently healthy bulls, the vaginas of a small proportion of heifers and cows suffering from vaginitis and low fertility rates, and from milk in some cases of mastitis in which it was confirmed as the aetiological agent of the condition. The organism is not usually present in virgin heifers under natural conditions but experimental inoculation into these animals will cause a vulvovaginitis. Similarly, inoculation of *M. bovigenitalium* into the teat canal of cows produces mastitis but the relative infrequency of this type of mycoplasmal infection compared with its incidence in the genital tract indicates that it is not a highly virulent organism.

M. bovirhinis has been associated mainly with the respiratory tracts of cattle and its role as a pathogen has not been clearly defined. The organism was originally isolated from the noses and lungs of animals suffering from a respiratory disease on a farm in the United Kingdom, and similar isolations have been made subsequently in other European countries and in the U.S.A. On most occasions the presence of the organism in the respiratory tract has been associated with predisposing factors, including concurrent bacterial and viral infections, intensive methods of rearing calves and with transport of animals. Under these conditions the role of *M. bovirhinis* as either a primary aetiological agent or as a secondary invader of the respiratory tract has not been defined. The organism has been isolated from other tissues in calves suffering from pneumo-enteritis and has also been reported occasionally as a cause of bovine mastitis.

M. agalactiae var. *bovis*, also known as *M. bovimastitidis*, should not be confused with *M. agalactiae* the cause of agalactia in sheep and goats. *M. agalactiae* var. *bovis* is associated with mastitis in cattle and in these diseased animals the organism has been identified in milk, blood, visceral organs, respiratory and genital tracts, and in arthritic joints. In addition, the organism has been isolated from the respiratory and genital tracts of apparently healthy cattle.

Other mycoplasmal species, including the T-strains which produce very small colonies on solid media and *A. laidlawii*, have been isolated from the genital tracts of cattle and are regarded with suspicion as a cause of infertility. Mycoplasmas have also been isolated from aborted bovine fetuses but their role as primary causes of abortions remains to be determined.

Goats and sheep

M. capri is the cause of contagious pleuropneumonia in goats and like *M. mycoides* infection in cattle, it is a contagious pulmonary disease spread by airborne infection. During the last thirty years, since the properties of the aetiological agent were clearly established, the disease has been reported from the Mediterranean area, the Middle East, Nigeria, Mexico, India, Burma, Mongolia, the U.S.S.R. and China.

The mortality rate may be extremely high but mild cases also develop and these are probably important sources of infection for other susceptible animals. Experimentally, the disease spreads among goats by inhalation. Subcutaneous or intramuscular inoculation causes the development of areas of severe haemorrhagic oedema sometimes leading to death, and intravenous inoculation produces an acute generalised inflammatory response. Sheep are also susceptible to experimental inoculation with *M. capri* although they are apparently resistant to natural infection. Cattle, rabbits and guinea-pigs are not susceptible but the organism is lethal to the developing chicken embryo.

An organism similar to *M. capri* has been identified as the cause of an arthritic condition in goats. Experimentally, this organism produced disease in goats, sheep and pigs after intravenous, intraperitoneal and conjunctival inoculation.

Oedema disease of goats is another mycoplasmal disease which has been reported from Greece and Turkey. The condition is characterised by areas of painful, subcutaneous oedema of the head region and many other parts of the body together with an acute nephritis. The mortality rate may be as high as 30 per cent or more.

An increasing number of mycoplasmal species is being isolated from goats. Some of these additional species are associated with oedematous lesions, polyarthritis and mastitis, while others appear to be non-pathogenic. The detailed study of the characteristic properties and antigenic structures of many of these species has not been carried out.

M. agalactiae causes contagious agalactia in sheep and goats. The infection is spread by ingestion and via the teat canal, causing infection of the joints, eyes and udders of lactating animals. The disease occurs particularly in countries surrounding the Mediterranean, in some other European countries, and also in Iran, Sudan, India, Pakistan, the U.S.S.R. and the Far East. Under natural conditions the organism occurs in discharges from the eyes, open joint lesions and in milk, contaminating the environment and leading to spread of infection by ingestion. Although the mortality rate is not usually high, the drop in milk production constitutes a serious economic problem. Mild cases may act as carriers for several months. Laboratory animals are not susceptible to infection with *M. agalactiae* but the organism is lethal to the developing chicken embryo.

Several additional species of *Mycoplasma* have been isolated from the respiratory tracts of sheep. A few of these appear to be pathogenic but the majority are either non-pathogenic or associated with respiratory disease related to other concurrent microbial infections.

Pigs

M. hyorhinis has been isolated from the turbinates of pigs suffering from atrophic rhinitis and has also been identified in the nasal cavities of normal pigs. It is probably transmitted by inhalation but intranasal inoculation does not cause disease. It has also been isolated as a secondary invader from the lungs of pigs suffering from virus pneumonia. Pigs of less than 6 weeks of age are more susceptible than adults, and after intraperitoneal inoculation, *M. hyorhinis* causes a severe pericarditis, peritonitis and arthritis. Infection is lethal to chicken embryos and is cytotoxic for swine kidney cells. The organism does not cause disease in laboratory animals.

M. hyopneumoniae (Syn.: *M. suipneumoniae*) is the cause of chronic pneumonia in pigs which may affect an animal for months or even years. The organism has a world-wide distribution and may affect as many as 40 per cent or more of pigs. There are no reliable serological or microbiological tests for the control of this disease. *A. granularum* is associated with the development of arthritis in pigs and it is probable that the organism occurs naturally in the upper respiratory tracts of these animals.

Dogs and cats

A number of mycoplasmal species have been isolated from these animals. *M. spumans* was originally obtained from semen and vagina, and evidence suggests that this infection may be associated with infertility. *M. maculosum* and *M. canis* have been identified in the throats and urogenital tracts of healthy dogs. *M. felis, M. gateae* and *M. feliminutum* have been isolated from saliva of healthy cats and in addition, *M. felis* has been associated with conjunctivitis and catarrh. *M. leonis* has been isolated on one occasion from the lungs and brain of a captive lion suffering from pneumonia.

Rats and mice

M. arthritidis is the cause of arthritis in rats and mice but the disease cannot readily be transmitted by contact exposure. Subcutaneous inoculation causes severe necrotic lesions in both species and intracerebral inoculation will produce pneumonia and encephalitis in mice only. *M. neurolyticum*, the cause of 'rolling disease' in mice, is transmissible by direct contact and is found in the conjunctiva and nasal mucosa of infected animals. Brain lesions are produced by an exotoxin which becomes attached to astrocytes but strains vary considerably in their virulence and capacity to produce exotoxin. The organisms can exist as latent infections in healthy animals and the clinical manifestation of disease is usually associated with some debilitating condition. *M. pulmonis* is usually associated with lung infections in older rats and probably only becomes established as a disease entity when other predisposing factors are present. Mice are more susceptible to this infection and disease can be spread by contact or nasal instillation, giving rise to chronic respiratory catarrh. The disease spreads rapidly through colonies of rats and mice but usually does not manifest itself until the animals have become debilitated by some other disease condition.

Poultry

Recent investigations have shown that mycoplasmas are frequently present in the tissues of chickens, turkeys and other species of birds. Some confusion has developed as to the precise role these organisms play in the production of chronic respiratory disease (CRD) of chickens and infectious sinusitis (IS) of turkeys. It is evident that the various species of organisms differ in their pathogenicity and several of them are probably commensals. *M. gallisepticum* is recognised as a pathogenic species and is known to be a cause of chronic respiratory disease in chickens, turkeys, partridges, pheasants and pigeons. Additional species have also been isolated from pigeons suffering from coryza. The common routes of infection with *M. gallisepticum* are by contact, particularly inhalation of infected droplets, and by egg transmission when the ovules of laying hens become infected probably by invasion with *M. gallisepticum* from adjacent infected air-sacs. The organism is also pathogenic for the developing chicken embryo.

A significant feature of CRD caused by *M. gallisepticum* is that predisposing factors, particularly concurrent infections with bacteria and viruses, are of importance in the development and severity of the disease. For many years it has been recognised that mycoplasmal infections may be more severe in the presence of concurrent infections with *Haemophilus gallinarum*. It has also been shown that respiratory disease caused by *H. gallinarum* infection alone, is acute and lasts for only 2–3 weeks, whereas *M. gallisepticum* by itself, produces a more protracted form of the disease. Similarly, a mixed infection of *M. gallisepticum* with either *Escherichia coli* or *Klebsiella pneumoniae* produces particularly severe cases of respiratory disease. Comparable results have been obtained with mixed infections of *M. gallisepticum* and Newcastle disease virus or infectious bronchitis virus which also enhance egg-borne infection with *M. gallisepticum*.

M. meleagridis is a cause of airsacculitis in turkeys and can be isolated from the respiratory and genital tracts of apparently healthy birds. A common natural habitat for the organism is the male genital organ, and infection is transferred from the male to the female, where it becomes established in the oviduct and infects the ovules. In this way, egg transmission constitutes an important route for the disease to spread from one generation to the next.

M. synoviae is a cause of infectious synovitis in chickens and turkey poults, occurring in younger birds during approximately the first 10 weeks after hatching. The organisms may also be present in the upper respiratory tracts without causing disease and infection can be spread either by contact and inhalation of infected droplets or by egg transmission.

M. gallinarum and *M. iners* are serologically distinct from each other and from *M. gallisepticum*, and frequently occur in the tissues of chickens and turkeys. These organisms are non-pathogenic under both natural and experimental conditions but are lethal to developing chicken embryos to the same degree as *M. gallisepticum*.

Other incompletely described species of *Mycoplasma* have been isolated from poultry, particularly *M. anatis* from ducks, and several species from pigeons which appear to be non-pathogenic. The confusing picture of the aetiological role of these organisms as causes of respiratory diseases in poultry has arisen from the fact that they occur naturally in poultry, that they differ widely in their pathogenic properties, and that the pathogenicity of these mycoplasmal infections may be enhanced by concurrent debilitating conditions produced by bacterial or viral infections.

Symptoms

Cattle

Contagious bovine pleuropneumonia may affect cattle of any age. The incubation period under natural conditions varies from 1–4 months and has occasionally been recorded as either shorter or longer than this period. The duration is partly related to the number of organisms inhaled, and experimentally it has been shown that the period may be as short as 1 week after inhalation of a large dose of organisms.

The first clinical indications of acute infection are an increased temperature of about 40°C followed by the development of a dry cough, listlessness and inappetence. Later, the cough usually becomes more severe, the animal shows signs of pain, standing with arched back and extension of the head and neck forwards and downwards, increased grunting respirations, salivation and nasal discharge. The body temperature may continue to rise to 41–42°C before decreasing prior to death due to asphyxia, which may occur within 2–6 weeks following the initial appearance of clinical symptoms. Pregnant cattle may abort during the acute phase of the disease, and some animals develop synovitis of the limb joints. Cattle which recover are extremely weak and emaciated. Many infected animals develop milder forms of the disease which may be either symptomless or associated with only a slight temporary rise in body temperature and some loss of condition.

M. bovigenitalium infections causing mastitis are associated with symptoms of swollen udders, a sudden decrease in milk secretion and a slight rise in body temperature.

Goats and sheep

Contagious pleuropneumonia infection in goats commences with an incubation period of about 4 days to 4 weeks before clinical signs develop. These consist of a rise in body temperature to about 41°C, a mucopurulent nasal discharge, coughing, laboured breathing, salivation, diarrhoea and rapid loss of condition. Many pregnant animals will abort during the acute phase of the disease, and deaths occur some 10–14 days after the initial development of symptoms. The mortality rate in a group of animals may be as high as 90 per cent or more. Some cases of mycoplasmal infection in goats are characterised by arthritis, giving rise to swellings of leg joints and severe lameness followed by recumbency before death, or by development of acute subcutaneous oedematous swellings particularly of the head, neck and limbs.

Contagious agalactia affects goats and sheep of any age. After experimental infection there is an incubation period of 5–7 days before the appearance of clinical symptoms but under natural conditions the period may be longer. The first signs of disease include a rise in body temperature, listlessness and inappetence. Death may supervene at this stage or the disease may continue to develop in localised areas including the joints, especially of the lower limbs causing lameness, the eyes which develop a purulent discharge and the udders of lactating animals. In these latter cases the milk yield decreases and is replaced by small quantities of purulent secretion and the development of fibrosis in the udder. The mortality rate may be low and does not usually rise to more than 10–15 per cent.

Pigs

Mycoplasmal infection may cause symptoms of lameness due to arthritis of the limb joints. The majority of cases recover after a prolonged period of lameness and loss in weight. Occasionally, a generalised infection with *M. hyorhinis* and other mycoplasmal species may develop from a localised infection of the turbinates in cases of atrophic rhinitis, and this will lead to symptoms associated with inflammation of the serous surfaces and lameness. Infection with *M. hyopneumoniae* gives rise to symptoms of coughing, deterioration in condition and the severity of the disease will depend upon concurrent infections.

Poultry

Chronic respiratory disease of chickens and turkeys caused by *M. gallisepticum* is characterised by a nasal discharge, shaking of the head, coughing, swelling of the infraorbital sinuses and tracheal rales. In addition, affected birds suffer from inappetence, loss of condition, reduced egg production and lowered fertility. The mortality rate is usually low. Similarly, turkeys suffering from infectious sinusitis develop swollen infraorbital sinuses, nasal discharge, shaking of the head, conjunctivitis with lachrymation, dyspnoea, coughing and loss of condition. The mortality rate is also low. Infection with *M. synoviae* is characterised by lameness due to infection and inflammation of the joints and consequent loss of condition. The mortality rate is usually low.

Rats and mice

Mice infected with *M. neurolyticum* suffer characteristic symptoms of rolling or turning and sometimes display other spastic nervous symptoms followed by paralysis and death. Many affected animals recover after several weeks. *M. arthritidis* causes lameness in rats and mice consequent upon the development of arthritis in the limb joints with severe oedematous thickening in the area of the tibiotarsal or radiocarpal joints. Ulceration may occur. *M. pulmonis* is associated with symptoms of chronic respiratory catarrh in mice and rats, and the mortality rate is usually low. The disease manifests itself in mice by laboured respirations, rhinitis, ruffled fur and loss of condition. Some animals may develop a middle ear infection which becomes clinically apparent with signs of imbalance and circling movements. Affected rats usually suffer from more severe nasal catarrh than mice.

Lesions

Cattle

The characteristic lesions of contagious bovine pleuropneumonia occur in the lungs. In acute cases these show varying degrees of hepatization of the lobules which are separated from each other by grossly thickened interlobular septa, giving the so-called 'marbling' appearance which may involve either one or both lungs (Plate 27.1d, facing p. 267). The local lymphatic glands from which *M. mycoides* can be isolated, are enlarged, oedematous and often contain areas of necrosis. It has been suggested that these lesions may be the result of an Arthus-type reaction occurring in the glands draining the lungs. In some cases the thorax may contain several litres of blood-stained pleuritic fluid and in others this may be practically absent (Plate 27.1c, facing p. 267). The pleura shows oedematous thickening and its surface is covered with a layer of fibrin which may also extend over the surfaces of the diaphragm and pericardium. Post-mortem examination of more protracted cases reveals areas of the lungs which have necrosed and become surrounded by fibrous tissue. These sequestra contain viable *M. mycoides* organisms.

Goats and sheep

Lung lesions associated with contagious pleuropneumonia of goats are similar to those seen in cases of the bovine disease, including areas of hepatization and thickened interlobular septa. In more protracted cases the development of infected sequestra does not take place and recovered cases show only areas of extensive fibrosis from which the causal organism usually cannot be isolated.

Lesions of contagious agalactia may involve the joints, eyes and udder. Joint lesions consist of oedema of the periarticular connective tissue but the synovia usually remain normal or only slightly inflamed. Ocular lesions consist of keratitis which may be severe and associated with iritis and purulent conjunctivitis. Lesions in the udder develop as an interstitial mastitis followed in severe cases by fibrosis.

Pigs

Lesions are associated with arthritis of the limb joints and sometimes fibrous inflammation of the serous surfaces, including the peritoneum, pericardium and pleura. The organism can usually be recovered from pleural and pericardial exudates. Infections with *M. hyopneumoniae* produce lesions of chronic pneumonia which may become extensive.

Poultry

Lesions in chickens and turkeys caused by *M. gallisepticum* may involve both the upper and lower respiratory tracts. The infraorbital sinuses are congested, oedematous, contain large quantities of clear or purulent fluid and are infiltrated with lymphocytes and large mononuclear cells. The trachea is often similarly affected particularly in the upper region. In more severe cases associated with other concurrent respiratory infections, the inflammatory reaction extends to the lower region, and consists of accumulations of caseous material in the bronchi and the development of pneumonic areas in the lungs. Lesions in the air sacs are often widespread but commonly affect the posterior thoracic and abdominal air sacs. The linings of the air sacs become thickened, oedematous and covered with caseous exudate which accumulates in large quantities within the air sac cavities. Inflammation of the joints and synovitis may also develop.

Egg-borne infections with *M. gallisepticum* in chicken eggs produce lesions in the embryo similar to those seen in the air sacs, trachea and lungs of chickens, including large quantities of exudate within the air sacs, occlusion of the trachea with caseous material and consolidation of the lungs. In addition, there may be congestion and necrosis of the liver, kidneys and joints.

Infection with *M. synoviae* is characterised by synovial lesions of the hocks and feet associated with purulent exudates. The spleen is also enlarged and congested.

Rats and mice

Mice infected with *M. neurolyticum* may develop necrotic lesions in the brain associated with the action of the neurotoxin on astrocytes which become swollen. *M. arthritidis* causes the development of severe swelling of the tibiotarsal joints due to the accumulation of large quantities of purulent exudate. Other joints are affected less frequently.

Diagnosis

Cattle

Isolation of the causal organism. M. mycoides can be isolated from infected tissues using medium containing penicillin and thallium acetate. The isolate can then be identified by serological methods using standard antisera for the agglutination and complement-fixation tests, or the supernatant fluid from a broth culture can be used for carrying out a precipitation test. Growth and metabolic inhibition tests are additional methods used for identification of newly isolated strains. *M. bovigenitalium* can be identified microscopically in stained preparations of milk from cases of mastitis and the organisms can also be isolated from these samples.

The economic importance of contagious bovine pleuropneumonia has led to a variety of immunological methods being used for the diagnosis of this disease, particularly the complement-fixation, agar gel diffusion, rapid slide agglutination, fluorescent antibody and allergic skin tests. At the present time there is no single method which is completely reliable for the detection of all forms of this disease.

Complement-fixation test. This is the most sensitive and reliable serological test for the detection of both clinical cases of contagious bovine pleuropneumonia and carrier animals because complement-fixing antibody titres persist longer than agglutinins. For the detection of individuals in the incubative stage of the disease, the test needs to be repeated at intervals of 7–14 days. It is particularly reliable for the diagnosis of acutely infected cattle but less satisfactory for detecting chronic cases. Complement-fixing titres do not necessarily give an accurate record of resistance because they may be demonstrable in susceptible animals and conversely, may be undetectable in resistant individuals. Various modifications of the test have been devised in an attempt to improve the reliability and sensitivity of the method. For example, it has been found that the sensitivity can be increased by preserving serum samples with phenol, and that serum titres may be increased fivefold by incorporating normal bovine serum in the test.

The complement-fixation test has also been used for detecting serum antibodies in cattle suffering from mastitis caused by *M. bovigenitalium.*

Agar gel test. The agar gel double diffusion test is a particularly useful serological method for the diagnosis of acute forms of contagious bovine pleuropneumonia but is not so reliable for identifying chronic cases. It is also used for detecting infection in the tissues of slaughtered animals. The test can be carried out using a known *M. mycoides* hyperimmune serum and unknown antigen derived from lung, pleural exudate or other tissues, and this method can also be applied to tissues which have been fixed in formalin for at least one month. The primary antigen concerned in the reaction is galactan. For carrying out surveys on the incidence of the disease in cattle slaughtered for human consumption, strips of filter paper are dipped in pleural exudate and then forwarded to a laboratory to be used in the agar gel test. For the detection of serum antibodies by this method a known antigen is prepared from a concentrated suspension of *M. mycoides* which has been frozen and thawed three times.

During the acute stage of the disease, soluble antigen derived from *M. mycoides* becomes detectable in the serum of the host at the time when precipitin titres begin to decrease. This decline in antibody level is probably due to combination of antibody with antigen in the serum. At this stage of the disease it is of value to apply the precipitin test for the detection of antigen using a known antibody, as a supplementary test to the one used for the detection of antibodies. Specific antigen may be detectable in serum for long periods after the acute stage of the disease has passed.

Rapid slide serum agglutination test. This is a useful method for testing large numbers of animals in field surveys under conditions where laboratory facilities are not available. It consists of a rapid agglutination test using concentrated antigen either unstained or coloured with methyl violet or alcian blue. The limitations of the method are that it will identify approximately 75 per cent of acute cases but only about 35–40 per cent of chronic cases of the disease, because the presence of antigen in the serum during the later stages of the disease reduces the agglutinin titre.

Rapid slide whole blood agglutination test. This consists of mixing on a white tile drops of blood with a concentrated suspension of *M. mycoides* antigen stained with haematoxylin. It has the advantage that it is simple to carry out on large numbers of animals in the field without ancillary laboratory facilities, but the test is not wholly reliable because of the production of false positive and negative reactions. It is, however, suitable for screening purposes and for identifying infected herds and has been used for this purpose in African countries.

Indirect haemagglutination test. To carry out this test, washed, tanned red blood cells are coated with *M. mycoides* antigen and used in a haemagglutination test against cattle sera. The method requires laboratory facilities and is not wholly reliable for detecting infected animals.

An alternative method is to use galactan prepared from *M. mycoides* which will sensitize red blood cells directly without the need of a coupling agent. These modified red cells can then be used for detecting antibody in the sera of infected animals. Latex particles can be used in place of erythrocytes. The test is more sensitive than the complement-fixation test during the early stages of the disease but is less sensitive during the chronic stages.

Growth inhibition and metabolic inhibition tests. These are additional methods which can be used under conditions where laboratory facilities are available but are not applicable to field surveys.

Fluorescent antibody test. This recently developed

technique is used for the detection of *M. mycoides* in the tissues. The indirect method is to be preferred because it reduces the possibility of non-specific reactions. It can be satisfactorily applied to tissues which have previously been fixed in formalin for as long as 40–50 days.

Allergic (skin) test. This method is not as reliable as other tests for the detection of contagious bovine pleuropneumonia because of the frequency of non-specific reactions. It consists of the intradermal inoculation into the side of the neck of 0·1 ml of antigen which may be prepared by ultrasonic disintegration of *M. mycoides*, and measuring the thickness of the skin which develops at the site during the following 24 hours. It has the advantage that it is simple to carry out and can be used as a field test on large numbers of animals. Results are most reliable when applied to apparently recovered animals or to those not affected with the advanced, acute form of the disease. The antibodies associated with the allergic reaction are distinct from those involved in the complement-fixation and other serological tests and do not affect the results of these latter tests.

Goats and sheep
The diagnosis of contagious pleuropneumonia in goats is based largely on the nature of the disease and post-mortem lesions. *M. capri* can be isolated with difficulty from affected organs in chronic cases, provided that cultures are taken from the periphery of lesions where viable organisms are more likely to be present than at the centres. In acute cases, branching viable organisms are distributed widely throughout the tissues of the body and can be seen microscopically by dark ground illumination in pleural exudates.

Contagious agalactia may be diagnosed by isolating *M. agalactiae* from udder secretions, joint fluids or blood. Less frequently the organism may be cultured from the eyes and nose. Serological tests are not satisfactory because complement-fixing antibody titres show marked fluctuations and agglutinins may not be detectable.

Pigs
The presence of *M. hyorhinis*, *A. granularum* and *M. hyopneumoniae* in normal pigs complicates the diagnosis of infection in relation to the aetiology of disease. Diagnosis is based on symptoms, lesions, the isolation of organisms and the history of the particular disease problem being investigated, particularly in relation to other concurrent infections. Serological tests are not reliable diagnostic methods.

Rats and mice
M. pulmonis infections are diagnosed largely by the symptoms and lesions of infectious catarrh. The organisms can be isolated from the nasal passages and middle ear during the early stages of the disease and sometimes from the lungs and joints. Diagnosis of *M. arthritidis* infections in rats is based on the recognition of characteristic lesions in the joints and legs; and *M. neurolyticum* in mice is characterised by the symptoms of rolling and imbalance. This latter organism can be isolated from infected brain tissue and brain sections will show lesions of necrosis and abnormal morphology of astrocytes.

Poultry
Disease caused by *M. gallisepticum* can be diagnosed by observing the symptoms and lesions and employing serological tests, particularly the rapid serum plate agglutination test, the tube agglutination test and the haemagglutination-inhibition test. Sometimes the rapid serum plate test, in particular, may give non-specific agglutination which has been attributed to adsorbed globulins on the mycoplasmas and their consequent reaction with antiglobulin factors in the serum. Other unidentified factors may also be responsible for these non-specific reactions. Because serum antibody titres become markedly reduced during storage at room temperature in the presence of clots, sera should be separated from clots and stored as briefly as possible at room temperature before being tested. *M. synoviae* infections can be diagnosed from the joint lesions in association with visceral lesions and the use of the rapid serum plate agglutination test. *M. meleagridis* infection causing disease in turkey poults is difficult to diagnose apart from the recognition of symptoms and lesions, and the isolation of the organism in the absence of *M. gallisepticum*.

Control and prevention

Cattle
The prevention and control of contagious bovine pleuropneumonia depends upon the diagnosis of infection, the slaughter of diseased animals, the prevention of the spread of disease by prohibiting the movement of animals from an infected to a non-infected locality, and the protection of susceptible individuals by vaccination. The efficacy of these combined measures varies from country to country largely according to the conditions of animal husbandry practised in each territory.

The most difficult problem continues to be the production of a reliable method of vaccination which can be applied in different countries under various conditions and which will give adequate protection. During the many years of experimentation, the four major problems relating to the preparation and use of vaccines that have to be considered are:

(1) The difficulties of cultivating and preserving the organisms in sufficient quantities in some tropical countries.

(2) The lack of immune response stimulated by a killed vaccine which is safe to use.

(3) The inadequate immune response stimulated by an extremely attenuated vaccine which is safe to use.

(4) The solid immunity provided by a vaccine prepared from a virulent or partially avirulent culture which is potentially dangerous but on balance, is economically satisfactory when applied in conjunction with other supporting measures for prevention and control.

Partially avirulent cultures for use as vaccines can be readily prepared by serial passage of the organisms in serum broth cultures or in fertile chicken eggs. From such experiments it has become apparent that the immunogenic properties of these vaccines are directly in proportion to the virulence of the organisms, and that it is necessary to use partially avirulent organisms to obtain a satisfactory degree of immunity. It has been found that when such a vaccine is inoculated into the tip of the tail, the subsequent spread of infection is sufficiently slow to allow the development of immunity without causing a mortality rate of more than 1 per cent. in a group of animals; but the resulting local reaction may cause sloughing of the lower part of the tail in the region of the inoculation site. The severity of this local reaction is less in territories where the disease is enzootic than in areas where animals have not been naturally exposed to infection. In East Africa, the use of a broth culture vaccine prepared from the partially avirulent egg passage T_1 strain of *M. mycoides* is proving valuable, because it confers an immunity of approximately 12 months duration and seldom causes a severe reaction at the site of inoculation in the tail.

Inoculation of more attenuated vaccines subcutaneously into the side of the neck has also been used, particularly in Nigeria, and this gives some immunity without causing a severe reaction at the site of inoculation. Another method which has been used is intradermal inoculation into the muzzle or tip of the ear of West African cattle which seem to tolerate these sites because of dense networks of lymph vessels within the dermis.

Notwithstanding the difficulties inherent in the use of vaccines, they have been employed to advantage in conjunction with other control measures, but further research is required to develop a more satisfactory procedure which can be adopted in all countries where contagious bovine pleuropneumonia occurs.

A more recent development has been a vaccine prepared from an avirulent strain of *M. mycoides* mixed with a suspension of bovine brain tissue. The latter ingredient enables the vaccinal strain to establish itself and to stimulate a stronger immunogenic response without causing a severe local reaction in the tail at the site of inoculation. The vaccine can also be freeze-dried and stored.

Goats and sheep
The control of contagious pleuropneumonia of goats is by slaughter of infected and in-contact animals together with thorough disinfection of premises. A limiting factor is the lack of a reliable serological test for the detection of infected individuals. Attempts to develop a satisfactory vaccine have not been successful. Contagious agalactia is similarly controlled by slaughter and disinfection; in addition, the complement-fixation test has been used for detecting infected individuals but is not always reliable. Vaccination has been attempted.

Pigs
There are no satisfactory methods presently available for the prevention of mycoplasmosis in pigs. *M. hyorhinis* is highly susceptible to lincomycin and tylosin and the therapeutic use of these drugs during the early stages of arthritis caused by *A. granularum* may be beneficial. Similarly, early treatment of *M. hyopneumoniae* infection with broad spectrum antibiotics may curtail the development of pneumonic lesions.

Rats and mice
Inadequate knowledge of the natural mycoplasmal carrier state in these animals and the circumstances which affect the spread of infection, have prevented the development of reliable methods for the control and prevention of mycoplasmosis other than the establishment of germ-free colonies. It is known that serum antibody titres increase as *M. pulmonis* infection becomes established in the respiratory tract, but there is practically no information on the use of serological tests for the control of this disease. Current information indicates that passive protection against *M. neurolyticum* infection in mice is of no practical value as a control measure.

Poultry
The difficulties of controlling *M. gallisepticum* infections are related to the need for a more reliable serological test to identify infected birds and to the problems concerning the prevention of egg transmission. Under practical farming conditions it is not possible to identify all diseased birds in an infected flock by serological methods and disease-free flocks cannot be easily established and maintained. On the other hand, the dipping of eggs in tylosin has proved to be a valuable and practical

method for controlling *M. gallisepticum* infection in hatching eggs. The use of antibiotics in breeding flocks, particularly chlortetracycline in preference to tylosin, cannot be relied upon to prevent egg infection occurring. Similarly, the incidence of egg infection is reduced but not prevented by vaccination of either laying hens or younger birds before they reach maturity.

Chlortetracycline has been used in attempts to control infection with *M. synoviae* and this treatment will prevent the development of clinical cases during the period of medication but will not eliminate infection.

Public health aspects

With the possible exception of *M. pulmonis*, the named mycoplasmal species which occur in man are distinct from those which are known to exist in animals. They include *M. pneumoniae* (Eaton's agent) causing pneumonia, other commensal strains which inhabit the throat and mouth (*M. pharyngitis, M. salivarium*), and *M. hominis, M. fermentans* and the so-called T-strains occurring in the urogenital tract. *M. fermentans* is a commensal, the T-strains have been associated with non-gonococcal urethritis, and recent evidence indicates that the probable role of *M. hominis* as a cause of this condition is minimal. As in animals, it is probable that many other species of *Mycoplasma* occur in man and await characterisation and identification.

L-Phase of bacteria

In 1935 Klieneberger recorded the existence of various bizarre forms of a strain of *Streptobacillus moniliformis* which she termed L-forms — the letter L referring to the Lister Institute where these observations were made. Since that time similar L-forms have been described which were derived from a variety of bacterial species, and it has also become more acceptable to refer to these unusual bacterial forms as L-phase instead of L-form.

Morphology

L-phase may be described as independent growth variants of bacteria that have no cell wall, are capable of multiplication and possess a potential capacity to revert to their parental bacterial form, although some strains show little tendency to reversion and are referred to as stable L-phase.

The various morphological appearances of L-phase bacteria have been described as large bodies, granules and elementary corpuscles. The large bodies vary in size from about 1–50 μm and display considerable pleomorphism. Granules are smaller than large bodies, measuring 0.1–1.0 μm in size, and occur singly or in groups either inside or outside

large bodies. Elementary bodies are the smallest individual particles and usually measure less than 0.5 μm.

Cultivation

A satisfactory basal medium consists of meat digest broth made up as a soft gel by the incorporation of agar (1.0 per cent or less), with the inclusion of serum (10–20 per cent), a relatively high concentration of sodium chloride or sucrose to give osmotic stability, and the addition of penicillin to either promote the induction of L-phase or to prevent reversion of L-phase to the parental bacterial form. Varieties of this basal type of medium have been found appropriate for the cultivation of particular strains of L-phase, and after repeated subcultivation the growth of some strains can be maintained in the absence of serum in the medium. Anaerobic conditions enhance the growth of some L-phase. Several strains have been cultivated in embryonated eggs and tissue cultures.

Colonial formation is similar to that shown by *Mycoplasma* in the development sometimes of the so-called 'poached egg' appearance, and also in the characteristic feature that the dividing organisms in the centre of the colony penetrate into the substance of the solid medium. The different microenvironments which surround the organisms when growing on various media can affect the characteristic features of morphology and multiplication.

In vitro induction of L-phase

The development of L-phase from parent bacteria consists in the loss of that part of the cell wall giving rigidity to the bacteria, under conditions which do not cause lysis of the resulting L-phase organisms and enable multiplication to take place. The absence of the cell wall may come about either from dissolution by various substances, particularly lysozyme, or from inhibition of synthesis by penicillin, bacitracin, vancomycin and other antibiotics. It has also been observed that induction of L-phase may take place in the presence of specific bacterial antibody and complement.

In vivo induction of L-phase and pathogenicity

An evaluation of the possible pathogenic role of L-phase depends in part on the ability to observe the development and maintenance of L-phase under *in vivo* conditions in the absence of parental bacteria and in association with pathological conditions. To cultivate L-phase from tissues under conditions which prevent reversion to the bacterial form, media may be used which will induce the development of L-phase, but it is impossible by this method to ensure that all L-phase colonies which develop are derived from similar L-phase colonies in the tissues and not from parental bacteria. Conversely, attempts to cultivate L-phase organisms from tissues on customary bacteriological media without the incorporation of an inducing agent, will usually result in the development of only the parental bacterial form of the organism. To confirm the presence of L-phase in tissues it is necessary to use more sophisticated methods, including the cultivation of both unfiltered and filtered materials on ordinary bacteriological media and L-phase media with and without the incorporation of penicillin.

The few experiments of this nature which have been carried out give no precise picture of the possible pathogenic role of L-phase. There is evidence, however, that some species of L-phase organisms can produce endotoxins and exotoxins similar to those developed by the parental strains of bacteria. It is also possible that the existence of L-phase *in vivo* may represent a latent form of infection in 'carrier' hosts which either have developed specific antibodies against the parental bacteria or are being subjected to antibiotic therapy. In both these circumstances, L-phases may represent important stages in the life cycles of organisms which develop under adverse conditions preventing the growth of parental bacteria.

Further reading

BARBER T.L. AND FABRICANT J. (1971) A suggested reclassification of avian mycoplasma serotypes. *Avian Diseases*, **15**, 1.

BARDEN, J.A. AND PRESCOTT, B. (1973) Chemical and serological properties of *Mycoplasma hyorhinis* fractions. *Infection and Immunity*, **7**, 937.

CASSELL, G.H., LINDSEY, J.R. AND BAKER, H.J. (1974) Immune response of pathogen-free mice inoculated intranasally with *Mycoplasma pulmonis*. *Journal of Immunology*, **112**, 124.

DUTTA S.K., DIERKS R.E. AND POMEROY B.S. (1965) Electron microscopic studies of the morphology and the stages of the development of *Mycoplasma gallinarum*. *Avian Diseases*, **9**, 241.

EATON, M.D. (1965) Pleuropneumonia-like Organisms and Related Forms. *Annual Review of Microbiology*, **19**, 379.

FREUNDT E.A. (1960) Morphology and classification of the PPLO. *Annals of the New York Academy of Sciences*, **79**, 312.

FURNESS, G. AND DE MAGGIO, M. (1973) The growth cycle of *Mycoplasma mycoides* var. *mycoides*. *Journal of Infectious Diseases*, **127**, 563.

GHAZIKHANIAN, G. AND YAMAMOTO, R. (1974) Characterization of pathogenic and non-pathogenic strains of *Mycoplasma meleagridis*. I. Manifestations of disease in turkey embryos and poults. II. In ovo and in vitro studies. *American Journal of Veterinary Research*, **35**, 417, 425.

GOIS, M., KUKSA, F., FRANZ, J. AND TAYLOR-ROBINSON, D. (1974) The antigenic differentiation of seven strains of *Mycoplasma hyorhinis* by growth-inhibition, metabolism-inhibition, latex-agglutination, and polyacrylamide-gel-electrophoresis tests. *Journal of Medical Microbiology*, **7**, 105.

GOURLEY, R.N. (1973) Significance of Mycoplasma Infections in Cattle. *Journal of the American Veterinary Medical Association*, **163**, 905.

GOURLAY, R.N., LEACH, R.H. AND HOWARD, C.J. (1974) *Mycoplasma verecundum*, a new species isolated from bovine eyes. *Journal of General Microbiology*, **81**, 475.

HAYFLICK L., Ed. (1967) Biology of the mycoplasma. *Annals of the New York Academy of Sciences*, **143**, 1.

HAYFLICK L. Ed. (1969) *The Mycoplasmatales and the L-phase of Bacteria*, 1st Edition, pp. 731. Amsterdam: North-Holland.

HOLMGREN, N. (1974) An indirect haemagglutination test for detection of antibodies against *Mycoplasma hyopneumoniae* using formalinised tanned swine erythrocytes. *Research in Veterinary Science*, **16**, 341.

KAKOMA, I., MASIGA, W.N. AND WINDSOR, R.S. (1973) Detection of immunoconglutinin in cattle with contagious bovine pleuropneumonia: evidence of autoimmunity. *Research in Veterinary Science*, **15**, 101.

KENNY G.E., Chairman (1973) Workshop on the Mycoplasmatales as agents of disease. *Journal of Infectious Diseases*, **127**, Supplement, S1.

KLIENEBERGER E. (1935) The natural occurrence of pleuropneumonia-like organisms in apparent symbiosis with *Streptobacillus moniliformis* and other bacteria. *Journal of Pathology and Bacteriology*, **40**, 93.

KLIENEBERGER-NOBEL E. (1962) *Pleuropneumonia-like organisms (PPLO) Mycoplasmataceae*, 1st Edition, pp. 157. London: Academic Press.

LANGFORD, E.V. AND LEACH, R.H. (1973) Characterization of a mycoplasma isolated from infectious bovine keratoconjunctivitis: *M. bovoculi* sp. nov. *Canadian Journal of Microbiology*, **19**, 1435.

LEACH, R.H. (1967) Comparative studies of Mycoplasma of bovine origin. *Annals of the New York Academy of Sciences*, **143**, 305.

LEACH, R.H. (1970) The occurrence of *Mycoplasma arginini* in several animal hosts. *Veterinary Record*, **87**, 319.

MARAMOROSCH, K. [Editor] (1973) Mycoplasma and mycoplasma-like agents of human, animal and plant diseases. *Annals of the New York Academy of Sciences*, **225**, 532.

MOROWITZ H.J. AND MANILOFF J. (1966) Analysis

of life cycle of *Mycoplasma gallisepticum*. *Journal of Bacteriology*, **91**, 1638.

OGATA, M., WATABE, J. AND KOSHIMIZU, K. (1974) Classification of acholeplasmas isolated from horses. *Japanese Journal of Veterinary Science*, **36**, 43.

POTGIETER, L.N.D. and ROSS, R.F. (1972) Identification of *Mycoplasma hyorhinis* and *Mycoplasma hyosynoviae* by immunofluorescence. *American Journal of Veterinary Research*, **33**, 91

POWER, J. AND JORDAN, F.T.W. (1973) The virulence of *Mycoplasma gallisepticum* for embryonated fowl eggs. *Research in Veterinary Science*, **14**, 259.

ROBERTS, D.H., WINDSOR, R.S., MASIGA, W.N. AND KARIAVU, C.G. (1973) Cell-mediated immune response in cattle to *Mycoplasma mycoides* var. *mycoides. Infection and Immunity*, **8**, 349.

ROSENDAL, S. (1974) Canine mycoplasmas. II. Biochemical characteristics and serological differentiation. *Acta Pathologica et Microbiologica Scandinavica*, **82B**, 25.

ROSS R.F. AND DUNCAN, J.R. (1970) *Mycoplasma hyosynoviae* Arthritis. *Journal of the American Veterinary Medical Association*, **157**, 1515.

ROSS, R.F. AND KARMON, J.A. (1970) Heterogeneity among strains of *Mycoplasma granularum* and identification of *Mycoplasma hyosynoviae*: sp.n. *Journal of Bacteriology*, **103**, 707.

STIPKOVITS, L., ROMVARY, J., NAGY, Z., BODON, L. AND VARGA, L. (1974) Studies on the pathogenicity of *Acholeplasma axanthum* in swine. *Journal of Hygiene*, **72**, 289.

STONE, S.S. AND RAZIN, S. (1973) Immunoelectro

phoretic analysis of *Mycoplasma mycoides* var. *mycoides. Infection and Immunity*, **7**, 922.

Subcommittee on the Taxonomy of Mycoplasmatales (1972). Proposal for the Minimal Standards for Descriptions of New Species of the Order Mycoplasmatales. *International Journal of Systematic Bacteriology*, **22**, 184.

SURMAN, P.G. (1973) Mycoplasma aetiology of keratoconjunctivitis ['pink-eye'] in domestic ruminants. *Australian Journal of Experimental Biology and Medicine*, **51**, 589.

TAN, R.J.S. AND MILES, J.A.R. (1974) Incidence and significance of mycoplasmas in sick cats. *Research in Veterinary Science*, **16**, 27.

TANAKA T. AND WOODS D.A. (1970) Electron microscopic studies of *Mycoplasma pulmonis* (Negroni strain). *Journal of General Microbiology*, **63**, 281.

THOMAS, L.H. AND HOWARD, C.J. (1974) Effect of *Mycoplasma dispar, Mycoplasma bovirhinis, Acholeplasma laidlawii* and T-mycoplasmas on explant cultures of bovine trachea. *Journal of Comparative Pathology*, **84**, 193.

TIMMS, L. AND CULLEN, G.A. (1974) Detection of *M. synoviae* infection in chickens and its differentiation from *M. gallisepticum* infection. *British Veterinary Journal*, **130**, 75.

VARDAMAN, T.H., REECE, F.N. AND DEATON, J.W. (1973) Effect of *Mycoplasma synoviae* on broiler performance. *Poultry Science*, **52**, 1909.

WHITELOCK O v ST., Ed. (1960) Biology of the pleuropneumonia-like organisms. *Annals of the New York Academy of Sciences*, **79**, 305.

MYCOLOGY

CHAPTER 28

Structure, classification and diagnosis of Pathogenic Fungi

Morphology and nomenclature

The fungi constitute a very large heterogeneous group of organisms having many different morphological forms. These range from the unicellular yeast bodies of, say, *Cryptococcus*, which are wholly transformed at maturity into the developmental stage, to the more common mycelium forming types of fungi such as *Aspergillus* in which the filamentous growth is differentiated into vegetative and reproductive portions.

Although a single fragment of the filament or **hypha** of a fungus may grow and produce a new colony the main method of reproduction is by means of specialized cells, called spores, of which unlimited numbers may be produced. When the conditions for germination are suitable the fungal spore enlarges and produces through a thin part of the cell-wall (**germ pore**), a cylindrical tube-like filament called the **germ-tube**. As growth proceeds, the germ-tube elongates and eventually branches again and again to form long filamentous, hollow structures called **hyphae** (Fig. 28.1). The hyphal walls are rigid structures composed of cellulose and chitin which enclose the multi-nucleate protoplasm. As the hyphae continue to grow by apical elongation they rebranch and intertwine to form a dense closely-knit mat or mesh of growth known as the **mycelium**. This represents the colony and gives the fungus its characteristic appearance. In addition to the surface growth, which is virtually unlimited in extent, many of the hyphal elements extend into the depths of the substrate forming the vegetative mycelium which is responsible for absorbing further food for growth after it has been rendered soluble by means of exo-enzymes. Other specialised hyphae extend upwards from the surface of the colony forming the aerial mycelium which not only gives the colony its characteristic fluffy or granular appearance but also bears the spores that are responsible for reproduction.

In most species of higher fungi, the *Mycomycetes*, the hyphae are divided by numerous transverse walls or septae into a long chain of uninucleate or multinucleate cells. These are readily distinguished microscopically from the non-septate or **coenocytic hyphae** of the lower fungi, the *Phycomycetes*, which permit the uninterrupted flow of protoplasm through their hollow core. In *Rhizopus*, as well as in some other species of fungi with coencytic hyphae, a number of root-like filaments termed **rhizoids** may project from the surface mycelium into the substrate, and their presence and distribution in a culture often serve as a useful diagnostic feature (Fig. 28.4).

In some species of higher fungi the hyphae may be so closely interwoven as to form a compact mass or **stroma**, or variously combined to give rise to tissue-like aggregations which make up the large 'fruit-bodies' such as the **sclerotium** of ergot of rye. In the *Basidiomycetes*, the fleshy gills of mushrooms

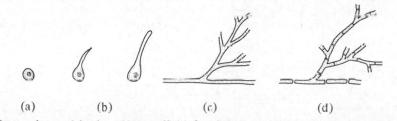

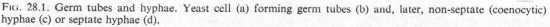

(a)   (b)   (c)   (d)

FIG. 28.1. Germ tubes and hyphae. Yeast cell (a) forming germ tubes (b) and, later, non-septate (coenocytic) hyphae (c) or septate hyphae (d).

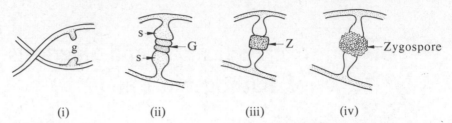

(i)　　　　　(ii)　　　　　(iii)　　　　　(iv)

FIG. 28.2. Conjugation and formation of zygospores: (i) approximation of gametes (g); (ii) formation of gametangia (G) supported by suspensors (s); (iii) gametangia fuse to form zygote (Z); (iv) which matures to produce a spherical, thick-walled sexual spore, the zygospore.

and toadstools are also composed of closely packed masses of hyphae.

The unit of reproduction is the spore, of which there are two main types: the **perfect spore** which results from a sexual process and the **imperfect spore** which arises from an asexual process. Although it varies in size, shape, number and septation as well as in the manner in which it is formed, the spore is used probably more than any other structure as a criterion for classifying the fungi. Indeed, the four main groups of fungi the *Phycomycetes*, the *Ascomycetes*, the *Basidiomycetes* and the '*Fungi imperfecti*' are differentiated by their methods of spore formation.

In the *Phycomycetes*, perfect spores may be produced when the tips of two suitable adjacent hyphae come together and form short side branches called **suspensors**. At the point where the suspensors meet and fuse a **gametangium** is formed. This, in turn, enlarges and secretes a thick horny wall which forms the resting-spore or **zygospore** (Fig. 28.2). Alternatively, a perfect spore may be formed when a 'female' portion of a hypha is fertilized by a 'male' portion. The resulting sexual spore is termed an **oospore** (Fig. 28.3), and the structure which contains it is the **oosphere**.

In addition to this sexual method of reproduction, the *Phycomycetes* produce long, non-septate modified aerial filaments called **sporangiophores** which terminate in a large thin-walled spherical cell or **sporangium** within which are contained large numbers of asexual spores, the **sporangiospores**. Two types of sporangiospores have been described, **aplanospores** which are non-motile spores containing

several nuclei, and **zoospores** which are usually uninucleate motile spores possessing one or more **flagellae**. When the spores reach maturity the sporangium ruptures or **dehisces** and the sporangiospores are released to initiate new hyphae and a new fungus. The size and shape of the spores and the shape of the **columella** or tip of the sporangiophore, together with the type of collar produced by the attached remnants of the ruptured sporangium, are important diagnostic features of *Mucor* and other *Phycomycete* species (Fig. 28.4).

In higher forms of fungi, having septate hyphae, sexual spores are formed in an enlarged specialised cell in the mycelium called an **ascus**. Fusion of nuclei in the ascus mother cell is followed by meiosis and mitosis giving rise, usually, to eight haploid nuclei around each of which an **ascospore** is formed. Thus, there are usually eight spores (ascospores) within each ascus and each is formed as a result of true sexual union (Fig. 28.5). Fungi capable of producing ascospores are called *Ascomycetes* which include not only many true fungi such as *Penicillium* and *Aspergillus* but also more primitive forms such as the yeast *Saccharomyces*.

Most *Ascomycetes*, other than the atypical unicellular yeast members of the group, have an asexual phase of development which is similar in many ways to that of *Phycomycetes*. However, as in all higher fungi, the specialised aerial hyphae are septate and the spores they bear are developed externally. In some species, e.g. *Aspergillus*, the modified hyphae, the **conidiophore**, ends in a small terminal expansion which is sometimes referred to as the **conidiophore vesicle**. From the surface of the

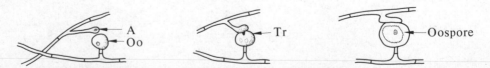

FIG. 28.3. Formation of oospore as a result of fertilization of a specialized female sex structure, oogonium (Oo) by the transfer of the nucleus (Tr) of a nearby male structure, the antheridium (A).

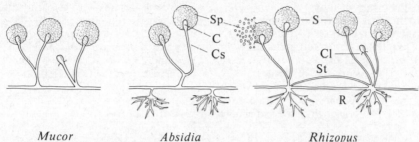

Mucor   *Absidia*   *Rhizopus*

FIG. 28.4. Growth habitat of *Phycomycetes*. Showing expanded tip or columella (C) of coencytic sporangiophore (CS) bearing large sporangiophore vesicle or sporangium (S) containing numerous asexual sporangiospores (Sp).

Also shown are the rhizoids (R) of *Absidia* and *Rhizopus*, the collar of a ruptured sporangium (Cl) and a stolon (St) or runner.

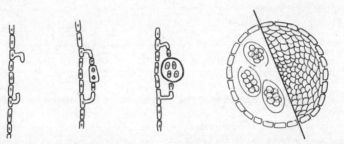

FIG. 28.5. Development of cleisthothecium containing asci (each with eight ascospores) of *Aspergillus*.

vesicle project numerous fleshy goblet or club-shaped structures called **sterigmata** (sing. **sterigma**) from each end of which arises a long chain of exogenous unicellular or multicellular asexual spores called **conidiospores** or **conidia** (Fig. 28.6). In *Penicillium*, however, the conidiophore is also septate but there is no terminal vesicle. Instead, the conidiophore produces a number of long lateral branches along its length and each ends by abstriction in several finger-like projections from which chains of asexual spores

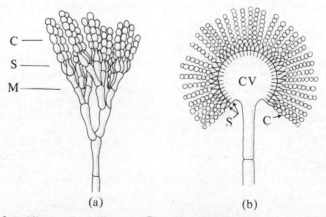

(a)   (b)

FIG. 28.6. Formation of conidia. (a) *Penicillium* spp. Branching conidiophore bearing metullae (M) sterigmata (S) and conidia (C). (b) *Aspergillus* spp. (optical section). Conidiophore with conidiophore vesicle (CV) bearing two rows of sterigmata (S) and conidia (C).

(conidiospores) give the structure its characteristic brush-like appearance.

The third major group of fungi, *Basidiomycetes*, include mushrooms and toadstools, as well as the rusts and smuts which do great economic damage to cereal crops. Despite their marked differences in morphology all members of the *Basidiomycetes* are characterized by the formation of large, fleshy unicellular structures called **basidia** on each of which about four spores (**basidiospores**) are borne exogenously (Fig. 28.7). Although they are externally

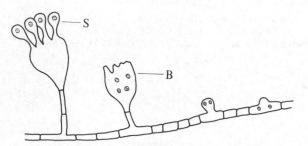

FIG. 28.7. *Basidiomycetes*. Showing the development of four exogenous sexual spores (S) on a basidium (B).

placed, most workers in this field are agreed that the basidiospores are perfect spores and that true sexual union takes place in the basidium. In this respect they are, therefore, quite different from the exogenously developed conidiospores of *Ascomycetes* or the sporangiospores of *Phycomycetes*.

The fourth main group of fungi is, in effect, an artificial group containing those fungi in which there is no sexual stage of development or where, perhaps, no sexual development has yet been observed. For this reason they have been termed *Fungi imperfecti* and include many yeast and yeast-like organisms as well as many pathogenic and non-pathogenic species of mycelial fungi. That this is an unsatisfactory method of classification is underlined by the fact that many workers believe that several species of *Fungi imperfecti* are in fact *Ascomycetes* in which the sexual stage of development has been lost during evolution, or has not yet been identified. A further difficulty stems from the fact that *Fungi imperfecti* form only asexual spores and tend, therefore, to lack the many constant morphological features of the perfect fungi which are essential for accurate diagnosis.

Fungi imperfecti form several different types of asexual spores or **thallospores**. As the name implies these are reproductive spores that develop from the sequestration of unmodified hyphae in contrast to the asexual spores produced by abstriction of the specialised sporangiophores and conidiophores in other types of fungi. The different types of thallospores may be defined as follows:

(1) When a unicellular yeast such as *Cryptococcus* matures the cell enlarges and, if the conditions are favourable for growth, it germinates by a process of budding from one pole of the mother cell. In most instances the budding spore or **blastospore**, which is a form of thallospore, is constricted at its base and detaches from the mother cell to reproduce by further budding (Fig. 28.8).

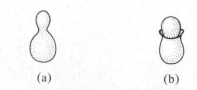

(a)   (b)

FIG. 28.8. Asexual budding of yeasts: (a) blastospore developing on narrow base, e.g. *Cryptococcus*; (b) blastospore developing on broad base, e.g. *Pityrosporum*.

(2) The surface colonies of yeasts and yeast-like organisms are soft, bacterial-like and consist almost entirely of many thousands of deep-staining unicellular organisms. In addition to their surface colonies, yeast-like organisms including *Candida* (*Monilia*) form a vegetative type of growth whereby elongated germ-tubes project downwards from the mother cells into the substrate of the medium. Abstrictions at their growing points give rise to a number of branched chains of attached cells resembling true hyphae and are termed **pseudohyphae**. In the case of *C. albicans*, segmentation of individual cells may occur along or towards the tip of the growing pseudohyphae producing spherical structures which enlarge greatly and form thick-walled resting spores called **chlamydospores** (Fig. 28.9). These usually remain viable after the remainder of the mycelium has died and disintegrated.

(3) A third type of thallospore, the **arthrospore**, is formed by disarticulation or segmentation of a septate hypha into a series of thick-walled rectangular structures which tend to round off and become oval or pillow-shaped when the hypha fragments or is damaged. The presence of arthrospores is a feature of many species of *Fungi imperfecti* and they are frequently formed by **dermatophytes** (ringworm fungi) when parasitizing skin or hair.

Other structures produced by dermatophytic fungi include **microconidia** and **macroconidia**. The former are very small asexual spores of various shapes and sizes which occur either singly alongside the hyphae ('en thyrse'), in clusters ('en grappe') or in long chains (Fig. 28.10). The latter, macroconidia or fuseaux, are much larger imperfect spores which are usually elongated, multi-septate, fusiform or spindle-shaped structures with thick and sometimes wrinkled,

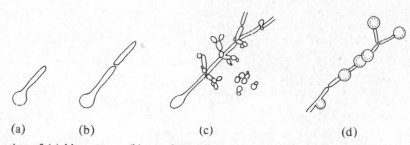

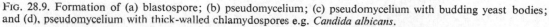

FIG. 28.9. Formation of (a) blastospore; (b) pseudomycelium; (c) pseudomycelium with budding yeast bodies; and (d), pseudomycelium with thick-walled chlamydospores e.g. *Candida albicans*.

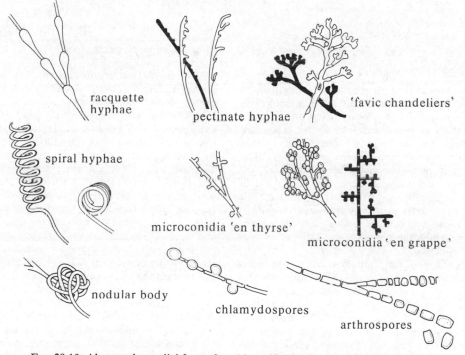

racquette hyphae

pectinate hyphae

'favic chandeliers'

spiral hyphae

microconidia 'en thyrse'

microconidia 'en grappe'

nodular body

chlamydospores

arthrospores

FIG. 28.10. Abnormal mycelial forms found in artificial cultures of dermatophytes.

wart-like walls (e.g. *Microsporum canis*) or long, thin, multiseptate, smooth-walled, cigar-shaped spores as seen in cultures of some *Trichophyton spp.* The third type of ringworm, *Epidermophyton*, is characterized by the formation of a few oval or pear-shaped fuseaux with only a few septae. Fuseaux are produced in primary cultures of most ringworm species but they are often few in number and difficult to find (Fig. 28.11). Furthermore, they may be difficult to maintain as a constant feature of the strain since the dermatophytes are extremely unstable in sub-culture and generally develop a **floccose** or fluffy appearance in place of the normal granular type of growth.

Because of these difficulties in handling dermatophytes, other microscopic structures are often used to identify ringworm species as well as some other members of the *Fungi imperfecti*. These include spiral or coiled hyphae, '**racquet hyphae**' composed of a chain of individual elongated hyphal cells expanded at one end resembling a tennis racquet, **pectinate bodies** resembling the teeth of a comb, or with irregular projections along one side of the hyphal element like antlers or stag-horns – the so-called '**favic chandeliers**'.

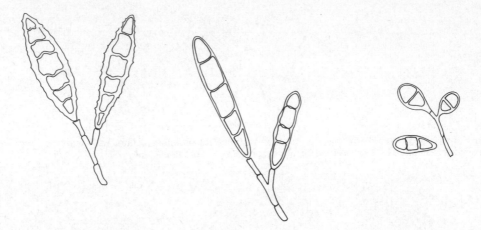

Microsporum   Trichophyton   Epidermophyton

FIG. 28.11. Types of macroconidia found in cultures of ringworm fungi.

Classification

The plant kingdom is divided into a number of phyla one of which, the *Thallophyta*, includes all plants and plant-like organisms below the level of the *Bryophyta* (mosses and liverworts). They are characterized by the fact that the thallus is not differentiated into roots, stems or leaves. The irregular plant masses of the *Thallophyta* are in turn divided into two main groups: the algae, which contain chlorophyll and are able to produce their own food, and fungi, which do not contain chlorophyl and must, accordingly, lead a parasitic, saprophytic or symbiotic relationship with other organisms.

The sub-groups of fungi are *Eumycetes* (true fungi) and *Pseudomycetes* (false fungi). The latter includes *Myxomycetes* (slime moulds) which are of no veterinary importance and the *Schizomycetes* (or bacteria) in which *Actinomyces*, *Nocardia* and, possibly, *Dermatophilus* are classed. The *Eumycetes* are classified into two main families, the *Phycomycetes* or lower fungi and the *Mycomycetes* or higher fungi, according to the type of colony they produce, the type of mycelium if present, the type of spore and the method of spore development.

The *Phycomycetes* which contain the genera *Mucor*, *Absidia* and *Rhizopus* are identified by the fact that they have non-septate hyphae and produce asexual spores within a swollen structure called a sporangium. The *Mycomycetes* on the other hand form septate hyphae, if present, (yeasts do not produce hyphae) and include the *Ascomycetes*, *Basidiomycetes* and *Fungi imperfecti*. *Ascomycetes* are characterized by the production of sexual spores, ascospores, usually eight in number lying

within an enlarged cell or sac called an **ascus**, while the asexual spores (conidia) are formed on specialized septae called conidiophores. *Basidiomycetes* are identified by their characteristic septate, binucleate hyphae and the exogenous development of their four sexual spores on each club-shaped basidium. In some species, e.g. mushrooms, compact masses of mycelia form gills on which the basidia, basidiophores and basidiospores are formed. *Fungi imperfecti* include a number of pathogenic species which may be difficult to identify with accuracy not only because they do not appear to produce sexual spores but because the characteristics of their asexual spores vary greatly with changes of temperature, constituents of the cultural media and even within the strain of fungus itself. This has given rise to a great deal of confusion in the literature regarding the relationship of individual species of *Fungi imperfecti* to pathogenic processes in man and animals. Difficulties in nomenclature are legion and there are numerous conflicting claims for the same fungus as, for example, among the dermatophytes where about 1000 names have been given for the 350 known species.

Apart from the fact that members of the *Fungi imperfecti* range from the simplest type of unicellular yeast, e.g. *Cryptococcus* to the commoner types of fungi which produce both an aerial and vegetative septate mycelium, e.g. dermatophytes, they also include a number of **dimorphic fungi**. By dimorphism is meant the ability of a fungus to show a yeast-like parasitic phase of development with the formation of soft surface colonies when grown on artificial media at 37°C, and a mycelial saprophytic phase with aerial septate hyphae and asexual spores in cultures incubated at room temperature (20–22°C). The phenomenon is largely confined to a group of fungi, e.g. *Blastomyces spp.* and *Histoplasma farciminosum*, which cause systemic infections of man and animals, but is never found in plant fungi.

The classification of fungi is, therefore, complex and little benefit will be derived in a textbook of this nature by giving details of all the relationships possible between the 200 000 species of fungi, particularly since the four main classes which include the fungi of veterinary importance, contain no fewer than 3–4000 genera. Nevertheless, some knowledge of the main differences between the pathogenic fungi is necessary and the simplified form of classification shown in Fig. 28.12 should prove helpful.

Pathogenic fungi

Fungi which cause mycoses of man and animals are many and diverse, but most of the important pathogens are imperfect forms and are classified as *Fungi imperfecti*. These include a wide variety of organisms ranging from yeasts, e.g. *Cryptococcus neoformans* causing human European blastomycosis or torulosis, and yeast-like organisms, e.g. *Candida albicans* responsible for moniliasis or 'thrush' in man, animals and birds, to the dimorphic fungi such as *Histoplasma farciminosum* of epizootic lymphangitis of horses, and true fungi including the dermatophytes or ringworm moulds. The *Basidiomycetes* do not contain species pathogenic for animals although mushrooms, toadstools and some other species may be poisonous when ingested by man. *Phycomycetes*, or mucor-like moulds have often been found in association with disease processes in man and animals but their causative role is often obscure and difficult to assess. *Ascomycetes* are seldom pathogenic although some members of the group such as *Aspergillus* are frequently responsible for respiratory and other disease conditions in mammals and birds.

In general, pathogenic fungi fall readily into two distinct groups, the one comprising the superficial and cutaneous infections and the other the deep-seated or systemic infections. The former are usually characterized by sudden onset of an acute illness after a short incubation period. This is usually followed by a decrease in severity of the condition and spontaneous healing of the lesions. In systemic mycoses, on the other hand, the incubation period may be prolonged, the onset of clinical symptoms slow and insidious, and the course of the disease is one of increasing severity which often terminates in death. Most mycoses induce an allergic state and may contain endotoxins which are liberated when the cells of the invading fungus are damaged or disintegrate. Fungal infections are seldom contagious although there are a number of notable exceptions including superficial mycoses such as ringworm and certain systemic infections including equine epizootic lymphangitis. Most mycotic diseases are exogenous in origin and are usually contracted individually from saprophytic species in the environment rather than by contact with affected patients.

Laboratory diagnostic methods

Diagnostic procedures in mycology are very similar to those employed in bacteriology and the same general rules apply regarding the selection, collection and despatch of suitable specimens to the laboratory. For the accurate identification of the causative agent of a mycotic infection, great care must be taken in the choice of specimen and the clinician must ensure that the material is taken from an active focus of infection and from a portion of the lesion where the fungus is likely to be present in quantity and in a state of active development. Prior to collecting the specimen, the affected area should be lightly sponged with 70 per cent alcohol to remove surface contaminants. Skin scrapings should be taken from the active periphery of the lesion by means of a scalpel blade or the edge of a glass slide. Hairs from suspected cases of ringworm should be plucked from the lesion and not cut by scissors. Suspected material should always be obtained as fresh as possible and despatched to the laboratory in suitable containers. These vary from dry sterile tightly-stoppered bottles for pus, exudates, secretions, body fluids or tissues, to envelopes or glass slides wrapped tightly together, for hair, wool, or skin-scrapings.

Laboratory diagnostic methods include direct examination of the specimen for the presence of spores or vegetative organisms, isolation and identification of likely pathogens including animal inoculation and, occasionally, serological tests such as immunofluorescence and agar-gel diffusion. In routine mycological examinations artifacts such as oil droplets, pigment granules, vegetable fibres and debris must be distinguished from fungal elements, and every effort must be made not to confuse contaminant fungi with those associated with the disease condition.

Direct examination

Wet preparations of pus, secretions, exudates, skin-scrapings, fetal stomach contents, etc. may be examined directly by light microscopy on a clean glass slide with a small coverslip carefully applied to prevent air-bubbles. In many cases it is an advantage when observing hyphae or spores to suspend the material in lactophenol cotton blue, to obtain contrast.

Gram's and other staining methods are often useful in mycology since many of the yeasts or yeast-like organisms such as *Pityrosporum* and *Candida*

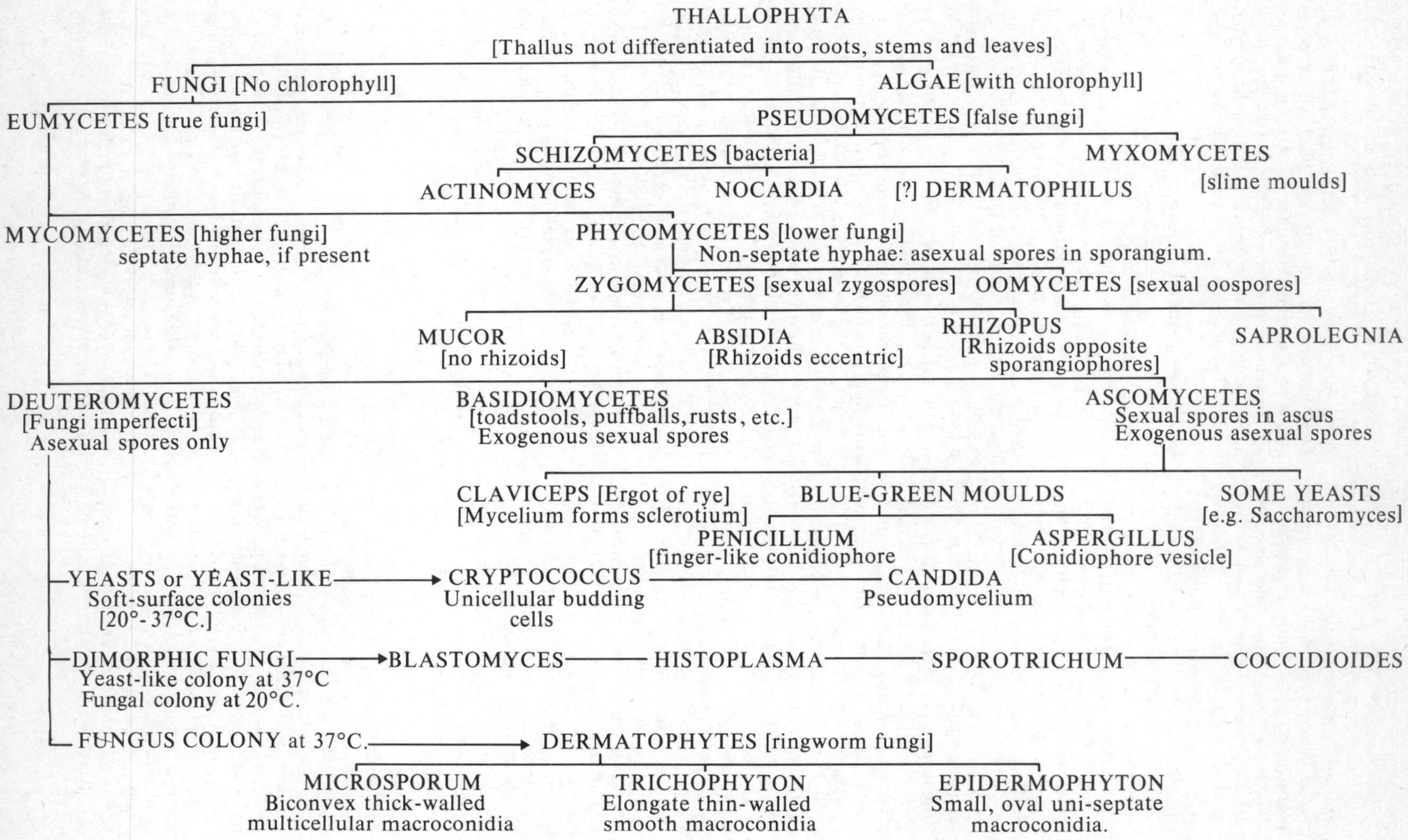

THALLOPHYTA
[Thallus not differentiated into roots, stems and leaves]

ALGAE [with chlorophyll]

FUNGI [No chlorophyll]

EUMYCETES [true fungi]

PSEUDOMYCETES [false fungi]

MYXOMYCETES [slime moulds]

SCHIZOMYCETES [bacteria]
ACTINOMYCES
NOCARDIA
[?] DERMATOPHILUS

MYCOMYCETES [higher fungi] septate hyphae, if present

PHYCOMYCETES [lower fungi] Non-septate hyphae: asexual spores in sporangium.

ZYGOMYCETES [sexual zygospores]
OOMYCETES [sexual oospores]

MUCOR [no rhizoids]
ABSIDIA [Rhizoids eccentric]
RHIZOPUS [Rhizoids opposite sporangiophores]
SAPROLEGNIA

ASCOMYCETES
Sexual spores in ascus
Exogenous asexual spores

BASIDIOMYCETES
[toadstools, puffballs, rusts, etc.]
Exogenous sexual spores

CLAVICEPS [Ergot of rye] [Mycelium forms sclerotium]

PENICILLIUM [finger-like conidiophore]
BLUE-GREEN MOULDS
ASPERGILLUS [Conidiophore vesicle]
SOME YEASTS [e.g. Saccharomyces]
CANDIDA Pseudomycelium

DEUTEROMYCETES
[Fungi imperfecti]
Asexual spores only

YEASTS or YEAST-LIKE
Soft-surface colonies
[20°–37°C.]

CRYPTOCOCCUS Unicellular budding cells

DIMORPHIC FUNGI
Yeast-like colony at 37°C
Fungal colony at 20°C.

BLASTOMYCES
HISTOPLASMA
SPOROTRICHUM
COCCIDIOIDES

FUNGUS COLONY at 37°C.

DERMATOPHYTES [ringworm fungi]

MICROSPORUM
Biconvex thick-walled
multicellular macroconidia

TRICHOPHYTON
Elongate thin-walled
smooth macroconidia

EPIDERMOPHYTON
Small, oval uni-septate
macroconidia.

FIG. 28.12. The outline of a classification of the fungi.

give a strong positive reaction and are readily identified in smear preparations. *Actinomyces, Nocardia* and *Dermatophilus spp.* also stain Gram-positive and some are acid-alcohol fast when stained by Ziehl-Neelsen. Acid-fast staining methods are of value in studies of systemic mycoses to eliminate mycobacterial infections since tuberculous granulomas may be confused with chronic fungal lesions.

Histological examination of tissue sections is also useful in diagnostic mycology since hyphal elements are clearly visible in preparations stained by Gram, Claudius, Giemsa and haematoxylin-eosin. One of the most important technical advances made in modern mycology was the adaptation of the periodic-acid-Schiff stain (PAS) for the detection of fungi in pathological specimens. The two methods mostly employed are Kligman's modification or a combination of the PAS and Gomori's Aldehyde-Fuchsin stain known as Gridley's modification. This latter method has the advantage of staining equally the spores and hyphae in infected tissues. By the PAS method of Kligman, the hyphae stain bright red or magenta against a green or blue background whereas with Gridley's modification the hyphal elements appear dark bluish-purple in contrast to the light yellow colour of the tissue background. In many instances, however, the simpler haematoxylin-eosin staining method is adequate and has the advantage of showing details of the tissue reaction as well as the organisms.

Fluorescent antibody staining has not been used to the same extent as in bacteriology or virology but recent evidence indicates that it may be used to advantage for the rapid and accurate diagnosis of ringworms and mycotic dermatitis of cattle and sheep. In ringworm diagnosis a simple, non-serological fluorescence technique is helpful in eliminating artefacts in specimens prepared for direct microscopy. In this procedure the mounting fluid consists of 1 part of 1:1000 acridine orange and nine parts of 20 per cent KOH. When viewed under a fluorescence microscope, the hyphae, spores and yeast-bodies fluoresce brightly against a darkened background.

The classical method of examining hair, fur or wool for the presence of ringworm infection is to mount the suspected specimen on a slide in 10–20 per cent KOH, cover it with a cover-glass, clear by heating for about 30 minutes and observe it with a dry objective for the presence of arthrospores outside (ectothrix) or inside (endothrix) the hair shaft. The detection and identification of certain dermatophytes is greatly facilitated by direct examination of affected hairs by means of ultra-violet rays. Light from a mercury-vapour lamp, filtered through sodium-barium-silicate glass containing nickel oxide — the so-called Wood's lamp —

causes the externally arranged ectothrix spores of most *Microsporum*, e.g. *M. canis* and *M. audouinii*, as well as a few *Trichophyton spp.* such as *T. quinckeanum*, to produce a bright greenish-yellow fluorescence when viewed in a darkened room. In other types of ringworm where the arthrospores are distributed within the hair shaft (endothrix) the Wood's lamp yields only rays outside the visible spectrum and there is no fluorescence. The technique is particularly useful in the selection of hairs for microscopical and cultural examination from cats and other animals where typical ringworm lesions are often difficult to detect. It is emphasized, however, that hair-shafts contaminated with oily-based lotions used to treat the condition may cause non-specific fluorescence.

Cultural examination

In the great majority of cases of suspected mycotic infections a confirmatory diagnosis is only possible after the causative fungus has been isolated and cultivated successfully in synthetic media, and its growth characters studied in specially prepared mounts. As one might expect, a wide range of solid and fluid media has been devised for studying the growth and development of fungi, but it is outside the scope of this present text to do more than mention those that are useful in veterinary mycology.

In general mycology, organic media comprising carrot, potato, hair, pieces of wood or extracts of these substances are particularly useful for the isolation of fungi, and in animal mycology extracts of malt and beer-wort have proved valuable. At present, however, most medical and veterinary mycologists prefer to use semi-natural media or synthetic media because they are readily available and of standard quality. In most laboratories all materials from suspected cases of mycotic infections are cultured for fungi whether or not there is evidence of their presence in direct microscopical examinations.

Isolation. Before culture plates are inoculated with the suspected material it is often an advantage to pre-treat the specimens to liberate the spores or free the fungus from bacterial contamination. This can be done in the case of hair, wool or skin scrapings by keeping the specimens dry for several weeks to allow the bacteria to die out. If time permits, pure cultures of dermatophytes or *Dermatophilus* can be obtained by this simple method. Alternatively, the specimens can be treated by frequent brief washes in ether, acetone, alcohol, other bactericidal substances, or suitable antibiotics can be incorporated in the growth media prior to pouring the plates. The possibility of isolating *Trichophyton spp.* from animal hairs is greatly enhanced if cyclohexamide (0·1 mg/ml) is added to the agar base in order to depress the growth of contaminant moulds.

Media. Plates or slopes of standard mycological media, e.g. malt agar or Sabouraud's glucose or maltose agar, are inoculated with the specimen and incubated in a moist chamber at room temperature. In addition, plates of mycological and bacteriological agar as well as blood agar should be inoculated and incubated at 37°C because many yeasts and some pathogenic species of fungi grow better in conditions of higher pH and temperature. Incorporation of penicillin (20 units/ml), streptomycin (100 μg/ml) or other substances in the media will reduce bacterial contamination and aid recovery of the fungus.

Malt agar is probably the most useful general purpose medium but Sabouraud's glucose or maltose agar is preferred by some workers as the standard medium for cultivating dermatophytes, although nutrient agar is generally regarded as being best for the isolation of *Trichophyton discoides.* Blood agar is recommended for growing yeasts or yeast-like organisms, and for stimulating the production of macroconidia in *Trichophyton spp.* Beer wort agar is especially useful for the isolation of yeasts, while Raulin's is a helpful selective medium for separating yeasts from contaminating bacteria because of its low pH [*c.* 3·0]. In some laboratories Littman Oxgall agar is employed for the primary isolation of dermatophytes and corn (maize) meal agar is invaluable for stimulating production of the characteristic chlamydospores of *C. albicans.*

Growth requirements. Most fungi grow and develop best in the presence of 1–4 per cent carbohydrate and when incubated in the dark in a warm, moist aerobic atmosphere. Compared with bacteria, fungi are large, robust structures which usually prefer a more acid pH for growth. They develop surface colonies more slowly than the majority of bacteria and the growth usually extends into the substrate of the medium. Fungi, like plants, require a source of nitrogen for the synthesis of protein and protoplasm, carbohydrates for energy, and other essential elements including potassium, magnesium and iron. Some species also require fats, vitamins and trace elements. In general, pathogenic species grow well on simple synthetic or organic media but the less pathogenic varieties tend to be more fastidious and require more complex media for satisfactory isolation and growth. The majority of fungi will grow over a wide range of temperatures (— 10° to 60°C) but others are more selective. Pathogenic species can be grown between 10° to 40°C but the optimal temperature is about 25° to 30°C, rather than 37°C. Thermophilic species such as *Aspergillus fumigatus,* which causes respiratory disease in birds and mammals, grow well at body temperature and their spores are very resistant to higher temperatures. The morphological characters of fungi, on which a diagnosis is usually based, are largely dependent upon the degree of humidity and temperature of incubation. If the humidity is allowed to fall below 90 per cent many primary cultures will fail to develop the characteristic spores. Unlike bacteria all fungi, other than *Actinomyces bovis,* require free oxygen for satisfactory growth.

Cultural characters. The majority of fungi do not lend themselves to the use of biochemical and other bacteriological techniques for their identification. Instead, they are usually classified morphologically according to the appearance of the colony, the type of spore produced and the method of spore formation.

The type of colony may be one of three forms:
(1) the regular, raised, soft, often non-pigmented bacterial-type growth of yeasts, composed of unicellular budding forms, e.g. *Cryptococcus,*
(2) similar, soft, bacterial-type surface colonies of yeast-like organisms consisting of unicellular budding forms on the surface of the medium and hyphal elements (pseudomycelium) penetrating the depths of the medium, e.g. *Candida,*
(3) a typical mould colony consisting of a vegetative mycelium in the substrate and aerial hyphae producing asexual spores which give the colony its fluffy or granular appearance, e.g. *Mucor* and *Aspergillus.* Yeast or yeast-like organisms may produce white or pigmented surface colonies whereas the typical mould colony is often deeply pigmented on one or both surfaces.

In order to identify the organism, suspect colonies are removed from the primary plate cultures and each is re-seeded on a suitable medium to obtain pure growths. Although experienced workers can recognise many species by the colonial characters it is generally necessary to make wet preparations for studying the morphological features of the developing fungus before a positive diagnosis can be made. Since both the colonial characteristics and the morphology of the fungus are profoundly influenced by physical and chemical factors, it is important to standardise the constituents of the different media used as well as the time, temperature and humidity of incubation. Cultures should be maintained with care because fungi change their growth characters readily and may develop sterile hyphae without spores after only a few serial transfers. Occasionally, however, it may be possible to induce an isolate to restore its specific properties by varying one or more of the conditions under which it is being maintained or simply by transferring it to an entirely different type of culture medium.

It is often convenient to examine the morphology of a primary or secondary culture by suspending a small portion of the growth in a drop of lactophenol cotton blue and carefully teasing the structures apart with fine dissecting needles on a glass slide. A cover-glass is then carefully applied and the preparation is examined under low and high power dry objectives in the light microscope. Semi-permanent slide-mounts can be made if evaporation is prevented by sealing the edges of the coverslip, which must be dry, to the glass slide by means of nail varnish. A more satisfactory but slower method, which is particularly suitable for observing the development of spores and hyphae, is by the block-slide culture technique. This is done by pouring sufficient agar medium into a sterile petri-dish to form a layer of 1–1·5 mm deep. When the medium is set, two or three small (5–10 mm²) blocks of agar are cut out with a sterile scalpel-blade and carefully placed on a sterile glass slide. The fungus culture to be studied is inoculated around the edges of the agar-block, a sterile cover-glass of suitable size is carefully placed in position on top of the block and the slide is incubated in a moist chamber at the appropriate temperature. When sufficient growth has extended outwards on to the cover-glass it is carefully removed from the agar-block, mounted in a drop of lactophenol cotton blue on a clean slide and examined microscopically for details of fungal development. Apart from clarity of the preparations, the technique is particularly suitable for observing the growth characteristics of a culture over a period merely by removing and examining one of a series of coverslip preparations at the appropriate time. Semi-permanent mounts can again be made by ringing the cover-glass with a good quality nail varnish.

The fermentation reactions of yeasts and yeast-like organisms in fluid carbohydrate media can be readily investigated by the usual bacteriological methods. With strains of *Candida*, however, the production of gas is often best studied when the tubes are sealed immediately after inoculation by means of sterile molten paraffin-wax carefully layered, and allowed to set on the surface of each 'sugar'. After incubation, the extent to which the wax plug is displaced above the surface of the medium is an indication of the amount of gas produced by fermentation.

Animal inoculation.
Biological examinations are seldom necessary in diagnostic mycology because accurate identification of a fungus can usually be accomplished more easily and quickly by routine cultural methods. In certain circumstances, however, animal inoculation tests are helpful and justifiable to assist isolation and assess the pathogenicity of a particular isolate. For example, cultures and infected exudates of *Coccidioides immitis* and *Histoplasma capsulatum* are pathogenic for mice and cause demonstrable infection 1–2 weeks after intraperitoneal injection. Moreover, rabbits and mice injected intravenously with suspensions of *C. albicans*, but not other *Candida* species, succumb to a fatal infection with typical lesions in the kidneys. Laboratory animals have also proved useful for isolation of pathogenic fungi from soil and other materials, and for studies of the tissue phase of dimorphic fungi such as *Blastomyces dermatitidis* and *Sporotrichum schenckii*.

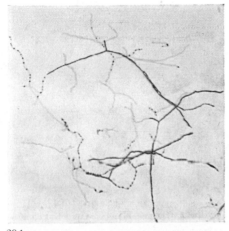

29.1a

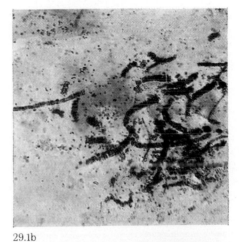

29.1b

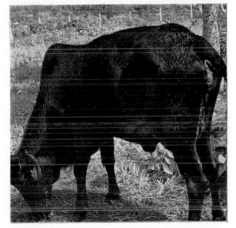

29.1c

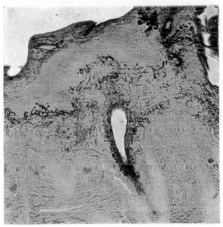

29.1d

29.1a   Gram-stained film made from an aerobic glucose broth culture inoculated with pus from the thoracic cavity of a dog, showing the slender branching filaments of *Nocardia spp*, × 645.

29.1c   A typical case of bovine streptothricosis. Dry, powdery, raised exudative lesions are widely distributed over the surface of the body including the face, ears, neck and escutcheon.

29.1b   Gram-stained preparation of exudate from the skin of a cow severely affected with streptothricosis. Notice the broad Gram-positive filaments with evidence of fragmentation into coccal forms (zoospores), × 645.

29.1d   Section through the skin of a sheep suffering from lumpy wool disease. Large numbers of deeply staining branching filaments are found in the deeper dermal layers and around the wool follicles. Claudius' stain, × 54.

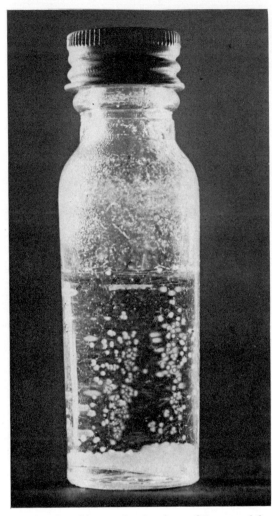

29.2a   A 4-day-old serum broth culture of *Dermatophilus dermatonomus*. Bright yellow fluffy colonies adhere to the surface of the glass or settle at the foot of the tube. The medium remains clear.

29.2b, c   Raised yellow wax-like convoluted colonies of *D. dermatonomus* on the surface of serum agar plates after 10 days' aerobic incubation at 37°C. The diameter of the colonies is approximately 10 mm.

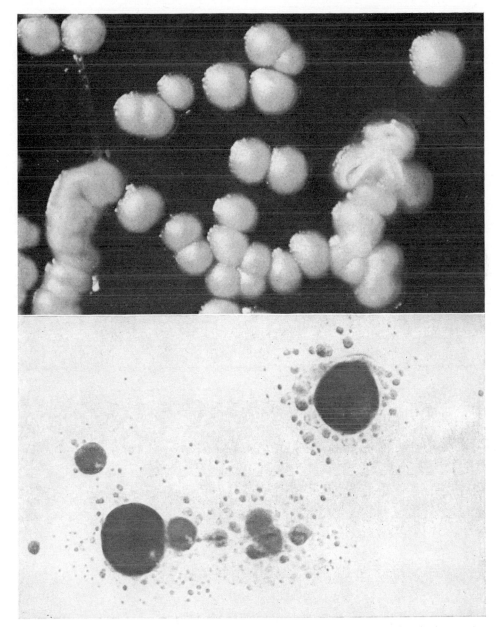

29.3a   Recent isolates of *D. dermatonomus* may produce regular domed non-pigmented colonies on the surface of serum plates incubated for 3-5 days in air plus 10 per cent added CO_2. The colonies are friable and firmly adherent to the medium. Their diameter is slightly smaller than that of a typical *Staphylococcus albus* colony.

29.3b   Surface colonies of *D. dermatonomus* on 2 per cent agar. The small satellite colonies are formed by the motile coccal forms of the organism.

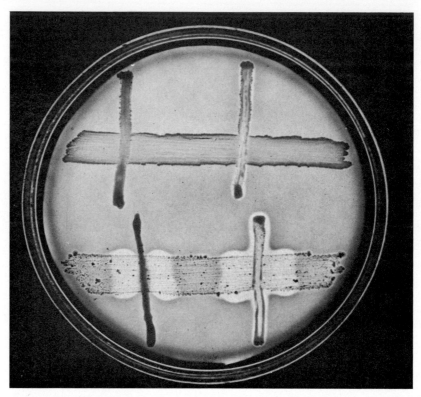

29.4 An increased haemolytic effect is obtained on 4 per cent sheep blood agar by drawing cultures of *Corynebacterium equi* downwards across a horizontal streak culture of *D. dermatonomus* (lower), but not *D. congolensis* (upper). After 48 hours' incubation at 37°C in 10 per cent CO_2.

CHAPTER 29

Dermatophilus

The *Pseudomycetes* or 'false fungi' are divided into the *Myxomycetes* (slime moulds) and *Schizomycetes* or bacteria. *Eubacteriae*, a class of unicellular or mycelial organisms with rigid cell walls, flagellate motility when present, and the possible formation of endospores or conidia, are sub-divided into two groups of non-photosynthetic microorganisms. The unicellular organisms are termed *Eubacteriales* whilst the mycelial members are placed in the order *Actinomycetales*. The *Actinomycetales* consist of two families, the *Actinomycetaceae* and the *Mycobacteriaceae* of which the former comprises several genera including *Actinomyces* and *Nocardia*.

Although *Nocardia* spp. produce a Gram-positive mycelium which may break up into rods and coccoid forms (Plate 29.1a facing p. 294), the characteristics of the genus do not include all the properties shown by the causative agent of 'mycotic dermatitis'. For this reason, a new family, *Dermatophilaceae*, has been proposed. This will include the single genus *Dermatophilus* of which the type species is likely to be *Dermatophilus congolensis* van Saceghem.

'Streptothricosis'
Mycotic dermatitis of cattle, or bovine streptothricosis, is an exudative eczema which causes a considerable amount of illness in cattle throughout central and certain other parts of Africa and, consequently, is responsible for severe damage to hides and considerable economic loss to the skin trades in these territories. The pathogenesis of the disease is still obscure and the causal organism *Dermatophilus congolensis* van Saceghem is very similar in character, if not identical, to the causative agents of mycotic dermatitis of cattle, goats and horses described in the U.K., Australia, the U.S.A. and elsewhere; and of a similar condition of sheep popularly known as 'lumpy wool disease'. It was proposed in 1958 that the genus *Dermatophilus* should include three species namely, *D. dermatonomus* associated with lumpy wool of sheep, *D.*

pedis with strawberry-foot-rot of sheep and *D. congolensis* with bovine streptothricosis. However, experimental evidence indicates that these diseases can be transmitted from one species of animal to another with comparative ease and that the morphology, staining reactions, cultural and biological characters of the causal organisms are so similar that they cannot be used to differentiate one species from another.

Mycotic dermatitis of cattle
Mycotic dermatitis or cutaneous streptothricosis has been recognised as a serious skin disease of cattle since it was first described in the Belgian Congo in 1910–13. It is prevalent in many parts of tropical Africa, particularly in West Africa, and sporadic outbreaks have been reported from Australia, New Zealand, India, the U.S.A. and the U.K. The disease in horses was first described in 1937, in England.

The causative organism, *Dermatophilus congolensis*, has been variously described as *Actinomyces congolensis*, *Nocardia* species, *Sporotrichum* species and *Streptothrix bovis*. Although it is undoubtedly a Gram-positive filamentous organism which gives rise to motile coccal forms typically arranged in two to eight parallel rows within the branching parent filaments, there is still considerable confusion about its classification. However, there is now general agreement that the first 3 generic names (*Actinomyces*, *Nocardia* and *Sporotrichum*) are no longer valid, and since the term *Streptothrix* had already been used in 1839 for a member of the *Hyphomycetes*, the citation *Streptothrix bovis* has no standing either. Nevertheless, the retention of the names 'streptothricosis' and 'mycotic dermatitis' for the disease in cattle is considered to be justified on the grounds of their common usage, although the causal organism may be neither a streptothrix nor even a fungus.

The symptoms vary according to the site, extent and degree of the lesions. In the majority of cases the back appears to be the main predilection site particularly on the 'hump' and 'saddle', and the early lesions frequently form an inverted triangle on each side of the back immediately behind the hump. Other parts commonly affected include the face, neck, dewlap, flanks, udder or scrotum, escutcheon, axilla and groin. The earliest lesion is that of an eruptive eczema which causes thickening of the skin and the formation of numerous exuding pimples. At the base of each tuft of affected hairs an extensive serous exudate appears which forms a thick crust or scab on drying. Hairs in the vicinity become matted together by the dry exudate, stand erect and form the characteristic 'paint-brush' effect. In the smooth-haired parts of the body such as the face and escutcheon the lesions may be flat or wart-like. In the early stages of the disease the lesions are firmly attached to the underlying tissues and their removal, which causes acute discomfort to the animal, leaves a raw bleeding area. Older lesions can be detached painlessly and leave a moist pink patch on the skin covered with a greyish sticky exudate. In long-standing cases the lesions extend over much of the surface of the body causing large patches of moist, evil-smelling eczema or masses of white or buff-coloured powdery crusts which crumble readily when handled (Plate 29.1c facing p. 294). Secondary bacterial invaders entering the eczematous lesions may give rise to an extensive cellulitis and death of the affected animal. In many cases, however, the lesions are limited to certain areas and invariably regress during the dry season. In temperate climates bovine cutaneous streptothricosis is a benign condition but in many tropical countries it can cause marked debilitation of severely affected animals and may prove fatal. The disease in some overseas territories is of considerable economic importance because of its damaging effects on the hides.

There is no doubt that the onset of cutaneous streptothricosis in tropical Africa is closely associated with the rainy season and much significance has been attached to the higher incidence and greater activity of biting-flies and ticks during the wet months of the year. The damage caused to the skin by prolonged wetting is doubly important since the moist spongy nature of the keratinized epithelium probably facilitates the introduction of the organisms by biting insects, provides a suitable substrate for their development and greatly assists the spread of the motile zoospores to adjacent hitherto uninfected parts of the body. Although several workers have postulated a relationship between the onset of streptothricosis and the presence of tick-bites or scratches from thorns, others have pointed out that the injuries thus inflicted are not related to the triangular area of the back which they believe to be the main site of the primary lesions of strepto-

thricosis. Instead, they consider that there is a very close relationship between the early lesions of streptothricosis and the areas favoured for attack, the hump and saddle, by small blood-sucking flies of the genus *Siphona* (*Lyperosia*) which make their appearance in very large numbers with the onset of the rains. The species mostly involved are *S.minuta* and, occasionally, *S.thirouxi*. They also stress that the triangular area on the back is one of the few parts of the body beyond the reach of the animal's tail, horns or tongue. An additional feature of considerable epidemiological importance is the marked resistance of the causative organism to drying and its ability to survive for long periods in the hair and hides, on dried crusts and, possibly, the soil.

Lumpy-wool of sheep

Mycotic dermatitis or lumpy-wool of sheep was first described in South Africa in 1928, and in the following year it was reported from Australia. Other disease conditions of sheep with which *Dermatophilus* is associated include an inflammatory swelling of the feet and lower limbs, known in Scotland as Strawberry foot-rot, and lesions of the hairy parts of the face and scrotum of sheep in Scotland and Kenya.

The distribution of the lesions of lumpy-wool is very variable but is mostly confined to the wool-covered skin of the dorsal part of the body, especially the lumbar region and flanks, as well as the brisket of tups. Lesions are occasionally present on the hairy-parts of the face, ears, scrotum and legs. The earliest signs of infection are small localised areas of hyperaemia which may persist for 7–14 days, followed by papule formation and exudation leading to the development of heaped up scabs about 0·5 cm in diameter. In chronic infections the dried exudates bind bundles of wool fibres together giving them a golden-yellow to brown colour. Matting of the wool fibres sometimes extends a long way up the fleece depending upon the age of the lesion. The clinical disease may persist for 1–3 weeks in sheep in the U.K. and for 2–3 months in Africa but a proportion of the flock may be affected indefinitely. The disease is of economic importance because affected fleeces are usually down-graded and lose a considerable part of their value.

Little is known about the epidemiology of lumpy-wool disease but it is generally agreed that there is a close relationship between the appearance of the disease and the onset of mild wet weather. The source of the infection and the means by which it is transmitted under natural conditions is not understood.

Strawberry foot-rot

Strawberry foot-rot was described in sheep in

North-East Scotland in 1946. Affected animals show numerous small, heaped scabs on the skin of the leg between the coronet and hock or elbow. Removal of the scabs reveals a raw surface with numerous bleeding points giving a superficial resemblance to a strawberry. Although a Gram-positive branching filamentous organism called *Rhizobium* species and, later, *Polysepta pedis* has been isolated from typical cases of strawberry foot-rot, most microbiologists prefer to classify it in the genus *Dermatophilus* of the recently created family *Dermatophilaceae*. On the other hand, not all workers are agreed that the agents of cutaneous streptothricosis (*D. congolensis*), lumpy wool (*D. dermatonomus*) and strawberry foot-rot (*D. pedis*) are each worthy of specific rank, and recent biological and biochemical studies suggest that they are all strains of the single species. *D. congolensis*.

Laboratory diagnosis

Examination of stained smears of scabs from lesions in all three diseases reveals the presence of short lengths of strongly Gram-positive branching filaments and clusters of numerous coccal forms resembling staphylococci (Plate 29.1b, facing p. 294). Smears prepared from the moist areas after removal of the scab generally contain abundant hyphae, coccoid zoospores, epithelial cells and leucocytes. Such lesions are particularly suitable for isolation techniques. In sections, the organisms are widely distributed in the superficial sero-fibrinous areas of the epithelium and are most clearly demonstrated by Gram or Claudius' staining methods (Plate 29.1d).

Despite the abundance of hyphal and coccal forms in the acute lesions, *Dermatophilus* may be difficult to isolate if bacterial contamination is severe. The method recommended by some workers is to soak small fragments from the underside of a scab in a small amount of sterile distilled water, and leave for 2–4 hours at 30–35°C in an atmosphere of air plus 10 per cent CO_2 (e.g. in a candle jar) to allow liberation of the motile zoospores. A small loopful from the surface of the water, containing the zoospores, is then inoculated on to blood agar plates which are incubated overnight at 37°C. However, a simpler and more reliable method is to macerate finely the crust material with the edge of a dry glass slide, shake off the gross particles and lightly scatter the powdery material from the end of the slide, by scraping it with a scalpel blade, over the surface of a number of blood agar plates which are incubated for 24 hours at 37°C in 10 per cent CO_2. The use of a hand lens greatly facilitates identification and, with care, a number of tiny adherent waxy,

domed colonies can be removed by means of a sterile wire and subcultured in broth or enriched agar media. In glucose or serum broth, small fluffy spherical colonies form at the bottom of the medium or attach to the walls of the container. (Plate 29.2a, between pp. 294–5). The media remains clear or slightly turbid. Stained smears of fluid cultures show that the organism consists of Gram-positive branching filaments (3–5 µm in diameter) which divide transversely into numerous narrow segments and then two to three times longitudinally, producing rows of up to eight cells across. These cells ultimately round off and are released as motile zoospores with four to six long polar flagellae. On solid media, such as blood agar, raised wax-like yellow or orange coloured colonies develop which assume a dry, rough uneven appearance when subcultivated (Plates 29.2b–c & 29.3a–b, between pp. 294–5). The colonies may or may not be surrounded by a narrow zone of complete lysis and sheep strains grown on ruminant blood agar plates usually produce an enhanced haemolytic effect in association with *Streptococcus agalactiae* or *Corynebacterium equi*, but not with *C. ovis* (Plate 29.4, facing p. 295).

Dermatophilus is susceptible to penicillin and many other antibiotic and antiseptic agents. Most strains are also sensitive to bacteriocin-like substances formed by many skin staphylococci. The biochemical characteristics of *Dermatophilus* are not well defined but, in general, most strains give the following reactions irrespective of the host species from which they are isolated. Acid production, without gas, is obtained with glucose, maltose, trehalose, dextrin, mannose and laevulose, but not with lactose, mannitol, dulcitol, inositol and galactose. Casein, urea and gelatin are hydrolysed, catalase is formed, but negative reactions are obtained with the nitrate reduction, methylene blue, MR-VP and indole tests.

Treatment

Numerous unsuccessful attempts have been made to find an effective method of treatment for mycotic dermatitis of cattle and sheep, but when recovery occurs it is mostly spontaneous and is invariably associated with a spell of drier weather. External treatments including the use of arsenicals, copper sulphate, quaternary ammonium compounds, and formalin have no curative value because the majority of hyphae are inaccessible in the follicle sheaths. Although a number of persistent infections have been effectively cured with large doses of streptomycin combined with penicillin, and even by intravenous iodide therapy, these methods are generally impracticable in large flocks and herds.

CHAPTER 30

Phycomycetes

The *Phycomycetes* are characterized by non-septate (coenocytic) hyphae, asexual spores (sporangiospores) produced in unlimited numbers within a thin-walled sporangium, and sexual zygospores and oospores. (Plates 30.1a–b, facing p. 302) Members of the group are ubiquitous saprophytes, (e.g. bread mould), but a few are believed to be associated with disease conditions of animals. In the veterinary field two sub-classes of Phycomycetes, the *Zygomycetes* and *Oomycetes*, are considered to be of some importance.

Zygomycetes includes the family *Mucoraceae* which is characterized by sexual zygospores and sporangia bearing a clearly defined columella, and includes three important species *Mucor*, *Absidia* and *Rhizopus*. One essential difference between these three genera is that species of *Mucor* do not possess root-like rhizoids in the pseudomycelium. In *Rhizopus*, rhizoids are found directly opposite the base of the aerial sporangiophores whereas in *Absidia* they are found opposite but between the sporangiophores (Fig. 28.4). The second sub-class of *Phycomycetes* is termed *Oomycetes*, and includes the genus *Saprolegnia*. Members of this genus are characterized by the formation of sexual spores (oospores), within an oosphere, and elongated club-shaped (clavate) sporangia opening by a single pore at the tip or side.

Mucormycosis
Although the term mucormycosis should be restricted to mycoses caused by species of *Mucor* it is still generally used for infections associated with any member of the family *Mucoraceae*, be they species of *Mucor*, *Rhizopus* or *Absidia*. The organs most frequently affected are the lymph nodes and alimentary tract and the infections, which are often of a granulomatous or ulcerative character, may become generalized with fatal consequences.

The natural hosts are man and many species of domestic animals including horses, cattle, pigs, dogs, cats, rodents and birds. Susceptible animal hosts probably acquire the infection by inhaling or ingesting spores from heavily contaminated soil, manure, fruit or mouldy hay and straw. There is good evidence that chronic debilitating conditions may predispose to this type of infection and in human patients mucormycosis is frequently associated with diabetes mellitus or leukaemia. In diabetics, mucormycosis may give rise to meningoencephalitis or acute bronchial or lobar pneumonia frequently terminating in death after a brief illness of 2–10 days. Cases of ocular mucormycosis and ulcerative colitis have occasionally been described in non-diabetic patients also, and superficial skin lesions infected with *Mucor* have been described in otomycosis.

In animals, mucoraceous fungi may be associated with respiratory infections of birds and sheep and with placental lesions of cattle. *Absidia spp.*, including *A. corymbifera* and *A. ramosa*, cause a pseudotuberculosis-like disease of guinea-pigs and have also been observed in cases of ulcerative colitis and generalized granulomatous conditions of swine, placental lesions of cattle, and nasal lesions in horses. Species of *Rhizopus* have been reported in placental tissues of cattle and swine. Members of all three genera have been isolated from external otitis of dogs.

Unfortunately, symptoms of mucormycosis are seldom seen until there is general debility or the animal dies, when the lesions may be observed during post-mortem examination. It is equally unfortunate that fungal infections are usually not suspected until histopathological investigations reveal the presence of numerous coenocytic hyphal elements throughout the affected tissues (Plates 30.1c and 30.1d, facing p. 302), by which time the tissues have been processed in fixatives and fresh material is no longer available for cultural examination. The distribution of the granulomatous lesions may be localized or generalised and in cattle, swine and guinea-pigs lesions have been observed in the liver, spleen, lungs and kidneys as well as in most of the carcase lymph nodes. The ulcerative type of lesion is usually confined to the alimentary tract especially in younger animals.

Because of their ubiquitous nature, it is often very difficult to assess the pathogenic significance of a particular isolate but in recent years there is strong circumstantial evidence to suggest that mucors are responsible for placentitis and abortion in cattle. Aborted calves generally show a number of superficial skin lesions heavily infected with fungi while examination of wet impression smears of the stomach contents usually reveals considerable numbers of coenocytic hyphal elements.

In aquaria, species of *Saprolegnia* may invade the epidermal tissues of fish causing severe lesions with fuzzy outgrowths on the head and gills, and occasionally on the body and tail. In cases of ulcerative dermal necrosis of salmon, secondary skin lesions caused by *Saprolegnia* are frequently seen on the head and other parts of the body.

A provisional diagnosis of mucormycosis may be possible by demonstration of coenocytic hyphae in wet impressions of fetal calf stomach contents, skin or bowel scrapings and in stained sections of affected organs. For confirmatory diagnosis the fungus must be isolated and identified by its morphological characteristics (Chapter 28).

There is no specific treatment but systemic potassium iodide may be attempted.

CHAPTER 31

Ascomycetes

The *Ascomycetes* are characterized by septate mycelia, the formation of sexual spores (ascospores) within a sac (ascus) several of which are usually enclosed in a fruiting body called an ascocarp. In addition to the sexual phase typified by the ascospore, many of the *Ascomycetes* produce numerous asexual spores (conidiospores or conidia) from specialized aerial hyphal branches (conidiophores). In *Aspergillus* the conidiophores terminate in a vesicle with one or more rows of sterigmata from which the conidia are formed (Fig. 28.6 and Plate 31.2a. between pp. 302–3).

The *Ascomycetes* are a very large group of fungi most of which are non-pathogenic although a number are frequently present as contaminants of various disease processes in man and animals. Notable exceptions are certain species of *Aspergillus*, e.g. *A. fumigatus* which can cause severe respiratory disease in a variety of hosts, and the food poisoning moulds such as *Claviceps purpurea* of ergot of rye.

Aspergillosis

Most species of *Aspergillus* are common and ubiquitous saprophytic moulds of dust, soil and rotting plant or animal matter. Some are also abundant on hay, straw and grain which have become heated during storage and are frequently present in the air. Together with *Penicillium* and *Mucor* they are the most frequent contaminants of laboratories. At least one member of the group, *Aspergillus fumigatus*, can give rise to mycoses of the respiratory tracts of animals and birds, but especially of very young domesticated chickens and water fowl. Adult aquatic birds such as penguins in zoological gardens are particularly prone to the infection during the early weeks of captivity. Man is also susceptible and pulmonary aspergillosis is an occupational disease of agricultural workers and others who are often exposed to high concentrations of spores. In other circumstances, the role of *Aspergillus* in human infections is mainly of a

secondary nature and fungal growth is not infrequently observed in pulmonary lesions caused by malignant growths or tuberculosis. Secondary infections also occur after prolonged antibiotic or corticosteroid therapy and after transplant and open heart surgery. Apart from pulmonary conditions, *Aspergillus* species may be associated with lesions in the skin, external ear, nasal sinuses and, occasionally, in the bones and meninges: but the ears and nails are probably the commonest sites of infection. Allergies associated with inhalation of spores have frequently been reported in human patients, while toxicosis of animals due to ingestion of food contaminated by toxic fungal metabolites have given rise to severe economic losses.

Whatever may be the pathogenic status of *Aspergillus* for human subjects there can be no doubt that *A. fumigatus* and some other members of the genus are responsible for a number of severe infections of domestic animals. These include bovine mycotic abortion, equine guttural-pouch mycosis and other respiratory disorders. Of these, avian aspergillosis is undoubtedly the most important as well as being the most prevalent.

Avian aspergillosis

Avian aspergillosis occurs in all parts of the world but Australia and many tropical countries are relatively free from the disease. Birds of almost all species and ages may be affected and the commonest route of infection is probably by inhalation.

In the acute form of aspergillosis, such as brooder pneumonia, many of the affected chicks die suddenly within the first 24–48 hours of the disease. The symptoms, if present, are generally those of anorexia, listlessness, high temperature, increased respirations, diarrhoea and sometimes convulsions. The clinical picture and post-mortem findings of brooder pneumonia are similar to those of pullorum disease (bacillary white diarrhoea). At autopsy many of the carcases show a number of small, discrete, miliary-type, yellow-white granulomata scattered throughout the lungs, similar to those found in pullorum disease. Characteristically, the air sacs are involved and small firm nodules are invariably present attached to the membranous lining of the anterior thoracic sacs. These are largely composed of tightly packed masses of hyphae and spores. (Plates 31.1b & d, between pp. 302–3) In older birds the lesions vary in size from a pin-head up to that of a pea, while in the more chronic form in adults the fungus tends to grow on the mucous membranes of the bronchi and air sacs, often completely filling the cavities with a dense dark-green fluffy mass of hyphae and spores. In some birds the radiating hyphae in chronically infected air sacs give rise to the formation of a fatty or caseous-type exudate which fills the cavity in the manner of a plaster-cast. In many birds the infection becomes generalized and lesions may be found in the liver, spleen, kidneys, muscles and brain.

An accurate diagnosis of aspergillosis is virtually impossible while the patient is alive, whereas at autopsy the history of the outbreak together with the appearance and distribution of the lesions, the presence of septate hyphae in stained sections of affected tissues and the appearance of the characteristic fungal structures in direct wet impression smears and in cultures of fungal isolates, usually enables a confirmatory diagnosis to be made (Plates 31.1a & c, between pp. 302–3).

The cultural characters of *Aspergillus* can be conveniently studied on blood agar or most types of mycological media after incubation at 25–37°C. The colonies develop quickly and appear first as white, fluffy, low filamentous growths, later becoming granular as the colony spreads across the medium, and the colour changes to dark green as the conidia are produced. It is stressed, however, that *Aspergillus*, of which there are more than 200 species, are common laboratory contaminants and accurate identification of *A. fumigatus* is often difficult. (Plates 31.2b–f between pp. 302–3) Despite the fact that the genus *Aspergillus* belongs to the family of *Ascomycetes* a number of species including *A. fumigatus* and *A. niger* have not been shown to form a perithecium (flask-shaped ascocarp with a pore) with asci containing ascospores, whereas others such as *A. nidulans* and *A. glaucus* do have this method of forming sexual spores. Moreover, *A. fumigatus* and *A. glaucus* form only one row of goblet-shaped sterigmata whereas *A. niger* and *A. nidulans* produce two rows. There are many other distinguishing features of the aspergilli but for accurate species identification it is often necessary to enlist the help of a reference laboratory.

Penicillium species are readily distinguished from aspergilli by the fact that they do not form conidiophore vesicles and their conidia-bearing sterigmata arise from finger-like branching processes of the conidiophores.

Bovine mycotic abortion

In recent years, about twenty species of moulds including *A. fumigatus* and other aspergilli, *Mucor*, *Absidia*, *Rhizopus* and *Penicillium* have been found associated with a placentitis of cattle. The infection is characterized by gross thickening and focal necrosis of the affected cotyledons and a number of large, circular lesions are sometimes present on the skin of the fetus. Abortions usually occur during the second half of pregnancy. The disease can be readily diagnosed by the demonstration of hyphal elements in wet impression smears of the stomach contents mounted in lactophenol cotton blue. The fungus can also be isolated from the stomach contents.

Little is known about the pathogenesis of mycotic abortion but it is generally considered that the most likely source of infection is mouldy hay and straw, and that the animal probably becomes infected by inhalation of the spores. It is also possible that infection of the placenta results from haematogenous spread from the primary lesion in the lungs.

Most cases of mycotic abortion seem to occur when the cattle are housed during the winter monhts especially in those years when there has been a wet harvest. Recent evidence suggests that infected cattle do not show clinical symptoms before the abortions occur and that the infection does not persist in the uterus thereafter.

Other conditions

Aspergillosis in adult cattle usually gives rise to numerous small encapsulated lesions in the affected lungs, but in cattle and especially calves and lambs exposed to heavy aerosols of spores from mouldy hay and straw, a more acute infection may occur in which there are a large number of yellow-white miliary nodules. In horses, the proximity of the guttural pouch to the carotid vessels and glossopharyngeal and vagus nerves is probably responsible for the symptoms of epistaxis or pharyngeal paralysis which are often characteristic of mycotic infection. Most fungi grow well in eggs and there are reports, the first being from Italy in 1729, of green-mould of eggs which is probably due to *Aspergillus*.

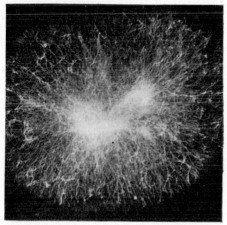

30.1a

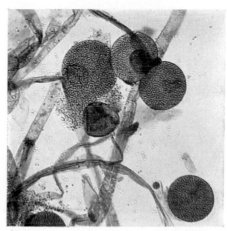

30.1b

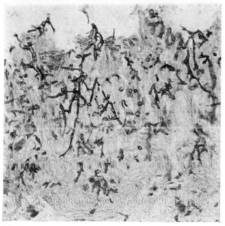

30.1c

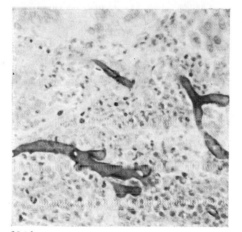

30.1d

30.1a   Young culture of *Mucor spp*. The aerial mycelium is characteristically white and fluffy.

30.1c   Section through the intestinal wall of a scouring piglet showing numerous branching coenocytic hyphae of *Rhizopus*, × 106.

30.1b   Portion of a slide culture of *Mucor* mounted in lactophenol cotton blue. The coenocytic sporangiophore bears a large sporangium and rupture of its wall releases the asexual sporangiospores, × 106.

30.1d   The same as Plate 30.1c viewed at higher magnification, × 350.

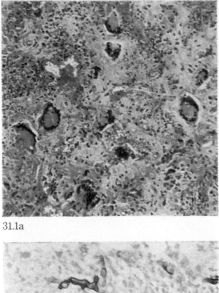

31.1a

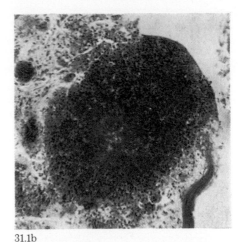

31.1b

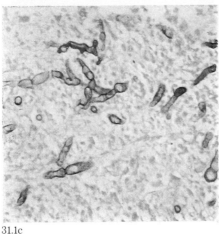

31.1c

31.1d

31.1a Section through a granulomatous lesion in the liver of a calf affected with aspergillosis, showing 'giant-cells' and a few hyphal elements. Haematoxylin eosin stain, × 130.

31.1c Section through a large tumour-like mass in the wall of the small intestine of an adult pig. The septate hyphae were identified in culture as those of *Aspergillus fumigatus*. Periodic acid-Schiff stain, × 280.

31.1b Section through a nodule in the lung of a penguin dying from pulmonary aspergillosis. The central pale area of necrosis contains numerous branching hyphal elements of *A. fumigatus*. Haematoxylin eosin stain, × 133.

31.1d Section prepared from a small nodular lesion in the lung of a penguin dying from pulmonary aspergillosis, showing branching hyphal elements of the causative fungus. Periodic acid-Schiff stain, × 170.

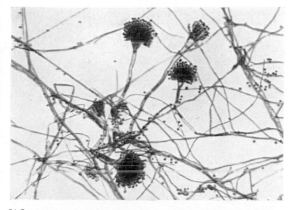

31.2a

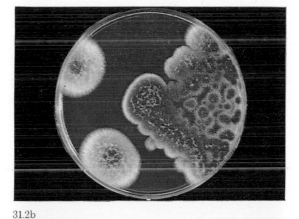

31.2b

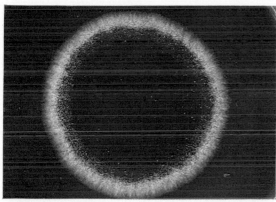

31.2c

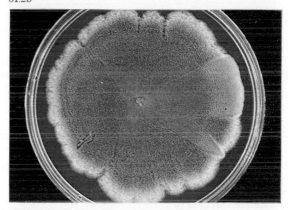

31.2d

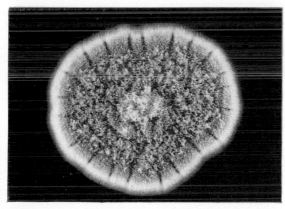

31.2e

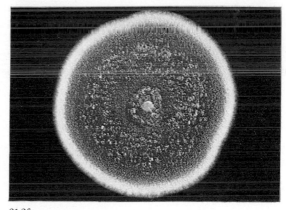

31.2f

31.2a Slide culture of *Aspergillus spp.* mounted in lactophenol cotton blue, showing specialised septate hyphae (conidiophores) each bearing an expanded conidiophore vesicle on which asexual spores (conidia) are produced externally, ×230.

31.2c Colony of *Aspergillus niger* after 5 days' incubation. The older central area contains deeply pigmented conidia and is surrounded by a pale peripheral zone of younger undifferentiated mycelium.

31.2b Typical growth of *Aspergillus fumigatus* on Sabouraud's maltose agar, showing grey-green pigmentation.

31.2d-f Single colonies of three species of *Penicillium* growing on the surface of Sabouraud's maltose agar.

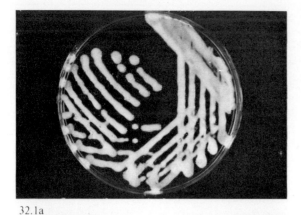

32.1a

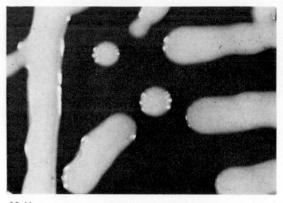

32.1b

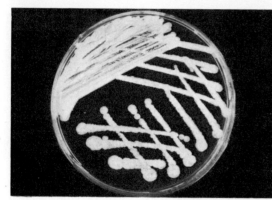

32.1c

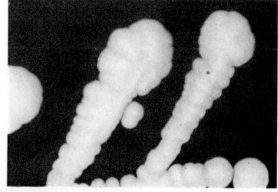

32.1d

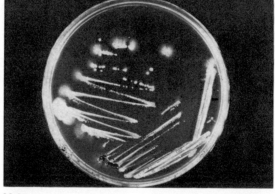

32.1e

32.1a   Colony development of *Cryptococcus neoformans* on Sabouraud's glucose agar after 4 days' incubation at 37°C.

32.1b   A detail from Plate 32.1a. The surface growth of *C. neoformans* is mucoid and cream to light brown in colour.

32.1c   Culture of *Candida albicans* on Sabouraud's agar after 7 days' incubation at 37°C.

32.1d   A detail from Plate 32.1c, showing the characteristic creamy type of growth.

32.1e   Culture of *Candida tropicalis*. Some of the surface colonies are surrounded by a mycelial fringe.

CHAPTER 32

Fungi imperfecti

Included in the *Fungi imperfecti* are those organisms which do not have a sexual stage of development and cannot be placed among the previously described classes. The group is a large one and includes a wide variety of fungi ranging from the yeasts and yeast-like organisms such as *Cryptococcus* and *Candida* to the dimorphic species, e.g. *Blastomyces*, *Histoplasma*, *Sporotrichum* and *Coccidiodes*, and the dermatophytes or ringworm group, including *Microsporum*, *Epidermophyton* and *Trichophyton*. From time to time a perfect or sexual stage is discovered in fungi hitherto believed to be capable of producing only asexual spores and these species are generally removed from the 'fungi imperfecti' and reclassified in the *Ascomycetes*.

YEASTS AND YEAST-LIKE ORGANISMS

Cryptococcaceae

The yeasts are a large group of organisms with forms related to all three of the main classes of fungi. Their natural habitat is probably the soil and some are plant pathogens whereas others are important causes of diseases of man and animals. The yeasts are mostly unicellular organisms which reproduce vegetatively by a process of budding and the spore which develops from the 'mother cell' is termed a blastospore. Some produce a mycelium or pseudomycelium whilst a few form arthrospores and, occasionally, thick-walled spores known as chlamydospores.

It is emphasised that not all yeasts are classified in the *Fungi imperfecti* and some, such as brewer's yeasts (*Saccharomyces cerevisiae*) of the family *Endomycetaceae*, reproduce sexually by the formation of ascospores, 1–8 per ascus, and are included in the *Ascomycetes*. A second group of yeasts produce aerial spores called ballistospores which are forcibly projected into the air and include many of the pink yeasts, e.g. *Sporoblastomyces roseus*. A third and important group are the 'imperfect'

yeasts which have neither ascospores nor ballistospores but reproduce vegetatively. One of the families, *Cryptococcaceae*, contains many pathogenic forms including *Cryptococcus neoformans* and *Candida* (*Monilia*) *albicans*. The division of the family into genera is largely based on the morphology of the asexual spores and on the presence or absence of a mycelial or pseudomycelial growth. Most of the species are distinguished, like bacteria, by the fermentation of sugars and other biochemical characters.

Cryptococcus

Cryptococcosis, sometimes called European blastomycosis or torulosis is a sporadic, non-contagious, chronic, commonly fatal systemic infection which may involve the lungs, skin or other parts of the body but has a marked predilection for the brain and meninges. The disease affects man, monkey, horse, ox, pig, dog, cat, cheetah, and ferret; and is world-wide in its distribution. The causative organism, *Cryptococcus neoformans*, has been isolated as a saprophyte from soil, fruit and milk but the most common source of the fungus is believed to be old accumulations of pigeon droppings. Recently, *C. neoformans* has been isolated from the intestinal contents of pigeons but it does not appear to multiply within the pigeon because of its high body temperature.

In man, *C. neoformans* may initiate a primary pulmonary infection which spreads haematogenously to involve a wide variety of organs and tissues. The most common clinical manifestation of cryptococcosis is a slowly developing meningitis which may extend over many years, often with long remissions, but ultimately proving fatal in all untreated cases.

C. neoformans has been isolated from myxoma-like lesions in the lungs and nasal passages of horses showing persistent respiratory symptoms and nasal discharge, as well as from a lesion on the lips. In cattle, there are several reports of cryptococcal mastitis and in one outbreak no fewer than 106 of

235 cows became infected in one herd during a 12-months period. The first signs of infection are severe swelling and firmness of the udder and enlargement of the regional lymph nodes. In most cases, the milk yield is markedly reduced and the milk is visibly abnormal. Generalised infections are rare but metastasis to the lungs has occasionally been reported following accidental infection of the udder via the teat canal. In dogs, cryptococcosis usually involves the central nervous system causing incoordination, hyperaesthesia and nasal discharge. Oral and cutaneous lesions are also frequently reported and subcutaneous granulomas have been described around the ears, face and feet. In cats, particularly older cats, cryptococcosis is usually associated with a chronic nasal and ocular discharge. Proliferative lesions have been observed in the nose, lungs and central nervous system and granulomas have been described in the lungs. Extension of the infection from the nasal cavity to the optic nerves frequently results in blindness.

Diagnosis is made by demonstrating the presence of *C. neoformans* in wet mounts of suspected exudates, secretions, spinal fluid or tissues from lesions. Direct microscopical examination of specimens mounted in undiluted Giemsa's stain or India ink under a cover glass shows *C. neoformans* as a large (5–20 µm in diameter) spherical, thick-walled, single-budding yeast surrounded by a wide, refractile, gelatinous capsule. A definitive diagnosis is obtained by immunofluorescence, cultural and biological tests. Primary isolates grow well on Sabouraud's glucose agar, malt agar, blood agar or other laboratory media at 22°–37°C (Plate 32.1a facing p. 303). In young cultures the surface growth is white or cream-coloured but later it becomes pale brown, mucoid and runs down slope cultures to collect at the bottom of the tube (Plate 32.1b, facing p. 303). It lacks the ability to ferment sugars and it differs from other yeast-like fungi in being urea-positive. It also differs from other fungi producing yeast-like cells in affected tissues, (e.g. *Blastomyces dermatitidis* and *B. brasiliensis*) by its single bud, its wide transparent capsule and its failure to produce a mould-like growth at room temperature. It is the only member of the genus that is pathogenic for mice. Following intraperitoneal or intracerebral inoculation, budding, encapsulated yeasts are clearly visible in wet-mount preparations of gelatinous abdominal masses, lungs and brain. Fatal infections are usually produced in pigeons and chick embryos by intracerebral and intravenous inoculation, respectively.

Most antimicrobial substances are ineffective in spontaneous cases of cryptococcosis but amphotericin B (100 mg/day), although toxic, has cured a small number of human infections.

Pityrosporum

The sub-family *Cryptococcidae* includes the genus *Pityrosporum* of which the type species is *P. ovale*. These are Gram-positive oval or flask-shaped, non-mycelial asporogenous yeasts without fermentative ability, first described in 1873 in a case of psoriasis in man. In 1952, the genus was redefined to include two species, *P. ovale* and *P. pachydermatis*, together with two candidate members *P. orbiculare* and *P. canis*.

P. ovale, the 'bottle-bacillus', is most commonly found associated with dandruff scales and is believed to be a contributory cause of seborrhoeic dermatitis and other disorders of the human skin. In animals, *P. pachydermatis* has been observed in skin lesions in the rhinoceros, in ulcers of the conjunctiva of dogs and in healthy and diseased external ears of dogs and cats. The pathogenic role of *Pityrosporum* species in these conditions is not well understood but most workers believe that their status is usually that of a highly specialised saprophyte.

Films prepared from affected canine tissues and stained by Gram's method show the yeasts as positively staining oval or flask-shaped, double-contoured, budding cells approximately 2–3 × 4–8 µm. The single blastospore develops on a broad base at one end of the mother cell. Following the release of the fully mature blastospore many of the yeast bodies show small lateral projections immediately below the transverse septum, resembling a protoplasmic collar of residual 'scar' tissue (Fig. 28.8 and Plates 32.2a & c facing p. 310).

Compared with other members of the genus, *P. canis* grows well on blood agar, malt agar and on various other fluid and solid media without added oleic acid or olive oil. Primary cultures on 10 per cent. horse blood agar develop tiny, raised, non-haemolytic surface colonies within 48 hours of incubation at 37°C. On Sabouraud's glucose agar and malt agar a relatively heavy growth is obtained within 48 hours of small, circular, domed, white or buff colonies which reach full size (2–3 mm) by the 5th day (Plates 32.2b & d, facing p. 310). Later, the colonies become dry and brittle, whilst the surface resembles frosted glass and acquires a dimpled appearance not unlike the skin of an orange. In glucose broth, most strains grow poorly but invariably form a characteristic, fine, lace-like, flaky growth on the surface of the medium which settles to the foot of the tube with gentle agitation leaving the supernatant clear. Good growth occurs on Dorset's egg media and all strains hydrolyse urea within 7 days.

Fluid carbohydrate media are not fermented and all strains produce pale pink or orange-coloured colonies on MacConkey's lactose bile salt medium. On most solid media growth of *P. canis* is enhanced

TABLE 32.1. Characteristics of *Pityrosporum* species.

Character	P. ovale	P. orbiculare	P. pachydermatis	P. canis
Host	Man	Man	Rhinoceros	Dog
Commonest site	Scalp and skin lesions	Shoulder, upper trunk and arms	Skin lesions	External ear
Cell shape	Oval	Spherical	Egg-shaped	Oval
Size (μm)	2–3 x 4–6	2–5	2–3 x 3–5	2–3 x 4–8
Budding	Broad base	Narrow base	Broad base	Broad base
Cultivation	Difficult	Difficult	Difficult to maintain	Easy
Substances required for growth	Oleic acid	Olive oil and fats	Not known	None
Colony	Buff, domed 2 mm diameter	Buff, domed 2 mm diameter	Cream to yellow. Doughy consistency. Smooth surface	Dry, frosted glass, dimpled surface. Domed 2–3 mm diameter

in the vicinity of a horizontal streak culture of staphylococcus.

Cultures applied to the scarified skin surface of mice, rabbits and guinea-pigs or inoculated into mice intravenously do not produce any reaction.

The principal characteristics of the *Pityrosporum* group are summarised in Table 32.1.

Monilia (Candida)

One order of the *Fungi imperfecti*, the *Moniliales*, is divided into four families but only one of these, the *Moniliaceae*, is of importance in veterinary mycology, and includes the genus *Monilia* or *Candida*. The more important species belonging to this genus are *C. albicans*, *C. parapsilosis*, *C. tropicalis*, *C. krusei* and *C. stellatoidea*.

Unlike the true yeasts of *Cryptococcus*, members of the genus *Candida* have a slightly more complex type of development. They are readily grown on conventional bacteriological media at 25–37°C and produce smooth, creamy, bacteria-like surface colonies that become furrowed and roughened after prolonged incubation (Plates 32.1c–e, facing p. 303). The vegetative portion, however, contains elongated buds that penetrate the depths of the media but remain attached to the parent cells. After repeated subdivisions the elongated buds produce chains of attached cells known as pseudohyphae. Buds are produced which serve as spores at the points of constriction of the cells of the pseudohyphae. One member of the group, *C. albicans*, produces characteristic thick-walled resting spores (chlamydospores) on the pseudohyphae, when cultivated on nutritionally poor media (e.g. corn-meal agar). This feature readily distinguishes *C. albicans* from all other candidae.

Candidiasis

Candidiasis (moniliasis) is an acute, subacute or chronic infection caused by *C. albicans* which occurs in small numbers saprophytically on the mucous membranes of the respiratory, gastrointestinal and urinogenital tracts of many healthy humans and animals. Although they are usually non-pathogenic in healthy individuals, they may become invasive and behave as opportunistic virulent pathogens in patients suffering from a variety of unrelated disorders such as malignant disease and nutritional deficiencies or in those treated intensively with antibiotics.

In man, *C. albicans* causes superficial infections of the skin (cutaneous candidiasis) and mucous membranes (oral and vaginal 'thrush'). Oral candidiasis mostly occurs in patients in the terminal stages of a wasting disease or in babies during the first few days of life following infection during birth. Vaginal candidiasis occurs particularly during pregnancy and in diabetes. Weakening of the body defence mechanisms may also give rise to bronchopulmonary infections, secondary intestinal infections and, less frequently, meningitis, endocarditis and pyelonephritis. Infection may involve the nails and lead to chronic paronychia and onychia.

Data regarding candidiasis in animals other than birds are scanty and generally unsatisfactory, but there are a number of reliable reports of the disease in pigs, dogs, cattle and various rodents. On the other hand, avian candidiasis is of particular importance and the veterinary literature contains several detailed accounts of the naturally occurring disease in fowls, turkeys, ducks, geese, guinea-fowl and pigeons.

Avian candidiasis (moniliasis or 'thrush')

Although moniliasis had been described in fowls (1912) and geese (1921) in Germany, the first major epidemic of avian moniliasis was reported from the U.S.A. in 1932, in a flock of young turkeys, and in the following year losses of 10 000 chicks were recorded in a commercial hatchery. Since then, severe outbreaks associated with high mortality have been recorded in many other countries of the world including the U.K.

In affected birds characteristic lesions develop in the upper alimentary tract, particularly on the inner lining of the crop. In acute cases they appear as tiny, discrete yellow-white or grey-white pustules loosely adherent to the mucous membrane, whereas in chronic infections the crop wall may be thickened and covered by a corrugated false membrane of yellowish-grey necrotic material resembling 'turkish-towelling'. Necrotic exudate may occur in the gizzard and intestines whilst abscesses or miliary nodules may be present in the lungs and liver. The necrotic tissue consists of proliferating stratum

consisting of Gram-positive budding yeast-like bodies. Agar-slope cultures clearly show the pseudohyphae extending downwards into the medium. *C. albicans* can be identified by the formation of chlamydospores on 'corn-meal' agar and by various biochemical tests (Table 32.2). For example, it assimilates glucose, maltose, sucrose and galactose, produces acid with abundant gas in glucose, maltose and galactose but does not utilise citrate as a sole source of energy. It is highly pathogenic when inoculated into rabbits and mice by the intravenous route and produces lesions in the kidneys, liver and spleen (Plate 32.3, between pp. 310–11).

Other disease conditions
C. albicans and some other species of candidae have been responsible for stomatitis and gastric ulcers in pigs during antibiotic supplement feeding, in

TABLE 32.2. Differential characters of *Candida* species.

	C. albicans	C. tropicalis	C. pseudo-tropicalis	C. krusei	C. parapsilosis	C. stellatoides
*Glucose	AG	AG	AG	AG	AG/A	AG
Maltose	AG	AG	—	—	—	AG
Sucrose	A	AG	AG	—	—	—
Lactose	—	—	AG	—	—	—
Chlamydospores on corn meal agar	+	—	—	—	—	—
Colonies on blood agar after 10 days at 37°C.	Medium, dull grey, circular, smooth	Large, grey, surrounded by mycelial fringe	Small	Small, round or irregular, flat or heaped	Small, brilliant white	Star-shaped
Growth on Sabouraud's agar after 48 hrs. at 37°C.	Creamy	Variable	Variable	Flat-dry	Creamy	Creamy
Surface growth in Sabouraud's broth after 48 hrs. at 37°C.	None	Narrow film with no bubbles	None	Thick film	None	None

*Production of acid (A) and gas (G) after 48 hours at 37°C in broth with 2 per cent carbohydrate (sugar).

corneum cells together with large numbers of hyphal elements and yeast bodies. The underlying tissue is usually smooth, reddened and inflamed. Moniliasis generally occurs in young birds and the acute form of the disease is characterized by rapid deaths and high mortality. There are no characteristic symptoms, however, and a definitive diagnosis is usually based on the post-mortem findings.

The causative organism, *C. albicans*, can be readily isolated on malt agar or blood agar with or without added antibiotics, or via Raulin's medium. Surface growth appears within 24 hours of incubation as soft, white or cream-coloured colonies

long-standing cases of canine external otitis and in bovine mastitis, particularly after prolonged antibiotic therapy. Other diseases include oral thrush in young animals, rumenitis of cattle and bovine mycotic abortion.

No satisfactory treatment is known but the addition of nystatin to the drinking water (150 000 units/gallon) was successful in curing an outbreak of candidiasis in partridges. Nystatin, or 1 per cent crystal violet, may be applied locally to accessible lesions and oral amphotericin B and iodides have been used successfully in the treatment of severe visceral infections in human patients.

CHAPTER 33

Pathogenic dimorphic fungi

Some half-dozen important systemic mycoses of man and animals are caused by certain members of the *Fungi imperfecti*. In the parasitic phase the causative fungi are characterized by the absence of a mycelium and in almost every instance they occur in the affected tissues of the host as single yeast-like cells which multiply by budding. All species can be grown in artificial cultures. At room temperature they produce a mycelial colony whereas at 37°C on suitable media they readily revert to the parasitic phase. This type of fungus is said to be dimorphic or to exhibit dimorphism; and the group includes *Sporotrichum*, *Blastomyces*, *Coccidioides* and *Histoplasma* (Fig. 33.1).

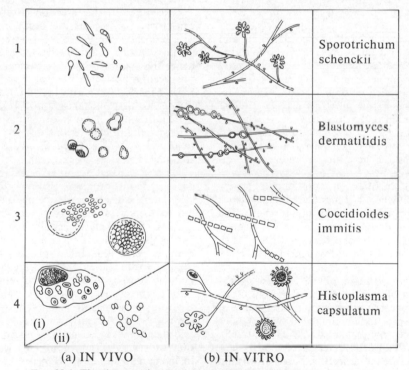

	(a) IN VIVO	(b) IN VITRO	
1			Sporotrichum schenckii
2			Blastomyces dermatitidis
3			Coccidioides immitis
4 (i) (ii)			Histoplasma capsulatum

FIG. 33.1. The tissue and culture phase of some dimorphic fungi.
1. (a) Small cigar-shaped budding yeast cells.
   (b) Clusters of conidia on conidiospores.
2. (a) Single budding yeasts in tissue smear.
   (b) Numerous microconidia and chlamydospores.
3. (a) Spherules: one showing release of endospores.
   (b) Hyphae forming arthrospores.
4. (a) Yeasts (i) within macrophage and (ii) yeasts lying extracellularly.
   (b) Hyphae bearing microconidia and tuberculate chlamydospores.

Sporotrichosis

Sporotrichosis is a chronic, non-contagious granulomatous infection of the skin, lymphatics and, less commonly, the internal organs of animals and man. The causative organism, *Sporotrichum schenckii* is a member of the order *Moniliales* of the *Fungi imperfecti*. The disease in man was first described in the U.S.A. in 1898 and the first account of natural infection of animals was in rats in Brazil in 1907. Since that time sporotrichosis has been confirmed in dogs, horses, donkeys, mules, cattle, camels and poultry but the number of cases is far outnumbered by those in man.

The organism grows saprophytically on many types of decaying plants, on wood and in the soil. The disease occurs most commonly among gardeners and agricultural workers when the fungus is introduced into the skin of the extremities through trauma caused by plant thorns or splinters of wood. The initial lesion begins as a small subcutaneous nodule at the site of injury, gradually enlarges, becomes indurated and breaks down to form an indolent ulcer. The infection spreads to the lymph nodes by way of the lymphatics which become thickened and cord-like. Later, multiple subcutaneous nodules and abscesses are formed along the lymphatics and the lymph nodes which are enlarged, become necrotic and ulcerate. In animals, nodules appear at the site of trauma after an incubation period of 3–12 weeks; the hair over the lesion falls out leaving a moist exudate which eventually dries to form a scab. In horses, the presence of nodules along the thickened lymphatics, which usually ulcerate and discharge pus, closely resembles the condition of epizootic lymphangitis caused by *Histoplasma farciminosum*. Dissemination of the infection to the internal organs is uncommon but when it occurs there is no evidence of ulceration or of lymphatic involvement. The clinical disease in dogs is very similar but involvement of the bones, liver and lungs with fatal consequences is probably more frequent than in other hosts.

The small Gram-positive, spindle- or cigar-shaped yeast-like bodies of *S. schenckii* may be difficult to demonstrate in pus or tissues from affected animals. Pus or other suspect tissue inoculated on to Sabouraud's agar and incubated at 22–28°C usually produces moist, flat, leathery cream-coloured to dark brown colonies within a week but never develop a cottony aerial mycelium. Microscopical examination of the surface growth reveals thin, septate branching hyphae bearing clusters of pear-shaped conidia (2–4 × 2–6 μm) which radiate from the tips of lateral unbranched conidiophores. The parasitic yeast-phase can be induced *in vitro* by growing the organism on brain-heart infusion agar at 37°C. Mice are susceptible to intraperitoneal inoculation and develop peritonitis, or orchitis in males inoculated intratesticularly. Oval or cigar-shaped yeast bodies can generally be demonstrated both extracellularly and intracellularly in macrophages.

Sporotrichosis of animals responds remarkably well to iodide therapy. Potassium iodide may be administered orally or sodium iodide intravenously to the point of producing symptoms of iodism.

Blastomycosis

This is a chronic, non-contagious infection of dogs, horses and man caused by *Blastomyces dermatitidis*. It is characterized by the formation of suppurative and granulomatous lesions in any part of the body but with a predilection for the lungs, skin and bones. In man, blastomycosis is generally a cutaneous infection whereas in dogs and other animals it is usually systemic as a result of a primary infection of the lungs with subsequent haematogenous dissemination to the skin, bones, brain, kidneys and other organs.

The source of the infection is unknown and the causative organism has only occasionally been found as a saprophyte in the soil. It is essentially a disease of the Eastern half of the U.S.A. and Canada, hence the synonym North American blastomycosis, but recent reports indicate that it might be present in Latin America and parts of Africa. Canine blastomycosis was first recognised in 1913, as a chronic debilitating and highly fatal disease associated with extensive pulmonary lesions. In 1948 the disease was reported in a mare which showed a series of long-standing abscesses in the region of the anus and vulva and marked debility for several weeks before death. The infection was also reported in 1959, in a sea-lion. The disease is now being found with increasing frequency in dogs, particularly in areas where man is most likely to acquire the infection. Thus, blastomycosis should be suspected in dogs showing nodules in the skin, and respiratory distress. Radiographs of the chest cavity may reveal non-calcified nodules or consolidation of the lungs and enlargement of the bronchial and mediastinal lymph nodes. Blastomycotic mastitis has been reported in dairy cows in South Africa.

A diagnosis can be made by microscopic examination of pus, tissue scrapings or autopsy material in unstained wet films. If necessary, the specimen can be cleared in 10 per cent potassium or sodium hydroxide under a cover-glass. In wet mounts of suspected tissues the causative yeasts occur in the parasitic phase and are seen as thick-walled spherical cells about 8–16 μm in diameter, lying freely or within phagocytes (Plate 33.1a, between pp. 310–11). Budding forms bear only single blastospores attached by a wide septum to the parent cell. For confirmatory diagnosis the organism is cultivated in suitable media both at 22°C and 37°C. After 1–3 weeks of incubation wrinkled, creamy or waxy colonies are formed on blood agar plates at 37°C, consisting of budding yeast cells morphologically identical to those seen in infected tissues. On Sabouraud's glucose agar at 22°C, however, the colonies are initially like those of the yeast form but eventually become covered with a white, fluffy aerial mycelium which becomes tan or dark brown with age. The mycelial growth consists of closely packed septate hyphae bearing large numbers of spherical or pear-shaped conidia and, eventually, many smooth and thick-walled chlamydospores, 7–18 μm in diameter. Infected material from the lesions can be inoculated intraperitoneally into guinea-pigs or mice, and the yeast-like budding forms are later seen by microscopical examination of material from the peritoneal exudate of the infected animals.

The prognosis in systemic blastomycosis is usually grave and most cases terminate in death once the infection becomes disseminated. Iodide therapy or slow intravenous administration of amphotericin B have proved successful but in the latter method of treatment great care must be taken to avoid kidney damage and shock.

Coccidioidomycosis

This is an extremely infectious but non-contagious disease of man, monkeys, horses, cattle, sheep, dogs, cats and rodents. Indeed, the majority of individuals living in endemic areas for any length of time probably acquire the infection. Fortunately, coccidioidomycosis is mostly an acute but benign self-limiting pulmonary disease although at other times it may result in a chronic, progressive, fatal disseminated infection involving cutaneous, subcutaneous, visceral and osseous tissues. The disease was first recognized in the 1890s and is presently endemic in arid parts of the southwestern States of the U.S.A., through Central America into Venezuela and parts of Bolivia, Paraguay and Argentina. Animal infections have also been reported from Hungary. The causative organism, *Coccidioides immitis*, has been isolated from soil in endemic areas and the infection is probably transmitted by inhalation of dust heavily laden with infectious arthrospores or introduced into the skin following trauma. There seems little doubt that the highest incidence of infection in man occurs during the dry and dusty months of the year and that the incidence is lowest during wet weather.

Of the domestic animals, dogs and cattle appear to be the most important hosts. In dogs, the onset of infection is insidious and the course of the disease varies from 2–5 months. Despite the fact that the dissemination rate in dogs is several times that of man and much more extensive than in cattle, the majority of infections are subclinical and the patient makes an uneventful recovery. Nevertheless, there are reports of granulomata of the lungs, pleura, heart, liver, spleen or kidneys and, occasionally, involvement of the bones and joints. Cattle infections are usually benign and asymptomatic. In the majority of cases the granulomatous lesions are limited to the bronchial and mediastinal lymph nodes or, occasionally, the lungs.

Precipitins and complement-fixing antibodies are produced in severe primary infections and hypersensitivity to *C. immitis* antigens appears during the first or second week of the illness. The coccidioidin skin test (0·1 ml of a 1/100 dilution of coccidioidin injected intradermally) produces an area of erythema and induration. Positive results are usually obtained in patients 20–48 days after exposure to the infection or within a few days of the clinical symptoms developing. However, patients with disseminated infections usually fail to react to the coccidioidin test. In animals, the intradermal injection of 0·1 ml of undiluted coccidioidin may induce an area (at least 5 mm wide) of oedema or induration within 48 hours.

Skin-scrapings, sputa, exudates or biopsy tissues are best examined in wet mounts mixed with lacto-phenol cotton blue, or 10 per cent. potassium hydroxide if it is necessary to clear cellular debris in the preparation. In infected tissues the fungus appears in several phases, as round, thick-walled bodies (20–100 μm in diameter) termed spherules or sporangia, which contain a few to several hundred globular or irregularly shaped endospores varying from 2–5 μm in diameter. When the large, mature spherules rupture, the endospores are released and in turn develop into spherules. Occasionally, when pus or exudates are allowed to stand at room temperature for several days, hyphal elements are seen protruding from the wall of the spherules.

The organism is readily cultivated on blood agar, Sabouraud's glucose agar or Littman oxgall agar forming white surface colonies, at first moist and membranous but later becoming cottony and mottled with the development of an abundant aerial mycelium which changes from white to buff with age. There is little difference in the colonial characteristics at 22°C or 37°C. The hyphae segment into barrel-shaped arthrospores which fragment readily in older cultures and are easily airborne. Thus, cultures of *C. immitis* are highly infective and should be handled with great care and only by highly-trained personnel.

Infected tissues and cultures are pathogenic for mice and cause demonstrable infection 1–2 weeks after intraperitoneal inoculation. Serological tests, including complement-fixation, immunofluorescence and agar gel diffusion, have proved useful for diagnostic purposes.

The disease in dogs and cattle is usually benign but in cases of disseminated infection intravenous amphotericin B therapy may prove helpful.

Histoplasmosis

Histoplasmosis caused by *Histoplasma capsulatum* is the most frequently occurring systemic fungus disease of man and dogs in the Mississippi valley and central States of the U.S.A. Natural infections also occur in cows, horses, cats, rodents and other animals but the disease is not of importance in these species. Histoplasmosis has a world-wide distribution and occurs sporadically in most countries as a disseminated and highly fatal progressive granulomatous disease particularly of the reticuloendothelial tissues or, more usually, as a localized, benign often asymptomatic infection involving the lungs. The infection is non-contagious and is usually acquired by inhalation of infected dust from the soil.

Although acute canine histoplasmosis is almost always fatal after a course of 2–5 weeks, the disease in other animals is usually diagnosed only after post-mortem examination. However, a histoplasmin intradermal test may prove helpful in diagnosing the infection in dogs with a chronic cough or dysentery, especially in endemic areas. Radiographic examination may reveal calcified pulmonary lesions and enlargement of the bronchial and mediastinal lymph nodes.

H. capsulatum is dimorphic with a yeast-like parasitic phase in infected tissues and a mycelial saprophytic phase in artificial cultures. The yeast bodies appear as small, capsulate oval cells (1–3 μm in diameter) and are usually found within the macrophages. They are rarely present extracellularly and seldom show budding. When clinical specimens are cultivated on Sabouraud's glucose agar at 22°C, slowly growing mycelial colonies develop which are white at first but change to tan with ageing. The fine, cottony aerial hyphae bear small lateral conidia (2–3 μm in diameter) and later large spherical chlamydospores measuring up to 7–15 μm across. The chlamydospores are covered by small regularly spaced spines projecting from the outer surface of the thick wall and are diagnostic of *H. capsulatum*. Conversion of the mycelial to the yeast-like phase is readily accomplished by cultivating the organism at 37°C in glucose blood agar or other enriched media. The colonies that are produced at this higher temperature are moist wrinkled and creamy, and consist of budding yeast cells. The conversion to the yeast phase also occurs in mice inoculated intra-peritoneally or in monolayer cell cultures such as HeLa cells.

Progressive systemic histoplasmosis is usually fatal and there is no satisfactory treatment. In other forms of the disease intravenous administration of 0·1 per cent solution of amphotericin B in 5 per cent glucose may prove effective depending upon the patient's ability to tolerate the drug.

Epizootic lymphangitis

Epizootic lymphangitis, sometimes called pseudo-glanders or Japanese farcy, is a chronic, contagious mycotic infection of equidae characterized by granulomata and suppurating ulcers on the skin with inflammation of the associated lymph nodes and cording of the lymphatics. The causative organism is *Histoplasma farciminosum*, previously known as *Cryptococcus farciminosus*, *Saccharomyces farciminosus* or *Zymonema farciminosum*.

The disease is enzootic in horse-breeding areas bordering the Mediterranean particularly in Italy and North Africa, in African territories between the equator and the Sahara and in parts of Asia including Pakistan, India, Burma, Indonesia, China and the U.S.S.R. In South Africa a number of serious outbreaks occurred during the Boer War and the disease was introduced into the U.K. by returning army horses but was eradicated in 1906 by a policy of slaughter. Epizootic lymphangitis is still notifiable in the U.K. under The Diseases of Animals Act, 1950. In World War II major epizootics were recorded in Italy, India and Burma.

The disease occurs naturally in horses and mules. Donkeys are less susceptible but several cases were reported from Zanzibar in 1957. Although there are a few doubtful records of cases occurring in pigs, camels and man, attempts to infect other animal species have failed. The onset of clinical infection is insidious and difficult to control and new cases appear weeks or even months after the disease seems to have been eradicated. The source and method of transmission of the infection is not understood but the incidence is high only when large numbers of horses are collected together. The causal organism is very resistant to environmental conditions, and contaminated saddlery and grooming utensils may be responsible for transferring infection to saddle sores, minor wounds or abrasions of the skin. Infection of wounds and the conjunctiva by flies which become contaminated while feeding on open lesions of affected animals may be responsible for natural transmission of the disease, and biting flies which pierce the skin in order to suck blood may also play a part. It has also been suggested that infection by ingestion or inhalation with subsequent haematogenous spread may be possible. Although *H. farciminosum* has only been found in association with infected horses it seems likely that it has a saprophytic phase which, like that of *H. capsulatum*, occurs in the soil.

Epizootic lymphangitis is characterized by chronic

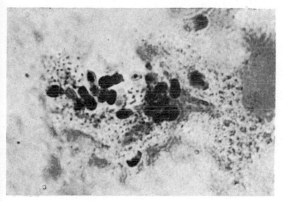

32.2a

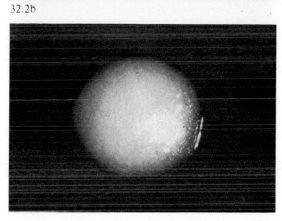

32.2b

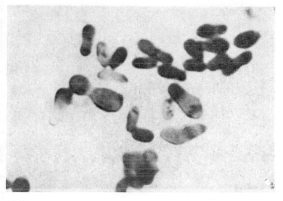

32.2c

32.2d

32.2a   Stained film of exudate from the external auditory meatus of a dog suffering from acute otitis. The yeast bodies of *Pityrosporum* are Gram-positive and the blastospores develop on a broad base. Gram stain, × 850.

32.2c   Stained film of a culture of *Pityrosporum* showing different stages of blastospore development. Ziehl-Neelsen stain, × 1250.

32.2b   Primary culture of *Pityrosporum canis* on malt agar plate (3 in diameter) incubated at 37°C for 3 days.

32.2d   A detail from Plate 32.2b showing the pitted surface of the regular domed colony of *Pityrosporum*.

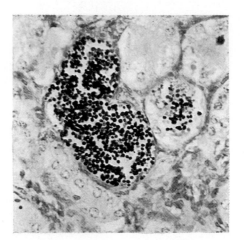

32.3

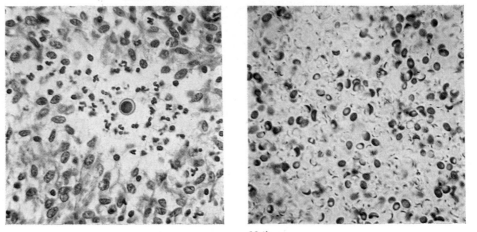

33.1a
33.1b

32.3 Section through the kidney of a mouse dying 5 days after intravenous inoculation of a broth culture of *C. albicans*. Large numbers of yeast bodies are present in the renal tubules. Gram stain, ×280.

33.1a Blastomycosis in the dog. Section of affected lymph node showing a single yeast cell with a thick wall. Periodic acid-Schiff stain, ×350 (Courtesy of Mrs S. T. Smith).

33.1b Epizootic lymphangitis. Stained film prepared from conjunctival discharge of a horse, showing large numbers of thin-walled ovoid yeast cells of *Histoplasma farciminosum*. Claudius' stain, ×645.

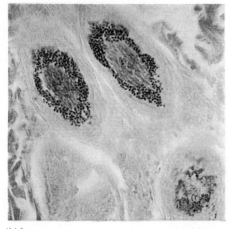

34.1a

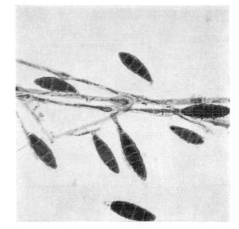

34.1b

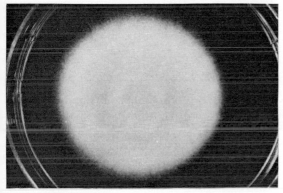

34.1c

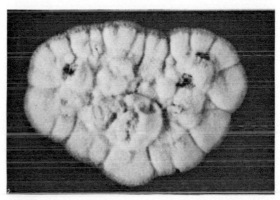

34.1d

34.1a Section of skin showing medium-sized spores of *Trichophyton mentagrophytes* forming a sheath around two infected hairs. The third hair follicle is unaffected. Claudius' stain, ×280.

34.1c *Epidermophyton floccosum* forms a slowly developing colony with abundant short fluffy non-pigmented aerial hyphae.

34.1b Needle mount from slide culture of *Microsporum gypseum*, showing the large multiseptate thick-walled ellipsoid macroconidia (fuseaux) which are characteristic of many species of *Microsporum*. Lactophenol cotton blue stain, ×280.

34.1d *Trichophyton verrucosum* is characterized by a slow-growing heaped glaborous colony which becomes corrugated or cerebriform and is covered with a white or yellow-white surface down of low aerial hyphae.

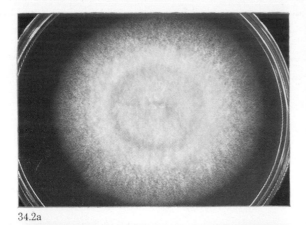

34.2a

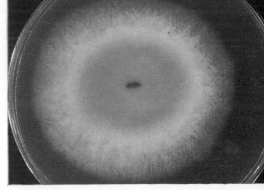

34.2b

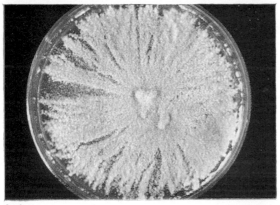

34.2c

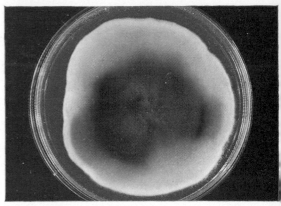

34.2d

34.2e

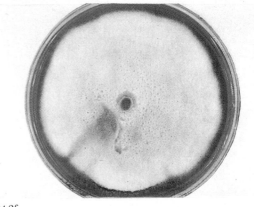

34.2f

Colonies of ringworm fungi

34.2a *M. canis*: Young rapidly growing surface colony with a white fluffy aerial mycelium.

34.2b The reverse is typically yellow and the central area tends to develop an orange-brown pigmentation after prolonged cultivation.

34.2c *T. mentagrophytes*: A rapidly growing surface colony with a downy surface. Pigmentation varies from white, through light tan to salmon pink.

34.2d The reverse may be colourless, yellow, tan, pink or reddish brown.

34.2e *M. gypseum*: The colony is characteristically flat, with a powdery cinnamon-brown surface and irregular border.

34.2f *T. rubrum*: The flat fluffy white colony produces a reddish-brown pigment which diffuses rapidly through the medium.

suppurating lesions on the exposed surface of the skin associated with the lymphatic vessels, particularly of the limbs and neck. The infected lymphatics become dilated at intervals and form lines of hard abscesses ('cording') which rupture to give ulcers from which blood-stained pus is discharged for several weeks. The granulating ulcers have a concave, bright red, glistening surface. After a prolonged period (2–3 months) of intermittent ulceration, scab formation and sloughing, the lesions become smaller until finally only a scar remains. Primary infection of the lungs may occur and lesions may also appear on the mucous membranes of the nostrils, extending inwards along the nasal septum to the pharynx, larynx and trachea. Ocular involvement results in a watery discharge from the affected eyes, conjunctivitis and the formation of papules on the conjunctiva or nictitating membrane.

Advanced cases showing typical 'cording' of the lymphatics on the neck, shoulders and limbs together with slow, progressive ulceration can readily be diagnosed in endemic areas but must be differentiated from farcy or glanders and ulcerative lymphadenitis of horses. Thus, the microscopic demonstration of thin-walled spherical, oval or pear-shaped yeast-like bodies in pus, preferably from an unopened abscess, or in nasal or conjunctival discharges may be necessary for confirmation. These can readily be seen in wet preparations or by staining thin films by Claudius, Gram or Giemsa (Plate 33.1b, between pp. 310–11).

The causal organism can be isolated, with some difficulty, by inoculating pus from unruptured cutaneous nodules on Sabouraud's agar or Hartley digest agar (pH 7·4) containing 10 per cent horse serum. The tubes must be tightly sealed before being incubated at 37°C. The colonies of *H. farciminosum* appear as tiny grey flakes after 2–8 weeks of incubation but grow readily when subcultivated on a number of mycological media. The mycelial saprophytic phase can be induced by growing the fungus on blood agar medium at 37°C in an atmosphere containing 15–20 per cent CO_2.

Most infected animals show well marked allergic reactions to intradermal inoculation of culture filtrates of the organism and the fact that some mild cases recover spontaneously within 4–6 weeks suggests that some immunity can develop. It is not known, however, if animals can become immune without showing clinical symptoms of the disease. Autoclaved extracts of *H. farciminosum* treated with a mixture of alcohol and ether for 24 hours are suitable antigens for complement-fixation and precipitation tests. There is evidence that complement-fixing antibodies appear in the serum a few days before the onset of clinical illness and the method might prove useful for detecting infected animals early in an outbreak.

There is, unfortunately, no effective means of treatment although local treatment including disinfection or cauterization of open lesions and surgical removal of affected lymphatic cords may be beneficial. Intravenous iodide therapy was used successfully in a number of cases by some early workers.

The disease is best controlled by isolation and slaughter but this is not practicable in most endemic areas. Wherever possible infected stalls, equipment and saddlery should be thoroughly disinfected, open wounds must be protected from flies and steps taken to avoid saddle galls and other injuries to the skin. The use of communal feeding and watering troughs should be discontinued. There can be no doubt that when animals are individually owned and stabled, the disease remains sporadic and epizootics do not occur.

Rhinosporidiosis

Rhinosporidiosis is a chronic, non-fatal mycotic infection of man, horses, mules and cattle caused by *Rhinosporidium seeberi*. The disease is endemic in warmer countries such as India, Egypt and Ceylon, but occurs sporadically in other parts of the world including Turkey, South Africa, Japan, the U.S.A., Brazil, Uruguay and Argentina. The infection has occasionally been reported from Poland, Italy and the United Kingdom. It is characterized by the development of nasal, less frequently ocular, polyps due to infection of the mucous membranes. In man, infection of the mucous membranes leads to the formation of polyps of the nose, eyes, ears or larynx and, occasionally, of the vagina, penis, rectum and skin.

The source of infection is not known and the causal organism has not been cultivated in the laboratory, nor has it been transmitted to man or animals by experimental infection. A report that *R. seeberi* has been cultured on cell cultures in Parker's Medium 199 has not been confirmed. It has been suggested that the infection is carried by dust or water and, even, that it is primarily a disease of fish and that man and animals are accidental hosts.

In animals the polyps may either be pedunculated or sessile and are seldom larger than 2–3 cm in diameter. The appearance of the lesion is a distinctive pink colour and careful examination of the surface of the polyps shows minute white spots of sporangia. The lesions are lobulated, soft to the touch and bleed readily.

Examination of wet mounts prepared from the friable polypoid mass reveals the presence of numerous large globular sporangia which measure from 200–300 μm in diameter. Their large size differentiates the sporangia of *R. seeberi* from the smaller 'spherules' of *C. immitis* to which they bear a superficial resemblance. Although the sporangia of *R. seeberi* may appear empty they are usually filled with numerous endospores measuring 5–8 μm in diameter which eventually escape from the sporangium by means of a special pore.

In human cases successes have been claimed by the administration of antimony compounds together with surgical excision or cautery. Prognosis is good although recurrence may follow incomplete removal.

CHAPTER 34

Dermatomycoses

Dermatomycoses, commonly called ringworms, are fungal infections of the skin and its appendages caused by three related genera of filamentous *Fungi imperfecti* namely, *Trichophyton*, *Microsporum* and *Epidermophyton*. In human patients *Trichophyton* generally affects the skin, hair and nails, *Microsporum* attacks the skin and hair whilst *Epidermophyton* which is almost entirely restricted to man attacks skin and nails. Although some infections may be acquired from animals, dermatomycoses due to *Microsporum audouinii* and some of the species of *Trichophyton* are contracted by contact with human hosts. In animals, almost all ringworms are due to species of *Microsporum* or *Trichophyton* and the genus *Epidermophyton* is not represented.

The parasitic activity of the dermatophytes is restricted to the keratin-bearing tissues (e.g. skin, hair, feathers, nails, horns) which they are capable of breaking down and utilizing as their sole source of nutriment. They do not invade the underlying living tissues that form the keratin or the deeper tissues and organs of the body. The infection starts in the stratum corneum where the spores (arthrospores) germinate and give rise to long, thread-like branching septate hyphae which spread as a mycelium through the whole depth of the horny layer and extend radially into adjoining areas of the skin. In hair-infecting species, the hyphae grow down the hair follicles, enter the shaft of the hair and parasitize the superficial layers of newly keratinized cells just above the root bulb (Plate 34.1a, between pp. 310–11). According to the species of fungus, septation of the hyphae may result in the formation of large numbers of thick-walled arthrospores within the hair shaft (endothrix type) or in rows or mosaics along the outer surface of the hairs (ectothrix type). These asexual arthrospores are the only spores formed during the parasitic phase. However, in artificial cultures the growth of ringworm fungi is more diversified and other spore forms develop such as macroconidia (fuseaux) and microconidia. The morphology of the macroconidia is probably the most important single character for delineating the three genera of dermatophytes. Other structures which indicate that the culture is that of a dermatophyte and which may assist in identification are racquet hyphae, spiral hyphae, pectinate hyphae, nodular organs and chlamydospores (Figs. 28.10 and 28.11).

The ringworm group of fungi can be divided into three categories:

(1) anthropophilic dermatophytes which are pathogenic only for man, e.g. *M. furrugineum*, *T. concentricum* and *E. floccosum*, or are mainly human parasites but occasionally infect animals, e.g. *M. audouinii*, *T. megninii*, *T. rubrum*, *T. schöenleinii*, *T. tonsurans* and *T. violaceum*,

(2) zoophilic dermatophytes which are fundamentally animal pathogens but sometimes cause disease in man, e.g. *M. canis*, *T. equinum*, *T. mentagrophytes* and *T. gallinae*, and

(3) geophilic dermatophytes such as *M. cookei* which are free living soil fungi that parasitize man or animals under certain conditions.

Man, and many species of animals and birds are susceptible to infection with ringworm fungi and the most usual route of infection is by penetration of intact skin or, more commonly, of skin subjected to minor trauma by rubbing, scratching or prolonged moistening. Since dermatomycoses are highly contagious the main source of infection is the infected animal or infected hairs, feathers, scabs, harness, grooming equipment, stalls, soil and other debris contaminated by the highly-resistant arthrospores from the lesions. Many species of ringworm fungi are world-wide in their distribution, e.g. *M. canis*, *T. mentagrophytes* and *T. verrucosum* but others including *M. nanum*, *M. distortum*, *T. megninii*, *T. gourvilii*, *T. simii* and *T. yaoundei* occur, or are endemic, in certain areas only. The main geographical distribution of the species causing ringworm in animals is shown in Table 34.1.

Laboratory diagnosis
The clinical signs of ringworm are not pathogno-

TABLE 34.1. Dermatophytes affecting animals.

Host		Species	Main distribution	Remarks
DOG	++	M. canis	Worldwide	Accounts for 70% of all dog cases
	+	M. gypseum	France, U.S.A.	Accounts for 20% of all dog cases.
	++	M. audouinii	Europe, U.S.A.	Worldwide in man.
	++	M. distortum	U.S.A., Australia	
	[+]	M. vanbreuseghemii	U.S.A.	Also in squirrel
	—	T. mentagrophytes	Europe, U.S.A.	Accounts for 10% of all dog cases
	—	T. gallinae	France	Very rare. Also rare in man.
	—	T. rubrum	Europe	Common, worldwide in man.
	+	T. quinckeanum	Germany	Common in mice. May form favic scutula.
	—	T. verrucosum	U.K.	Rare
	[+]	T. schöenleinii	Europe	Common, worldwide in man.
	++	T. simii	India	Mostly in poultry. Rare in man.
CAT	++	M. canis	Worldwide	Inconspicuous lesions. Accounts for 98% of cat cases.
	+	M. gypseum	Europe, U.S.A.	Accounts for 1% of all cat cases.
	—	T. mentagrophytes	Europe, U.S.A.	Accounts for 1% of all cat cases.
	+	T. quinckeanum	Worldwide	Forms favic scutula
	[+]	T. schöenleinii	Europe	Common in man
	—	T. violaceum	Europe	Occurs in man.
HORSE	+	M. gypseum	Europe. E. Africa	
	++	M. equinum	Europe U.S.A.	May be same fungus as M. canis
	—	T. equinum	Worldwide	Commonest species in the horse
	—	T. mentagrophytes	Europe	Second commonest species in the horse
	+	T. quinckeanum	Germany	May be worldwide
	[+]	T. schöenleinii		
	—	T. verrucosum	Brazil, U.S.A., U.K.	Rare in horses. Common in cattle
	—	T. bullosum	Syria, Sudan, Libya	
OX	—	T. verrucosum	Worldwide	Commonest species in cattle
	—	T. mentagrophytes	U.K., U.S.A., Canada	Uncommon in cattle
	—	T. megninii	Europe, Africa	Mostly in man.
	—	T. rubrum	Europe	Worldwide in man
	—	T. papillosum	Syria and Morocco	
	—	T. violaceum		Worldwide in man
	[+]	T. schöenleinii		Worldwide in man
SHEEP	++	M. canis	Czechoslovakia	
	—	T. mentagrophytes	France	Crusted lesions on head. Wool not affected.
	—	T. verrucosum	Europe. U.S.A.	Crusted lesions on head. Wool not affected.
	—	T. rubrum	Europe	Worldwide in man
	+	T. quinckeanum	Czechoslovakia	
GOAT	—	T. verrucosum	N. Africa	
	—	T. langeroni	N. Africa	Congo and Ruandi Urundi in man.
PIG	+	M. nanum	U.S.A. Australia. Africa	Commonest ringworm of pigs. Dark scabby lesions
	+	M. gypseum	U.S.A.	
	—	T. mentagrophytes	Scotland	Circular reddened areas
	—	T. verrucosum	Europe	Scales and blisters
POULTRY	+	M. gypseum	Italy	
	++	T. simii	India	Common in chickens. Also affects man.
	—	T. gallinae	Europe. U.S.A. S. America	Commonest species but rare. Lesions resemble scutula of favus of man.
LABORATORY ANIMALS	++	M. canis	Rabbit, guinea-pig, hamster	
	++	M. audouinii	Guinea-pig	
	+	M. gypseum	Guinea-pig, mouse, rat	
	++	M. distortum	Guinea-pig, mouse, rat	
	—	T. mentagrophytes	Guinea-pig, mouse, rabbit, rat.	
	+	T. quinckeanum	Guinea-pig, mouse, rabbit, rat.	Mouse favus.
	—	T. violaceum	Mouse	
	[+]	T. schöenleinii	Mouse	

++ = Bright fluorescence
+ = Weak fluorescence
[+] = Very poor fluorescence or none } When viewed with Wood's lamp.
— = No fluorescence

monic and the lesions often resemble those of other skin conditions. Thus for accurate diagnosis it is usually necessary to examine the skin or hairs by means of Wood's lamp, to demonstrate the presence of spores and hyphae in wet mounts of hairs or skin scrapings, and to isolate and identify the causative fungus in artificial culture. Under the filtered ultraviolet rays of Wood's lamp, hairs infected with *M. canis* and certain other species of fungi fluoresce with a brilliant yellow-green hue (Table 34.1). Even minimal infection may be detected in this way and suspected hairs can be plucked individually from the site of infection and sent to a laboratory for final identification. It is important to note that many species of dermatophytes do not fluoresce and that negative results with Wood's light does not eliminate the presence of ringworm infection. Moreover, a variety of substances such as petroleum jelly, salicylic acid and various lotions and ointments used in treatment of ringworm may show non-specific fluorescence and for this reason great care must be exercised in the interpretation of results.

Samples taken for laboratory diagnosis should include material from all parts of the lesion. Scales and crusts should be scraped with a blunt scalpel and affected hairs plucked from the lesion and never cut or broken. A preliminary cleansing of the lesion with 70 per cent alcohol helps to reduce bacterial contamination. The specimens are wrapped in small packages or envelopes of folded paper, and bacteria but not fungal spores are partially eliminated after a few weeks by such storage. They should not be kept in screw-topped bottles since the retention of

moisture tends to increase the numbers of contaminating bacteria and saprophytic fungi.

For direct microscopic examination small fragments of skin-scrapings or hairs including the hair bulb, are placed in a drop of 10–30 per cent potassium hydroxide on a clean slide, a cover-glass is added and the preparation is left to 'clear' at room temperature. Hydrolysation and partial digestion of the keratin by potassium hydroxide may be hastened by gently heating the preparation over a low flame. Although staining is usually unnecessary in routine diagnostic work the alkali may be replaced with a solution of lactophenol cotton blue and the wet mount re-examined. When infected tissues are examined first by a low power (16 mm) objective and then by using a high dry (4 mm) objective, the appearance of the mycelial fragments and the size, shape and distribution of the spores permits a diagnosis of ringworm and serves as a guide to the genus of dermatophyte involved. Thus, *Microsporum canis* and *Trichophyton mentagrophytes* are seen as small-spore ectothrix infections, *T. verrucosum* and *T. equinum* as large-spore ectothrix infections and *T. violaceum* and *T. sudanense* as large-spore endothrix infections. In favus due to *T. schoënlenii* the infection is also endothrix but is distinguished from the others by the presence of a number of characteristic air-bubbles in the hair. A number of fungi including *E. floccosum*, and *T. simii* do not attack the hair stalk (Fig. 34.1).

For confirmation, the suspected material should be cultured on artificial media such as Sabouraud's glucose agar or malt agar to which chloramphenicol (0·05 mg/ml) and cyclohexamide — 'Actidione'

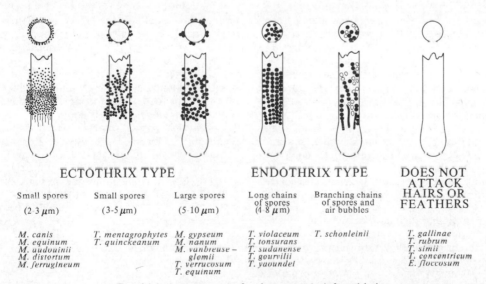

ECTOTHRIX TYPE			ENDOTHRIX TYPE		DOES NOT ATTACK HAIRS OR FEATHERS
Small spores (2·3 µm)	Small spores (3-5 µm)	Large spores (5·10 µm)	Long chains of spores (4·8 µm)	Branching chains of spores and air bubbles	
M. canis	*T. mentagrophytes*	*M. gypseum*	*T. violaceum*	*T. schonleinii*	*T. gallinae*
M. equinum	*T. quinckeanum*	*M. nanum*	*T. tonsurans*		*T. rubrum*
M. audouinii		*M. vanbreuse-glomii*	*T. sudanense*		*T. simii*
M. distortum		*T. verrucosum*	*T. gourvilii*		*T. concentricum*
M. ferrugineum		*T. equinum*	*T. yaoundei*		*E. floccosum*

FIG. 34.1. Arrangement of arthrospores in infected hairs.

(0·5 mg/ml) have been added to suppress bacterial contamination and overgrowth by saprophytic moulds. The malt agar at pH 5·4 can be made more selective by incorporating 0·036 per cent potassium tellurite and the bacterial contamination further reduced by immersing the specimen in 70 per cent ethyl alcohol for 2–3 minutes prior to inoculation. The fragments are then firmly embedded in the surface of the agar medium and the plates are incubated at 22°C or, preferably, at 28°C for 2–3 weeks. The cultures are examined every 3–4 days for evidence of growth around the implanted tissues, and material from the edge of any likely colony is transplanted to fresh medium in order to obtain a pure culture.

Pure cultures of the isolated fungus are examined microscopically by removing a small portion of the aerial growth with the point of a firm inoculating wire and transferring to a drop of lactophenol cotton blue on a clean slide. The mycelial growth is then teased apart with dissecting needles, a cover-glass applied and the preparation examined microscopically. Primary cultures should be examined as soon as reasonable growth is obtained since they are generally unstable and the characteristic spore-producing growth is quickly replaced by a white, sterile cotton-wool-like mycelium that cannot be used for identification of the species. However, these pleomorphic changes can be delayed if the culture is grown on a peptone agar such as Sabouraud's conservation medium.

In the dermatophytes, as in all *Fungi imperfecti*, the genera and species are differentiated according to the gross colony characteristics and the microscopical morphology of the hyphae and asexual spores (macro- and microconidia). Unfortunately, these properties vary considerably depending upon the source and type of cultural media employed and it is very difficult to give precise descriptions for any one species. In general, most dermatophyte species form large regular or irregular spreading surface colonies whose filamentous structure is rapidly obscured by a fluffy (*M. distortum*), velvety (*M. audouinii*) or powdery (*M. gypseum*) covering of aerial hyphae and spores. On the other hand, some species including *T. verrucosum*, *T. violaceum* and *T. schöenleinii* produce slow-growing, compact, heaped, bacteria-like colonies which are initially smooth and waxy but later become corrugated or cerebriform and covered with a white or yellowish-white surface down as the aerial mycelium develops. Most dermatophyte colonies are whitish-grey in colour but rapidly acquire a degree of pigmentation commonly pink, buff, pale lemon yellow or yellow-green (*M. canis*) but others may be claret-coloured (*T. megninii*), rusty (*M. nanum*), lilac or purple (*T. violaceum*). In a few species the pigment may diffuse

into the medium as in *M. canis* (lemon yellow), *T. equinum* (yellow) and *T. rubrum* (reddish-purple). In every case, the texture and colour of the growth should be observed on both the upper and lower surfaces of the colony (Plates 34.2a–f and 34.1c & d, between pp. 310–11).

One of the most useful features for distinguishing species of dermatophytes is the morphology of their macroconidia (fuseaux). These are very large elongated structures which are formed at the tips of certain hyphae and, when mature, are divided by visible transverse septa into several segments. In *Microsporum* they are large (up to 28 μm wide in *M. distortum*, and 190 μm in length in *M. audouinii*), spindle or boat-shaped structures with pointed ends and often thick warty walls (*M. canis*, *M. distortum* and *M. audouinii*), thin warty walls (*M. gypseum*) and, occasionally, thick smooth walls in some cultures of *M. audouinii* (Plate 34.1b, between pp. 310–11). An important exception in this group is *M. nanum*, a pathogen of swine, which produces large numbers of ovoid or pear-shaped smooth or rough thin-walled macroconidia with only one or two septa. The macroconidia of *Trichophyton* species tend to be smaller (up to 12 μm wide in *T. mentagrophytes* and 85 μm long in *T. simii*) cylindrical or cigar shaped thin-walled spores, whilst those of *Epidermophyton* are usually club or pear-shaped and divided into only a few segments. Unfortunately, some species including *M. ferrugineum*, *T. concentricum* and *T. sudanense* do not produce macroconidia in artificial cultures whereas others such as *T. schöenleinii* and *T. violaceum* do so irregularly.

Spherical, pear-shaped or elongated microconidia may be numerous, few in number or absent but, if present, are usually borne singly along the sides of the hyphae (*M. gypseum*) or in bunches, 'en grappe', as in *T. mentagrophytes*. Thick-walled chlamydospores may occur singly along the length of the vegetative hypha bulging to one side or at its end. They are abundant in *T. verrucosum*, which rarely produces microconidia, and are also found in *T. equinum*, *M. audouinii* and some other species of *Microsporum*. Other morphological features of diagnostic importance are racquet hyphae, spiral hyphae and convoluted segments of hyphae forming the so-called nodular organ. In a few species such as *T. schöenleinii* and *T. gallinae* the presence of irregularly swollen hyphal elements called 'antler hyphae' or the 'favic chandeliers' is considered to be of some diagnostic importance.

Ringworm in animals

Dogs and cats

The commonest causal agent, *M. canis* (syn. *M.*

felineum, M. lanosum) is believed to be endemic in many dog and cat populations throughout the world and is probably transmitted directly from animal to animal. Other ringworm fungi including *T. mentagrophytes* and *T. quinckeanum* occur in rats and mice which may act as a source of infection for cats, and cases of *T. verrucosum* infection have been reported in dogs in contact with infected cattle. In general, lesions of ringworm in dogs usually appear as thick circular scaly patches up to 3 cm in diameter on any part of the body. In some instances the lesions may be distributed generally over the body whilst in others an exudative form known as 'wet eczema' may occur. Affected areas may show broken stubs of hair or may be completely hairless, and vesicles or pustules may appear at the periphery of the sore where the infection is most active.

In cats, the clinical signs are generally more variable than in dogs and are often inconspicuous with only a few broken hairs over the nose and face and on the ears. In severe infections, or in cases of *T. quinckeanum* infection, a more inflammatory reaction may develop leading to erythema, bare crust-covered lesions or, occasionally, the formation of small favic scutula on the head and body. Although the lesions of cat ringworm are often very difficult to detect with the unaided eye, the fact that over 90 per cent of cases are due to *M. canis* enables this ectothrix type of infection to be readily diagnosed by fluorescence under Wood's light. The colony of *M. canis* grows rapidly and may be fluffy, cottony, velvety or powdery. The pigmentation changes with age from white, pink, pale yellow to brownish-yellow, and a greenish-yellow pigment diffuses through the medium. The reverse of the colony is mostly bright yellow, changing later to dull orange brown.

An important diagnostic feature of *M. canis* is the presence of large numbers of multi-septate, boat-shaped macroconidia with thick warty walls and pointed ends. Microconidia are present in limited numbers but racquet hyphae are almost always produced. Older cultures may show large numbers of chlamydospores.

Cattle

Cattle of all ages are susceptible to ringworm but calves and young stock are most commonly affected when housed indoors especially in overcrowded pens during the winter months of the year. The most frequent cause is *T. verrucosum var. discoides* but *T. mentagrophytes* and, occasionally, *T. megninii*, *T. violaceum* and *T. rubrum* are encountered.

After an incubation period of about 3–4 weeks, the hair in the affected area falls out and large, circular, discrete or confluent raised scaly lesions appear on the head (eyes, ears, muzzle), neck and, less frequently, the back, flanks, escutcheon and limbs. Although natural recovery generally occurs 2–4 months from the time of first appearance of the disease, a number of old-standing lesions may become confluent and develop thick yellow-brown asbestos-like scabs. Cattle recovered from the disease are highly resistant to reinfection for many months or years.

T. verrucosum and *T. mentagrophytes* are both of the ectothrix type. The former gives rise to irregular chains of large spores (5–8 μm) on the surface of the affected hairs whereas the latter produces long chains of smaller spores (3–5 μm). *T. verrucosum* grows slowly and the surface colony is irregular in shape with little evidence of an aerial mycelium. In some strains the membranous-type colony becomes powdery or velvety and tends to wrinkle. The pigmentation may be white-grey, pink, buff or pale yellow whilst the reverse surface is either pink or unpigmented. The colonies of *T. mentagrophytes* mature within 10 days and are usually flat and granular, but sometimes velvety or powdery. The aerial growth is white to grey, pale pink, buff, lemon yellow, lilac or purple. The reverse surface is reddish-brown or pale yellow.

Neither species produces many macroconidia, and microconidia are normally absent in *T. verrucosum* but abundant in *T. mentagrophytes*. Favic chandeliers are often present in the former and nodular bodies, pectinate and racquet-hyphae and chlamydospores are usually found in the latter.

Horses

The commonest cause of ringworm in horses is *T. equinum* which is almost entirely restricted to the equidae. Young horses are the most frequently affected and transmission to horsemen can occur. *M. equinum* is also a common cause of epidemic equine ringworm but recent evidence suggests that *M. equinum* and *M. canis* should be classified as the same species. Other causal parasites include *T. mentagrophytes* and, not infrequently, *T. verrucosum* which may be contracted from infected hairs, scabs or from buildings, fences and grooming equipment contaminated by infected cattle.

The infection is usually characterized by the appearance of oval or irregular, focal, inflamed, oedematous lesions, loss of hair and, finally, raised, circumscribed bare plaques covered by a thick 'soft crust' measuring about 2–3 cm in diameter. The lesions may occur on any part of the body but the main predilection sites are probably the withers, saddle and girth regions. The incubation period for *T. equinum* and *M. equinum* is about 7–10 days but *T. verrucosum* grows more slowly and may take several weeks to develop. In most horses, the clinical disease persists for 8–12 weeks, or longer, and may be accompanied by severe itching. *M. gypseum* is unusual in that it causes a favic type of infection in which yellow masses of spores accumulate beneath the raised scabs or scutula. The disease is now rare but seems to be more common in warm rather than temperate climates.

The commonest species, *T. equinum,* is of the ectothrix type and forms irregular chains of large spores outside the hair. The colony is flat, velvety to powdery and, initially, is white with a bright yellow periphery. Later the surface pigment changes to cream or tan. The reverse side is at first yellow, then pink and, later, reddish-brown. Small numbers of smooth, cigar-shaped macroconidia may be present, numerous microconidia are seen 'en thyrse' and there may also be racquet hyphae and chlamydospores.

Other domestic animals

In contrast to cats, dogs, cattle and horses, there are comparatively few records of ringworm of sheep, goats and pigs. Small encrusted lesions have been observed on the face and head of affected sheep but the wool is rarely involved. In the case of *T. verrucosum* infection of sheep and goats the foci are mostly found around the ears, horns, nose and eyelids but lesions may also occur on the tail, back, neck and chest. In young animals confluent, crusted lesions on the lips may resemble contagious pustular dermatitis.

In pigs, *T. mentagrophytes* causes circular, reddened areas, especially on the neck and trunk. The lesions are sometimes covered with brown or reddish-brown crusts but there is usually no loss of hair. With *T. verrucosum* the tissue changes appear as scales or blisters rather than crusts and are mostly located on the back, loins and outer aspects of the thighs. Most cases of *M. nanum* infection occur in adult swine, particularly sows. The lesions are either diffusely distributed over the animal's body or restricted to the pinna of the ears or abdomen. The skin of the affected areas is reddened and may become uneven, but there is no loss of hair and the foci appear as dark brown scurfy patches, about 4 cm in diameter covered with numerous small reddish-brown scales.

Ringworm or favus of poultry occurs particularly in chickens and turkeys and is caused by *T. gallinae.* Infection produces thick white crusts on the comb, wattles and other featherless parts of the head. The base of the neck and the cloacal region may occasionally be affected. The infection may also spread to the skin in other parts of the body and involve the base of the feathers giving rise to circular favic lesions resembling the scutula of favus in man. In very severe infections the entire head is covered with scabs and powdered scales, there is marked loss of feathers, emaciation and sometimes death. Fowl favus is highly contagious and may spread to pigeons and other species of birds. Cases have also been recorded in man and dogs. The colony of *T. gallinae* is flat or raised, fluffy or velvety and is white, grey or pink in colour. The reverse surface is pink or occasionally red and the pigment may diffuse into the medium. Thin-walled cigar-shaped macroconidia are present in variable numbers and chlamydospores may also be found.

There are a number of reports from India of *T. simii* infection of poultry and, less frequently, of man and dog. Cultures grow rapidly and produce velvety colonies with a granular surface and fluffy margin. The surface pigment is buff but the reverse is pink or salmon in colour.

Treatment

The oral administration of griseofulvin, an antifungal substance produced by the mould *Penicillium griseofulvum,* is highly beneficial in the treatment of most forms of ringworm in dogs and cats. The minimal daily dosage required is 20–40 mg/kg body weight continued for 10 days or longer if possible. Griseofulvin is absorbed into the blood-stream and is deposited in the keratin precursor cells where it inhibits fungal growth at the point of lowest penetration on the hair shaft and lays down a barrier which persists and thereby prevents further invasion by the fungus. Unfortunately, griseofulvin is fungistatic rather than fungicidal so that spread of infection to other parts of the body or to incontact animals may occur even during treatment. Clipping of the hair for some distance from the affected areas and the topical administration of antifungal ointments or dips helps to remove infected hairs and debris and stimulates the growth of healthy new hair.

Oral administration of griseofulvin has given good results in cattle but its use in large animal practice is limited by the high cost of treatment. There is, unfortunately, no other reliable method of treatment of cattle, horses and other farm animals and it is doubtful if any of the innumerable traditional methods of treatment is either effective in curing the condition or in influencing the course of the disease. Substances that have been widely used include salicylic acid, benzoic acid, sulphur-containing compounds such as ichthammol, tars, paraffin, engine oil and creosote. Daily applications of a 20 per cent solution of sodium caprylate to lesions from which the crusts have been removed is effective, as is tincture of iodine or Lugol's solution applied 2 or 3 times per week until the lesions heal. Badly affected cattle may be given intravenous sodium iodide therapy at weekly intervals but treatment should be discontinued if symptoms of iodism appear. In many instances, however, the animals will recover spontaneously in 3–4 months' time if the disease is allowed to run its course. Thorough cleansing and disinfection of stables and byres and the use of a blow-lamp on non-inflammable walls and partitions may ensure that infection does not recur.

CHAPTER 35

Mycotoxicoses

The term mycotoxicoses is the collective name for that group of diseases caused by toxic metabolites of moulds (i.e. mycotoxins) which cause disease in tissues distant from the site of mould growth as a result of the ingestion of contaminated animal foodstuffs under customary conditions of husbandry. With few exceptions (e.g. ergotism) the study of these diseases was not extensively undertaken until the last decade following the discovery of aflatoxin produced by the mould *Aspergillus flavus*. The following chapter gives a brief outline of some of the important established features relating to mycotoxicoses in animals and the subject is discussed under different groups of fungi and the various disease entities related to them.

Claviceps

Disease entity

Ergotism in cattle, sheep, pigs, horses, poultry and man.

Ergotism in man was one of the first of the mycotoxicoses to be described. Outbreaks of this disease were recorded in the fifteenth century and its association with the ingestion of fungal growths on rye was suggested in the eighteenth century. The causal fungi *Claviceps purpurea* and *Claviceps paspali* are parasites of cereals and grasses, and the mycelia develop as hard masses known as ergots or 'sclerotia' which grow in the ovaries of the flowers and replace the grain or seed in the ears. Development of these dark coloured horn-like structures (2–4 cm in length) is favoured by mild, damp weather conditions which prolong the period of maturation of the grain or seed and allow extensive development of the mycelia in the affected plants. The ergot remains dormant over the winter and germinates in the spring, producing ascospores which are discharged into the air and dispersed by the wind. The mould produces a number of alkaloids derived from lysergic acid of which ergometrine, ergotamine and ergotoxine are the most important. They have vasocon-strictor properties on arterioles by stimulating the neuromuscular junction of sympathetic nerves and thereby causing restricted blood supply to the extremities of the body.

Following ingestion of food heavily contaminated with sclerotia, the characteristic symptoms of ergotism are lameness associated with the restriction of blood supply and the development of gangrenous lesions of the feet especially of the hind limbs, and less frequently the tips of the ears and the tail. Additional symptoms include persistent diarrhoea, convulsions, agalactia and abortion in cattle and sheep in an advanced stage of pregnancy. The condition known as 'paspalum staggers' which occurs in South America, South Africa and Australia is caused by the fungus *Claviceps paspali*.

Among poultry, the symptoms of ergotism include lethargy followed by loss of appetite, thirst, diarrhoea, paralysis and death which takes place in severe cases within 48 hours of the onset of these symptoms. Post-mortem lesions consist of gastroenteritis and degenerative changes in the heart, liver and kidneys.

There is no satisfactory treatment other than the removal of the source of ergot. Because the sclerotia develop only in seedling grasses, pastures should be kept well grazed or mowed in the late summer.

Ergot poisoning in man usually results from consumption of ergot-contaminated rye bread.

Aspergillus

Disease entities

(1) Aflatoxicosis affecting many species of animals.

(2) Aspergillotoxicoses associated with hyperkeratosis in cattle, malt sprout poisoning in cattle, and a haemorrhagic syndrome in poultry.

Aflatoxicosis

The study of this condition caused by certain strains of *Aspergillus flavus* began in 1960 when thousands of turkey poults in the United Kingdom died from a disease which was initially termed 'Turkey X disease' and is now referred to as aflatoxicosis. The condition was acute and affected birds showed symptoms of inappetance, lethargy, a rapidly developing weakness, convulsions and death within 5–7 days of the onset of symptoms. Post-mortem lesions consisted mainly of haemorrhage or necrosis of the liver and congested kidneys. Subsequent investigations have shown that a wide variety of animal species are susceptible to aflatoxicosis, particularly turkey poults, ducklings and rainbow trout. A few species including horses, sheep and cats do not appear to be very susceptible. Some of the characteristic symptoms of the disease which have been reported in various animal species include jaundice in pigs and dogs, tenesmus and eversion of the rectum in calves and subcutaneous oedema in guinea-pigs. Lesions in all animals are associated typically with the liver which is the organ most susceptible to the action of aflatoxin, and they include fatty changes, cirrhosis, haemorrhages and microscopically there is proliferation of bile-duct epithelial cells and fibrosis. In addition, it is now known that aflatoxin is a highly potent hepatocarcinogen and the development of liver tumours has been studied in rats, ducks and rainbow trout after prolonged feeding of either small quantities of aflatoxin or contaminated foodstuffs. Similar studies are also being made on the possible role of aflatoxin as the aetiological agent of human liver tumours in some tropical countries.

The original outbreaks of aflatoxicosis in turkey poults were caused by the incorporation of groundnut meal which contained aflatoxin derived from contamination with *A. flavus*. Subsequent studies of this mycotoxin showed that it consisted of four compounds labelled B_1, B_2, G_1 and G_2, where the letters B (blue) and G (green) refer to the colour of fluorescence under ultra-violet light. Toxigenic strains of *A. flavus* can be recognised in fluid cultures incubated for 10 days at 25°C. If toxin is present the fluid will fluoresce when viewed under Wood's light. Although all strains of *A. flavus* are not toxigenic, aflatoxin has been identified in a wide variety of foodstuffs including maize, cottonseed and palm kernels, but under natural conditions groundnuts constitute the most important contaminated commodity. Toxin production usually occurs subsequent to harvesting and during either the drying of the product, oil extraction or storage when the humidity is suitable for generation of *A. flavus* spores which have infected the kernels of groundnuts through damaged shells. The optimum conditions for growth and production of aflatoxin by the organisms are a temperature of 30°C and a relative humidity of 80–85 per cent. Thus, the most satisfactory method for preventing aflatoxicosis is to ensure satisfactory

harvesting, processing and storage methods which prevent the development of conditions suitable for the growth of *A. flavus* and aflatoxin production.

Aspergillotoxicoses

A condition of hyperkeratosis in cattle may be caused by toxic strains of *A. chevalieri*, *A. clavatus* and *A. fumigatus*. The condition arises from the feeding of foodstuffs in which toxigenic strains of these fungi have proliferated. The disease usually occurs in the winter and acutely affected animals develop symptoms of depression, salivation, incoordination of the limbs, muscular tremors, a rise in body temperature to about 39°C, increased pulse and respiratory rates followed by congestion of the mucous membranes, fetid diarrhoea, prostration and death. Chronic cases show signs of depression, lachrymation, salivation, followed by gross thickening of the skin on the cheeks and neck due to overproduction of the keratin layer. Post-mortem lesions usually include ulceration of the mouth, haemorrhages and oedema of the gastrointestinal tract and other organs.

Malt sprout poisoning in cattle is another mycotoxic condition which has been described as arising from the feeding of sprouted malt infected with *A. oryzae* or *A. clavatus*. Affected animals develop an unsteady gait, a drop in milk production and a marked hypersensitivity to external stimuli. The condition may be fatal. Post-mortem lesions include ulceration of the abomasal mucosa and emphysema of the lungs.

A haemorrhagic syndrome in poultry is a disease entity which develops as a mycotoxicosis caused by strains of *A. clavatus*, *A. flavus* and certain other moulds including *Penicillium purpurogenum* and species of *Alternaria*. It arises from contamination of foodstuffs with these fungi which develop under favourable conditions of temperature and humidity in the litter of poultry houses during the winter, and especially as the result of the scattering of broiler mash in the immediate vicinity of food and water troughs. Signs of disease include depression, paleness of the comb and wattles, and blood-stained diarrhoea affecting as many as 50 per cent of birds and causing a mortality rate of 5–10 per cent. Post-mortem examination reveals extensive congestion and haemorrhages in many tissues, including the gastrointestinal tract, particularly the proventriculus and gizzard, the liver, kidneys, lungs, skin and muscles. Preventive measures include the incorporation of good quality ingredients in the mash and the storing of foodstuffs under dry conditions for as short a time as possible before use. Satisfactory ventilation of broiler houses to reduce the moisture content of the litter is also necessary.

Pithomyces

Disease entity

Facial eczema in sheep and cattle.

This condition is caused by sporidesmin, a mycotoxin present in spores of the saprophytic fungus *Pithomyces charterum* (syn: *Sporidesmium bakeri*). The disease occurs particularly in the North Island of New Zealand and in the Victoria area of Australia during the late summer and autumn in sunny weather following rain. The fungus exists in dead material at the base of rye grass pastures. In warm, moist conditions the spores proliferate, produce sporidesmin and because of their sticky surfaces they adhere to the growing grass. Ingestion of this mycotoxin initially causes inappetence, lethargy, loss in weight and diarrhoea. A few days later these symptoms are followed by the development of jaundice, oedematous inflammation and photosensitization of those areas of the skin which are not protected by the wool or hair from sunlight, particularly the lips, ears and vulva. Affected animals seek the shade and irritation of the skin causes shaking of the head and rubbing of the affected parts. Sporidesmin is primarily a hepatotoxin causing liver cirrhosis, inflammation of the bile ducts leading to fibrosis and an obstructive jaundice. The condition of photosensitization arises from the build-up of phylloerythrin (a breakdown product of chlorophyll) in the peripheral blood due to failure of the damaged liver to excrete it. Preventive measures include the practice of hard summer grazing to reduce the amount of moist, dead material at the base of pastures in late summer and autumn, and more recently the application of fungicides to pastures has been practised.

Fusarium

Disease entities

Gastroenteritis in animals and Barley Scab disease.

Species of the mould *Fusarium* are the cause of a condition known as 'scab' which affects grain crops, particularly maize, oats and barley. The organisms exist as saprophytes in the soil, they are particularly resistant to cold weather and will grow slowly at temperatures as low as -8 to $-10°C$. The optimum temperature for growth is about $24°C$ although toxin production will take place at lower temperatures of $2-4°C$. Various toxic conditions have been described in animals as a consequence of eating grains severely infected with *Fusarium* species, especially *F. sporotrichiella*, *F. culmorum* and *F. graminearum*. Symptoms may include vomiting in pigs due to the emetic action of the mycotoxin which has been demonstrated in animals with simple stomachs. In addition, pigs may develop an oestrogenic syndrome involving squamous cell metaplasia and shedding of vaginal and cervical mucosa. Dairy cattle show symptoms of inappetence, decreased milk production, and severe cases develop scouring, a staggering gait and occasionally an acute, fatal haemorrhagic enteritis. Horses are also susceptible to the mycotoxin and develop nervous symptoms, incoordination of the limbs, tachycardia, cyanosis and occasionally lesions on the lips and buccal cavity similar to those produced by the mould *Stachybotrys*. Provided the disease in animals is not too advanced, recovery will take place rapidly following the withdrawal of infected grain from the diet. Man is also susceptible to this condition which mainly affects the central nervous system.

Stachybotrys

Disease entities

Stachybotryotoxicosis in horses, cattle, sheep, pigs and poultry.

Toxigenic strains of *Stachybotrys alternans* (syn: *S. atra*) may develop rapidly in damp straw and hay causing a black or sooty discolouration and for this reason is sometimes referred to as 'sooty fungus'. The optimum conditions for growth are a temperature of $20-25°C$ and a humidity of $60-100$ per cent. The spores and mycelia are destroyed by a temperature of $80°C$ for 1 hour at a low humidity and are highly susceptible to the lethal action of disinfectants. They are destroyed by the thermal decomposition of manure, but survive passage through the intestinal tract.

The disease in animals commonly has a seasonal incidence commencing when they are housed in the autumn and reaching a peak in February and March. Typically, the mycotoxin causes stomatitis with necrosis and fissures in the commissures of the mouth, accompanied by salivation and enlargement of the submaxillary lymph glands. Several days or weeks later, systemic reactions develop which include a rise in body temperature, diarrhoea, a marked extension together with secondary infection of the buccal necrotic areas, thrombocytopenia, leukopenia, a failure of the blood to clot and death. Occasionally an atypical acute form of the disease develops within 72 hours following the ingestion of large quantities of mycotoxin, and is manifest by a loss of reflex responses, hyperexcitability, blindness and death. Lesions consist of extensive areas of haemorrhage and necrosis throughout the intestinal tract. A unique feature of the necrotic areas is that there are no zones of reaction delineating them from the surrounding normal tissue, indicating that there appears to be no tissue response. Moreover, no immune response develops and following recovery from the disease, animals of all ages remain susceptible to further intoxication. The mycotoxin is not excreted in the milk. Lesions in pigs consist of rhinitis and skin lesions on the snout, lips and teats.

In poultry the mycotoxin produces oral lesions similar to those of the diphtheritic form of fowl pox; the lesions which occur on those parts of the mouth where food tends to remain longest, develop as a degeneration of superficial epithelium and necrosis but without cellular infiltration of the submucosa which is associated with fowl pox.

Preventive measures include storage of roughage under dry conditions and the burning of suspected samples.

Man is also susceptible to this disease.

Penicillium

Disease entities

Yellow Rice disease in man; hepatitis in rats and mice; mycotoxicosis in cattle; haemorrhagic syndrome in poultry.

More than ninety toxic metabolites are known to be produced by *Penicillium* species but so far only a minority of these have been classified as mycotoxins capable of causing disease when fed at concentrations normally expected under natural conditions. The human condition termed Yellow Rice disease was described in Japan at the end of the last century. More recently it has been shown to be caused usually by the consumption of rice infected with toxigenic strains of *P. islandicum*, *P. citrinum* and *P. toxicarum*. The first of these can cause hepatitis and liver tumours in mice and rats, the second causes necrosis of renal tubular cells, and the third produces paralysis. Other mycotoxic conditions in animals associated with *Penicillium* species include disease in cattle related to the production of patulin, a neurotoxin produced by these organisms; an hae-

morrhagic syndrome in chicks, ducklings and turkey poults caused by *P. purpurogenum*, and several other less well defined conditions have been described. It is important to remember that under favourable conditions a variety of toxigenic species of *Penicillium* are potentially capable of producing mycotoxicosis in animals.

Micropolyspora

Disease entity

Farmers' lung affecting man and cattle.

Unlike the conditions already described in this chapter, Farmers' lung is not a true mycotoxicosis but develops as an immune hypersensitive reaction by the host against the infecting fungal spores. The disease in man develops in the lungs following the repeated inhalation from mouldy hay of the spores of *Micropolyspora faeni*. The spores are approximately 1 μm in diameter and penetrate the alveoli of the lungs. Following the development of precipitating antibodies in the serum, repeated exposure to these spores leads to an Arthus reaction occurring in the walls of the alveoli and the consequent respiratory distress characteristic of the disease. The condition has been described as an extrinsic allergic alveolitis and also as an allergic bronchiolo-alveolitis since there may also be bronchiolar lesions.

A similar condition has recently been described in cattle caused by the feeding of mouldy hay to housed animals and the consequent inhalation of large numbers of spores giving rise to symptoms of increased respiratory rate with an expiratory grunt, a rise in body temperature but no coughing. The lesions consist of cellular infiltration of alveolar interstitium by lymphocytes, plasma cells and other mononuclear cells together with the development of an obliterative bronchiolitis. Thus, the condition closely resembles the disease in man.

Further reading in mycology

ADAMS, S.E.I. (1974) Hepatotoxic activity of plant poisons and mycotoxins in domestic animals. *Veterinary Bulletin*, **44**, 767.

AINSWORTH G.C. (1949). List of fungi recorded as pathogenic for man and higher animals in Britain. *Transactions of the British Mycological Society*, **32**, 318.

AINSWORTH G.C. AND AUSTWICK P.K.C. (1955). A survey of animal mycoses in Britain: General aspects. *Veterinary Record*, **67**, 88.

AINSWORTH G.C. AND AUSTWICK P.K.C. (1959). *Fungal Diseases of Animals*. Review series, No. 6, Commonwealth Agricultural Bureaux, England.

AUSTWICK P.K.C. (1958). Cutaneous streptothricosis, mycotic dermatitis and strawberry foot rot and the genus *Dermatophilus* Van Saceghem. *Veterinary Reviews and Annotations*, **4**, 33.

BARRON C.N. (1955). Cryptococcosis in animals. *Journal of the American Veterinary Medical Association*, **127**, 125.

BLANK F. (1955). Dermatophytes of animal origin transmissible to man. *American Journal of the Medical Sciences*, **229**, 302.

BLAXLAND J.D. AND FINSHAM I.H. (1950). Mycosis of the crop (moniliasis) in poultry, with particular reference to serious mortality occurring in young turkeys. *British Veterinary Journal*, **106**, 221.

CARNAGHAN R.B.A. (1966). Mycotoxicosis. *Veterinary Annual*, **8**, 84.

CHODNIK K.S. (1956). Mycotic dermatitis of cattle in British West Africa. *Journal of Comparative Pathology and Therapeutics*, **66**, 179.

CONANT N.F., SMITH D.T., BAKER R.D. AND CALLAWAY J.L. (1971). *Manual of Clinical Mycology*, 3rd Edition. Philadelphia: Saunders.

DVORAK J. AND OTCENASEK M. (1969). *Mycological Diagnosis of Animal Dermatophytoses*. The Hague: W. Junk NV.

EDDS G.T. (1973). Acute aflatoxicosis: a review. *Journal of the American Veterinary Medical Association*, **162**, 304.

EMMONS C.W. (1955). Mycoses of animals. *Advances in Veterinary Science*, **2**, 47.

FORGACS J. AND CARLL W.T. (1962). Mycotoxicoses. *Advances in Veterinary Science*, **7**, 273.

FRASER G. (1961). *Pityrosporum pachydermatis* Weidman of canine origin. *Transactions of the British Mycological Society*, **44**, 441.

GEORG L.K. (1954). The diagnosis of ringworm in animals. *Veterinary Medicine*, **49**, 157.

GRIDLEY M.F. (1953). A stain for fungi in tissue sections. *American Journal of Clinical Pathology*, **23**, 303.

HARRISS S.T. (1948). Proliferative dermatitis of the legs (strawberry foot rot) in sheep. *Journal of Comparative Pathology and Therapeutics*, **58**, 314.

HESSELTINE C.W., SHOTWELL O.L., ELLIS J.J. AND STUBBLEFIELD R.D. (1966). Aflatoxin formation by *Aspergillus flavus*. *Bacteriological Reviews*, **30**, 795.

KLIGMAN A.M. MESCON H. AND DELAMATER E.D. (1951). The Hotchkiss-McManus stain for the histologic diagnosis of fungus diseases. *American Journal of Clinical Pathology*, **21**, 86.

LODDER J. AND VAN RIJ J.W. KREGER (1952). *The Yeasts: a taxonomic study*. Amsterdam: North Holland.

MADDY K.T. (1954). Coccidioidomycosis of cattle in the southwestern United States. *Journal of the American Veterinary Medical Association*, **124**, 456.

MARTIN-SCOTT I. (1952). The Pityrosporum ovale. *British Journal of Dermatology*, **64**, 257.

McPHERSON E.A. (1957). A survey of the incidence of ringworm in cattle in Northern Britain. *Veterinary Record*, **69**, 674.

MENGES R.W. AND GEORG L.K. (1957). Survey of animal ringworm in the United States. *Public Health Reports (Washington)*, **72**, 503.

MORNET P. AND THIERY G. (1955). Streptothricose cutanee des bovins. *Bulletin of Epizootic Diseases of Africa*, **3**, 302.

NISBET D.I. AND BANNATYNE C.C. (1955). A dermatitis of sheep associated with an organism of the genus *Actinomyces*. *Veterinary Record*, **67**, 713.

PIER, A.C. [Edit] (1973) An overview of the mycotoxicoses of domestic animals. *Journal of the American Veterinary Medical Association*, **163**, 1259.

RUNE J.S. AND CAZIER P.O. (1949). A review of histoplasmosis. *Journal of the American Veterinary Medical Association*, **122**, 78.

SAHAI L. (1938). Rhinosporidiosis in equines. *Indian Journal of Veterinary Science and Animal Husbandry*, **8**, 221.

SAUNDERS L.Z. (1948). Systemic fungous infections in animals: a review. *Cornell Veterinarian*, **38**, 213.

SCHULTZ K.C.A. (1955). Mycotic dermatitis (Senkobo skin-disease) of cattle in the Union of South Africa. *Bulletin of Epizootic Diseases of Africa*, **3**, 244.

SCHWABE C.W. (1954). Present knowledge of the systemic mycoses in dogs: a review. *Veterinary Medicine*, **49**, 479 and 490.

SKINNER C.E., EMMONS C.W. AND TSUCHIYA H.M. (1957). *Henrici's Moulds, Yeasts and Actinomycetes*, 2nd Edition. New York: John Wiley.

SINGH S. (1956). Equine cryptococcosis (Epizootic lymphangitis). *Indian Veterinary Journal*, **32**, 260.

SMITH H. (1948). Coccidiodomycosis in animals with report of a new case in a dog. *American Journal of Pathology*, **24**, 223.

WOGAN G.N. (1966). Chemical nature and biological effects of the aflatoxins. *Bacteriological Reviews*, **30**, 460.

WRIGHT D.E. (1968). Toxins produced by fungi. *Annual Review of Microbiology*, **22**, 269.

APPENDIX 1
DISEASES OF FISH

Diseases of fish

Fish farming for the production of human food has been practised in the Far East for thousands of years and for several hundred years in other countries. The current need to expand the world supply of food for the increasing human population has resulted in the development of intensive production of aquatic life under controlled conditions. For several years shellfish and shrimps have been produced on farms in association with rice paddies, and many countries have already developed freshwater farms for the intensive production of fish. Similar methods are also being applied to the rearing of saltwater fish in bays, river estuaries and saltwater reservoirs. Annual production rates of fish can be maintained at high levels in confined waters by supplementary feeding and maintaining water temperatures at optimum levels. Experiments are now being carried out on the employment of warm water used for cooling atomic reactors for rearing fish at optimum temperatures throughout the year. The economic value of fish farming as a source of human food can be appreciated when it is realised that only approximately 640 g of feed are required to produce about 460 g of fish meat, whereas 1 kilo or more of feed is needed for the production of similar weights of chicken or mammalian meats. Moreover, the use of supplementary feeding methods enables freshwater fish farms to yield a larger quantity of food per unit area than corresponding areas of farmland employed for rearing domestic mammals.

The use of artificial methods of intensive fish farming provides predisposing factors which can give rise to serious disease problems of epidemic proportions. The maintenance of water temperatures at relatively high levels, the rearing of large numbers of newly-hatched and growing fish in confined waters with supplementary feeding, and the risks of pollution are all factors predisposing to the development of nutritional diseases, microbial infections specific for fish and to contamination of fish with human pathogens. For example, it has been known for more than 20 years that during winter when fish are living in water temperatures below the optimum, bacteria may be present in the tissues. A subsequent rise in water temperature may result in either the development of a septicaemia causing disease or the production of antibodies and survival of immune fish. It has also been shown that the maintenance of healthy fish in confined waters during the winter and the subsequent development of resistance to infection in the spring is closely dependent upon satisfactory nutritional and environmental conditions being maintained during the preceding summer and autumn. At the present time, knowledge relating to microbial infections occurring under artificial conditions is limited to some few infections for which the causal agents and pathogenesis of diseases are known, and to others of undefined aetiology which require further investigation. It is important that veterinarians should be acquainted with the problems relating to the epidemiology and control of fish diseases in this growing industry.

Immunology

Although the immunological mechanisms of fish have not been studied to the same extent as those of mammals, it is evident that the cellular and humoral mechanisms are similar but less well developed, and that they play a significant role in the host's reaction to disease. The disposition of lymphoid tissue and the sites where antibody production takes place show some species variations. Lymphoid tissue commonly occurs in the thymus, spleen, pharyngeal submucosa and pronephros, and some of these tissues appear to act as filters in a manner comparable to the function of mammalian lymph nodes. The thymus is concerned with the production of lymphocytes similar to that which occurs in mammals, and in all young fish this organ is well developed and in some species it involutes with age as it does in mammals. Among elasmobranches and some other fish, however, the thymus does not involute but persists into adult life as a source of lymphocytes.

Antibody production takes place in these concentrations of lymphoid tissue, especially the pronephros and spleen, and the process is closely associated with plasma cells and lymphocytes. However, antibody production in fish is not so highly developed and IgM is the only immunoglobulin fraction which has so far been identified with immunological responses. Fish can produce bacterial agglutinins but under controlled conditions the rate of production is directly affected by the temperature of the water. For example, fish acclimatized to living in warm water have a greatly reduced metabolic rate when kept at a temperature of 5°C. At this temperature the fish will not produce agglutinins following the subcutaneous inoculation of bacteria. When the fish are subsequently transferred to water at a temperature of 10°C, agglutinin production can be detected after about 30 days; at 15°C it occurs after 2 weeks, and at a temperature of 25°C agglutinins are detectable after only 4 days. Under optimal conditions, high concentrations of antibodies may be developed against both living and dead antigens, and the specificities of these antibodies are similar to those produced in mammals. Experiments of this nature clearly illustrate the increased rate of immunological responses which take place at higher temperatures. At the same time, these higher temperatures are often conducive to the development of pathogenic micro-organisms in fish and their distribution from one host to another in contaminated waters. In addition, certain aspects of fish farming subject these animals to stress, and it has been demonstrated that stress can have a depressive effect on the development of immune responses in fish.

Bacterial diseases

Aeromonas infections

The classification of *Aeromonas* species is in some doubt but they are usually included in the family *Pseudomonadaceae*. They are rod-shaped organisms and most species are motile, aquatic and many are pathogenic to reptiles and fish.

Aeromonas punctata
This organism has been associated with a variety of primary and secondary infections in fish.

Synonyms: *Aeromonas hydrophila*, *Aeromonas liquefaciens*. Recent studies of the taxonomy of these organisms has led some authors to conclude that there is no justification for distinguishing between *A. punctata*, *A. hydrophila* and *A. liquefaciens*, and that all should be known as *A. punctata*. Similarly, it has been suggested that the anaerogenic strains

known as *A. formicans* or *A. caviae* should also be named *A. punctata*.

Morphology and staining. *A punctata* are rod-shaped organisms and most strains have polar flagella and are motile.

The organisms stain Gram-negative.

Cultural characteristics. The organisms produce β-haemolysis when grown on blood agar. This haemolysin is a toxin which is both lethal and cytotoxic. For most strains the optimum temperature for toxin production is 25°C, but some are actively toxigenic when grown at 37°C in media with pH 7·4–7·8. *A. punctata* ferments a variety of carbohydrates including glucose, with production of acid and gas but some strains are anaerogenic and produce acid, only. Fermentation of lactose is variable. The organisms produce indole and H_2S but not urease, the MR test is positive and the VP test variable.

Epidemiology and pathogenesis. The role of *A. punctata* as either a primary aetiological agent causing disease in fish or as a secondary invader associated with primary viral or fungal infections, has not been clearly defined. In some countries the organisms have been isolated from as many as 50 per cent of healthy pike, perch, bream, dace and other species, and the commonest sites of infection are the nostrils and, less frequently, the branchial cavity and intestines. The incidence of infection among healthy fish varies considerably with the quality of water. Organic pollution, especially with sewage, can cause an increased incidence of aeromonas infection in water and a lowered resistance of fish to infection with other species of microbes. This can result in the incidence of *A. punctata* infection being as high in apparently normal fish as in diseased fish, and this situation has been observed among healthy carp and those suffering from infectious abdominal dropsy or from inflammation of the swimming bladder. For these reasons, the isolation of *A. punctata* from pathological lesions may not necessarily indicate that the organism is the primary cause of a pathological condition. It is known that the virulence of these organisms varies, and that although inoculation of avirulent strains may cause no disease, injection of relatively small doses of virulent toxigenic cultures can prove fatal.

Diseases. *A. punctata* has been isolated from a variety of fish diseases, including the following:
(1) Red mouth disease of rainbow trout develops as a severe and progressive erosion of the upper jaw associated with *A. punctata* and other related species

which have been cultivated in the laboratory at 10°C on media containing a digest of fish muscle.

(2) Carp dropsy for which there is some evidence that the primary aetiological agent may be a virus followed by a secondary build-up of infection in the intestines with *A. punctata*.

(3) Pike pest is a disease of pike resembling carp dropsy which may be caused primarily by a virus followed by secondary infection with *A. punctata*.

(4) Septicaemia of warm water fish.

Aeromonas salmonicida

This organism is the cause of furunculosis in salmonid fish.

Morphology and staining. A. salmonicida are rod-shaped organisms measuring $1 \cdot 7$–$2 \cdot 0$ μm in length and $1 \cdot 0$ μm in width. They are non-motile and have a tendency to grow in pairs or chains.

The organisms stain Gram-negative.

Cultural characteristics. A. salmonicida is a facultative aerobe which requires arginine and methionine for growth. It can be cultured on trypticase-soy agar. Growth will develop within a temperature range of 6–$34 \cdot 5°C$ but the optimum temperature is 20–$25°C$. Growth develops on solid media as round, convex, semi-translucent colonies which tend to develop a brownish colour with age. Cultivation on rabbit blood agar results in the development of marked β-haemolysis after 48 hours' growth. Other characteristic properties include fermentation of glucose but not lactose and there is no production of indole, H_2S nor urease. Both the MR and VP tests are negative.

Epidemiology and pathogenesis. Furunculosis is a disease of trout and less commonly of salmon which has been known since the end of the last century. Under natural conditions the disease occurs during the summer months and some of the predisposing factors are a water temperature of 13–$19°C$, a reduced oxygen content, a low level of water in the rivers, and the aggregation of trout and salmon from the sea which are less resistant than those that have been in fresh water for some time. The disease also occurs in the spring when the water temperature may be 6–$8°C$ and fish have a lowered vitality. Although trout and salmon are the species most commonly affected, they show a marked resistance to the disease during their first year of life. Other species known to be susceptible and which are occasionally affected include carp, pike, tench and catfish.

Apparently normal fish can be temporary carriers of *A. salmonicida* in the kidneys for periods of several months but may ultimately suffer from a generalised and fatal infection. Infected fish discharge *A. salmonicida* into the water via excreta or from surface lesions, and it will be evident that an infected decomposing carcase may release large numbers of organisms into the environment and become a major source of disease. The spread of infection takes place by ingestion, contamination of surface wounds or is transmitted by infected eggs.

Symptoms and lesions. The acute form of the disease may be described as a generalised bacteraemia associated with enteritis and abdominal haemorrhage. The more chronic form develops as focal abscesses or ulcers in various organs, particularly the skin, fins and kidneys. Initially, these foci become infiltrated with lymphocytes, neutrophils and macrophages. Later, these cells tend to disappear, the lesions become necrotic and filled with reddish, opaque fluid, often breaking to the surface and producing ulcers (hence the name furunculosis). A generalised bacteraemia then develops followed by death which may occur as early as the fourth day after infection.

Diagnosis. The symptoms, lesions, breeds of affected fish, and the time of year of the outbreak (usually summer, but sometimes spring) are strongly suggestive of the disease. A final diagnosis can be made by isolating the causal organism from the blood and from various organs of acutely infected carcases. Bacterial agglutination tests have also been used for diagnosis. The disease must not be confused with Ulcer disease or Red Mouth.

Control and prevention. The disease has been effectively controlled and prevented by sulphamerazine therapy.

Chondrococcus infections

Chondrococcus columnaris and related species

Synonym: Cytophaga columnaris.
This organism is the cause of columnaris disease in salmon and trout, and related organisms have also been isolated from so-called Gill disease in eels and trout fry.

Morphology and staining. C. columnaris is a flexible rod measuring 4–8 μm in length and $0 \cdot 5$–$0 \cdot 7$ μm in width, which can develop spherical or ellipsoidal microcysts measuring $0 \cdot 7$–$1 \cdot 2$ μm in diameter. When in contact with infected tissues or scales they characteristically develop branching, fruiting bodies which may contain microcysts. Some strains fail to develop microcysts and these have been named *C. columnaris*.

The organisms stain Gram-negative.

Cultural characteristics. Relatively good growth can be obtained on 0·5–0·8 per cent agar containing 0·25–0·5 per cent bacto tryptose at pH 7·3. Colonies are yellow or golden yellow and flat with irregular stellate edges and show swarming. After 48 hours' incubation at 22°C the colonies vary in size up to a maximum of about 4 mm diameter, and are adherent to the agar and difficult to remove. There is no growth at 37°C.

Gelatin is rapidly liquefied, indole is not produced and nitrates are not reduced. The organism is catalase-positive, oxidase-positive and produces small quantities of H_2S. Sugars are not fermented.

Antigens and toxins. All strains of *C. columnaris* possess a common antigen and, in addition, there are type-specific antigens which enable the organisms to be divided into four distinct serological groups. The organisms also produce bacteriocins, similar to colicins, which have been used for typing.

Epidemiology and pathogenesis. Columnaris disease occurs among salmon, trout and other fresh-water fish in the United Kingdom, Europe, Canada, the U.S.A. and Japan. The incidence is affected by the temperature of the water and usually occurs during the summer months. Highly virulent strains can kill young salmon after only 24 hours following inoculation into water, but virulence may become greatly reduced after the organisms have been grown in the laboratory. Although less virulent strains may not cause death of infected fish which subsequently become carriers and disseminate infection, it is known that these less virulent strains can cause disease in water temperatures of 20°C, whereas highly virulent organisms do so at lower temperatures of about 15°C.

Gill disease occurs in eels and has recently become a serious condition affecting trout fry intensively reared in confined waters. A variety of factors which increase the susceptibility of the gills to microbial infections have been suggested. These include overcrowding of fish in tanks and an accumulation of metabolic products in water with insufficient circulation. It has also been suggested that mechanical irritation of the gills may be caused by suspended particles, including earth or dry feed, which predispose to bacterial infection with species of *Chondrococcus* and sometimes mixed infections with moulds belonging to the species *Saprolegnia*.

Symptoms and lesions. Columnaris disease caused by infection with virulent strains of *C. columnaris* often develops as greyish-white spots or areas of necrosis resembling mycotic lesions, which occur on the dorsal and lateral surfaces of the body, on the head, fins and less commonly on the gills. Some of these lesions will develop into shallow ulcers and become secondarily infected with fungi and aeromonas species. This stage of the disease is often followed by a generalized systemic infection and death.

Gill disease initially causes loss of appetite and sluggish movements of affected fry which tend to remain clustered around water inlets. The gills are noticeably congested and eventually become hyperplastic and unable to close. Microbial growths often form a layer of slime over affected lamellae causing anoxia and death.

Diagnosis. Typical lesions of columnaris disease developing during the summer months are often diagnostic. Confirmation can be obtained by isolating the organism and identifying the characteristic features. Direct smears from lesions show long, flexuous organisms which stain Gram-negative and can be readily isolated from early and late lesions but only rarely from liver and kidney. It is necessary to differentiate this disease from ulcerative dermal necrosis (UDN) which may be caused by a virus with secondary aeromonas infection and occurs during the colder months of the year, generally affecting only salmon and trout which have recently returned from the sea.

The symptoms and macroscopic lesions of gill disease may be diagnostic. Detailed examination of affected gills shows hypertrophy and fusion of the lamellae with concentrations of bacterial or fungal growth but no necrosis of the tissues.

Vibrio infections

Vibrio anguillarum and related species
These organisms cause acute septicaemic diseases in fish, especially rainbow trout and eels.

Morphology and staining. *V. anguillarum* are curved organisms, measuring 1·8–2·0 μm in length, and are motile by means of polar flagella. After prolonged cultivation in the laboratory they have a tendency to become pleomorphic and may develop as cocci or long filamentous forms.

The organisms stain Gram-negative.

Cultural characteristics. *V. anguillarum* requires a salt concentration of 2 per cent in the medium for optimal growth. Under these conditions it will grow on meat infusion agar containing 5 per cent defibrinated calf blood when incubated at 30°C. After 24 hours' growth the organisms produce β-haemolysis.

Epidemiology and pathogenesis. This can be a serious

disease of fish farms and affects a variety of species, particularly rainbow trout and eels. It usually occurs during the summer months and young fish are particularly susceptible.

Symptoms and lesions. In young fish the disease may be an acute septicaemia and cause a high mortality rate without the development of typical lesions. Some outbreaks are characterized by the development of a swollen abdomen resulting from the accumulation of ascitic fluid and also the development of surface ulcers.

Diagnosis. Fresh preparations made from ascitic fluid or surface ulcers show large numbers of *V. anguillarum* and the organisms can be cultured from these sites.

Nocardial infections

Nocardia asteroides
An important cause of disease among intensively reared fish and also in wild fish.

Morphology and staining. The organisms appear as filaments of varying length and about 1 μm in width which tend to break up into bacilli after growth on laboratory media.

N. asteroides stains Gram-positive and the majority of strains are also acid-alcohol-fast and stain by the Ziehl-Neelsen method.

Cultural characteristics. The organism grows aerobically on ordinary laboratory media as dry, white, nodular colonies which later turn yellow or pink in colour and become covered by a whitish layer of aerial hyphae. The optimal temperature for growth is 28–35°C.

Acid is produced from glucose and glycerol. No fermentation occurs in lactose, adonitol, arabinose, raffinose, sorbitol, xylose or inositol. Most strains reduce nitrate to nitrite.

Epidemiology and pathogenesis. *N. asteroides* is commonly found in soil and it is probable that infection of fish is derived from infected soil contaminating the water, or possibly from pelleted fish foods which usually contain plant ingredients. Experimentally, it is difficult to infect fish and usually the organisms remain localised at the site of inoculation. It is probable that overcrowding and increased water temperatures are predisposing factors leading to outbreaks of nocardiosis.

Symptoms and lesions. Affected fish tend to swim in circles on their sides or to have the appearance of 'chasing their tails'. The mortality rate is usually low but many fish develop a distended abdomen which contains large numbers of the causal organisms.
Diagnosis. Smears prepared from the abdominal region contain large numbers of filamentous *N. asteroides* organisms.

Other bacterial infections

Haemophilus
Haemophilus piscium can cause the development of surface ulcers on trout and is sometimes referred to as Ulcer Disease. The disease may occur concurrently with furunculosis.

Morphology and staining. The organisms usually occur as rods, measuring 2–3 μm in length and 0·5–0·7 μm in width. Sometimes they develop long filaments 10–12 μm in length. They are non-motile and stain Gram-negative.

Cultural characteristics. The organism is an aerobe and growth takes place on laboratory media which incorporates a peptic digest of fish tissue. The optimum temperature for growth is 20–25°C and no growth develops at 37°C. On fish extract agar the colonies develop to a size of 1–3 mm diameter, and are circular, convex and cream-coloured. On blood agar β-haemolysis is produced. The organisms do not require the V and X factors for growth.

Pasteurella
Pasteurella piscicida was described in 1968 as causing disease among perch during the summer months and has been isolated from the blood and organs of infected fish.

Morphology and staining. Occurs as non-motile, capsulated, short rods measuring approximately 1·0–1·5 μm in length. The organisms stain Gram-negative and show bipolar staining.

Cultural characteristics. The organisms grow on ordinary laboratory media including MacConkey's agar containing 0·5 per cent added salt. Optimum conditions for growth are a temperature of 17–31°C and pH 6·8. No growth occurs at 37°C. No haemolysis is produced on rabbit blood agar.

Acid is produced in glucose, fructose, maltose, mannose and sucrose. Other reactions include M.R.+, V.P.−, H_2S−, urease−. The organism is not pathogenic for mice.

Mycobacterium
There has been some confusion concerning the identification of the different strains of mycobacteria causing disease in fish. It is probable that the

commonest causes of tuberculosis are *Myco. fortuitum* in tropical and temperate waters, *Myco. marinum* (closely related to *Myco. kansasii*) in tropical waters and variants of these organisms. Factors predisposing to tuberculosis include over-crowding, lowered oxygen levels in the water and poor nutrition.

Infected fish become dull, sluggish, emaciated, and the mortality rate is variable. Mycobacteria occur in large numbers in the organs, particularly the liver, spleen and kidneys where they produce tubercular-like lesions.

Mycobacteria adapted to growing in fish have morphological and staining properties similar to *Myco. tuberculosis*. Culturally, some of these strains grow at temperatures of 25–30°C but not at 37°C. Growth at these lower temperatures is compara-tively rapid particularly on glycerol egg medium, and the colonies develop a yellow-orange colour.

Corynebacterium

Corynebacteria are the cause of a condition in salmon and trout known as Kidney Disease which has also been described under the names of 'Dee Disease' and 'White Boil Disease'. It is a chronic condition affecting the kidneys which develop characteristic pale coloured foci of infection, and there is evidence to suggest that the incidence is closely related to poor standards of nutrition and husbandry.

Viral diseases

In many respects, the aetiology, physiology and pathology of fish diseases closely resemble those found in other vertebrate hosts, and fish viruses have similar characteristics to those found in diseases of warm-blooded animals.

Since 1949, when poliovirus was shown to replicate in non-neural tissue in culture, there has been a spectacular increase in the volume of cell-culture research in human and animal virology. As a result of these advances it has been possible to utilize cell-culture methods to establish the viral nature of a number of important disease conditions of free-living and hatchery-reared fish.

Although several fish diseases are transmissible to experimental fish it is necessary for an understanding of the disease processes and the virus-cell relation-ships to be able to isolate, identify and characterize the causal viruses. Unlike the developing chick embryo, fertile fish eggs have little practical value in fish virology, but the use of cell cultures derived from cold-blooded vertebrates has greatly increased the scope and tempo of fish virus research.

As in animal virology, a wide range of primary and secondary cell cultures can be readily obtained from several species of teleost or bony fishes, and

an increasing number of continuous or established cell lines have been developed and stabilized in culture. The varying virus susceptibilities of these different cell systems has placed a series of useful hosts in the hands of fish virologists and are now a routine provision of many fish laboratories. Con-trary to widely held opinion, teleost cells can be readily cultivated in growth or maintenance media designed originally for human, animal and avian cells. The blood composition and osmolarity of freshwater fish are so similar to those of mammals that basic salt solutions, e.g. Earle's or Hanks' with added animal serum as a supplement are entirely suitable. In many cases, however, the temperature of incubation is critical and it is important to ensure that this does not rise too high, and should generally be kept below 18°C. Since microorganisms are commonly present in the viscera of fish it is frequently necessary to incorporate antibiotics in the growth medium to prevent contaminating organisms destroy-ing the developing monolayers.

The first continuous line of fish cells was establish-ed in 1962 from the ovaries of rainbow trout, and is known as RTG-2. The cells are fibroblastic in character and support the growth of infectious pancreatic necrosis virus (IPN) and viral haemor-rhagic septicaemia or Egtved virus. It is also of interest that certain mammalian viruses, e.g. togaviruses can be grown on RTG-2 cells. The second fish cell line (GF) to be developed was obtained from fin tissue of a saltwater fish, the yellow striped grunt. The IPN virus multiplies readily on GF cells but does not produce a cyto-pathic effect. The same virus can also be propagated on an epithelioid cell line (FHM) derived from the tail tissue of a freshwater fathead minnow. Other cell lines have been established from brown bullhead trout, goldfish and salmon. Unlike mammalian cell cultures, fish cell lines metabolize very slowly at low temperatures and can be kept for up to 18 months without trypsinization or refeeding.

Viruses have been isolated or strongly implicated in a number of fish diseases while others have been suspected from the appearance of virus-like particles in ultra-thin sections of tumours or other abnormal tissues. The following are among the more important viral diseases of fish.

Infectious pancreatic necrosis (IPN)

The first virus to be isolated in cell cultures and identified as the causal agent of disease in fish was obtained from young grossly normal hatchery-reared trout showing symptoms of frantic spiral swimming movements followed by periods of quiescence. This acute viral infection affects salmonids mainly in North America but also occurs in Europe. Histolo-gical examination reveals pancreatic necrosis, haemorrhages accompanied by necrosis in the musculature and intracytoplasmic inclusions. The virus, which produces cytopathic changes in cell cultures was tentatively placed in the picornavirus (rhinovirus) group but has recently been classified with the reoviruses (Chapter, 48).

Viral haemorrhagic septicaemia (VHS)

This disease occurs amongst European salmonids and is probably the greatest single cause of mortality in rainbow trout. Brown trout, brook trout and salmon are susceptible to experimental infection. In spontaneous outbreaks the mortality rate may be as high as 75 per cent, but in the natural hosts, e.g. grayling or whitefish the virus usually produces a mild or subclinical infection. The disease has not been reported in North America.

The acute form of the disease is characterized by slow, sluggish spiral swimming movements, by darkening of the skin, exophthalmia, anorexia, anaemia and ascites. The kidneys are swollen and haemorrhagic, and petechiae are scattered throughout the body, especially on the perivisceral fat, musculature, swim bladder, fins and meninges. In 1963, the causative agent was isolated on primary cell cultures of trout ovarian cells (RTG-2) and was subsequently shown to be strikingly similar to vesicular stomatitis virus and other rhabdoviruses (Chapter, 44).

Oregon Sockeye disease and Sacramento River Chinook salmon disease

These are highly fatal infections occurring most commonly in salmon under 6 months of age. The causal virus or viruses affect primarily haematopoietic tissues giving rise to exophthalmia and haemorrhages at the bases of the fins. Infected Sockeye salmon appear sluggish, darker than normal in colour and show marked abdominal distension. The stomach is filled with a milky fluid and there are petechial haemorrhages on the swim bladder, peritoneum and adipose tissues. A number of survivors have spinal deformities. Infected Chinook salmon are more darkly pigmented and show a characteristic dark red subdermal lesion at the back of the head, due to massive vascular damage.

At autopsy, the viscera are pale and the gall bladder is darker green than usual. Histologically, nuclear and cytoplasmic inclusions have been described and advanced necrosis is present in the kidneys and, sometimes, in the liver and pancreas.

The virions resemble rhabdoviruses in morphology and like Egtved virus they are sensitive to ether and pH 3, and are readily inactivated by heat.

Infectious haematopoietic necrosis (IHN)

In 1967, an epidemic was reported among Rainbow trout and Sockeye salmon in British Columbia and because of the histopathological changes and the fact that the causative agent affected primarily haematopoietic tissues, the disease was named infectious haematopoietic necrosis (IHN). Subsequent investigations clearly showed that the agents of IHN, Sockeye and Chinook diseases of salmon produce similar cytopathic effects in cell cultures and that all three viruses are morphologically indistinguishable from the bullet-shaped virions of rhabdoviruses. Moreover, reciprocal neutralization tests have shown that the three viruses are serologically related and there can be little doubt that the agents of Sockeye, Chinook and IHN are one and the same virus.

Lymphocystis

This benign viral disease affecting many species of marine and freshwater fish is especially prevalent in Great Lakes' walleyes and bluegills. The disease is characterized by granular, tumour-like masses on the skin and fins consisting of grossly hypertrophied lymphocystis cells, each measuring up to several millimetres in diameter. Characteristic intracytoplasmic inclusion bodies stain Feulgen-positive, as for DNA. The lesions develop slowly and persist for long periods but ultimately regress. The disease is seldom fatal but affected fish lose their market value.

The virus can be propagated in a number of fish cell cultures including a fibroblastic cell line derived from largemouth bass but other lines such as RTG-2 and FHM are refractory. Lymphocystis virus has similar properties to those of *Tipula* iridescent virus and is classified with the iridoviruses. (Chapter, 57).

Spring viraemia of carp (SVC)

An acute or chronic disease of European carp called infectious abdominal dropsy was thought for many years to be caused by *Pseudomonas fluorescens*, *Aeromonas punctata* or other bacteria, but these are now regarded as being only secondary invaders. In 1971, however, the acute form of carp dropsy was found to be caused by a virus of the rhabdovirus group and the condition has been renamed spring viraemia of carp (SVC). It is an acute disease associated with a high mortality. Naturally and experimentally infected fish show pallor of the gills, peritonitis, enteritis, oedema and petechial haemorrhages of the viscera.

The virions are typical bullet-shaped rhabdoviruses measuring 70×180 nm and developing from the cytoplasmic membranes of affected cells. The virus grows readily and produces cellular changes in primary monolayer cultures of carp ovary cells and in various fish cell lines including FHM and RTG-2, at an optimal temperature of 20–22°C. SVC is the fifth fish virus to be placed in the rhabdovirus group, the others being the European Egtved virus and the American viruses causing infectious haematopoietic necrosis, Sockeye and Chinook Salmon diseases, respectively.

Carp erythrodermatitis

In 1971, following the isolation and identification of SVC virus the subacute or chronic form of the infectious carp dropsy complex was renamed carp erythrodermatitis (CE). Although the causative agent of this condition is unknown recent evidence suggests that it is highly dermotropic, larger than 450 nm in diameter and sensitive to a number of chemotherapeutic agents. It enters the body through abrasions in the skin and is localized in the sub-epidermis where it gives rise to inflammation, haemorrhage and necrosis leading to ulceration of the skin. In the terminal stages of the disease a generalized oedema occurs.

Fish pox

This is a benign, localized epidermal hyperplasia affecting principally carp, but smelt, pike and perch are also susceptible. The disease is generally non-fatal and is characterized by proliferative cutaneous lesions affecting the fins, lips, eyes and, occasionally, other parts of the body. Sections of the characteristic papillary-like growths show the presence of intranuclear inclusions in the affected cells. There is no conclusive evidence that the causal agent has been isolated from cases of fish pox but a report in 1956 describes multinucleated 'giant-cells' and other cellular changes in inoculated tissue cultures derived from embryonic guppy (*Lebistes reticulatus*). Recent electron microscopy has confirmed the presence of viral particles in pox lesion tissue of carp which contain DNA and are morphologically indistinct from herpesviruses (Chapter 56).

Ulcerative dermal necrosis (UDN)

Ulcerative dermal necrosis of Atlantic salmon is a disease of returning adult fish which came into prominence in 1964 in South West Ireland, and has now spread to almost all British rivers. It would appear that UDN has occurred at roughly 30-year intervals since 1830, and generally lasts for about 3–5 years.

The disease is characterized by a progressive cytolytic necrosis of the skin of the head, giving rise to whitish, scaleless areas that are clearly visible while the fish are in water. As the ulcers develop they rapidly become infected with secondary fungi (*Saprolegnia parasitica*) or bacteria (*Aeromonas* spp., *Pseudomonas* spp. etc.).

Attempts to isolate the primary agent of UDN have failed, but it is widely believed that a virus is the cause. However, electron microscopy of affected tissues has failed to reveal the presence of virus-like particles although a number of workers have recently obtained evidence of transmission by means of bacteria-free filtrates.

Neoplasm-associated diseases

During recent years, a virus causation has been suspected for a number of tumours of fish. These include fish pox, a benign localised, epidermal hyperplasia particularly of carp (*vide supra*); epidermal non-invasive papillomas of young flathead sole; fibroepithelial tumours or 'Cauliflower disease' of the European eel and cod; superficial wart-like papillomas among intensively farmed Scandinavian salmon; highly vascularized papillomas of lips and oral epithelium in the Brown Bullhead; sarcomatous dermal nodules in walleye fish; and tumours of the kidneys and other organs of aquarium fish. In a number of these conditions presumptive evidence of an associated virus has been obtained by transmission experiments and with electron microscopy of smear preparations and ultra-thin sections. Most fish virologists believe that some at least of the many fish tumours will ultimately be proved to have a viral aetiology.

Clem's bluegill 'orphan' virus

The first fish 'orphan' virus was isolated in 1965 during investigations of a benign giant-cell disease of bluegills. It was observed that cultures of the GF line of grunt cells underwent spontaneous degeneration at the 65th passage level and that the cytopathic changes were readily transmissible from culture to culture.

The grunt fin agent (GFA), or Clem virus, multiplies in the cytoplasm and produces a cytopathic effect when inoculated into the CAR line of goldfish cells but does not replicate in RTG-2, KB and HeLa cells, nor in developing hens' eggs. It is heat-labile and is completely inactivated in serum-free media at 45°C for 15 minutes or 37°C for 1 hour. It is ether-sensitive but does not agglutinate red blood cells from mammals or fish. Electron microscopy of ultra-thin sections reveals dense, electron-opaque particles about 70 nm across and larger, immature, empty particles measuring 90–120 nm. in diameter. The nucleoid contains RNA. Attempts to induce disease in young experimental bluegills has proved unsuccessful and the virus is considered as an 'orphan', an agent without an associated disease. It is presently classified as a member of the Myxovirus group (Chapter 43).

Chemotherapy

A variety of chemotherapeutic substances have been used in attempts to control bacterial diseases of fish, particularly aeromonas diseases and other generalized infections causing high mortality rates. The substances employed have included mercury salts and malachite green as well as oxytetracycline, chlortetracycline, furazolidone, sulphamerazine, sulphasoxizole and other agents commonly used for the control of diseases in warm-blooded animals.

Preparations of mercury, including mercurous chloride, pyridylmercuric acetate and ethyl mercury phosphate, when added to water are absorbed by fish, and concentrations greater than 0·05 ppm. may be toxic and also a hazard to public health by rendering fish meat toxic for human consumption. These risks can arise either as a result of prolonged application of these preparations for the control of specific diseases or from the contamination of polluted waters with industrial effluents containing salts of mercury.

Chemotherapeutic substances used for the control of diseases in warm-blooded animals can be employed for the control of fish diseases either by addition of water or by injection. Relatively high concentrations of these substances can be obtained in the tissues but their general application to the control of disease is of limited value. As in mammals, these chemotherapeutic agents may reduce mortality rates but many individuals will remain carriers of the infective agents and potential sources of infection to other susceptible fish. Moreover, it has been found that their prolonged use may retard the growth of young fish.

Public health aspects

It is rare for species of bacteria which cause disease in man to be pathogenic for fish. However, fish may become infected with human bacterial pathogens and these organisms while not producing clinical disease, may remain viable in fish for variable periods of time and thus constitute a potential hazard to human health, either by contaminating fish meat or by constituting a risk to fish handlers. Reports on the variety of bacterial species pathogenic to man which have been isolated from fish in different parts of the world, emphasise the importance of pollution of waters, particularly with human sewage, as being one of the most serious factors responsible for increasing the incidence of these organisms in fish

Enteric pathogens, including salmonellae and shigellae, have been identified in fish from polluted waters, and under these circumstances fish act as temporary carriers, only. Experimentally, it has been shown that oral dosage of fish with large numbers of viable salmonellae results in excretion of these bacteria in faeces during the subsequent few days, and in most cases the infection is eliminated over a period of 7–14 days or more, and seldom continues for longer than 3 weeks. It has also recently been observed under natural conditions, that fish in polluted waters may have appreciable levels of serum antibodies to shigellae, salmonellae and E. coli, which would indicate that in this unhygienic environment repeated infection with these organisms and to some extent colonization of the bacteria in fish tissues, must take place to cause noticeable stimulation of antibody production. It is also noteworthy that molluscs living in in-shore polluted waters may carry enteric bacteria and are a risk to public health, especially when eaten raw.

Clostridium botulinum type E infections in fish constitute another potential hazard to human health. Surveys have shown that viable spores of this organism are distributed on the sea bed in different parts of the world, and it is also significant that toxin production is known to take place at temperatures as low as 5°C. There are reports of fish products having been incriminated as sources of human botulism associated with type E toxin, and the increasing potential risk to public health from modern methods of packaging fish and fish products which may encourage the growth of anaerobic bacteria have been emphasized, particularly in relation to human fish foods which are eaten raw. The toxin is susceptible to heat treatment and is destroyed during cooking.

A number of other bacterial species pathogenic for man have been identified in fish and fish products. Fish may be symptomless carriers of Leptospira icterohaemorrhagiae. The organism can penetrate gill tissue from infected water and colonise in the liver, kidney and muscle tissues. Similarly, Erysipelothrix insidiosa may occur in fish tissue and give rise to erysipeloid infection on the skin of fish handlers which takes the form of painful swellings of fingers and hands with greyish discolouration of the skin over the affected areas. Vibrio parahaemolyticus is a pathogen of fish and shellfish and is capable of causing human enteritis. Staphylococcus pyogenes has been isolated from fish products and it is probable that this type of infection is derived from fish handlers who are carriers of the organism and may contaminate the products during preparation. Other pathogens which may occur in fish products include Listeria monocytogenes, Mycobacterium fortuitum from tropical fresh water fish, Clostridium tetani and species of Nocardia and Pasteurella.

Further reading

ANACKER R.L. AND ORDAL E.J. (1959) Studies on the Myxobacterium Chondrococcus columnaris. I. Serological typing. Journal of Bacteriology, **78**, 25.

AVTALION, R.R. (1969) Temperature Effect on Antibody Production and Immunological Memory, in Carp [Cyprinus carpio] immunized against bovine serum albumin [BSA]. *Immunology*, **17**, 927.

AVTALION, R.R. WOJDANI, A., MALIK, Z., SHAHRA-BANI, R. and DUCZYMINER, M. (1973) Influence of environmental temperature on the immune response in fish. *Current Topics in Microbiology and Immunology*, **61**, 1.

CHILLER, J.M., HODGINS, H.O., CHAMBERS, V.C. AND WEISER, R.S. (1969) Antibody response in Rainbow Trout [*Salmo gairdneri*]. I. Immunocompetent cells in the spleen and anterior kidney. *Journal of Immunology*, **102**, 1193.

CHILLER, J.M., HODGINS, H.O. and WEISER, R.S. (1969) Antibody response in Rainbow Trout [*Salmo gairdneri*]. II. Studies on the kinetics of development of antibody-producing cells and on complement and natural hemolysin. *Journal of Immunology*, **102**, 1202.

CUSHING, J.E. (1942) An effect of temperature upon antibody production in fish. *Journal of Immunology*, **45**, 123.

HODGINS, H.O., WEISER, R.S. AND RIDGWAY, G.J. (1967) The nature of antibodies and the immune response in Rainbow trout [*Salmo gairdneri*]. *Journal of Immunology*, **99**, 534.

KINKELIN, P. DE, GALIMARD, B. AND BOOTSMA, R. (1973) Isolation and identification of the causative agent of "red disease" of pike [*Esox Lucius* L. 1766]. *Nature*, **241**, 465.

MARCHALONIS, J.J. (1971) Isolation and Partial Characterisation of Immunoglobulins of Goldfish [*Carassius auratus*] and Carp [*Cyprinus carpio*] *Immunology*, **20**, 161.

MARLSBERGER, R.G. AND CERINI, C.P. (1963) Characteristics of infectious pancreatic necrosis virus. *Journal of Bacteriology*, **86**, 1283.

MASON SMITH, A., POTTER, M. AND MERCHANT, E.B. (1967) Antibody-forming cells in the Pronephros of the Teleost *Lepomis macrochirus*. *Journal of Immunology*, **99**, 876.

MAWDESLEY-THOMAS, L.E., ed. (1972) *Symposium on Diseases of Fish* pp. 380. New York: Academic Press.

MAWDESLEY-THOMAS, L.E. (1972) Research into fish diseases. *Nature*, **235**, 17.

MURPHY, T. (1973) Ulcerative dermal necrosis [UDN] of salmonids. A review. *Irish Veterinary Journal*, **27**, 85.

PARISOT, T.J. (1958) Tuberculosis of fish. A review of the literature with a description of the disease in Salmonid fish. *Bacteriological Reviews*, **22**, 240.

PEARSON, W.E. (1971) Fish diseases. *Veterinary Annual*, **12**, 109.

ROBERTS, R.J., SHEARER, W.M., MUNRO, A.L.S. AND ELSON, K.G.R. (1969) The pathology of ulcerative dermal necrosis of Scottish Salmon. *Journal of Pathology and Bacteriology*, **97**, 563.

SMITH, W.W. (1940) Production of anti-bacterial agglutinins by carp and trout at 10°C. *Proceedings of the Society for Experimental Biology and Medicine*, **45**, 726.

STUART, M.R. AND FULLER, H.T. (1968) Mycological aspects of diseased Atlantic Salmon. *Nature*, **217**, 90.

Third Symposium on Diseases of Fish [Stockholm] (1968) *Bulletin officiel de la Société internationale de l' Epizoote*, **69**, 969 and 1349.

WILLOUGHBY, L.G. (1968) Atlantic Salmon disease Fungus, *Nature*, **217**, 872.

WOLF, K. (1965) Some recent developments and applications of fish cell and tissue culture. *Progress in Fish Culture*, **27**, 67.

WOLF, K. (1966) The fish viruses. *Advances in Virus Research*, **12**, 35.

APPENDIX 2
LABORATORY METHODS

APPENDIX 2

Laboratory methods

Serological Techniques

Bacterial agglutination tests

When a suspension of bacteria (i.e. antigen) is mixed with serum containing an optimal concentration of specific homologous antibody in the presence of an electrolyte, an antigen-antibody reaction takes place in which the antibody molecules join together the bacterial cells into clumps (i.e. agglutination), which settle to the bottom of the tube leaving a clear supernatant fluid. When no agglutination occurs the fluid appears uniformly opaque because the bacteria remain in even suspension.

An agglutination test is carried out by mixing in tubes a series of serum dilutions with constant amounts of antigen, incubating the mixtures at 37°C or 52°C in an incubator or waterbath, and then observing the amount of agglutination which has occurred in each tube.

The *titre* of an antiserum is the greatest dilution which will cause agglutination, visible to the naked eye, of a standard amount of antigen, and is a measure of the concentration of antibody in the serum. Thus, if the greatest dilution of serum causing agglutination is 1/500 in a volume of 1·0 ml, the titre of the serum can be expressed as 500 units of antibody per ml of antiserum. Provided that different batches of one type of antigen are standardised to the same concentration of bacteria per ml, the agglutination titres of all sera tested against different batches of that antigen can be compared directly one with another.

Agglutination tests can be used for estimating the concentration in sera of antibodies against particular bacterial antigens for the diagnosis of infectious diseases in animals (e.g. brucellosis, salmonellosis). Conversely, the test may also be employed for the identification of unknown organisms, in which a suspension of the bacteria to be identified is used as antigen in an agglutination test with known antisera (e.g. serotyping of salmonellae).

Preparation of bacterial antigens
O-antigens. The common method for preparing these antigens consists of growing the organisms on nutrient agar and suspending the growth in saline. The bacteria are then killed by one of the following methods:

(1) Heat (e.g. boiling in a waterbath to destroy flagellar antigens or to remove capsular material from *E. coli* and expose the O-antigen).

(2) Suspending in phenol saline to act as a preservative and prevent the growth of contaminants during storage.

(3) Alcohol — the growth from an agar slope is suspended in about 2 ml of saline, transferred to a clean test tube and 20 ml absolute alcohol added. The resulting precipitate of killed bacteria is removed after centrifugation with the minimum amount of alcohol, and suspended in saline to the required density. This method of preparation destroys flagella and leaves the O-antigen exposed for an agglutination reaction.

H-antigens. These can be prepared by culturing an actively motile strain of bacteria in nutrient broth for 18 hours and then adding formalin in the proportion of 10 drops of 40 per cent formaldehyde to 10 ml of broth culture. Alternatively, the growth from nutrient agar can be suspended in formol saline and will make a satisfactory H-antigen provided that the culture on agar was actively motile. The surface of the agar should be slightly moist to ensure active motility of the culture.

Doubling dilution method (Fig. A2.1)
(1) Using a graduated 5·0 ml pipette, place 0·8 ml saline into the first tube and 0·5 ml into each of the remaining tubes.

(2) Using a graduated 1·0 ml pipette, place 0·2 ml of serum to be tested in the first tube. Mix with the saline by sucking in and out of the pipette gently to avoid producing bubbles.

(3) Transfer 0·5 ml of this mixture to the second

337

	①	②	③	④	⑤	⑥	⑦	⑧		ⓒ
NaC1	0.8	0.5	0.5	0.5	0.5	0.5	0.5	0.5		0.5
Serum	0.2	0.5	0.5	0.5	0.5	0.5	0.5	0.5	→ 0.5 discard	
Antigen	0.5	0.5	0.5	0.5	0.5	0.5	0.5	0.5		0.5
Dilutions	$\frac{1}{10}$	$\frac{1}{20}$	$\frac{1}{40}$	$\frac{1}{80}$	$\frac{1}{160}$	$\frac{1}{320}$	$\frac{1}{640}$	$\frac{1}{1280}$		Control

(Volumes measured in mls.)

FIG. A2.1. Procedure for an agglutination test — doubling dilution method.

tube, mix with the 0·5 ml saline in this tube, and tranfer 0·5 ml to the third tube.

(4) Continue making these dilutions of serum in each successive tube. After mixing serum and saline in the last tube of the series, discard 0·5 ml of the mixture.

(5) Do not add serum to the control tube.

(6) Using a graduated 5·0 ml pipette, add 0·5 ml antigen to each tube including the control tube.

perpendicular position and drops counted at the rate of 1 per sec., this technique is an accurate method for measuring small volumes of fluids.

(1) Place 5, 8, 9 and 10 drops of saline into tubes 2, 3, 4 and the control tube (C), respectively.

(2) Place 18 drops of saline into a separate dilution tube and add 2 drops of serum. Mix gently by sucking in and out of the pipette to avoid producing bubbles. This is now a 1:10 dilution of the serum.

	①	②	③	④	ⓒ
NaCl	0	5	8	9	10
Serum $\left(\frac{1}{10}\right)$	10	5	2	1	0
Antigen	15	15	15	15	15
Dilutions	$\frac{1}{25}$	$\frac{1}{50}$	$\frac{1}{125}$	$\frac{1}{250}$	Control

(Volumes measured in drops)

FIG. A2.2. Procedure for agglutination test — drop dilution method.

(7) Incubate in a waterbath overnight at 37°C or 52°C and read the result on the following morning. The antigen in the control tube should remain evenly dispersed throughout the test.

Drop dilution method (Fig. A2.2)

This is a useful and rapid method applicable to the identification of unknown organisms when using specific antisera with known titres of (say) 1:250. All volumes are measured by drops delivered from a pipette made by drawing out a length of glass tubing to a narrow capillary which should be cut off evenly at the tip. When the pipette is held in a

(3) Add 10, 5, 2 and 1 drops of diluted serum to tubes 1, 2, 3 and 4, respectively. Do not add any to the control tube.

(4) Rinse the pipette thoroughly in saline.

(5) Add 15 drops of antigen to each tube, including the control tube (C).

(6) Incubate in a waterbath overnight at 37°C or 52°C and read the result on the following morning. The antigen in the control tube should remain evenly dispersed throughout the test.

Rapid slide agglutination method

This is a useful laboratory technique for rapidly

identifying the antigenic structure of an unknown strain of bacteria, and is commonly applied as a preliminary step in the serological identification of salmonellae and other groups of the family *Enterobacteriaceae*.

Loopfuls of known antisera are placed on a slide and with the aid of a straight wire, small quantities of bacterial growth from the culture to be tested are emulsified in the drops of antisera. Rapid agglutination observed under a hand lens or low power microscope will give some indication of the probable antigenic structure of the culture being examined, but because of the possibility of non-specific reactions occurring when using heavy suspensions of bacteria and low dilutions of antisera, all results should be confirmed by tube agglutination tests.

Agglutinin-absorption test
This test is used for the differentiation of two organisms which have a common antigen as well as their own specific antigens, and is based on the fact that antibodies which have combined with antigens on the surfaces of bacteria are 'absorbed' and can be subsequently removed from the serum by centrifugation and separation of the bacteria. In this way, an antiserum containing antibodies against a specific antigenic component can be prepared and used for the routine differentiation of one bacterial species from other antigenically related species.

Example
The flagellar antigens of *S. enteritidis* are gm and those of *S. dublin* are gp. Both organisms possess similar somatic antigens (9, 12).

When an antiserum prepared against the antigens gm of *S. enteritidis* is absorbed with the flagellar antigens gp of *S. dublin*, agglutinins to the factor 'g' will be absorbed from the serum which will then contain agglutinins to factor 'm', only. Conversely, absorption of a 'gp' antiserum with 'gm' antigens will remove factor 'g' agglutinins and leave only factor 'p' agglutinins in the serum.

In this way, single factor sera containing agglutinins to either factor 'm' or factor 'p' can be prepared and used for the differentiation of the two organisms *S. enteritidis* and *S. dublin*.

The general procedure for carrying out absorptions is to prepare a heavy suspension of washed bacteria from an agar culture and to add this to an equal volume of a high titred antiserum which has been previously diluted. (Dilution of the serum, beforehand, facilitates the thorough absorption of homologous antibodies). The mixture is then incubated at 37°C for 4 hours and the contents of the tube repeatedly mixed during this time. The bacteria are then removed by centrifugation. Sometimes it may be necessary to repeat the process with additional

preparations of antigen before absorption is complete. It should be noted that after each absorption the final dilution of the serum will be doubled.

Complement-fixation test
The complement-fixation test is one of the most useful serological techniques available in microbiology, and is based on the fixation of complement by antigen–antibody aggregates. Essentially, the procedure comprises two steps: (a) a primary reaction where antigen, antibody and complement are allowed to interact and (b) a secondary reaction in which red blood cells sensitized by specific red cell antibodies serve as an indicator system for the amount of complement fixed in the primary reaction. Absence of haemolysis indicates fixation of complement in the test system, and the result is positive.

Materials required
(1) *Diluent* — 'Veronal' buffer (VB) is used as diluent throughout the test. It contains Ca and Mg ions which allow full fixation of complement at high dilutions of serum. Sodium azide (0·08 per cent) should be added to VB for dilutions of antigens and antisera as these must be held for several days.

(2) *Sheep erythrocytes* — A 4 per cent suspension of freshly washed sheep red blood cells resuspended in VB.

(3) *Haemolytic serum* — a serum containing antibodies to sheep red blood cells which has usually been prepared in horses or rabbits.

(4) *Complement* — Obtained from pooled samples of guinea-pig sera. Complement is unstable and should not be diluted for use until immediately before being required in the test.

(5) *Antigen* — The technique to be described is suitable for viral antigens.

(6) *Antiserum to be tested* — This must be heated before use to 56°C for 30 minutes to inactivate complement.

Preparation of materials for test
Haemolytic system. This consists of sheep red cells sensitized with antibody contained in the haemolytic serum. The latter can be obtained from commercial sources with instructions giving the procedure to be followed for the sensitization of sheep red cells. This consists essentially of mixing optimal quantities of haemolytic serum (e.g. 5MHD) with sensitized red blood cells, incubating in a waterbath for 10–30 minutes, washing the cells in buffered saline and resuspending them to give a final concentration of 2 per cent. This suspension of antibody-sensitized red cells constitutes the haemolytic system ready for use.

Complement. This is obtainable from commercial sources as preserved guinea-pig serum. Because the complement is hypertonic it should be diluted immediately before use by adding 1 volume to 7 volumes of *deionised* water which is equivalent to a 1 in 10 dilution of fresh guinea-pig serum in saline.

Antigen. When a known antigen is being used it

should be prepared by diluting to optimal concentration in the diluent.

Titration of complement (Fig. A2.3a)
The minimal amount of complement required to haemolyse similar volumes of different preparations of haemolytic systems may vary. Before carrying out a complement-fixation test it is necessary to ensure that the amount of complement incorporated in the

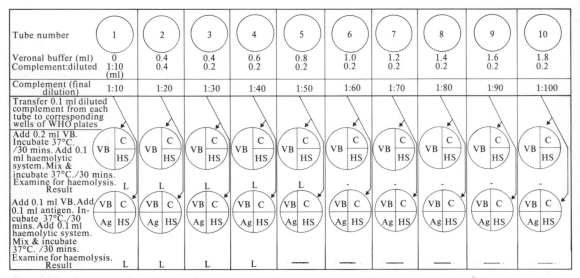

FIG. A2.3a. Procedure for titration of complement. C = complement, VB = veronal buffer, HS = haemolytic system, Ag = antigen, L = lysis, — = no lysis. The final volume of fluid in each well is 0·4 ml.

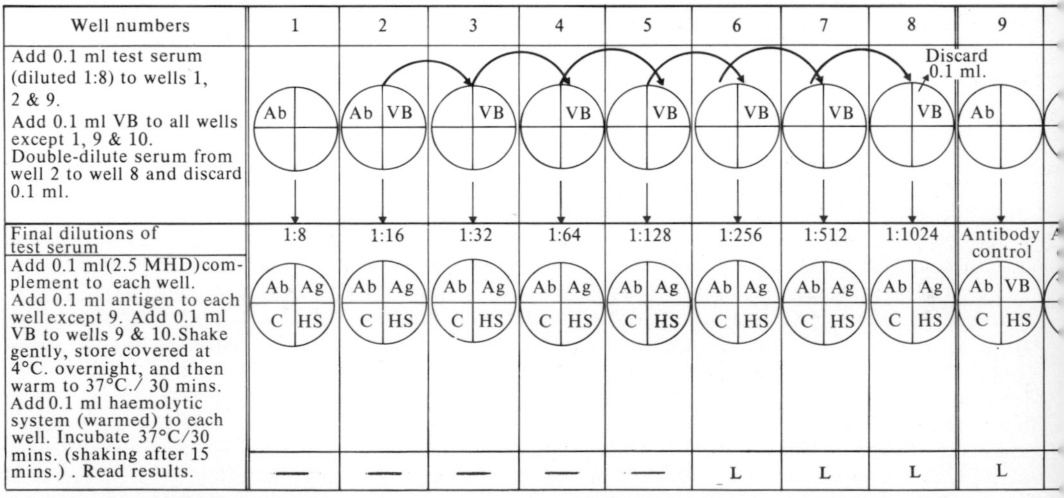

FIG. A2.3b. Procedure for complement-fixation test (test proper). C = complement, VB = veronal buffer, HS = haemolytic system, MHD = minimal haemolytic dose, Ag = antigen, Ab = antibody, L = lysis, — = no lysis. The final volume of fluid in each well is 0·4 ml.

test is sufficient to cause complete haemolysis of the haemolytic system and to leave available an excess sufficient to neutralize occasional anti-complementary activities of some test sera, without interfering with the final test result. The anti-complementary activities of test sera are thermostable and may be caused by bacterial or chemical contamination of the test serum or by an abnormally high concentration of γ-globulin. The titration of complement estimates the minimal haemolytic dose (MHD) which is the least amount of complement required to cause complete lysis of the haemolytic system under defined conditions, and for optimal results in the following example of a complement-fixation test using a viral antigen, 2·5 MHD are used in the final test.

Procedure

(1) Make up a 1:10 dilution of complement in VB.

(2) Prepare in tubes serial dilutions of complement in VB extending from 1:10 to 1:100.

(3) Working from tube 10 to tube 1, transfer 0·1 ml diluted complement from each tube to each of two corresponding upper and lower rows of wells in a clean perspex WHO plate.

(4) To each well in the upper row add 0·2 ml VB (This volume represents the patient's serum plus test antigen).

(5) To each well in the lower row add 0·1 ml VB followed by 0·1 ml test antigen.

(6) Incubate at 37°C for 30 minutes for short fixation or at 4°C overnight for long fixation.

(7) Add 0·1 ml warmed, freshly prepared haemolytic system to each well in both rows.

(8) Mix by gentle agitation.

(9) Incubate at 37°C for 30 minutes, shake occasionally.

(10) Reagitate to ensure that all cells are suspended and examine for haemolysis.

From the test recorded in Fig. A2.3a, the highest dilution of complement causing lysis of the haemolytic system in the presence of antigen is 1:40.

Thus, the titre of complement is 1:40, and 0·1 ml of this dilution contains 1 MHD.

Therefore, 2·5 MHD of complement are contained in 0·1 ml of $1/40 \times 5/2 = 1:16$ dilution.

For the following complement-fixation test, this preparation of complement should be diluted 1:16 before use.

Complement-fixation test (test proper) (Fig. A2.3b)
Procedure
(*A*) *Preparation of serum dilutions*

(1) Dilute the test serum 1:8 in VB and inactivate by heating to 56°C for 30 minutes.

(2) Add 0·1 ml of the serum to wells 1, 2 and 9.

(3) Add 0·1 ml VB to wells 2–8, inclusive.

(4) Mix serum and diluent in well 2 and transfer 0·1 ml to well 3. Mix and transfer 0·1 ml to well 4. Continue in this manner to well 8, and after mixing, discard 0·1 ml. This will give doubling dilutions of serum extending from 1:8 to 1:1024.

(*B*) *Completion of test*

(5) Add 0·1 ml complement (containing 2·5 MHD) to each well.

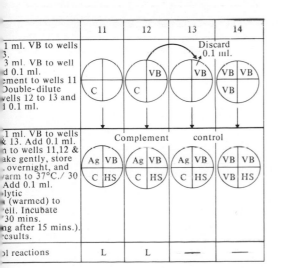

(6) Add 0·1 ml antigen at optimal dilution to each well, except 9 which is used as an antibody control test.

(7) Add 0·1 ml VB to wells 9 and 10. Well 10 is used as an antigen control test.

(8) Using wells 11–14, add 0·1 ml VB to wells 12 and 13, and 0·3 ml to well 14. Add 0·1 ml complement to wells 11 and 12. Mix complement with saline in well 12, transfer 0·1 ml to well 13, mix and discard 0·1 ml. Add 0·1 ml saline to wells 11, 12 and 13 and then add 0·1 ml antigen to wells 11, 12 and 13.

(9) Shake gently and incubate at 4°C overnight.

(10) Warm the plate at 37°C for 30 minutes.

(11) Add 0·1 ml of warmed haemolytic system (i.e. 2 per cent sensitized sheep red cells) to all wells, including controls.

(12) Incubate at 37°C for 15 minutes, shake and reincubate for a further 15 minutes.

(13) Read the test for haemolysis, store at 4°C for one hour and make a final reading.

Interpretation

Where complement has been fixed by the virus-antibody complex, there is no lysis, and the red blood cells sediment to the bottom of the well. Thus, in the example shown in Fig. A2.3b, the highest dilution of serum in which approximately 100 per cent of cells are remaining (1/128) is taken as the titre of that serum.

Staining methods
Loeffler's alkaline methylene blue stain (L.A.M.B.)

Reagents
Saturated solution of methylene blue in alcohol and an aqueous solution of potassium hydroxide.

Method
(1) Prepare film, dry in air and fix by passing through flame.

(2) Flood slide with stain and allow to act for 2–3 minutes.

(3) Wash in water, blot and dry.

(4) Examine under oil immersion.

Appearance
Vegetative bacteria are stained blue.

Polychrome methylene blue stain

Reagents
Methylene blue solution which has been allowed to oxidise by storing for several months.

Method
(1) Prepare film, dry in air and fix by passing through flame.

(2) Flood slide with stain and allow to act for 2–3 minutes.

(3) Wash in water, blot and dry.

(4) Examine under oil immersion.

Appearance
B. anthracis stains blue and capsular material pale pink (MacFadyean's reaction). *Note* The blotting paper should be burned after use in case it has become contaminated with anthrax spores.

Gram's stain

Reagents
(1) Methyl violet (0·5 per cent) in distilled water.

(2) Iodine (1·0 per cent), potassium iodide (2·0 per cent) in distilled water.

(3) Absolute alcohol.

(4) (a) Basic fuchsin (0·05 per cent) in distilled water, or

  (b) Neutral red (0·1 per cent), acetic acid 0·002 per cent) in distilled water.

Method
(1) Prepare film, dry in air, and fix by passing through flame.

(2) Flood with methyl violet and stain for 2 minutes.

(3) Wash in water.

(4) Flood with iodine solution and allow to act for 1 minute. (This will 'fix' methyl violet to Gram-positive staining organisms and inhibit its removal by alcohol or acetone.)

(5) Wash thoroughly in water.

(6) Flood with alcohol and gently rock slide until colour ceases to leave film (about 30 seconds). This will remove methyl violet (i.e. decolourise) from those bacteria which stain Gram-negative.

(Acetone may be used in place of alcohol for decolourisation, and should be applied for 3–5 seconds only).

(7) Promptly wash thoroughly in tap water.

(8) Counterstain with fuchsin or neutral red for 30 seconds.

(9) Wash in water, blot and dry.

(10) Examine under oil immersion.

Appearance
Bacteria which stain Gram-positive will be coloured violet. Bacteria which stain Gram-negative will be coloured pink. Dead bacteria which normally stain Gram-positive will not retain the methyl violet dye and will tend to stain Gram-negative. The reason for bacteria staining either Gram-positive or Gram-negative has not been fully explained. It may be that the higher acid content of the protoplasm in the

former enables them to retain basic dyes, particularly after treatment with iodine. It is also probable that the cell walls of Gram-negative bacteria allow basic dyes to diffuse out under the action of the decolouriser, but that the intact walls of Gram-positive bacteria prevent this diffusion as a result of the interaction between the iodine and the dye.

Ziehl-Neelsen's stain

Reagents
(1) Strong carbol fuchsin solution, containing basic fuchsin (1 per cent), phenol and absolute alcohol.
(2) Acid-alcohol solution containing concentrated HC1 (3 per cent) and alcohol (97 per cent).
(3) Loeffler's alkaline methylene blue or aqueous malachite green (1 per cent).

Method
(1) Prepare film, dry in air and fix by passing through flame.
(2) Flood slide with carbol fuchsin solution. Heat at intervals until steam rises without boiling the fluid. Allow to act for at least 5 minutes. (Stain must not be allowed to dry on the slide. Add more stain if required to keep surface of slide covered).
(3) Wash in water.
(4) Decolourise by flooding slide with acid-alcohol solution for at least 5 minutes, rock and pour off. Rinse in acid-alcohol.
(5) Wash in water.
(6) Counterstain with Loeffler's methylene blue or malachite green for 30 seconds.
(7) Wash in water, blot and dry.
(8) Examine under oil immersion.

Appearance
Acid-alcohol-fast organisms (e.g. mycobacteria) stain pink against a blue or green background.
Note. In cases where the operator suffers from colour blindness, acid-alcohol-fast organisms may be observed more readily against a yellow background, and films should be counterstained with picric acid in place of Loeffler's methylene blue or malachite green.

Differential stain for Brucella
This technique is a modification of Macchiavello's method and can also be used for distinguishing certain rickettsiae and chlamydiae.

Reagents
(1) Dilute carbol fuchsin solution (1:10 dilution of strong Ziehl-Neelsen's carbol fuchsin in distilled water).
(2) Acetic acid solution (0·5 per cent).

(3) Loeffler's alkaline methylene blue.

Method
(1) Prepare film, dry in air and fix by passing through flame.
(2) Flood slide with dilute carbol fuchsin solution and allow to act for 15 minutes.
(3) Wash in water.
(4) Decolourise by flooding slide with acetic acid solution for 10 seconds.
(5) Wash in water.
(6) Counterstain with Loeffler's methylene blue for 2 minutes.
(7) Wash in water.
(8) Examine under oil immersion.

Appearance
Brucella organisms stain pink against a blue background.

Leishman's stain

Reagents
This stain is usually purchased ready for use. It is prepared by heating methylene blue with sodium carbonate. This treated form of methylene blue is then mixed with water-soluble eosin. The precipitate which forms is dissolved in methyl alcohol to give Leishman's stain.

Method
(1) Prepare film, dry in air but do not fix by heat.
(2) Cover film with the stain and allow to act for 1 minute. (The methyl alcohol in the stain will fix the film).
(3) Add twice the volume of distilled water to the stain on the slide with the aid of a pipette. Mix the water and stain by repeatedly sucking in and out of the pipette. Allow the diluted stain to act for 10 minutes.
(4) Gently flood the slide with distilled water and allow the film to differentiate in the distilled water until it appears bright pink.
(5) Wash thoroughly in distilled water, blot off excess water and dry.
(6) Examine under oil immersion.

Appearance
Pasteurella organisms show characteristic blue bipolar staining. Red blood cells stain pink. This staining technique may also be used for the diagnosis of tick-borne fever in sheep.

Giemsa's stain

Reagents
This stain is similar to Leishman's stain, consisting

of methylene blue and eosin, and can be purchased ready for use.

Method

(1) Prepare film, dry in air but do not fix by heat.

(2) The film is fixed by flooding with methyl alcohol for 3 minutes.

(3) Pour off alcohol and cover the film with 1 part stain and 10 parts buffer solution (pH 7·0) for 1 hour. Alternatively, the slides may be inverted for 18–24 hours in stain diluted 1/100.

(4) Wash off stain with buffer solution and allow film to differentiate for 1 minute.

(5) Blot off excess buffer solution and dry.

(6) Examine under oil immersion.

Appearance

The capsules of *B. anthracis* stain a more intense reddish-mauve colour than they do with polychrome methylene blue. *Note*: The blotting-paper should be burned after use in case it has become contaminated with *B. anthracis* spores.

Albert's stain for volutin granules

Reagents

(1) Solution of toluidine blue (0·15 per cent), malachite green (0·2 per cent), glacial acetic acid (1 per cent), alcohol (2 per cent) and distilled water.

(2) Gram's iodine solution.

Method

(1) Prepare film, dry in air and fix by passing through flame.

(2) Flood slide with solution containing stains and allow to act for 3–5 minutes.

(3) Wash in water, blot and dry.

(4) Flood slide with iodine solution and allow to act for 1 minute.

(5) Wash in water, blot and dry.

(6) Examine under oil immersion.

Appearance

The bacteria stain green and the volutin granules appear blueish-black.

Neisser's stain for volutin granules

Reagents

(1) Solution of methylene blue (0·1 per cent), glacial acetic acid (0·5 per cent), alcohol (5 per cent) and distilled water.

(2) Gram's iodine solution diluted 1:10 in water.

(3) Gram's neutral red solution.

Method

(1) Prepare film, dry in air and fix by passing through flame.

(2) Flood slide with methylene blue stain and allow to act for 3 minutes.

(3) Wash off stain with dilute iodine, and leave the film covered with some of the solution for 1 minute.

(4) Wash in water.

(5) Counterstain with neutral red solution for 3 minutes.

(6) Wash in water, blot and dry.

(7) Examine under oil immersion.

Appearance

The bacteria stain pink and the volutin granules appear dark blue.

India ink for demonstration of capsules (wet film)

Reagents

India ink which has been shaken with glass beads.

Method

(1) Place loopful of ink in centre of clean glass slide.

(2) Mix a *small* amount of bacterial growth with the ink.

(3) Cover the mixture with a clean coverslip and press firmly between several layers of blotting paper.

(4) Examine under oil immersion.

Appearance

Bacterial capsules will appear as clear spaces between the refractile edges of the bacteria and the surrounding dark grey background of India ink. The method can be applied to the examination of cerebrospinal fluids, tissue extracts and has also been used for the identification of some yeasts.

India ink for demonstration of capsules (dry film)

Reagents

(1) Glucose solution (6 per cent)

(2) India ink

(3) Methyl alcohol

(4) Methyl violet solution (Gram's stain).

Method

(1) Emulsify a small amount of bacterial culture in a loopful of glucose solution at one end of the slide.

(2) Add a loopful of India ink and mix thoroughly.

(3) Spread the mixture over the slide as for a blood film.

(4) Dry in air.

(5) Fix the film by covering with methyl alcohol for 15 seconds.

(6) Drain and dry.

(7) Stain with methyl violet for 2 minutes.

(8) Wash in water, blot and dry.

Appearance

Bacterial capsules will appear as clear spaces surrounding the violet stained bacteria on a dark grey background of India ink.

Strong carbol fuchsin for demonstration of spores

Reagents

(1) Strong carbol fuchsin (Ziehl–Neelsen).
(2) Sulphuric acid solution (0·5 per cent.).
(3) Loeffler's alkaline methylene blue.

Method

(1) Prepare film, dry in air and fix by passing through flame.
(2) Flood slide with strong carbol fuchsin. Heat at intervals until steam rises without boiling the fluid. Allow to act for 5 minutes.
(3) Wash in water.
(4) Decolourise by flooding slide with sulphuric acid solution and allow to act for 1 minute.
(5) Wash in water.
(6) Counterstain with Loeffler's methylene blue for 2 minutes.
(7) Wash in water, blot and dry.
(8) Examine under oil immersion.

Appearance

Spores stain pink and vegetative bacilli stain blue.

Fontana's staining method for spirochaetes

Reagents

(1) Fixative solution comprising acetic acid (1·0 per cent) and formalin (2·0 per cent) in distilled water.
(2) Mordant solution comprising phenol (1·0 per cent) and tannic acid (5·0 per cent) in distilled water.
(3) Ammoniated silver nitrate solution prepared by adding ammonia (10·0 per cent) to 0·5 per cent solution of silver nitrate in distilled water until the precipitate which forms, dissolves and then reappears and persists after shaking.

Method

(1) Prepare the film and dry in the atmosphere.
(2) Cover the film with the fixative solution and allow to act for 2 minutes.
(3) Wash off the fixative solution with absolute alcohol, cover the film with alcohol and allow to act for 3 minutes.
(4) Drain off the alcohol and carefully burn off the remainder until the film is dry.
(5) Cover film with mordant solution, heat till steam rises and allow to act for 30 seconds.
(6) Wash thoroughly in distilled water and allow to dry.

(7) Cover film with ammoniated silver nitrate solution, heat till steam rises and allow to act for 30 seconds when the film becomes brown in colour.
(8) Wash thoroughly in distilled water, dry and mount in Canada balsam under a coverslip. (Immersion oil may cause the colour of the smear to fade).
(9) Examine under oil immersion.

Appearance

Spirochaetes appear dark brown in colour against a yellowish-brown background.

Lactophenol cotton blue for mycological specimens

Reagents

Phenol (pure crystals)	20 g
Lactic acid	20 ml
Glycerol	40 ml
Distilled water	20 ml

Dissolve by heating gently under a hot water tap. Add 0·05 g cotton blue.

Method

Used for the preparation of semi-permanent stained mycological specimens. Slide-culture mounts or small pieces of mycelium teased out on a clean slide in lactophenol cotton blue are sealed with nail varnish.

Gram-Claudius stain for mycological specimens

Method

(1) Stain in methyl violet (1 per cent aqueous solution) for 3–5 min.
(2) Treat with 2 parts of picric acid (concentrated aqueous solution) for 1 min.
(3) Wash in water and dry.
(4) Decolourise with clove oil.
(5) Wash off clove oil with xylol.
(6) Mount in xylol-balsam.

Appearance

Fungi and yeasts stain blue against a yellow background.

Haematoxylin and eosin staining technique for coverslip preparations.

Used for the examination of tissue reactions to microbial infections.

Method

(1) Wash coverslip preparation in warm (37°C) buffered saline.
(2) Fix in Dubosque (alcohol Bouin's) fluid for not less than 30 minutes.
(3) Wash in 70 per cent alcohol, absolute alcohol and then acetone (few seconds only).

(4) Re-wash in absolute alcohol and then 70 per cent alcohol.

(5) Wash thoroughly in running tap water and then in distilled water.

(6) Stain with Harris' acid haematoxylin for 30 seconds.

(7) Wash in running tap water.

(8) Pass briefly in lithium carbonate or sodium carbonate until the preparation is blue. This also removes picric acid.

(9) Wash in running tap water.

(10) Stain with eosin for 10 minutes.

(11) Wash thoroughly.

(12) Pass through fresh 70 per cent alcohol (or acetone).

(13) Pass through fresh absolute alcohol (or acetone/xylol).

(14) Pass through xylol.

(15) Mount in DePeX.

Acridine Orange for nucleic acid

Reagents

(1) 3 per cent HCl in 95 per cent alcohol.

(2) Citrate-phosphate buffer pH 3·8, consisting of 32·3 ml of 0·1M solution of citric acid plus 17·7 ml of 0·2M dibasic sodium phosphate solution.

(3) Acridine orange (0·1 per cent in distilled water).

Solutions 2 and 3 are prepared each week and stored at 4°C.

Method

(1) Dilute the Acridine Orange solution 1 in 10 with buffer.

(2) Place coverslip preparation in acid-alcohol to fix for 5 min.

(3) Rinse for 2 min in two changes of buffer.

(4) Stain with fresh 0·01 per cent. Acridine Orange for 4–10 min.

(5) Wash for 2 min in two changes of buffer.

(6) Mount in buffer.

(7) Ring coverslip with nail varnish.

Appearance

This dye has a marked affinity for the nucleic acids found in host cell-parasite relationships. When cells stained with this dye are viewed with u.v. light the RNA components fluoresce with shades of orange and red while DNA components take on shades of green. The method is of great value in studying the growth of animal viruses in their respective host cells. (Note: single stranded nucleic acid appears orange red and double stranded appears green). The method is applied to coverslip preparations of living cells, tissues and exudates.

Mann's method for staining inclusion bodies in tissue sections

Reagents

1 per cent methyl blue	35 ml
1 per cent aqueous eosin	45 ml
Distilled water	100 ml

Method

(1) Take the section to water.

(2) Leave the section in Mann's methyl-eosin for 30–60 mins.

(3) Wash and differentiate in tap water.

(4) Take the section to xylol and mount in DePeX.

Seller's stain for demonstrating Negri Bodies

Reagents

Stock solution:

(1)	Methylene blue	10 g
	Methyl alcohol (absolute acetone free)	1000 ml
(2)	Basic fuchsin	5 g
	Methyl alcohol (absolute acetone free)	500 ml

For use:

Mix 2 parts of solution (1) with 1 part of solution (2). Mix thoroughly but do not filter. Store in tightly stoppered container. The mixed stain improves after standing for 24 hours and keeps indefinitely if protected from evaporation.

Method

Prepare smears in the usual way. No fixation is necessary. Immediately, while the preparation is still moist, immerse it in the stain solution for 1–5 seconds. Rinse quickly in running water and dry in the air without blotting.

Sterilization

The essential requirement for practical bacteriology is the ability to be able to study a particular microbial species in pure culture. Thus, all equipment used for preparing, dispensing and storing media must be sterilized before use to prevent contamination from the atmosphere. Glassware is still extensively employed for these purposes but plastic disposable containers (e.g. Petri dishes for solid media) are being increasingly used for culture material and have the advantage that they can be purchased in sterile packs ready for use. In addition to equipment, the medium itself must also be sterile before use, so that no growth will take place except that derived from the inoculum of the particular microbial strain under examination. The following is a brief outline of the methods used for the sterilization of equipment and media in microbiological laboratories.

Dry Heat

Flaming:

A bunsen flame is commonly used for sterilizing wire loops, for heating spatulas used for searing the surfaces of organs prior to making cultures, and for sterilizing the mouths of test tubes and other glass containers when inoculating media.

Hot-air oven

An insulated cabinet which is heated usually by electricity to pre-set thermostatically controlled temperatures. Thus, the apparatus may be used as a drying oven when the temperature is controlled at a maximum of 80–100°C, or as a sterilizing oven for dry glassware when the temperature is maintained at a minimum of 160°C for 1–1½ hours. Before sterilization, flasks and test tubes should be dry and plugged with cotton wool, and pipettes should be wrapped individually in kraft paper or placed in pipette canisters. For cell cultures, cotton wool should not be used because it contains volatile oils which are toxic to living cells. Aluminium foil should be used for closing flasks and tubes employed for cell culture work.

Moist Heat

Vaccine bath

Used for the sterilization of sera and vaccines and consists of a thermostatically controlled waterbath. A temperature of 56°C for 1 hour is used repeatedly on successive days for sterilization of sera because at this temperature coagulation of the protein will not occur. For the sterilization of bacterial vaccines a temperature of 60°C maintained for 1 hour is commonly employed.

Inspissator

This is a water-jacketed container which is heated electrically under thermostatic control. It is used for the preparation of media containing serum or egg, and is usually operated at a temperature of about 80°C which allows solidification without the production of bubbles. Tubes of media are placed on sloping racks to provide a maximum surface area of solid medium. Drying of the media during inspissation is prevented by allowing steam to pass from above the level of water in the surrounding jacket into the container.

Steamer

This is essentially a metal box containing a small quantity of water which is boiled and the steam allowed to escape through a small hole in the conical lid. Above the level of water in the base of the steamer is a rack or perforated shelf on which are placed the flasks or bottles containing media to be sterilized. This method of heating to 100°C is particularly useful for the sterilization of sugars and other substances which would be decomposed by subjecting to higher temperatures. To ensure that both vegetative organisms and relatively heat-resistant spores are killed by steaming at 100°C, it is common practice to heat media to this temperature for 45 minutes on each of 3 successive days. This process is often referred to as 'Tyndallisation' and is based on the principle that the first steaming kills all vegetative organisms, and the spores which survive in the nutrient medium subsequently develop into vegetative organisms and are killed during the second steaming on the following day. A further steaming on the third day ensures that this process of sterilization is complete. Alternatively, it may be satisfactory to subject media to a single period of sterilization at 100°C for 1½ hours. This is usually lethal to most spores except those derived from thermophilic strains of organisms.

Boiling waterbath

This method can be used for sterilizing instruments, syringes, pipettes, etc. Boiling at 100°C for 10 minutes will kill vegetative organisms and some, but not all, types of spores.

Autoclave

This apparatus is essentially a closed container in which water is boiled under pressure and consequently the temperature rises above 100°C. It is the most useful and widely used method for sterilization because it is lethal to spores as well as to vegetative organisms.

A variety of models of autoclaves have been developed, either vertical or horizontal, and the steam is provided by heating water in the base of the autoclave or by a direct supply from a separate boiler. Some models have a steam jacket which heats the walls independently from the steam within the container itself, and this enables the contents to be dried after sterilization and before removal from the autoclave.

After loading the autoclave, the lid is closed and the source of steam turned on. With the escape valve open, steam is allowed to drive off all the air from the container; the valve is then closed and the pressure allowed to rise according to the setting on the pressure gauge. For most purposes a temperature of 120°C for 20 minutes (i.e. a pressure of approximately 15lb/in^2) is satisfactory, and the safety valve will maintain this temperature at a steady level. After this period the source of steam is turned off and when the pressure inside the autoclave has returned to atmospheric pressure, the valve is opened slowly and air allowed to enter. It is important not to open the valve before the pressure has returned to atmospheric level, otherwise liquids within the autoclave may boil over from their containers. Some models of autoclaves are fitted with automatic systems which control the whole process of heating-up, sterilization at a fixed temperature and pressure, and both cooling and drying in the case of steam-jacketed models.

Filtration
This is a useful method for removing bacteria from fluid substances which would be decomposed if sterilized by other methods. Filtration is widely applied to the sterilization of sera, toxins, antibiotic preparations and other labile substances. A variety of filters has been devised for these purposes.

Seitz filters
These consist of asbestos-type filter pads inserted in metal holders. The filter pads can be obtained in three grades of clarifying, normal and special, and each pad is discarded after use. The filters are manufactured in various sizes suitable for the filtration of small volumes of special fluids or large volumes of material during the preparation of media. Before filtration it is advisable to moisten the pad with saline to reduce the adsorptive capacity of the filter and to be able to effectively tighten the upper part of the metal holder on to the surface of the pad. Additional limitations to the method are that the pad causes a fall in pH of the filtrate which may also contain fibres derived from the pad.

Membrane filters
These are prepared from cellulose nitrate or cellulose acetate and are sometimes referred to as 'gradocol' or cellulose membrane filters. Their chemical composition can be varied so that the average pore diameter (APD) of these membranes can be graded to less than 20nm. These filters are increasingly employed in microbiological laboratories since they are less absorptive and allow more rapid filtration than Seitz filters, and are a useful means for estimating the sizes of viral particles.

Earthenware candles
Referred to as Berkefeld, Mandler or Chamberland filters, they are prepared from kieselgur or unglazed porcelain. They vary in porosity according to the granular size of the material used in their preparation, but the finer grade of porcelain candle will retain all but the smallest of viral particles. After use, these filters are cleaned and sterilised by brushing, boiling in distilled water and autoclaving.

Sintered glass filters
The glass filter mostly used is the grade No. 5 which has an APD of 1–1·5 μm and will retain most bacteria. The filter is cleaned by passing 2 per cent NaOH through it in the opposite direction to that in which it was last used. This is followed with N/1 HCl until the filter has a neutral pH, and is then washed thoroughly in distilled water. It should be dried slowly otherwise steam will be unable to escape sufficiently rapidly and consequently the fritted glass plate may be damaged.

Chemical disinfection
A wide variety of substances are used in microbiological laboratories for different purposes and the following are some of those most commonly employed.

Lysol
Used as a 3 per cent solution for the sterilization of discarded cultures and as a disinfectant for cleaning surfaces in a laboratory after accidental contamination of the environment with a living culture.

Phenol
Sometimes used in a strength of 0·3–0·5 per cent for the preservation of sera and vaccines.

Formaldehyde
A 0·5–10 per cent concentration of formaldehyde in water is a powerful disinfectant used for a variety of purposes. The stronger solutions can be used as disinfectants for general purposes and the weaker solutions for killing bacterial cultures, for the preparation of flagellar antigens, and for the 'fixing' of tissues.

Indicated Chloros (I.C.I. Ltd)
Chloros (sodium hypochlorite) containing potassium permanganate has the advantage of indicating the loss of available chlorine as the permanganate oxidises organic material, and in so doing loses its colour. The recommended strength for discard jars is 1–2 per cent. Perspex and glass may be disinfected in Chloros but metal instruments must not be exposed to hypochlorite solutions.

Merthiolate
This is the proprietory name for ethylmercurithiosalicylate and is often used in dilutions of about 1/10 000 for the preservation of antisera.

Mercuric chloride
Used in the laboratory in strengths of about 1/1000 as a disinfectant.

Chloroform
Used for the preservation of intestinal contents prior to testing for clostridial toxins, and also

occasionally for the preservation of sera and bulk media.

Ultraviolet irradiation and air filtration
These are methods used for the sterilization of confined atmospheres in sowing booths and inoculation hoods. The atmosphere is irradiated for several hours to reduce contamination in the environment before being used for the dispensing of media or the sowing of bacterial or tissue cultures. For the safety of operators the lamps are turned off when the booths and hoods are in use.

The microbial count in the atmosphere may also be controlled by filtration of the air entering a sowing booth which reduces contamination from the outside environment. In addition, inoculation hoods may be fitted with special incinerating equipment which kills organisms before they are expelled into the atmosphere of the laboratory. This apparatus is particularly useful for preventing contamination of the laboratory from cultures of highly pathogenic organisms which have been manipulated in the hood.

Cultivation of microorganisms

General Considerations
The study of bacteria, their characteristic properties and their relationship to health and disease in animals and man, depends almost entirely on the ability to cultivate these organisms in the laboratory under precise conditions. A wide variety of bacteriological media has been devised for these purposes which includes the necessary nutrients for growth incorporated in either a fluid or solid base. Fluid media are of limited value because it is usually difficult to obtain pure cultures of a single bacterial species and to study its characteristic features apart from some biochemical reactions. On the other hand, a solid medium provides a surface on which individual bacterial colonies can be identified, their characteristic properties studied, and mixed cultures of two or more bacterial species can be separated and grown individually as pure cultures.

In addition to suitable nutrients in the media, other essential environmental factors must be controlled to ensure the growth of bacteria under artificial conditions.

Temperature
The optimum temperature for growth of most bacterial species capable of living in the tissues of animals and man is 37°C. Some species will grow at temperatures as high as 40°C, and the majority multiply more slowly at 20–25°C and remain viable for long periods at even lower temperatures of about 5°C. Organisms which develop within this wide temperature range of approximately 5–40°C

are termed *mesophilic*, as distinct from non-pathogenic *thermophilic* organisms which have optimal growth temperatures of 55°C or higher. Thus, for the study of microorganisms associated with disease in animals and man, cultures are grown in *incubators* which are thermostatically controlled at temperatures of about 37°C.

Hydrogen-ion concentration
The majority of microbial species capable of living in animal and human tissues grow most satisfactorily in an environment with a neutral or slightly alkaline reaction of pH 7–7.4. A pH meter is used for adjusting microbiological media to the optimal reaction.

Gaseous environment
Microbial species vary according to their atmospheric requirements for optimal growth and survival, and are categorised as follows:

Obligate aerobes: organisms that can grow in the ordinary atmosphere.

Obligate anaerobes: organisms that can grow in the absence of O_2.

Facultative anaerobes: organisms that can modify their metabolism to grow as either aerobes or anaerobes.

Microaerophiles: organisms that can grow in a reduced O_2 tension provided by mixing the normal atmosphere surrounding the cultures with CO_2 to reduce the concentration of O_2.

To provide suitable atmospheric conditions for growth on solid media of obligate anaerobes or microaerophiles, a common practice is to employ an *anaerobic jar* (McIntosh and Fildes jar). The modern type of anaerobic jar consists of a cylindrical metal container with an airtight lid in which the cultures are placed. The lid is perforated by two tubes with taps and on the inside contains a catalyst which enhances the combination of O_2 with H_2 to form water. For the growth of anaerobic cultures (e.g. clostridia), about three-quarters of the air in the jar is evacuated through one of the tubes by means of a vacuum pump after the cultures have been placed inside and the lid screwed down. The tap is then closed and hydrogen is allowed to enter the jar through the other tube. This tap is then closed and the jar placed in a bacteriological incubator at 37°C. At this temperature the action of the catalyst results in the rapid and maximum combination of the remaining O_2 with H_2 to form water and the consequent production of a satisfactory anaerobic environment.

For the growth of microaerophilic organisms (e.g. brucellae) some of the air in the jar is replaced by CO_2 to provide a lowered oxygen tension for optimal growth conditions of these organisms.

Bacteriological and mycological media

A wide variety of fluid and solid media has been devised for the isolation and study of the characteristic properties of bacteria and fungi, and can be classified under the following headings.

Ordinary media: various fluid and solid media which support the growth of a wide variety of organisms (e.g. nutrient broth, nutrient agar).

Enrichment media: contain substances which meet the growth requirements of more exacting organisms and contain blood, serum or other special ingredients (e.g. mycobactin for the growth of *Myco. paratuberculosis*).

Selective media: contain substances which inhibit the growth of all but a few types of organisms or selectively allows the growth of one type at the expense of others (e.g. sodium selenite broth for the isolation of salmonellae).

Indicator media: allow the differentiation and selection of organisms according to their characteristic properties of growth (e.g. MacConkey's agar for the differentiation of lactose fermenting *E. coli* from lactose non-fermenting salmonellae).

Before discussing the various types of media most commonly used for the diagnosis of animal diseases, it is important to stress that during the last quarter of a century the procedures for the routine preparation of media have been simplified and to a large extent standardised by the introduction and increased use of dehydrated media. Laboratories can now purchase a variety of dehydrated media suitable for the majority of diagnostic procedures and their preparation for use largely involves only the reconstitution in water of the dehydrated material.

Nutrient broth and Nutrient gelatin

Broth is a basal medium allowing bacterial growth to which can be added a variety of additional and ingredients for specific purposes, including 15 per cent gelatin to observe liquefaction by proteolytic organisms. Originally, nutrient broth was prepared by infusing minced lean meat in water overnight and then adding peptone to the infusion. Alternatively, the infusion can be treated with trypsin to produce peptone. At the present time, high quality deptones can be purchased for the preparation of broth medium and similarly, meat extracts (known as Lab. Lemco) are also available and widely used as the basis for a variety of bacteriological media.

Constituents: Lab. Lemco (10g), peptone (10g), sodium chloride (5g), water (1000 ml).

Peptone water

Constituents. A simple medium consisting of peptone (10g), sodium chloride (5g) and water (1000 ml).

Indications. Widely used as a basal fluid medium for the growth of pure strains of bacteria, for testing their biochemical reactions by adding various sugars to the media, and for indole production tests.

Glucose broth and Serum broth

Constituents. Nutrient broth with either 1.0 per cent glucose or 10 per cent serum added.

Indications. Promotes growth, especially of fastidious organisms by serum broth.

Cooked meat broth (Robertson's cooked meat medium).

Constituents. Minced lean beef is simmered for 1 hour in alkaline water to neutralize the lactic acid. The meat is then separated by filtration, dried by squeezing in a cloth and distributed into screw-capped bottles to a depth of at least 2 cm, covered by 10 ml nutrient broth and autoclaved.

Indications. Particularly useful for the cultivation of anaerobic organisms (e.g. clostridia, *Sphaerophorus*) which will grow when this medium is incubated under normal atmospheric conditions because of the anaerobic environment within the layer of chopped meat due to the presence of unsaturated fatty acids. Also used for the storage of both aerobic and anaerobic cultures.

Agar

Agar is the solidifying agent most commonly used in the preparation of bacteriological media. It is derived from certain species of seaweeds (e.g. *Gelidium corneum*) occurring particularly off the coasts of Japan and New Zealand, and is composed mainly of a carbohydrate which has no effect on the growth of the great majority of bacterial species cultivated in the laboratory. For this reason, agar can be used as a gel and the growth of bacteria can be controlled by ingredients incorporated in the medium with the agar. An additional advantage is that agar melts at about 95–98°C and solidifies on cooling to a temperature of about 40–42°C. This means that heated agar in the fluid state can be cooled to about 50°C to allow for the addition of blood, serum or egg without causing the coagulation of protein; and that the agar subsequently remains as a gel when incubated at 37°C — the temperature usually employed for the growth of pathogenic and saprophytic organisms.

Modern preparations of agar are so refined that they do not need to be clarified by filtration before incorporation into the medium and can be used for many purposes at a strength of 1·0 per cent instead of 2–3 per cent. For special purposes a semi-solid or 'sloppy agar' consisting of only 0·1 per cent agar, can be employed for anaerobic cultures or for use with Craigie tubes when cultivating motile bacteria.

Nutrient agar

Constituents. Similar to nutrient broth but with the addition of agar (1 per cent) to form a gel.

Indications. Extensively used as a basal medium supporting the growth of many bacterial species for antigen production and other purposes. A variety of additional substances may be added to facilitate the isolation of particular bacterial species from inocula containing a mixture of different organisms, and also to encourage the growth of fastidious species.

Glucose agar

Constituents. Nutrient agar with 1 per cent glucose added.

Indications. Enhances the growth of many bacterial species. Glucose is a reducing agent and can be used in this medium for the growth of stab cultures of anaerobes.

Serum agar

Constituents. Nutrient agar with 1 per cent serum added.

Indications. Used as either slopes or plates for the growth of fastidious organisms.

Blood agar

Constituents. Sterile nutrient agar to which is added defibrinated, oxalated or citrated whole blood to give a final concentration of 5–10 per cent. Horse or sheep blood is commonly employed but other species of blood may be incorporated for special

reasons, and the concentration may be increased for particular purposes. A relatively thick layer of blood agar has the advantage of delaying dessication of the medium during incubation but results in a marked opacity which increases the difficulty of observing haemolytic reactions. Haemolysis can be observed more readily when a thin layer of blood agar is superimposed on a layer of nutrient agar.

Indications. For the observation of haemolytic reactions and for encouraging growth of fastidious organisms.

Crystal violet blood agar

Constituents. Blood agar with the addition of crystal violet to a concentration of 1:500 000 (i.e. 1 ml of 0·02 per cent aqueous solution per 100 ml of medium).

Indications. For the isolation of streptococci. Crystal violet inhibits the growth of staphylococci and some other bacterial species.

Edwards' modified blood agar

Constituents. Sheep blood agar with the addition of crystal violet (1:150 000), thallous acetate (1:3000) and aesculin (1·5 per cent).

Indications. For the isolation and identification of streptococci from cases of bovine mastitis.

Heated blood agar (chocolate agar)

Constituents. Prepared by heating a mixture of 10 per cent whole blood with melted nutrient agar at a temperature of 80°C for 5–10 minutes when the fluid turns brown. The medium is then poured into plates and allowed to set. The heating of the blood causes rupture of the erythrocytes and liberation of their contents into the medium.

Indications. Used for growing fastidious organisms, including *Haemophilus* (requiring the X factor) and *Campylobacter* species.

Loeffler's inspissated serum medium

Constituents. A mixture of 3 parts serum and 1 part glucose nutrient broth which is inspissated at 80°C for 2 hours.

Indications. Useful for enhancing the growth of fastidious organisms and especially for demonstrating proteolytic activity by 'pitting' of the surface of the media (e.g. *C. pyogenes*).

MacConkey's bile salt agar

Constituents. Peptone (20g), sodium taurocholate (5g), lactose (10g) neutral red (0·075g), agar (15g), water (1000ml).

Indications. Particularly useful for the isolation of enteric organisms because many other bacterial species are inhibited by sodium taurocholate. This medium also has the advantage that it enables a distinction to be made between lactose non-fermenting colonies of salmonellae (pale colour) and lactose fermenting colonies of *E. coli* (pink colour). The medium can also be used for differentiating between *Yersinia pseudotuberculosis* which grows on MacConkey's agar and *Past. multocida* which does not grow on this medium.

MacConkey's brilliant green bile salt agar

Constituents. As for MacConkey's bile salt agar with the addition of 0·4g brilliant green per litre of medium.

Indications. Useful for obtaining pure cultures of salmonellae from mixed inocula because the brilliant green inhibits the growth of *E. coli.*

Desoxycholate citrate agar (DCA)

Constituents. Lab. Lemco (20g), peptone (20g), lactose (40g), neutral red (0·1g), agar (90g), water (4000ml). To 100 ml of this solution is added 5 ml aqueous solution A containing sodium citrate (17 per cent), sodium thiosulphate (17 per cent), ferric ammonium citrate (2 per cent), followed by 5 ml aqueous solution B containing sodium desoxycholate (10 per cent). This medum has a clear pink colour.

Indications. Useful for the isolation of salmonellae which grow as pale coloured colonies. Colonies of *E. coli* are pink due to the fermentation of lactose.

Selenite broth

Constituents. Anhydrous sodium hydrogen selenite NaHSeO$_3$ (4g), disodium hydrogen phosphate (9·5g), sodium dihydrogen phosphate (0·5g), peptone (5g), lactose (4g), water, (1000 ml). It should be noted that sodium selenite is a highly toxic substance.

Indications. For the isolation of salmonellae.

Tetrathionate broth

Constituents. 50 per cent aqueous solution of sodium thiosulphate (10 ml), 1:1000 aqueous solution

brilliant green (1 ml), 25 per cent aqueous solution potassium iodide with a 20 per cent aqueous solution iodine (2 ml), 10 per cent aqueous solution ox bile (5 ml), calcium carbonate (5g), nutrient broth (90 ml).

Indications. For the isolation of salmonellae.

Serum dextrose antibiotic agar

Constituents. Peptone (10g), meat extract (5g), sodium chloride (5g) inactivated horse serum (50 ml), dextrose (10g), actidione (100 mg), polymyxin B (6000 units), bacitracin (25 000 units), agar (15g), water (1000 ml).

Indications. For the isolation of brucella organisms.

Albimi agar

Constituents. Albimi agar (1000 ml), ethyl violet (1:800 000), actidione (100 mg), polymyxin B (6000 units), bacitracin (25 000 units).
   (*Note.* Albimi agar is supplied by Albimi Laboratories, Brooklyn, New York).

Indications. For the isolation of *Campylobacter.*

Albimi broth

Constituents. Albimi broth (28 g), ethyl violet (1:800 000), actidione (100 mg), polymyxin B (5000 units), bacitracin (15 000 units), water (1000 ml).
   (*Note.* Albimi broth is supplied by Albimi Laboratories, Brooklyn, New York).

Indications. For the isolation of campylobacter.

Lowenstein-Jensen medium

Constituents. Anhydrous potassium dihydrogen phosphate KH$_2$PO$_4$ (2·4 g), magnesium sulphate Mg SO$_4$ (0·24 g), magnesium citrate (0·6 g), asparagine (3·6 g), glycerol (12 ml), 2 per cent aqueous solution of malachite green (20 ml), fresh egg fluid (1000 ml), water (600 ml). The medium is dispensed in 5 ml volumes in screw-capped bottles and solidified in an inspissator at 80°C for 1 hour.

Indications. For the isolation and cultivation of tubercle bacilli. The medium contains glycerol and may be inhibitory to the bovine type of tubercle bacillus (cf. Stonebrink's medium).

Stonebrink's medium

Constituents. Anhydrous potassium hydrogen phosphate KH$_2$PO$_4$ (7 g), disodium hydrogen phosphate Nu$_2$HPO$_4$. 2H$_2$O (4 g), sodium pyruvate (12·5 g), 2 per cent aqueous solution of malachite green (40 ml), fresh egg fluid (2000 ml), water (1000 ml). The medium is dispensed in 5 ml volumes in screw-capped bottles and solidified in an inspissator at 80°C for 1 hour.

Indications. Especially useful for the isolation of the bovine type of tubercle bacillus because it does not contain glycerol which may be inhibitory to the growth of this organism.

Dorset's egg medium

Constituents. Nutrient broth (25 ml), fresh egg fluid (75 ml). Dispensed and inspissated as for Stonebrink's medium.

Indications. Used for maintenance of stock cultures including tubercle bacilli.

Finlayson's medium

Constituents. Egg yolk (60 ml), egg albumen (15 ml), glycerol (4 ml), heat-killed *Myco. phlei* (1 ml), 1 per cent aqueous solution of Congo red (1 ml), saline (19 ml). Dispensed and inspissated as for Stonebrink's medium.

Note. Mycobactin may be used in place of *Myco. phlei* organisms.

Indications. For the isolation of *Myco. paratuberculosis.*

Korthof's medium

Constituents. Peptone (0·8 g), sodium chloride (1·4 g), potassium chloride (0·04 g), calcium chloride (0·04 g), sodium bicarbonate (0·02 g), potassium hydrogen phosphate (0·24 g), disodium hydrogen phosphate (0·88 g), water (1000 ml). To each 100 ml volume of this solution is added sterile inactivated blood serum (8 ml) and sterile haemoglobin solution (0·8 ml).

Note. Rabbit serum is generally used and should be tested beforehand to ensure that it does not contain leptospiral agglutinins. A haemoglobin solution is prepared by adding an equal volume of distilled water to a blood clot and repeatedly freezing and thawing to haemolyse the red blood cells.

Indications. For the growth of *Leptospira.*

Stuart's medium

Constituents. A complex medium without peptone but including sterile, inactivated rabbit serum with L-asparagine, NH$_4$Cl, MgCl$_2$.6H$_2$O, NaCl, thiamine hydrochloride, phosphate buffer (pH 7·6), phenol red and distilled water.

Indications. For the isolation of *Leptospira.* A large inoculum is required to establish satisfactory growth.

Dinger's medium

Constituents. Sterile inactivated blood serum (10 ml), 3 per cent nutrient agar (6 ml), water (100 ml).

Indications. A useful semi-solid medium for the growth of *Leptospira.*

Lactose-egg yolk-milk agar

Constituents. Lactose (4·8 g), egg yolk suspension (15 ml), milk (60 ml), 1 per cent aqueous solution neutral red (1·3 ml), agar (4·8 g), meat infusion broth (100 ml). Neomycin sulphate (250 μg/ml) may be added to inhibit the growth of other bacterial species, particularly when isolating *Cl. welchii* from contaminated inocula containing *E. coli* and aerobic sporing organisms. The addition of sodium thioglycollate (0·1 per cent) is recommended to enhance the growth of strict anaerobes.

Indications. For the isolation of clostridia. Also used for demonstrating the Nagler reaction which develops as zones of opalescence due to the action of lecithinases, especially those present in the alpha toxin of *Cl. welchii.* The development of clear zones around colonies is indicative of proteolytic activity and lactose fermentation is shown by a pink colouration surrounding the colonies.

Hoof agar

Constituents. Ground sheep hoof (20g), Lab. Lemco (1·5 g), peptone (5 g), agar (12 g), water (1000 ml).

Indications. Special medium for the growth of *Sphaer. nodosus*

Sabouraud's glucose agar

Constituents. Glucose (40 g), peptone (10 g), agar (15 g), water (1000 ml). Adjust to pH 5·4.

Indications. The acid pH makes this a suitable medium for the isolation and cultivation of fungi and also for studying the dermatophytes.

Note. Maltose may be substituted for glucose.

Corn meal agar

Constituents. Corn (maize) meal (40 g), agar (15 g), water (1000 ml).

Indications. For the growth of *Candida albicans* and particularly for the development of chlamydospores which are of diagnostic importance.

Malt extract agar

Constituents. Commercial malt extract (20 g), agar (20 g), distilled water (1000 ml).

Indications. General purpose medium for fungi and especially useful for the growth of yeasts.

Raulin's medium

Constituents. A complex medium containing sucrose, tartaric acid, ammonium nitrate, potassium carbonate, ammonium phosphate, magnesium carbonate, ammonium sulphate, zinc sulphate, ferrous sulphate and distilled water.

Indications. Has low pH (3·0) and used for separation of yeasts from contaminating bacteria.

Sugar media

Sugars are used as 1·0 per cent solutions in peptone water to test fermentative reactions of bacteria, and

Polysaccharides. Starch, dextrin, inulin, glycogen.

Alcohols. Glycerol, erythritol, adonitol, dulcitol, mannitol, sorbitol, inositol.

Glucosides. Salicin, aesculin.

A small inverted tube (Durham tube) is placed in the medium to detect the formation of gas, and one of the indicators shown in Table A2.1 is added to detect the formation of acid.

Miscellaneous tests

Proteolysis test (Using gelatin medium)

Procedure. Organisms are inoculated as a stab culture into the following medium: nutrient broth (1000 ml) containing 12 per cent gelatin, to which is added either a solution of albumen (10 g) in 50 ml water or 50 ml. serum to clarify the medium. This medium is fluid at 37°C.

Interpretation. Liquefaction caused by proteolysis is observed by removing the culture from the incubator and cooling for 30 minutes at 4°C before observing the reaction. A positive reaction may take several days to develop. It is necessary to compare the result with incubated uninoculated control media.

Indole test

Procedure. Incubate culture in peptone water for 2–4 days. Add 0·5 ml xylene, shake and stand for

TABLE A2.1.   Showing the reactions of indicators at different pH ranges.

Indicator	Concentration used in medium	Colour change	pH range
Andrade	1 per cent. solution of sod. hydroxide in acid fuchsin	pink → yellow	5 → 8
Phenol red	5 per cent of 0·2 per cent solution	yellow → red	6·8 → 8·4
Bromthymol blue	1 per cent of 0·2 per cent solution	yellow → blue	6·0 → 7·6
Bromcresol purple	1 per cent of 0·4 per cent solution	yellow → blue	5·2 → 6·8

litmus milk (milk + 2.5 per cent alcoholic litmus solution) to test for lactose fermentation and clotting. The following are some of the sugars in common use.

Monosaccharides

  Pentoses. Arabinose, rhamnose, xylose.

  Hexoses. Glucose (dextrose), fructose (laevulose), galactose, mannose, sorbose.

Disaccharides. Sucrose (saccharose) lactose, maltose, trehalose.

Trisaccharides. Raffinose.

1 minute. Add 0·5 ml of Ehrlich's or Kovac's reagent which contain *p*-dimethylaminobenzaldehyde in a mixture of concentrated HCl with either ethyl or amyl alcohol.

Interpretation. The development of a red colour indicates the presence of indole which has been formed by the bacterial decomposition of tryptophane. A yellow colour indicates a negative reaction.

Hydrogen sulphide production test

Procedure. Introduce dried strips of filter paper impregnated with a 10 per cent. solution lead acetate above nutrient broth or peptone water cultures and incubate.

Interpretation. The production of H_2S is indicated by blackening of the filter paper. An alternative method is to incorporate 0·1 per cent lead acetate in nutrient agar. Subsequent production of H_2S by a culture will be indicated by the development of black colonies.

Methyl red (MR) test

Procedure. Inoculate culture to be examined into 5 ml of glucose phosphate peptone water medium containing peptone (5 g), dipotassium hydrogen phosphate (5 g), glucose (0·5 per cent), water (1000 ml). Incubate for 48 hours at 37°C or for 5 days at 30°C. Add 5 drops of methyl red reagent containing methyl red (0·1 g), ethanol (300 ml), water (200 ml), mix and examine.

Interpretation. A red colouration is positive and indicates an acid pH of 4·5 or less resulting from the fermentation of glucose. A yellow colouration is negative.

Voges-Proskauer (VP) test

Procedure. Inoculate culture to be examined into 5 ml of glucose phosphate peptone water medium as for the Methyl Red test, and incubate for 48 hours at 37°C or for 5 days at 30°C. Add 1 ml of 40 per cent potassium hydroxide and 3 ml of 5 per cent *a*-naphthol in absolute ethanol, mix and examine.

Interpretation. A positive reaction, denoted by the development of the pink colour after 2 minutes which becomes crimson in 15–30 minutes, is due to the formation of acetyl methyl carbinol ($CH_3.CO.-CHOH.CH_3$) or butylene glycol ($CH_3.CHOH.CHOH.CH_3$).

Catalase test

Procedure. Either remove a small quantity of culture from an agar slope and place into a small volume of hydrogen peroxide in a tube, or pour a small quantity of hydrogen peroxide over the surface of an agar slope culture of the organism to be tested. Blood agar should not be used in this test.

Interpretation. The presence of the enzyme catalase in the culture is demonstrated by the immediate release of oxygen from hydrogen peroxide.

Urease test using Christensen's medium

Procedure. Christensen's medium consists of peptone (1g), sodium chloride (5 g), dipotassium hydrogen phosphate (2 g), aqueous 1:500 solution of phenol red (6 ml), agar (15 g), water (1000 ml). To this medium is added glucose to give a final concentration of 0·1 per cent, and 100 ml of a 20 per cent urea solution. The whole medium is prepared as slopes.

The medium is heavily inoculated with the culture to be tested, incubated at 37°C, and examined after 4–6 hours and again after 24 hours' incubation.

Interpretation. A positive reaction (i.e. production of urease with consequent formation of ammonia and an alkaline pH), ($NH_2.CO.NH_2 + H_2O \longrightarrow 2NH_3 + CO_2$) is indicated by the development of a purple-pink colouration of the indicator incorporated in the medium.

Nitrate reduction test

Procedure. Inoculate culture to be examined into 5 ml of peptone broth containing 0·1 per cent potassium nitrate and incubate at 37°C for 4 days. Add 1 ml of solution containing 8g sulphanilic acid in 1000 ml of 5N acetic-acid and mix. Add drop by drop a solution containing 5g *a*-naphthylamine in 1000 ml of 5N acetic-acid.

Interpretation. A positive reaction resulting from the breakdown of nitrates to nitrites is indicated by the development of a red colour, and is due to the formation of the nitrate reductase enzyme by the bacteria.

Optochin test

Procedure. Discs of filter paper, 5 mm in diameter, are impregnated with a 1:4000 solution of optochin (ethyl hydrocuprein hydrochloride), dried and placed on an inoculated blood agar plate.

Interpretation. The growth of pneumococci is inhibited in a zone of 5–10 mm around the impregnated disc of filter paper. *Str. viridans* is not inhibited.

Cell culture reagents

Basic salt solutions (BSS)
These are isotonic solutions of inorganic salts and glucose buffered with phosphates, to which serum and other biological products are added for the growth or maintenance of cells.

All cell culture media are based on a simple

balanced salt solution of which Hanks' saline and Earle's saline are the most widely used.

Hanks' BSS

Solution A (stock)

NaCl	40·0 g	
KCl	2·0 g	Dissolve in 200 ml
$MgSO_4.7H_2O$	0·5 g	deionised H_2O
$MgCl_2 \cdot 6H_2O$	0·5 g	

$CaCl_2$	0·7 g	Dissolve in 30 ml deionised H_2O

Mix the two solutions and make up to 250 ml with deionised H_2O

Add 0·5 ml chloroform as a preservative, and store at 4°C. (The solution is stable for at least 1 year).

Solution B (stock)

$Na_2HPO_4.12H_2O$	0·76 g	Dissolve in 200 ml
KH_2PO_4	0·30 g	deionised H_2O and
Dextrose	5·60 g	make up to 250 ml with deionised H_2O

Add 0·5 ml chloroform and store at 4°C.

Working solution (with lactalbumin hydrolysate supplement)

Solution A	50 ml
Solution B	50 ml
Deionised H_2O	870 ml

Add 0·4 per cent phenol red 5 ml.

Add lactalbumin hydrolysate (5 g/litre).

Distribute into bottles and autoclave at 10 lbs pressure for 15 minutes.

Before use adjust pH as desired with 4·4 per cent solution of $NaHCO_3$.

Primary cell cultures initially require a medium with a low buffering capacity and for this purpose Hanks' BSS is preferred. When the culture is growing satisfactorily, the medium is replaced with one containing Earle's BSS.

Modified Earle's BSS (10 x concentrated).

NaCl		80·0 g
KCl		4·0 g
$CaCl_2$		2·0 g
$MgSO_4.7H_2O$		2·0 g
NaH_2PO_4		1·4 g
Glucose		10·0 g
Penicillin-streptomycin		1·0 ml
Phenol red (1 per cent) solution		9·0 ml
Deionised H_2O	to	1000 ml

Sterilize by filtration through sintered glass (porosity 5) or membrane filter. Dispense and store at 4°C.

The medium is best stored without sodium bicarbonate which is added (5 per cent of 4·4 per cent

$NaHCO_3$) to the 'working strength' BSS (1 ×), just before use. Earle's BSS has a better buffering capacity than Hanks' BSS and, therefore, is of value where the cell population is likely to produce large amounts of acid.

Biological additives

Cells will survive only for short periods in BSS and for longer periods the fluid is supplemented with serum, lactalbumin hydrolysate (LAH) or yeast extract which encourage cell growth.

Serum. Almost all cell culture media contain serum. Freshly-drawn blood from young calves is allowed to clot and the serum separated by centrifugation (3000 rev/min for 10 minutes). The supernatant is sterilized by filtration and the pooled sera are inactivated at 56°C for 30 minutes, and stored at −30°C to prevent deterioration of heat-labile glutamine which is present in normal serum.

The concentration of serum added to the BSS varies from about 10–20 per cent for growth media to 2–5 per cent for maintenance media.

Lactalbumin hydrolysate (LAH). This is a protein supplement which is usually prepared as a 5 per cent stock solution in BSS, without sodium bicarbonate or dextrose. It is sterilized by autoclaving at 15 lbs pressure for 15 minutes and stored at 4°C. When required for use it is added in 10 ml amounts to each 90 ml of medium. Example:

Earle's BSS (1 ×)	84 ml
Calf serum	5 ml
5 per cent LAH solution	10 ml
Antibiotics	1 ml

Antibiotics. Penicillin and streptomycin are incorporated in most media and a mixture of both is prepared as one solution.

One mega-unit of penicillin plus 1 g of streptomycin are dissolved in 100 ml PBS and stored at 4°C in 1 ml amounts. The addition of 1 ml of the mixture to 100 ml of medium will give a final concentration of 100 units penicillin and 100 µg streptomycin per ml.

Nystatin (Mycostatin) may be used at a concentration of 25 µg/ml to counteract fungal and yeast contaminants.

Kanamycin will reduce PPLO (mycoplasma) contamination from continuous cell-lines if it is incorporated in the maintenance medium for 4–6 weeks at a concentration of 100 µg/ml.

Solutions for cell disaggregation

Trypsin. Dissolve 1 g of 1:250 trypsin in 400 ml Hanks' BSS (without lactalbumin) by agitation with a magnetic stirrer for 30 minutes at 37°C. Add 4·4 per cent sodium bicarbonate solution to bring the pH to 7·8. Filter and store at −20°C.

Versene. Dissolve 0·1 g of versene in 10 ml of deionised water. Dispense in 0·5 ml amounts in bijou bottles, autoclave at 10 lbs pressure for 15 minutes and store at room temperature. For use, add 0·4 ml of a 1 per cent solution to 20 ml of phosphate buffered saline (PBS) without calcium or magnesium.

Index

Page numbers of principal references are shown in **bold** print.
Page numbers of figures are shown in *italics*.

A

B

C

G

H

I

M

N

T

U

V